THE BIOLOGY OF HUMAN LONGEVITY

THE BIOLOGY OF HUMAN LONGEVITY

Inflammation, Nutrition, and Aging in the Evolution of Life Spans

Caleb E. Finch

Davis School of Gerontology and USC College
University of Southern California

ELSEVIER

AMSTERDAM • BOSTON • HEIDELBERG • LONDON
NEW YORK • OXFORD • PARIS • SAN DIEGO
SAN FRANCISCO • SINGAPORE • SYDNEY • TOKYO

Academic Press is an imprint of Elsevier

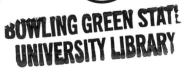

Academic Press is an imprint of Elsevier
30 Corporate Drive, Suite 400, Burlington, MA 01803, USA
525 B Street, Suite 1900, San Diego, California 92101-4495, USA
84 Theobald's Road, London WCIX 8RR, UK

This book is printed on acid-free paper. ♾

Library of Congress Cataloging-in-Publication Data
Finch, Caleb Ellicott.
   The biology of human longevity : inflammation, nutrition, and aging in the evolution
of lifespans / Caleb E. Finch.
      p. cm.
   Includes bibliographical references and index.
   ISBN-13: 978-0-12-373657-4 (hard cover : alk. paper)
   ISBN-10: 0-12-373657-9 (hard cover : alk. paper)
   1. Longevity–Physiological aspects. 2. Aging–Physiological aspects. 3. Inflammation.
4. Nutrition. I. Title.

QP85.F466 2007
612.6'8–dc22   2007004576

British Library Cataloguing-in-Publication Data
A catalogue record for this book is available from the British Library.

ISBN: 978-0-12-373657-4

For information on all Academic Press publications
visit our Web site at www.books.elsevier.com

Printed in China
07 08 09 10   9 8 7 6 5 4 3 2 1

CONTENTS

Chapter 3
Energy Balance, Inflammation, and Aging

PREFACE

Aging is a great scientific mystery. For 4 decades, I have been fascinated by the possibility of a general theory addressing genomic mechanisms in the continuum of development and aging in health and disease. While a Yale undergraduate in Biophysics, I was fortunate to be mentored by Carl Woese, who suggested that if I wanted to tackle a really new problem in little-trodden scientific territory, I should think about aging: "It is even more mysterious than development." About 5 years later as a graduate student at "the Rockefeller," I began work on neuroendocrine aspects of aging guided by Alfred Mirsky (McEwen, 1992). Mirsky was a major conceptualizer of differential gene expression in cell differentiation and development, including postnatal growth and maturation. Eric Davidson and Bruce McEwen, prior Mirsky students, were also key debaters in developing my thoughts on aging.

In writing my PhD thesis, I tried to read everything published on biological and medical aspects of aging up to 1969. I chanced across two remarkable articles by Hardin B. Jones (Jones, 1956, 1959). These papers, rarely cited at that time or since, showed the importance of cohort analyses to understanding aging. James Tanner also noted cohort effects in growth and puberty during the last 150 years (Tanner, 1962). Some readers of my thesis thought my attentions had strayed from my experiments by the emphasis I gave them:

> Tanner suspects that puberty occurs earlier because of decreased exposure to disease in childhood. Jones analyses has actually shown that the mortality of cohorts as children can be used to predict the mortality of these same cohorts as adults. If both conclusions prove true, there may be a common site of action of the environment on the organ systems governing the length of mature life. (Finch, 1969, p. 11.)

I was also was fortunate to learn some pathology as a graduate student at the Rockefeller by two masters of "in-the-gross" necropsy, Robert Leader and John Nelson, who taught me first-hand to use tweezers and scalpel and to see clues to pathology from the texture and color of tissues and fluids. "Old" John Nelson's vast experience in rodent pathology helped me understand McCay's observations that caloric restriction suppressed chronic lung disease (Chapter 3). Peyton Rous made a chilling comment after my thesis lecture (to the effect of): "Finch, I don't see why you are wasting your time on a subject like aging—everyone knows aging is only about vascular disease and cancer." Rous may yet be proved right, but to no chagrin in view of the thriving subject that has emerged and that may give a broad understanding of shared processes in many aspects of aging.

During the past 35 years, my research has remained focused on brain mechanisms in aging. The turn toward inflammation began with molecular studies of Alzheimer disease about 15 years ago. My lab and others discovered that inflammatory mechanisms were activated in Alzheimer disease (AD). Moreover, we showed that some glial inflammatory changes in AD also occur to lesser degrees during normal aging and can be detected before midlife. Furthermore, caloric restriction, which increases rodent life span, also retarded brain inflammatory changes. During this same decade, it became clear that vascular disease also involves slow inflammatory processes and that anti-inflammatory drugs reduce the risk of heart disease and possibly of Alzheimer disease as well. In the last 5 years, I have developed a major collaboration with Eileen Crimmins, a USC demographer whose work also showed the importance of inflammation in human health. Our papers address the questions of 4 decades back and have given the rationale for a new set of animal models being developed in collaboration with my close colleagues Todd Morgan and Valter Longo. Inflammation–diet interactions could explain the recent evolution of human longevity with caveats of its future potential.

My inquiry necessarily leads to a broad range of evidence usually not considered "on the same page" by highly focused researchers of specific diseases. The examples illustrate key points and cannot be comprehensive. I will try to indicate the level of certainty in evidence being considered and not try to explain "too much."

ACKNOWLEDGMENTS

I am grateful for the detailed comments and information given by Dawn Alley (NIA), Steve Austad (U Texas, San Antonio), David Barker (Oregon State U, MRC Southampton), Andrej Bartke (Southern Illinois U), Barry Bogin (U Michigan, Dearborn), Eileen Crimmins (USC), Greg Drevenstedt (USC), Rita Effros (UCLA), Doris Finch (Altadena, CA), Luigi Fontana (Washington U), Roger Gosden (Weill-Cornell Medical College), Michael Gurven (UC Santa Barbara), Shiro Horiuchi (Rockefeller U), Tom Johnson (U Colorado, Boulder), Marja Jylhä (U Tampere), Hillard Kaplan (U New Mexico), Edward Lakatta (NIA), Gary Landis (USC), Valter Longo (USC), George Martin (U Washington), Christopher Martyn (Winchester, UK), Edward Masoro (U Texas San Antonio), Roger McCarter (Penn State), Richard Miller (U Michigan, Ann Arbor), Charles Mobbs (Mount Sinai, NYC), Vincent Monnier (Case Western Reserve), Todd Morgan (USC), Wulf Palinski (U California, La Jolla), Kari Pitkänen (U Helsinki), Scott Pletcher (Baylor), Leena Räsänen (U Helsinki), Karri Silventoinin (U Helsinki), Craig Stanford (USC), Aryeh Stein (Emory U), John Tower (USC), and Paulus van Noord (Utrecht). And I am especially grateful to Eileen Crimmins and Valter Longo, who read all the chapters. Expert editorial assistance was provided by Jacqueline Lentz (USC), Bernard Steinman (USC), and Swamini Wakkar (USC); Bernard also masterfully developed the figures. The research from my lab was supported by the National Institute on Aging, the Alzheimer's Association, the John Douglas French Foundation for Alzheimer disease, the ARCO/William F. Kieschnick Chair in Neurobiology of Aging, the Ellison Foundation for Medical Research, and the Ruth Ziegler Fund. Lastly and firstly, I could not have completed this project without the unvarying support of Doris Finch, who was always ready to relight the scholar's lamp at flagging moments.

CHAPTER 1

Inflammation and Oxidation in Aging and Chronic Diseases

PART I

1.1. OVERVIEW

Human life spans may have evolved in two stages (Fig.1.1A). In the distant past, the life expectancy doubled from the 20 years of the great ape-human ancestor during the evolution of *Homo sapiens* to about 40 years. Then, since the 18th century, life expectancy has doubled again to 80 years in health-rich modern populations, with major increases in the post-reproductive ages (Fig. 1.1B) and decreases in early mortality (Fig. 1.1C). During these huge demographic shifts, human ancestors made two other major transitions. The diet changed from the plant-based diets of great apes to the high-level meat-eating and omnivory that characterizes humans. Moreover, exposure to infections increased. The great apes abandon their night nests each day and rarely congregate closely for very long in large groups. As group density and sedentism increased in our ancestors, so would their burden of infections and inflammation have increased from exposure to pathogens in raw animal tissues and from human excreta.

I propose that the growth of meat-eating and sedentism selected for gene variants adaptive in host defense and adaptive for high fat intake. Some of these genes may have favored the increased survival to later ages that enables the

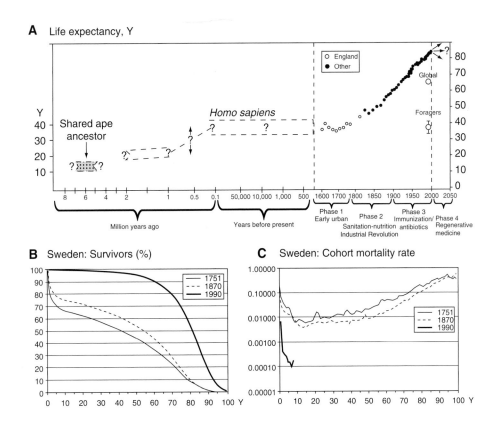

FIGURE 1.1 Evolution of the human life span. A. Life expectancy from 6 million years ago (MYA) to present. Left panel is simplified from Fig. 6.1. The shared ancestor of chimpanzee and human is predicted to have had a life expectancy at birth (qo) of 10 to 20 y, approximating that of wild chimps (Section 6.2.1). The range of q_0 from 30 to 40 y in early, but anatomically modern *H. sapiens* is hypothesized here to approximate that of current human foragers (Gurven and Kaplan, 2007) (Section 6.2.1; Fig. 6.1, legend) and pre-industrial Europe, e.g., England (Right panel). Life expectancy may have increased during the increase of brain size after 1.8 MYA (see Fig. 6.1 legend). Early *Homo* as a species was established by 1.8 MYA (Section 6.2) (Right panel). The major increase of life span speculatively began during later stages in evolution of *H. sapiens*, 0.5 to 0.195 MYA (see Fig. 6.1 legend and Section 6.2.2). Right panel, adapted from Oeppen and Vaupel (2002), Suppl. Fig. 5 and framed by historical markers of my interpretation. Data for England 1571–1847 from *op. cit.*; mean 36.2 y [30.6-41.7 y, 95% CI] calculated from Paine and Boldsen (2006), p.352 and (Wrigley and Schofeld, 1997). Global average life expectancy at birth in 2006: 64.8 y (weighted average, The World Factbook (CIA, 2006). B. Survival curves for Sweden showing the progressive increase in life span and rectangularization of the survival curves from 1751 to present. From Human Mortality Database. C. Mortality rate curves and aging (semi-log scale) for Sweden 1751, 1870, 1990, showing the historical trends for progressive downward shift of the entire mortality curve (See Fig. 2.7).

uniquely human multi-generational caregiving and mentoring. Many such genetic changes had probably evolved by the time of the Venus of Willendorf (cover photograph), 21,000 years ago in the Upper Paleolithic. Her manifest obesity may be viewed as adaptive in times of fluctuating food, with few ill consequences during the short lifespans of the pre-modern era, at the least, fewer than in the modern era of rampant chronic obesity. However, the most recent and rapid increases in life span cannot be due to the natural selection of genes for greater longevity.

I emphasize the plural lifespans, because many concurrent human life history schedules can be recognized in the world today that differ by the rate of growth, age of puberty and sexual maturation, the schedule of reproduction, and life expectancy. Evolutionary biologists recognize the huge plasticity of life history schedules, which vary between populations and respond rapidly to natural or artificial selection (Section 1.2.8). In the not too distant past, human life histories and lifespans may have been outcomes of natural selection, whereas changes in the last 200 years are clearly driven by culture and technology.

I propose that the evolution of the human life span depended on the genetic modulation of synergies between inflammation and nutrition. These dyadic synergies are both substrates and drivers of specific chronic diseases and dysfunctions (Fig. 1.2A). Many aspects of aging are accelerated by infections and inflammation, while drugs and nutritional interventions that slow aging may act by attenuating inflammation and oxidative damage. The current lab models selected for fecundity in atypically clean environments with unlimited food and no stress from predators may not represent aging processes in the bloody, dirty, invasive, and stingy environment of natural selection. Host defense and somatic repair processes are evolved to survive the relentless assaults by microorganisms, parasites, and other predators that are omnipresent in the natural environment.Understanding gene-environment (G x E) interactions in the inflammation-nutrition synergies is fundamental to human aging, past, present, and future. No single gene or mechanism is likely to explain human aging and its evolution, because natural selection acts mainly through successions of small quantitative gene effects. Many gene variants show trade-offs in balancing selection, epitomized by the sickle-cell gene in resistance. A broad theory of aging may emerge by mapping the nutrition-inflammation synergies of pathological aging changes (Fig. 1.2) and their role in oxidative damage.

Because host defense and repair require energy, homeostatic energy allocation strategies were evolved for eco-specific contingencies. High infectious burdens and poor nutrition attenuate somatic repair and growth (Fig. 1.2B). Homeostatic resource allocation involves insulin-like metabolic pathways that operate throughout development and adult life (Fig. 1.3). Insulin-like signaling pathways were recently shown to influence aging in many species. Many aspects of aging at the molecular and cell level can be attributed to 'bystander' damage from locally generated free radicals in the immediate microenvironment. DNA, lipids, and proteins are vulnerable to bystander oxidative damage from ROS produced by activated macrophages and from spontaneous reactions with glucose and other sugars. In turn, oxidatively damaged molecules interact with, and can stimulate, inflammatory processes.

A

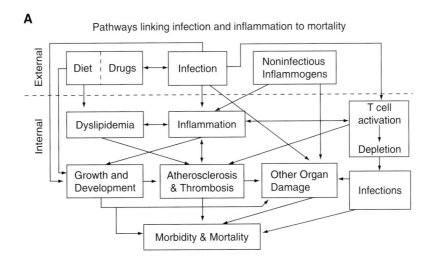

B

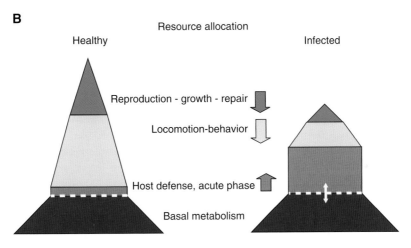

FIGURE 1.2 A. Pathways linking infection and inflammation in aging. Adapted from (Crimmins and Finch, 2006a); drawn by Aaron Hagedorn (USC). B. Energy allocation pyramid in health and during infection, showing energy reallocations during infections, which may cause acute and chronic energy deficits. Human basal metabolism is increased 30% by systemic infections (sepsis) and 15% by sickle cell disease (Lochmiller, 2000). The acute phase inflammatory responses decrease appetite and induce lethargy (sickness behavior). Fever burns energy and increases basal metabolism 25–100% (Roe and Kinney, 1965; Waterlow, 1984): For each 1°C of temperature elevation during fever, human basal metabolism is increased by 10–15%. It is unknown how much energy is consumed by immune cell proliferation and the increased production of CRP and other acute phase proteins. The major reallocation of energy during inflammation comes at the expense of voluntary activity and growth (Chapter 4).

This analysis of the complex interactions in the aging of humans and animal models is guided by three "Queries" about inflammation, nutrition, and oxidant stress during aging.

(QI)   Does bystander damage from oxidative stress stimulate
        inflammatory processes?
(QII)   Does inflammation cause bystander damage?
(QIII) Does nutrition influence bystander damage?

These Queries are not posed as testable hypotheses because in each domain, multiple outcomes are expected from the trade-offs present throughout natural selection. Consequently, many exceptions are expected in the direction and degree of these associations.

The evidence shows that inflammatory and oxidant damage accumulated by long-lived molecules and cells promote the major dysfunctions of aging that, in turn, drive the acceleration of mortality during aging. Later life dysfunctions of the vasculature, brain, and cell growth may be traced to prodromal (subclinical) inflammatory changes from early in life. These processes are examined across the stages of life history, from oogenesis, fetal and postnatal development, and adult stages into senescence.

This inquiry considers aging as a process that is *event-related*, rather than *time-related*, from fertilization to later ages (Finch, 1988; Finch, 1990, p.6). Degenerative changes that eventually lead to increased mortality risk can be analyzed as bystander events from agents acting 'without and within.' External agents include infections and physical trauma. Internal agents include free radicals produced by macrophages in host defense and subcellularly by mitochondria through normal metabolism. Most long-lived molecules inevitably accumulate oxidant damage during aging. Arterial aging demonstrates many bystander processes which stimulate inflammatory pleiotropies (multiple targets of a process) and which are major risk factors for mortality from heart attack and stroke. Diabetes and infections cause oxidative damage and accelerate arterial changes through complex recursive pathways (Fig. 1.2A).

The theory of inflammation and oxidative stress in aging draws from the free radical immunological and inflammatory theories of aging and the Barker theory of fetal origins of adult disease (Chapter 4). Free-radical causes of cancer and of aging 'itself' were hypothesized by Denham Harman in 1956 to involve genetic damage (Harman, 1956, 2003). Then, in the next decade, Roy Walford's immunological theory of aging extended the importance of somatic cell variation from mutations and other autogenous aging changes to autoimmune reactions, in which somatic cell neoantigens caused pathological aging (Walford, 1969). Since then, the free radical hypothesis was extended to many aspects of aging through mechanisms that involve oxidant stress (Bokov et al, 2004; Harper et al, 2004; Schriner et al, 2005; Stadtman and Levine, 2003; Beckman and Ames, 1998). Damage from inflammation is now well recognized in aging processes and chronic diseases and is mediated by

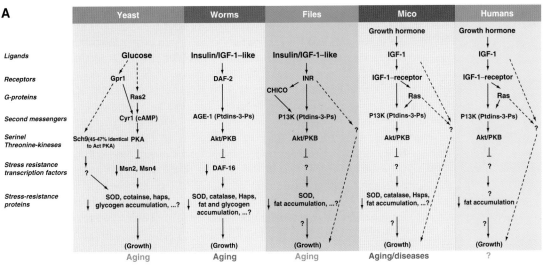

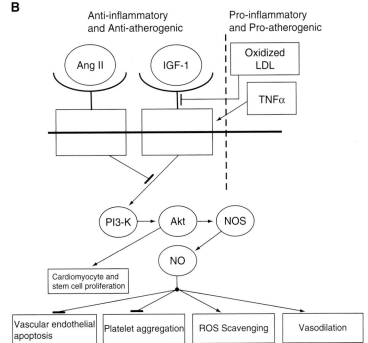

FIGURE 1.3 For legend see page 8.

free radicals and many specific inflammatory peptides (Beckman and Ames, 1998; Ershler and Keller, 2000; Finch and Longo, 2001; Finch, 2005; Franceschi et al, 2005; Wilson et al., 2002). Inflammation was already recognized in arterial disease a century ago by Rudolf Virchow (Bokov et al, 2004) (Section 1.5.3). One aspect of immunosenescence in Walford's theory has been recognized as the depletion of naive T-cells and the acquisition of memory T-cells that are present in unstable arterial plaques. Most recently, Barker's 'fetal origins of adult disease' identifies maternal nutritional influences on adult vascular and metabolic diseases (Chapter 4). I will argue that exposure to infection and inflammation during development also have major importance to outcomes of aging.

While the 'aging' risk factor in the chronic diseases is well recognized demographically, aging changes are often neglected in the disease mechanisms. There are many disconnects between the field of 'basic' aging and the biomedical fields of chronic diseases (Alzheimer, cancer, diabetes, vascular disease, etc.). I argue most age-associated diseases interact throughout with 'normal aging processes.' Many of the same molecules, cells, and gene systems that are altered during aging are considered separately by research in Alzheimer, cancer, and arterial diseases. Major shared mechanisms in aging and disease may be found to stem from roots in the common soil of aging. Shared mechanisms in aging are emerging in the genetics of aging, the insulin-like signaling pathways of metabolism in yeast, flies, worms, and mammals that influence longevity (Fig. 1.3A). Insulin signaling also operates in human arterial disease (Fig. 1.3B). These convergences of aging processes imply ancient genomic universals in life span evolution. It is time to reach for a more general theory that encompasses 'normal aging' and 'diseases of aging' in the context of evolution and development. However, we should not expect that gene regulation of longevity and senescence will operate by the strict gene regulatory circuits that govern early development (Davidson, 2006; Howard and Davidson, 2004).

FIGURE 1.3 Insulin-like metabolic signaling pathways in longevity and vascular disease. A. Yeast, worms, flies, and mice share metabolic pathways with conserved elements that modulate life span. From (Longo and Finch, 2003). B. Insulin/IGF-1 pathways in vascular disease. Redrawn and adapted from (Conti et al., 2004). IGF-1 strongly promotes the survival of vascular smooth muscle cells, whereas Low plasma IGF-1 is associated with many cardiovascular risk factors (Section 1.6.5). This sketch suggests cardioprotective (positive) and atherogenic-inflammatory (negative) limbs of the response (left and right sides) (Conti et al., 2004; Che et al., 2002). *Positive:* IGF-1 binding increases nitric oxide production via a PI3K-Akt cascade, which increases vasodilation and ROS scavenging, while inhibiting platelet aggregation and endothelial apoptosis (Isenovic et al. 2002, 2004; Conti et al., 2004; Dasu et al., 2003). Additionally, activation of IGF-1 receptor and Akt stimulates the proliferation of cardiomyocytes and stem cells (Linke et al., 2005; Catalucci and Condorelli, 2006). *Negative:* Oxidized LDL directly inhibits IGF-1 receptor levels in vascular smooth muscle cells (Scheidegger et al., 2000). However, TNFα may synergize with IGF-1 receptor through the Gab1 subunit to enhance adhesion and other inflammatory proatherogenic activities (Che et al., 2002).

Next is an overview of this book. Chapter 1 has two parts: Part 1 reviews human aging and age-related diseases for a diverse readership, emphasizing inflammation and major experimental models. An overview of inflammation and oxidant stress in host defense suggests a classification of bystander damage. Mechanisms of inflammation are outlined, including the energy costs. Part 2 reviews in more detail inflammation in arterial and Alzheimer disease. These details are critical to understanding human aging and the role of insulin-like metabolic pathways. Many inflammatory processes emerge during 'normal' or usual aging, but in the absence of specific diseases. The slow creep of inflammation from early years may drive the accelerating incidence of chronic diseases. This hypothesis is supported by evidence that many diseases benefit from drugs with anti-inflammatory and anti-coagulant activities (Chapter 2) and by energy (diet) restriction, which can have anti-inflammatory effects (Chapter 3).

Chapter 2 examines environmental inflammatory factors in vascular disease and dementia with a focus on infections, environmental inflammogens, and drugs that modulate both vascular disease and dementia. Infections and blood levels of inflammatory proteins are risk factors for future coronary events and possibly for dementia. When early age mortality is high, the survivors carry long-term infections that impair growth and accelerate mortality at later ages ('cohort morbidity phenotype'). Chronic infections, which are endured by most of the world's human and animal populations, cause energy reallocation for host defense. Infections and inflammation may impair stem cell generation, with consequences to arterial and brain aging. Diet may introduce glycotoxins that stimulate inflammation. Some anti-inflammatory and anti-coagulant drugs may protect against coronary artery disease and certain cancers, and possibly also for Alzheimer disease. These 'pharmacopleiotropies' implicate shared mechanisms in diverse diseases of aging.

Energy balance, inflammation, and exercise are addressed in Chapter 3. Diet restriction, which can slow aging and increase life span, also alters insulin-like signaling. Moreover, diet restriction attenuates vascular disease and Alzheimer disease in animal models, again suggesting common pathways. Diet restriction in some conditions has anti-inflammatory effects and may attenuate infections. Conversely, hyperglycemia is proinflammatory in obesity and diabetes. Exercise and energy balance influence molecular and cellular repair, in accord with evolutionary principles.

Chapter 4 considers developmental influences of infections, inflammation, and nutrition on aging and adult diseases. Birth size, overly small or excessively large, can adversely affect later health through complex pathways. Developmental influences attributed to maternal malnutrition in the Barker hypothesis are extended here to infections. Fogel's emphasis on malnutrition as a factor in poor health can also be extended to include consequences of infection and inflammation. I argue that infection and inflammation compromise fetal development by diverting maternal nutrients to host defense, with consequences to development that influence adult health and longevity.

Chapter 5 reviews genetic influences on inflammation, metabolism, and longevity in animal models and humans. Mutations in insulin-like metabolic pathways shared broadly by eukaryotes can also influence longevity. These metabolic pathways (Fig.1.3A) also interface with inflammation. Certain mutations of insulin signaling that increase the worm life span also increase resistance to infections. The human apoE alleles influence many aspects of aging and disease; the apoE4 allele shows population differences in frequency and effects that may prove to be exemplars of gene-environment interactions during aging.

The last chapter considers the evolution of human life span from shorter-lived great ape ancestors that ate much less meat and lived in low density populations. Human longevity may have evolved through 'meat-adaptive genes' that allowed major increases of animal fat consumption and increased exposure to infection and inflammation not experienced by the great apes. The book closes by discussing environmental trends and obesity, which may influence future longevity.

1.2. EXPERIMENTAL MODELS FOR AGING

Aging and senescence in yeast, fly, worm, rodent, monkey, and human are reviewed with details referred to in later chapters. Lab models are referred to by their common names: fly (*Drosophila melanogaster*); monkey (rhesus, *Macaca mulatta*); mouse (*Mus musculus*); rat (*Rattus norvegicus*); worm (roundworm, nematode *Caenorhabditis elegans*); yeast (baker's yeast, *Saccharomyces cerevisiae*). Other related species may have different life histories (Finch, 1990) and are identified by full name where discussed.

At the population level, humans and these models share the characteristics of finite life spans determined by accelerating mortality. These species share the characteristic of female reproductive decline and oxidant damage in many cells and tissues during aging. Each species has a canonical pattern of aging that persists in diverse environments (Table 1.1) (Finch, 1990). Insulin-like metabolic signaling influences life span, as shown by mutants (Fig. 1.3A) (Chapter 5), suggesting a core of shared mechanisms in aging. However, lab flies and worms differ importantly from mammals by the absence of tumors during aging. The recent discovery that the adult fly gut has replicating stem cells that replace the epithelium with 1 week turnover (Ohlstein and Spradling, 2006) could give a basis for tumor formation in longer-lived species, such as honeybee queens.

1.2.1. Mortality Rate Accelerations

All individual organisms have finite life spans, it is simple to say. The core issue in aging is to resolve environmental effects on endogenous aging processes. The hugely complex gene x environment interactions collectively result in mortality risks that define the statistical life span. Here, we face the immense challenge of moving the level of causal analysis from populations to the indi-

TABLE 1.1 General Characteristics of Aging (Canonical Patterns of Aging)

	Mortality Acceleration[a]	Reproductive Decline[b]	Slowed Movement[c]	Cardiac/Vascular Dysfunctions[d]	Abnormal Growths[e]	Oxidative Damage[f]	Brain Neuron Loss During Aging[g]
yeast	+	+	not relevant	not relevant	0	+	not relevant
fly	+	+	+	+	0	+	yes
worm	+	+	+	not relevant	0	+	not likely
mouse, rat	+	+	+	+	+	+	sporadic except in disease
monkey	+	+	+	+	+	+	"
human	+	+	+	+	+	+	"

a. see Table 1.2
b. yeast, budding diminishes; fly and worm, egg production diminishes before death; mammalian ovary becomes depleted (Finch, 1990).
c. spontaneous locomotion: fly (Finch, 1990, p. 65); worm, *idem*, p. 560; mammals (Slonaker, 1912) and common knowledge.
d. fly, slowed pulse and lower threshold for fibrillation (Section 5.6.3, Fig. 5.7) *and* vascular changes in other insects *ibid* p.65; rodent, loss of arterial elasticity, myocardial fibrosis, and atheroma (Sections 1.2.2 and 2.5); monkey, coronary artery disease induced by fat (Clarkson, 1998); human, Sections 1.2.2 and 1.5, Fig. 1.4 and 1.6.
e. fly and worm, no tumor observed in wild-type. The presence of dividing stem cells in the adult fly gut (Ohlstein and Spradling, 2006) might lead to tumors in long-lived fly species that over-winter.
f. worm, fly, Section 1.2.4; rodent and human, Sections 1.2.4 and 1.6.2.
g. Section 1.2.2.

vidual. Time (age) is the best predictor of future longevity in populations. However, the multifarious aging changes that can be identified in individuals are much weaker predictors of longevity risk, the elusive 'biomarkers of aging' discussed below.

Senescence in populations of humans and many other species can be compared by the rate of mortality acceleration during aging (Fig. 1.1C) (Finch, 1990, pp. 13–16; Finch et al, 1990; Johnson et al, 2001; Nusbaum et al, 1996; Pletcher et al, 2000; Sacher, 1977). In humans and rodents, mortality accelerations arise soon after puberty (Fig. 1.1C). The lowest values of mortality, which occur in mammals at about puberty, are designated as initial mortality rates (IMRs) (Finch et al., 1990; Finch, 1990, pp. 13–16). The main phase of mortality acceleration is described by the exponential coefficient of the Gompertz equation (Table 1.2). In humans, flies, and worms, mortality rates decelerate at later ages (Finch, 1990, p. 15) and (Carey et al, 1992; Johnson et al, 2001; Vaupel et al, 1998). Mortality deceleration at later ages is less definitive in lab rodents (Finch and Pike, 1996). These complex curves may also be fitted by multi-stage Gompertz (Johnson et al, 2001) or Weibull equations (Pletcher, 2000; Ricklefs and Scheuerlein, 2002). The mortality acceleration in both equations is the strongest determinant of life span in most populations.

The Gompertz exponential coefficient is conveniently expressed as the 'mortality rate doubling time' (MRDT), which ranges 1000-fold between yeast and long-lived mammals (Table 1.2) (Finch, 1990, pp. 662–666). Yeast, worm, and fly show the most rapid senescence, while birds and mammals show gradual senes-

TABLE 1.2 Comparative Demography of Aging			
	Initial Mortality Rate (IMR)	**Mortality Rate Doubling Time (MRDT)**	**Maximum Life Span**
yeast[a]	0.2/d	10 d	>20 d
fly[b]	0.1/d	5 d	>60 d
mouse, rat[c]	0.1/mo	4 m	> 48 mo
human Sweden)[d]			
1751	0.0090/y	7–9 y	<100
1931	0.0008/y		>110 y

These organisms show exponential accelerations of mortality, approximating a straight line on a semi-logarithmic plot of mortality rates against age (Fig. 1.1B), as described by the Gompertz equation for mortality rates: $m(x) = A\exp(\alpha x)$, where α is the Gompertz coefficient, x is age, and A is the initial mortality rate, IMR. Mortality rate doubling time is calculated as $\ln 2/\alpha$ (Finch et al, 1990). Rodents fed ad libitum. *a*, yeast (Finch, 1990, p. 105) from data of (Fabrizio et al, 2004), chronologic model (non-dividing); *b*, fly B stock (Nusbaum et al, 1996); *c*, representative rodent strains (Finch and Pike, 1996); d, Swedish historical populations (Finch and Crimmins, 2004, 2005; Crimmins and Finch, 2006a, b), and unpublished. IMR is calculated differently by species according to conventions. For rodents and human, IMR is calculated at the age of sexual maturation (puberty), its lowest value. For worm and fly, IMR is calculated at age 0 (hatching). Also see Table 5.1 and Finch (1990), pp. 663–666.

cence. At the other extreme is the theoretical limit of '*negligible senescence*', with MRDTs of >100 years (Finch, 1990, pp. 206–247; Finch, 1998; Vaupel et al., 2004). Species of long-lived fish (Cailliet et al, 2001; De Bruin et al, 2004; Geuerin, 2004), turtles (Congdon, 2003; Henry, 2003; Swartz, 2003), and conifers (Lanner and Connor, 2001) have not shown reproductive aging and are candidates for negligible senescence; however, data are lacking to evaluate mortality rates. MRTDs within a species vary less than the 10-fold or more variations in IMR. Human populations show a remarkable 10-fold range of IMR variations (Table 1.2), which reflect the level of health allowed by nutrition, infections, and other environmental factors (Chapters 2, 3, 4). Experimental variations of MRDT include 2-fold difference by diet (diet restriction in rodents, Chapter 3) and genotype (*Age-1* worm mutant, Chapter 5). Curiously, rodent MRTDs do not vary much by genotype, despite quite different diseases of aging (Finch and Pike, 1996). Human MRTDs are fairly similar across populations, despite major differences in diseases and overall mortality (Finch, 1990; Gurven and Kaplan, 2007), e.g., Sweden (Table 1.2; Fig. 1.1C and Fig. 2.7). Male mortality is generally higher throughout life (Section 5.3).

1.2.2. Mammals

Mammalian aging follows canonical patterns that gradually emerge after maturation and progress across the life span in proportion to the species life span (Finch, 1990). The seeds of aging are found before birth in many tissues, e.g., arteries and ovaries, as discussed below. The occurrence of these aging patterns in at least 5 of the 28 orders of placental mammals implies shared gene regulatory systems evolved hundreds of million years ago that determine the level of molecular and cell turnover and repair in specific tissues. The canonical patterns of aging thus can be considered as genetically programmed aging.

The increasing incidence of diseases of aging corresponds to the acceleration of mortality during aging, as known in detail for humans and rodents. Arterial disease (heart attack, stroke) and cancer are *the* main causes of death across aging human populations (Fig. 1.4). Vascular deaths increase more or less exponentially after age 40, whereas breast cancer incidence plateaus after menopause. By age 65, vascular deaths exceed those from cancer in most populations (Horiuchi et al, 2003). In 1985, in Japan, Sweden, and the United States, for example, the total male deaths recorded for heart attack and stroke were 2-fold or more than for cancers, 3-fold more than for respiratory conditions, and 30-fold more than for infectious diseases (Fig. 1.4) (Aronow, 2003; Himes, 1994; Horiuchi et al, 2003). The relative proportion of heart attacks (ischemic heart disease) and stroke (cerebrovascular disease) vary between populations. However, by 2002 in the United States, cancer mortality appears to have overtaken vascular-related mortality for age 85 and younger, where about 5% more died of cancer than from heart disease (476,009 vs. 450,637) (American Cancer Society, 2006). The campaigns on prevention and intervention of vascular disease are having remarkable impact on vascular changes.

In rodents, the incidence of new pathologic lesions also increases exponentially (Bronson, 1990; Simms and Berg, 1957; Turturro et al, 2002), and roughly

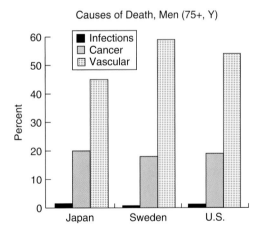

FIGURE 1.4 Circulatory diseases and cancer are the major cause of death in Japan, Sweden, and U.S. males aged 75+ in 1985. Circulatory diseases include ischemic heart disease and cerebrovascular disease. Very recently, cancer in the United States has risen to be the major cause of mortality before age 85, due to the remarkable success of the vascular disease campaigns. (Graphed from Table 4 of Himes, 1994).

paralleling the acceleration in mortality rates (Fig. 1.5). Diet restriction shifts the incidence of lesions to later ages and slows the acceleration of mortality (Chapter 3). The causes of death are often unresolvable, because multiple lesions are common at later ages (Fig. 1.5 and legend). The Berg-Simms colony founded in 1945 gives an unsurpassed documentation of age-related degenerative disease and mortality (Berg, 1976).

Despite the relatively primitive husbandry and hygiene, life span was in the current range. The pathology of aging (specific organ lesions and age incidence)

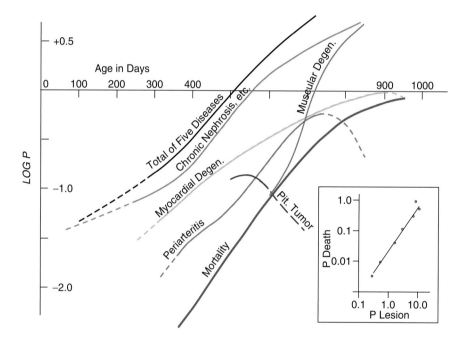

FIGURE 1.5 The incidence of new pathologic lesions in rats increases exponentially in parallel with accelerating mortality. Similarly, in C57BL/6NNia mice the percentage of mice with more than three lesions doubled every 6 months: 12 m, 20.4%; 18 m, 41.7%; 24 m, 75.9% (Bronson, 1990). This doubling rate is slower than that of mortality rate doubling of 3.6 m, calculated from the Gompertz slope (Finch and Pike, 1996). Although the Berg-Simms colony was founded in 1945 before laboratory animal infections were well controlled, their 'rat palace' at the College of Physicians and Surgeons (Columbia U) had little respiratory disease (<5% of rats). Rats were not selectively inbred, except to eliminate an 'eye anomaly' (Simms and Berg, 1957). Female life span: median 31 m, maximum 34 m; male life span: median 27 m, maximum 29 m (Berg, 1976).This level of health and longevity is remarkable for that time. (Redrawn from Simms and Berg, 1957.)

(Simms and Berg, 1957; Simms and Berg, 1962) has been confirmed in modern colonies (Bronson, 1990). Kidney lesions preceded tumors and cardiomyopathy; arterial calcification was occasional. In current colonies, kidney lesions and tumors also predominate, occurring in 80% of aging rodents across genotypes (Bronson, 1990; Turturro et al, 2002). Myocardial lesions are less common than in the Berg-Simms era and may vary; e.g., in aging C57BL/6 mice, myocardial degeneration ranged from 8% (Bronson, 1990) to 40% (Turturro et al, 2002), always less than tumors and kidney lesions. The arterial and myocardial pathology in early colonies is discussed in Section 2.5.2, together with improvements in hygiene and husbandry that increased life span with some parallels to the recent human improvements. Rodents in modern colonies on standard diets are not thought to die from arterial degeneration or thrombosis. This may be incorrect.

Rodent models for aging have been borrowed from existing lines that were originally developed for genetic studies of cancer and other chronic diseases, and of transplantation (immunogenetics). Rodents with delayed incidence of pathology until after 18 m were used as controls for early onset tumors, e.g., the relatively long-lived C57BL/6J and DBA/2J mice. All baseline stocks were selected for traits of fast growth and high fecundity, which is the rule for domestication for animals and plants. Infectious diseases were gradually minimized. The resulting models differ importantly from their feral origins, i.e., the true 'wild-types.' For example, wild-caught mice are smaller, mature later, and live longer than lab mice (Miller et al, 2002). Moreover, diet restriction has much less effect on life spans of wild-caught mice (Harper et al, 2006) (Chapter 3, Fig. 3.3). Immune functions also differ in 'unhygienic' feral mice and rats, with much higher levels of autoreactive IgG (Devalapalli et al, 2006). The modern lab rodents with unlimited access to food, low physical activity, and tendencies to obesity may thus be fine models for contemporary lifestyles. However, the limited exposure to infections is unlike the real world. It may be necessary to incorporate antigenic challenges in our aging animal colonies to understand the aging mechanisms at work in human populations, past, present, and future.

In humans, arterial degenerative aging changes result from two long-term processes: the inexorable progressive accumulation of arterial wall lipids (Fig. 1.6A) and arterial rigidity, both from starting early in life (Sections 1.2.6 and 1.6). The loss of elasticity increases blood pressure (Fig. 1.6B), independent of clinical hypertension syndromes. The atherosclerotic lesions can lead to clots (thromboses) that block blood flow with catastrophic effects. Mortality from ischemic heart disease and stroke increases exponentially with adult age (Fig. 1.6C). Systolic pressure elevations are major risk factors in heart attack and stroke and are as universal to human aging as menopause and bone thinning.

The loss of arterial elasticity and artery wall thickening (arteriosclerosis) are ubiquitous in mammals, while focal atherosclerosis is more prominent in humans and primates than rodents (Tables 1.1 and 1.4). The aorta and other central arteries become progressively thicker. The accumulation of oxidized lipids begins before birth

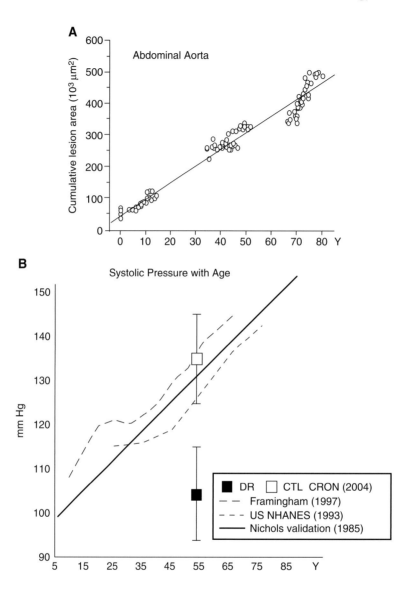

FIGURE 1.6 Arterial aging in humans. A. Arteries accumulate lipids progressively throughout life. The area of abdominal aorta surface covered by lipid-rich deposits (oil red O staining) increases progressively during postnatal life. (Redrawn from D'Armiento et al, 2001.) B. Increases of blood pressure with age (cuff pressure) are widely observed across human populations and are major risk factors in heart attacks and stroke. (Redrawn from O'Rourke and Nichols, 2005.) DR (diet resriction) and CTL (control) from CRON study of the Calorie Restriction Society (Fontana et al, 2004) (Section 3.2.3).

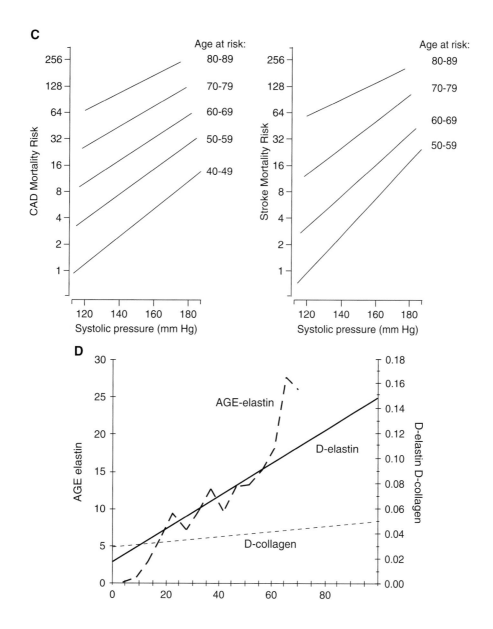

FIGURE 1.6 (continued) C. Mortality from coronary artery disease (CAD) and stroke increases exponentially with elevated systolic pressure. Aging (40–89 years) increases the risk over a 50-fold range at each blood pressure level. There is no apparent threshold or cut-off for protection against adverse effects of blood pressure elevations. (Redrawn from Lewington et al, 2002.) D. Progressive increase in the glycation of human aortic elastin with aging. (Redrawn from Konova et al, 2004.) The chemistry of these fluorescent products is uncharacterized. Elastin has a very long molecular life span in the adult aorta, as judged by the linear accumulation of racemized D-aspartate up through age 80 ("D-elastin") (Powell et al, 1992). Collagen, however, continues to turn over, as indicated by the smaller increase of D-aspartate ("D-collagen").

in microscopic cell clusters (Section 1.5.1). The numerous inflammatory changes include increased macrophages, free radical producing enzymes (NADPH oxidase), cell adhesion molecules (ICAM), cytokines (TGF-β1), and matrix metaloproteinases (MMP-2 and -9). These diffuse changes are generally independent of focal atheromas. Thus, oxidative damage (oxidized lipids) and inflammation are at work from the beginning in arterial aging (Queries I and II).

Arterial elasticity decreases progressively from alterations in collagen and elastin by inter-molecular AGE adducts (advanced glycation and glyco-oxidation end products) derived from glucose and other reducing sugars (Fig. 1.6D) (Section 1.4.4). AGE adducts contribute to arterial rigidity by intermolecular cross-links between collagen and other proteins. In turn, AGE may kindle local inflammation by activating scavenger receptors. Arterial elastin is very-long lived, as shown by accumulations of racemized D-aspartate (Fig. 1.6D). Racemization spontaneously converts normal L-amino acids to the D-isomers. In long-lived proteins, the accumulation of 'racemers' is a direct marker of age (Bada et al, 1974; Helfman and Bada, 1975). Because veins undergo less wall thickening, arterial aging is hypothesized to be driven by the repeated pressure waves at each pulse (Section 1.5.3.2). Blood flow patterns modify gene expression in atheroprone arterial regions.

New macroscopic atheromas appear throughout life. Lipid oxidation may be a key cause of atheroma initiation and progression (Queries 1 and 2). Inflammatory processes are active throughout atherogenesis and are intensified in atheroprone arterial zones. The developing atheromas are described as a complex wounding response with cell growth and cell recruitment; oxidation of lipids and proteins; cell death; and eventual calcification. Environmental influences from infections, diabetes, and stress can accelerate atheroma formation, whereas statins may facilitate atheroma regression (Chapter 2). The insulin/IGF-1 system that modulates life span in flies and worms is also at work in many aspects of atherogenesis (Fig. 1.3B). Animal models vary in susceptibility to arterial lesions. Macaques, chimpanzees (Finch and Stanford, 2004; Wagner and Clarkson, 2005), and rabbits (Yanni, 2004) are more vulnerable to atheroma induction by diet and stress than lab rodents (Moghadasian, 2002). The apoE-knockout mouse has extreme susceptibility to atheromas, in association with its extreme hypercholesterolemia (Rauscher et al, 2003).

The myocardium is altered during aging through inflammatory processes that can interact with arterial changes. Left ventricular stiffness increases progressively with aging (decreased 'compliance') and slows the diastolic of filling rate by up to 50% by age 80 (Brooks and Conrad, 2000; Lakatta and Levy, 2003a,b; Meyer et al., 2006). The stiffness is due to ventricular wall thickening and interstitial myocardial fibrosis, and possibly collagen cross-linking through nonenzymatic glycation. Fibrosis is very common during mammalian aging and deeply linked, if not intrinsic, to general inflammatory processes in aging (Thomas et al, 1992). TGF-β1 signaling pathways that regulate collagen synthesis are implicated in myocardial fibrosis. TGF-β1 deficiency (+/− heterozygote knockout) attenuated the age-related increase of left ventricular fibrosis, improved cardiac performance, and possibly increased life span (Brooks and Conrad, 2000). Myocardial stiffness is attenuated in humans during diet restriction in at least one study (Section 3.4.1). Conversely, transgenic mice with increased systemic TGF-β1 developed premature left ventricular fibrosis with increased levels of TIMPS (tissue inhibitor of metaloproteinase, also implicated in arterial aging) (Seeland et al, 2002).

Mitochondrial DNA changes in the myocardium also merit mention because of their interactions with ischemia and oxidative stress. Additionally, myocardial mitochondrial DNA deletions (mtDNA[4977], nt 8469–13,447) increase modestly after age 60 (up to 7 per 10,000 mitochondria). Ischemic hearts can have >200-fold more mtDNA deletions (Botto et al, 2005; Corral-Debrinski et al, 1992), which is attributed to the oxidative stress from ischemia. Because the DNA deletion impairs mitochondrial function and increases respiratory chain stress, a vicious cycle is hypothesized to cause further mitochondrial damage. Single base changes (point mutations) also increase with aging in a mutational hotspot (nt 16,025–16,055, control region) in cardiomyocytes, but not buccal epithelial cells, with indications of clonal expansion (Nekhaeva et al, 2002).

Besides these aspects of myocardial aging, there are many other aging changes, as well as compensatory mechanisms that go beyond this discussion. At the behavioral level, and of great importance to human aging, are complex social and psychological links to vascular disease and hypertension ('social etiology') (Berkman, 2005; Marmot, 2006; Sapolsky, 2005). Social stress also accelerates vascular changes in primates and rodents (Andrews et al, 2003; Henry et al, 1993). Complex social interaction during aging has not been defined in animal models.

Immunity declines in complex ways during aging: instructive immunity weakens concurrently with increased inflammation in most tissues and chronic diseases. Both changes may contribute to the decreased resistance to opportunistic infections, incidence and severity (Akbar et al, 2004; Miller, 2005; Pawelec et al, 2005; Weksler and Goodhardt, 2002). As examples, the elderly suffer 90% of the influenza deaths, while HIV has a shorter latency in the elderly, reviewed in (Olsson et al, 2000). The decreased resistance is associated with various dysfunctions of systemic and tissue immune mechanisms: the attenuation of adaptive (instructive) immunity and the hyperactivity of acute phase host defense processes. Aging of the adaptive immune responses may be very gradual in populations of humans and lab animals with low burdens of infection and inflammation, and good nutrition. Nonetheless, naive T cells progressively decrease at the apparent expense of memory T cells (CD4 and CD8) (Haynes, 2005; Linton and Dorshkind, 2004; Miller, 2005; Pawelec et al, 2002).

At birth, nearly all T cells express CD28, a major T cell-specific co-stimulator that binds to sites on antigen-presenting cells and activates IL-2 transcription, cell adhesion, and other critical T-cell functions. CD28 is progressively lost during aging (Merino et al, 1998; Pawelec et al, 2005; Trzonkowski et al, 2003). The loss of CD28+ T cells is attributed to chronic antigenic stimulation over the life span. Accelerated loss of CD28 T cells is observed in young HIV patients and is modeled in cultured T cells (Posnett et al, 1999). The CD8+ CD28− T cells are resistant to apoptosis and are considered 'fully differentiated.' During influenza inflections, the elderly have decreased cytotoxic T-cell activity in association with shifted cytokine profiles (T-helper type 2 dominance) (McElhaney, 2005).

Declines of thymus function begin before maturation (Krumbahr, 1939; Min et al, 2005; Steinmann, 1986). Infections and malnutrition in the early years can impair thymus development with later consequences to immunity (Moore et al, 2006; Savion, 2006). Striking examples come from West Africa. In rural Gambia, seasonal infections during childhood alter T-cell functions with correspondingly increased adult mortality (Moore et al, 2006). In Guinea-Bissau, a low small thymus is associated with increased mortality from infections (Aaby et al, 2002). These and other environmental effects on immunity during development are discussed in Section 4.6.2.

Between puberty and mid-life, adipocytes gradually replace the lymphocytic perivascular space. These gross changes are preceded by regression of the thymic epithelium and can be delayed by castration before puberty (Chiodi, 1940; Min et al, 2006). After maturation, the thymus continues to generate T cells throughout life, although at lower levels (Douek et al, 2000; Hakim et al, 2005). Immune homeostatic mechanisms decline during aging; e.g., T-cell recovery after chemotherapy is greatly reduced by age 50 (Hakim et al, 2005; Hakim et al, 2005). Extra-thymic aging changes include lower bone marrow production of lymphopoietic progenitor cells, possibly due to decreased growth hormone and IGF-1 (Hirokawa et al, 1986; Linton and Dorshkind, 2004). Most immunologists agree that thymic involution is multi-factorial and that immune aging is not reversed by simply restoring GH, IGF-1, or other hormones that change with aging (Chen et al, 2003; Min et al, 2006). The adverse effects of infections and malnutrition on thymic development may extend to other aspects of immunity.

The major shifts from virgin T cells to memory T cells during the life span are attributed to exposure to common infections, environmental antigens, and auto-antigens. Cytomegalovirus (CMV), an endemic ß-herpes virus that is a common infection in childhood, may be a general factor in the clonal depletion of CD28+ T cells (Koch et al, 2006; Pawalec et al, 2005). Up to 25% of the CD8 T cells in older healthy humans are CMV-specific (Khan et al, 2002) and are approaching replicative senescence (Fletcher et al, 2005). A proposed 'immune risk phenotype' of aging is characterized by (1) CMV-seropositivity; (2) inverted ratios of CD4:CD8 <1 (unlike the normal CD4 excess in healthy young adults); and (3) increases in 'fully differentiated' CD8$^+$ CD28$^-$ effector T cells, which have shortened telomeres and limited proliferation (Olsson et al, 2000; Pawelec et al, 2005). Elderly with ratios of CD4:CD8 <1 have 50% higher mortality in two populations: the Healthy Ageing Study (Cambridge UK) (Huppert et al, 2003) and the OCTO and NONA Longitudinal Studies (Jönköping, Sweden) (Wikby et al, 2005). These T-cell shifts decrease resistance to new infections. The greater vulnerability of elderly to influenza may be attributed to imbalances of central memory T cells over the effector memory T cells that mediate virus-specific IFN production (Kang et al, 2004). CMV-seropositive elderly who responded poorly to influenza vaccine also had more CD28$^-$ lymphocytes (Effros, 2004; Trzonkowski et al, 2003) and 2-fold higher IL-6 and TNFα (Trzonkowski et al, 2003). The higher cytokine production during aging in immune responses may extend to other classes of T-cells (O'Mahony et al, 1998) and may be a factor in the strong age trend for elevated cytokines (Section 1.8.1).

Besides CMV, many other infections influence the 'immune aging phenotypes.' Chronic immune activation can accelerate 'aging' of T-cell functions, as observed in infections by HIV (van Baarle et al, 2005) and nematode parasites (Borkow et al, 2000) (Section 2.7.1). As noted previously, childhood infections affect the thymus and impair immunity and increase mortality (Section 4.6). As another example, mice with genetically determined elevations of memory T-cells have shorter life spans and higher prevalence of tumors at middle age (Miller, 2005). Chronic immune activation also increases 'bystander' damage (Section 1.4.3) (Query II). We may anticipate that outcome of immune aging depends on gene-environment interactions with inflammatory gene variants, particularly the proinflammatory IL-6 and the antiinflammatory IL-10 (Caruso et al, 2004) (Section 1.3.2). The strong role of the antigenic environment on immune aging is included in the framework of Fig. 1.2A and extends to direct involvement of T-cells with unstable atheromas (Section 2.2.2).

Telomere erosion is implicated in immune aging in association with the reduced proliferation of T cells (Effros, 2004). In peripheral lymphocytes, telomeres shorten by 50 base pairs per year across the life span against initial telomere lengths at birth of about 15,000 base pairs (Hathcock et al, 2005). Telomeres are shorter in primed T-cell subsets, especially the 'effector memory' T cells (Akbar et al, 2004). Telomere loss may eventually activate gene regulatory programs leading to cell death (apoptosis) or a post-mitotic state (clonal senescence; considered equivalent to the Hayflick limit; see below). Telomerase reactivation is thought to be adaptive for clonal expansion without rapid clonal senescence. However, T cell proliferation does not always cause telomere erosion, because immune stimulation of B and T cell proliferation can induce telomerases (Akbar et al, 2004; Hathcock et al, 2005; van Baarle et al, 2005). Other evidence argues against telomere erosion as a general mechanism in immune aging (Miller et al, 2000); e.g., although mice have much longer telomeres than humans, mouse T cell proliferative aging is faster. Much is unknown about enzymes that mediate telomere replication, which differs between immune cell types and animal species.

In contrast to the decline of antigen-driven immunity, inflammatory processes in many tissues progressively increase during aging, e.g., muscle, fat, brain (Section 1.8.1). Inflammatory gene expression increases in these and other tissues. Blood IL-6 and C-reactive protein generally increase during aging in human populations, although much of the increase is associated with vascular disease. Tissue-specific macrophages are prominent in atheromas ('foam cells'), Alzheimer disease (microglia), and bone (osteoclasts). Apart from these degenerative diseases, studies of circulating macrophages from aging humans and rodents are puzzlingly inconsistent about the direction and type of aging changes (Finch and

Longo, 2001; Pawelec et al, 2002; Wu and Meydani, 2004). Despite blood IL-6 elevations, induction of IL-6 in response to LPS (gram-negative bacterial endotoxin) decreases with age in peritoneal macrophages (Stout and Suttles, 2005), but increases with age in brain microglia (Xie et al, 2003; Ye and Johnson, 1999).

Lastly, we should be mindful that decreased system-level and integrative functions ('organ reserves') contribute to mortality independently of specific immune subsystems. The declining 'vital capacity' of lungs (Janssens and Krause, 2004; Meyer, 2005) is strongly associated with survival in general and resistance to respiratory infections. In the Framingham Study, mortality risk at age 50–59 varied inversely with the lung vital capacity (Ashley et al, 1975; Finch, 1990, p. 563). Smoking, which decreases pulmonary volume and respiratory functions, increases vulnerability to influenza and pneumonia (Murin and Bilello, 2005). In the Cardiovascular Health Study of persons 65 years and older, smokers had a 50% higher risk of hospitalization for pneumonia and a 28% higher mortality in the 2.4 years after discharge (O'Meara et al, 2005). Moreover, CMV and other chronic infections may deplete the bone-marrow-derived endothelial progenitor cells that mediate vascular repair (Section 2.7.3). Thus, the decreased resistance to infectious disease should be analyzed in terms of systemic physiology and the ecological life history of exposure in infections and inflammogens (Chapters 2–4), which are subject to gene-environment interactions throughout the life history (Chapters 4 and 5).

Female reproductive senescence is due to the exhaustion of ovarian oocytes in all mammals examined (Finch, 1990, pp. 165–167; Gosden, 1984; vom Saal et al., 1994; Wise et al, 1999). Oocyte numbers are fixed during development by the cessation of primordial germ cell proliferation. Oocyte loss begins before birth and continues exponentially, like radioactive decay (Faddy et al, 1992). Recent evidence refutes the possibility of continuing *de novo* oogenesis from circulating stem cells (Eggan et al, 2006). Less than half of the original stock remains by puberty. The rate of oocyte loss is slowed by diet restriction, which alters hypothalamic controls of the gonadotrophins (Chapter 3, Fig. 3.17). Fecundity declines long before the failure of ovulation due to oocyte depletion, with marked reduction by age 35 years in women; lab rodents aged 8–12 months are culled as 'retired breeders' by production colonies. With the loss of ovarian follicles, the production of estrogens and progestins decreases sharply in human menopause, causing hot flushes, as also observed in macaques (Appt, 2004; Nichols and O'Rourke, 2005). Ovarian steroid loss is implicated in the post-menopausal increase of vascular disease and may interact with vascular inflammatory processes. In males, androgen levels show trends for decline, but more sporadically than in females. Estrogen replacement (hormone therapy), while controversial, appears to be health protective for some women (Section 2.9.4). Androgen replacements may benefit arterial disease, cognition, and glycemic control (Harman, 2005; Jones et al, 2005; Liu et al, 2004; Morley et al, 2005). The sharp rise of vascular disease during middle age is an example for the declining strength of natural selection during aging (evolutionary perspectives, below).

Bones and joints degenerate broadly during aging in mammals in processes that involve inflammatory regulators (Section 1.8). Osteoporosis (bone mineral resorption) occurs through an imbalance of production by osteoblasts versus resorption by osteoclasts. The inflammatory system is involved in bone resorption. First, osteoclasts are of macrophage/monocyte lineage. Then, bone resorption is stimulated by inflammatory cytokines (IL-1, TNFα) (Clowes et al, 2005; Tanaka et al, 2005). Osteoporotic bone loss accelerates after menopause and can be attenuated by estrogen replacement. In some contexts, estrogen has anti-inflammatory activities (Amantea et al, 2005; Thomas et al, 2003) (Section 2.10.4). Osteoarthritis is a focal, age-related inflammatory lesion in the joints that can be painful (Section 1.7). Mechanical pressures activate inflammatory cells and catabolic responses of the articular chondrocytes that cause matrix loss and accumulation of AGEs.

Brain-aging atrophic changes are manifest soon after maturation, in healthy humans by age 30 y and rodents aged 10 m (Finch et al, 1993; Teter and Finch, 2004). The volume of the brain as a whole shrinks by about 0.5%/year in normal humans across the adult age range, 20–98, and is accelerated by Alzheimer disease to about 1%/y (longitudinal MRI) (Burns et al, 2005; Fotenos et al, 2005). The volume of the hippocampus, which is critical to declarative memory, also shrank linearly in healthy elderly observed over 6 y (Cohen et al, 2006).

Neuron loss during aging is more limited than once widely presumed ('neuromythology') (Finch, 1976; Gallagher et al, 1996; Rasmussen et al, 1996; Teter et al, 2004; Tomasch, 1971). During normal human aging, the total number of cortical neurons does not change, but neuronal size shrinks. Small cortical neurons increase, while the numbers of large neurons decreases reciprocally (Terry et al, 1987) (Fig. 1.7A).

Synaptic loss parallels brain atrophy and neuron shrinkage, with progressive decreases in the presynaptic protein synaptophysin in the normal aging cerebral cortex (Fig. 1.7B) and dopamine D2 receptors in the cortex and striatum (Fig. 1.7C, D) (Morgan et al, 1987; Reeves et al, 2002; Suhara et al, 2002; Wong et al, 1997). Other receptors, however, may increase—e.g., dopamine D1 receptor (Morgan et al, 1987)—possibly as a compensatory response. The extent of synaptic loss approximates 1% loss per year after age 20. Rodent brains show similar changes in dopamine receptors, scaled to their shorter life span. By the mean life span, synaptic atrophy reaches 30–50%, independent of Alzheimer, stroke, or other clinical conditions in lab rodents and humans. Nonetheless, neuron cell death is minimal in cortex and possibly other brain regions to advanced ages, absent Alzheimer changes. Even at later ages, neuron loss in aging memory-impaired rats is modest or sporadic in brain regions afflicted by Alzheimer disease (Rasmussen et al, 1996; Rapp and Gallagher, 1996). However, sporadic neuron loss may arise from various stressors (Landfield et al, 1977; Meaney et al, 1988) or toxins (Section 3.2.3; Finch, 2004b). In rodents, D2 receptor loss in aging is attenuated by diet restriction (Chapter 3, Fig 3.17) while neuronal atrophy is reversed by nerve growth factors (Smith et al, 1999). The generality of synaptic atrophy during middle age in the absence of neuron loss distinguishes these changes from the subgroups at later ages that develop aggressive neurodegeneration during Alzheimer disease.

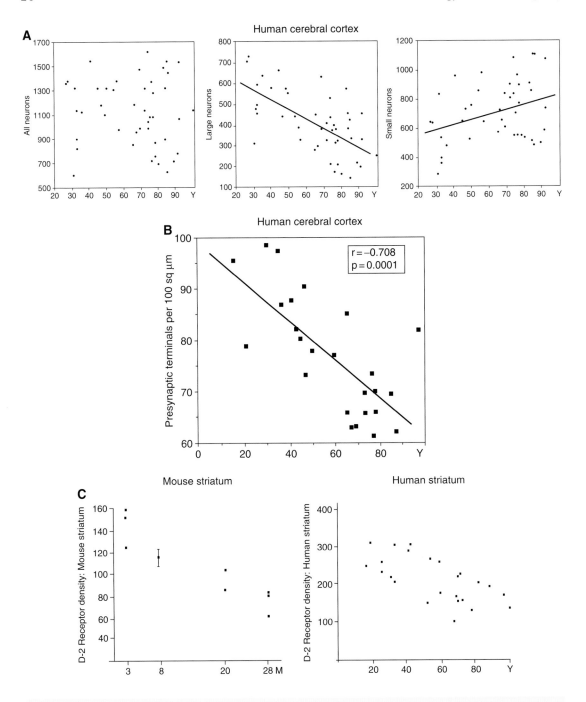

FIGURE 1.7 For legend see page 25.

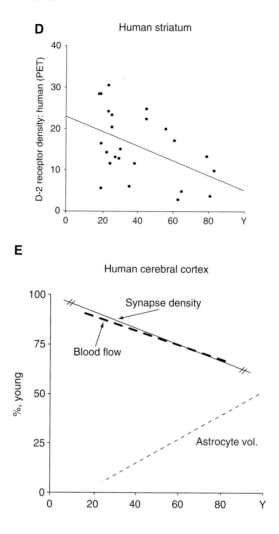

FIGURE 1.7 (continued) Normal brain aging: neuronal atrophy, glial hypertrophy, declining blood flow in brains without Alzheimer disease or ischaemic damage. A. Total cerebral cortical neuron numbers do not change. However, the numbers of small neurons increase inversely with decreased numbers of large neurons, apparently due to atrophy of large neurons (Masliah et al, 1993; Terry et al, 1987). B. Presynaptic terminal density (synaptophysin immunostaining) shows progressive decline of about 0.75%/y (Terry et al, 1987), possibly associated with neuronal atrophy. C. Dopamine (D2) receptor loss in human and mouse (ligand binding, postmortem), approximating 1%/y after age 20. (Redrawn from Morgan et al, 1987a.) D. *In vivo* D2 receptor sites (positron emission tomography/PET) in caudate of normal humans declined 1%/y after age 20 (Wong et al, 1997). E. Aging trends of synaptic density (panel B above), cerebral blood flow (Fig. 1.20) (Amano et al, 1982), and astrocyte volume in brains without Alzheimer disease or ischaemic damage (Hansen et al, 1987). Cerebral cortex from the same source and evaluated by the same criteria for health was used for studies of astrocyte volume and synaptic loss (Panel B).

Age-related synaptic atrophy (15–30%), while modest relative to Alzheimer disease, plausibly contributes to declines in complex brain functions. Memory capacity declines progressively in humans and rodents, with no evident pathology (Albert, 2002; Rajah and D'Esposito, 2005; Rosenzweig and Barnes, 2003; Woodruff-Pak, 2001). In the hippocampus, a seat of declarative memory, synapse loss is extensive. The hippocampus receives input from the cerebral cortex from the perforant pathway, which is much more damaged during Alzheimer disease than normal aging (Nicholson et al, 2004; Rosenzweig and Barnes, 2003). Some functional deficits may be linked to synaptic atrophy. The D2 receptor loss during aging (Fig. 1.7D) correlated with performance on tasks dependent on the frontal cortex, e.g., the Stroop Color-Word Test interference score (Volkow et al, 2000).

Other deficits may be due to the deterioration of myelinated pathways (white matter), which mediate high-speed exchanges between brain regions. Microglial activation may be a factor in white matter changes during middle age as seen by brain imaging (Bartzokis, 2004; Bartzokis et al., 2003, 2004, 2006; Burns et al., 2005) (Fig. 1.8B). ApoE4 carriers have accelerated myelin deterioration (Bartzokis et al., 2006), consistent with the 'proinflammatory' associations of the E4 allele (Section 1.3). White matter inflammatory changes may contribute to the usual slowing of information processing and the decreased multi-tasking by middle age (Bashore, 1994; Madden, 2001; Verhaeghen and Cerella, 2002). Multi-tasking becomes progressively impaired during aging. A striking example is the impairments by middle age in memorizing words while walking an irregular course (Li et al, 2001). Multi-tasking depends on high-speed processing across multiple circuits, which slows progressively during normal aging (Bashore and Ridderinkoff, 2002; Maeshima et al, 2003; Ylikoski et al, 1993). These processes suggest why few professional athletes remain competitive over the age of 40 and why driving errors increase with aging (Campagne et al, 2004).

Skeletal muscle atrophy during aging ('sarcopenia'), a major factor in frailty (Dow et al, 2005), may be due to motor neuron aging. The atrophy of aging muscle resembles denervation atrophy and is partly reversed by electrical stimulation (Dow et al, 2005). The major role of motor neuron age in skeletal muscle aging was shown by a powerful transplantation experiment: when reinnervated in young rat hosts, the 32-month-old muscle grafts regained full contractile strength (Carlson et al, 2001). Aging muscle also accumulates mitochondrial DNA mutations in association with muscle fibers deficient in cytochrome oxidase (COX) (Brierley et al, 1998; He et al, 2002; Kopsidas et al, 2002). However, COX-deficient fibers are relatively rare (0.1–5%), and the deficiency does not extend through the entire fiber (Brierley et al, 1998; Frahm et al, 2005). Thus, muscle mtDNA mutations may contribute less to muscle aging than motor neuron impairments. Impaired axoplasmic flow by motor neurons in the sciatic nerve (Goemaere-Vanneste et al, 1988) and spinal projections (Frolkis et al, 1985; McQuarrie et al, 1989) could be major causes of the reduced neurotrophic support. Axoplasmic flow also decreases during aging in the central projections

(De Lacalle et al, 1996; Geinisman et al, 1977). Cell-level gene expression may identify global or cell-specific impairments in biosynthesis that could cause diverse manifestation of synaptic atrophy.

What may cause the atrophy of neurons during aging? My lab is studying the increase of glial inflammatory changes that are concurrent with neuronal atrophy, in healthy humans, rodents, and monkeys (Morgan et al., 1999; Finch et al., 2002). Astrocytes and brain macrophages (microglia, of bone marrow lineage) are activated by middle age (Fig. 1.8A). The increased volume of astrocytes mainly represents cell hypertrophy. The total number of astrocytes does not increase during normal aging (Bjorklund et al, 1985; Finch et al., 2002; Long et al, 1998), although there are more and larger fibrous astrocytes with thick, GFAP containing processes (Hansen et al., 1987). GFAP is a cytoskeletal protein (intermediate filament) that increases with aging (Nichols et al., 1993) in parallel with increased astrocyte volume (Fig. 1.7E). The age-related increase of GFAP expression can be considered as an inflammatory response (Morgan et al, 1999). GFAP transcription increases in response to oxidative stress and inflammatory stimuli, possibly through redox sensitive elements (NF-1/NF-κB) in the upstream promoter (Morgan et al, 1997b, 1999). Diet restriction attenuates the increase of GFAP transcription and protein levels with aging (Morgan et al, 1999) in parallel with attenuating synaptic atrophy during aging (Chapter 3). Many other brain changes during aging are associated with inflammatory processes (Section 1.8.1).

We hypothesize that glial activation during aging is an inflammatory response to oxidative damage that, in turn, causes synaptic atrophy (Rozovsky et al., 2005). Microglia activation during aging is attenuated by diet restriction (Chapter 3, Fig. 3.19). We are testing these concepts by growing cultures of astrocytes from aging rats, which show age deficiencies in support of neuronal outgrowth (Fig. 1.9). The age deficiencies are associated with increased expression of GFAP and are inversely associated with secretion of laminin and other extracellular substrates. Conversely, we can induce an age-like phenotype in young astrocytes by increasing the cell levels of GFAP, with correspondingly less support of neurite ourtgrowth. These results show the close links of GFAP expression to astrocytic support of neurite outgrowth over a 2-fold range (Rozovsky et al, 2005).

Alzheimer disease (AD) differs from these normal brain aging changes (Section 1.6) by severe neurodegeneration in memory circuits with remarkable selectivity. The hippocampal pyramidal neurons of the CA1 field are devastated, while nearby granule neurons are relatively unscathed. Neuronal vulnerability to endogenous or exogenous insults must ultimately depend on gene expression patterns acquired during cell differentiation.

AD is rare before age 60 and increases exponentially thereafter with a doubling rate of about 5 years (Fig. 1.10) (Kawas and Katzman, 1999; Mayeux, 2003). By age 80, the AD prevalence approaches 50% in some populations but may be less than 15% in others. These huge differences are unexplained.

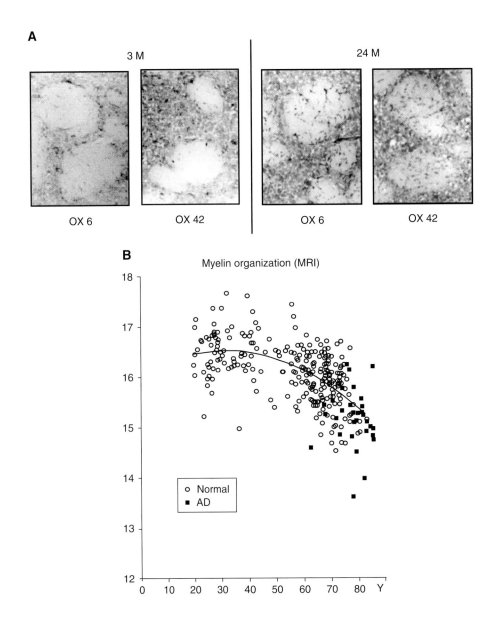

FIGURE 1.8 White matter (myelinated pathway) aging. A. Microglial activation in cortico-striatal myelinated tracts of aging F344 rats. Note the increased immunostaining (dark area) in 24 m markers of microglial activation; MHC-2, antigen of activated macrophage/microglia; CR3, complement receptor. (From Morgan et al., 1999.) B. Myelin integrity declines with aging in the corpus callosum (subcortical white matter) of normal brain (o) after age 50, with greater deterioration in Alzheimer disease (■). Determined from the transverse MRI relaxation rate signal (R2), a measure of myelin integrity (Bartzokis et al., 2004).

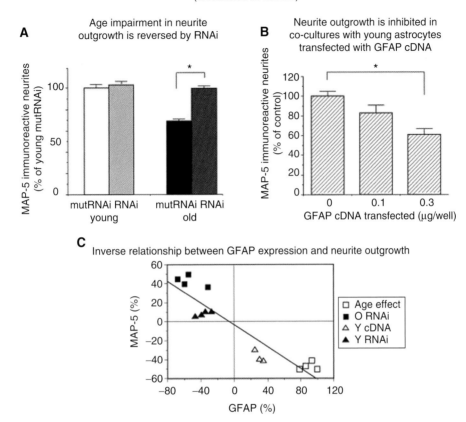

FIGURE 1.9 Astrocyte aging influences the growth of embryonic neurons. In the heterochronic glial-neuronal model, astrocytes are cultured from young adult and old rat cerebral cortex and then over-lain with embryonic (E18) cortical neurons (Rozovsky et al, 2005). Neuronal outgrowth on old astrocytes is markedly slower relative to growth on young astrocytes. The age effect on neurite outgrowth is reversed by downregulating GFAP, an astrocyte cytoskeletal protein that increases with aging (Nichols et al, 1993) in parallel with increased astrocyte volume (Fig. 1.7E). The age-related increase of GFAP expression can be considered an inflammatory response during aging, and is attenuated by diet restriction (Morgan et al, 1999) (Fig. 3.17B, Section 3.5.2). The lower panel summarizes experiments that manipulated GFAP bidirectionally in young and old astrocytes, with corresponding inverse effects on neuriote outgrowth (MAP-5 marker).

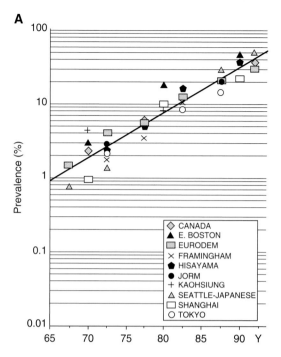

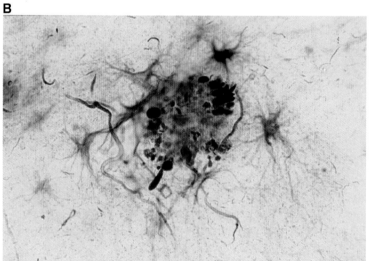

FIGURE 1.10 Alzheimer disease. A. Alzheimer prevalence increases after age 65 with a doubling time of about 5 y, which is faster than the Gompertz mortality rate doubling time of 8 y. Populations vary widely in dementia prevalence by 80 y (Kawas and Katzman, 1999). B. Senile (neuritic) plaque of Alzheimer brain showing abnormal neurites and activated glia. Courtesy of Christian Pike (USC).

A characteristic of AD is extensive deposits of extracellular senile plaques containing fibrillar $A\beta_{1-42}$ (Fig. 1.10B) and intraneuronal aggregates of neurofibrillary tangles containing hyperphosphorylated tau. A major hypothesis is that AD is driven by excess production of the 42 amino acid long amyloid β-peptide ($A\beta_{1-42}$) (Section 1.6). The diagnosis of Alzheimer disease is made by a threshold density of plaques, tangles, and neuron loss in the cerebral cortex and hippocampus. The diagnosis may be adjusted for age because of the increase of neurofibrillary tangles during aging. Non-demented elderly show accelerating increases of tangles to levels that overlap with early clinical AD (Braak and Braak, 1991; Price and Morris, 1999) and also show modest cortical atrophy with aging (Anderton, 1997; Launer et al, 1995). At very advanced ages, plaque and tangle accumulations may overlap with criteria for AD.

Amyloid accumulation in animal models is slowed by anti-inflammatory drugs (Chapter 2) and diet restriction (Chapter 3). Rodents are valuable experimental models to study human AD transgenes because they do not accumulate brain amyloid deposits during aging. Amino acid substitutions in the rodent $A\beta$ sequence (Johnstone et al, 1991) render it less able to aggregate into fibrils and possibly less toxic (Boyd-Kimball et al, 2004). In other vertebrates, the $A\beta$ sequence is remarkably conserved—fish to primates to humans. Aging dogs and macaques accumulate $A\beta$ deposits that resemble senile plaques of AD. However, aging chimpanzees, our closest ancestor, have negligible AD-like changes during aging (Section 6.3) (Finch and Stanford, 2004). The chimpanzee does not have a common risk factor in AD, the apoE4 allele, which evolved in humans.

1.2.3. Cultured Cell Models and Replicative Senescence

Unlike cancer cells, diploid somatic cells typically have a finite capacity for propagation during serial culture, shown first for skin fibroblasts (Hayflick and Moorhead, 1961). After a finite number of subcultures (population doublings), cell division ceases and cultures are considered senescent. The 'Hayflick' phenomenon extends to many cell types, including vascular endothelia and lymphocytes (Campisi, 2005; Cristofalo et al, 2004; Hayflick, 2000). Although the end-phase cultures are considered 'senescent,' post-replicative cells survive many months if media are refreshed (Matsumura et al, 1979). In fact, senescent cultures are highly resistant to apoptosis. Resistance to apoptosis may link back to the insulin pathways that modulate life span (Fig. 1.3), because senescent cell cultures have decreased endocytic uptake of the IGF-binding protein IGFBP-3 (Hampel et al, 2005). It is cogent to Query I that senescent cultures of fibroblasts and other cell types show increased inflammatory factors including COX-2, IL-1, MMP-3, collagenase, TIMP-1 (tissue inhibitor of metaloproteases) (Han et al, 2004; Parrinello et al, 2005; West et al, 1989; Zeng et al, 1996). These same changes arise in atheromas and, moreover, are blocked in senescing cultures by the COX-2 inhibitor NS398 (Han et al, 2004) (Chapter 2). Inflammatory factors secreted by replicatively senescent cells are implicated in focal tissue remodeling in the progression of pre-malignant cells (Campisi, 2005).

Individual cell variations in replicative potential are associated with variable telomere length (Martin-Ruiz et al, 2004). It is not known if telomere heterogeneity causes the daughter cell differences in proliferative potential, which range from 0 (growth arrest) to 15 or more replications (Matsumura et al, 1985). Somatic cell replicative heterogeneity may contribute to the remarkable differences of individual life span in twins and in highly inbred worms (Finch and Kirkwood, 2000) (Section 5.2).

Contrary to earlier conclusions, adult age up to 92 years does not change the Hayflick limit of skin fibroblasts (Cristofalo et al, 2004; Goldstein et al, 1978; Smith et al, 2002). However, cells from embryos or children have 2-fold higher Hayflick limits (Martin, 1970). Thus, the major effect of age on the cell senescence model is before maturation. *In vivo* exposure to oxidative stress may be a factor in the reduced proliferation of cells from diabetics (Goldstein et al, 1979). Moreover, the standard protocol of culturing cells for aging studies in ambient air (20% oxygen) is grossly unphysiological. When mouse cells were 'aged' at 3% oxygen, closer to the tissue levels, their replicative potential was greatly increased (Parrinello et al, 2003). Nonetheless, even under the standard culture conditions, in species comparisons, resistance of cultured fibroblasts to oxidative stress correlates with life span (Kapahi et al., 1999). We may anticipate fruitful further analysis of species differences in resistance to oxidative stress that might, in turn, inform about *in vivo* vulnerability to bystander effects from inflammatory processes.

1.2.4. Invertebrate Models

The fly and worm models are enabling highly successful studies of genetic influences because their gene regulatory systems of early development are known in detail (Davidson, 2006; Giudice, 2001; Grant and Wilkinson, 2003). Mutations modify longevity in association with altered mortality rate accelerations (Chapter 5). Some mutations that modify aging involve insulin-like signaling pathways and fat depots (Fig.1.3A). These convergences suggest the importance of energy regulation to aging, as well as to development. The energy-regulating gene circuits have persisted during descent from shared ancestors more than 650 million years ago. Although the causes of death in fly and worm are not well defined, the causes do not include tumors or other abnormal growth during aging.

The lab worm *C. elegans* naturally grows among the roots of plants. Propagation by self-fertilization eliminates more genetic variation than is possible with inbred laboratory mice (Johnson et al, 2005). Free-living larva hatch about 24 h after fertilization, followed by rapid development through larval stages (L1-L4) and maturation by 72 h. If food is limited, or population density is high, the larval development may be arrested for up to 2 m in the dauer larval stages. Dauer larvae cease feeding and utilize fat depots; body movements decrease, but stress resistance increases (Kimura et al, 1997). With improved conditions, dauer larvae complete maturation and proceed to normal life spans.

Worm life history has four stages lasting 2–3 w (Huang et al, 2004): I, active egg production by self-fertilization in the first 4 d (Bolanowski et al, 1983; Herndon et al, 2002), followed by several post-reproductive stages: II, post-reproductive, with vigorous movements; III, dwindling movement leading to the cessation of feeding; and IV, morbidity with little movement and accelerating mortality. Most eggs are produced during the first 4 days (Croll et al, 1977; Johnson, 1987; Klass, 1977).

While life spans in different genotypes and environments are well documented, less is known about the cellular changes and the pathology of aging. Cell death is not obvious during aging, despite the lack of somatic cell replacement. *C. elegans* is famous for its almost invariant cell number. Neurons look normal in ultrastructure studies throughout life, including neurons of slowed and decrepit worms (Herndon et al, 2002). However, muscle cells deteriorate in the body wall and in the pharynx, which grinds up bacteria that are the diet (Herndon et al., 2002). Lipids, lipofuscins (aging pigments), and lysosomal hydrolases accumulate in muscle and intestine cells (Bolanowski et al, 1983; Epstein et al, 1972; Garigan et al, 2002; Herndon et al, 2002), implying defects in catabolic pathways. Old worms are less resistant to pathogenic bacteria and show shorter latent period after infection (Kurz et al, 2003; Laws et al, 2004). Moreover, aging worms become constipated from bacterial packing in the intestine, which may induce oxidative damage. The usual diet of the bacteria *Escherichia coli* strain OP50 is considered by some to be mildly toxic; life spans are longer on heat-killed bacteria or other media (Section 2.3.2, Section 5.5.2). Long-lived mutants in insulin-like signaling (*age-1*) have delayed constipation (Section 5.5.2).

Although these worms are isogenic, constitutive variations in the levels of gene expression arise during development that influence later outcomes of aging (Finch and Kirkwood, 2000). Individual worms vary in the duration of these stages and in rates of aging. This extensive variability may be considered to extend variations present at younger ages in egg laying, feeding, and spontaneous movements (Finch, 1990, p. 560; Finch and Kirkwood, 2000). Individual declines of pharyngeal pumping and body movement were strongly correlated with life span in wild-type and longevity mutants (Chapter 5). For example, when fast pumping is maintained one day longer, the odds ratio for death by or later than a specified date is 1.7-fold greater (Huang et al, 2004a). The levels of expression of a stress-protective gene (hsp-16.2) in young worms predicted future life span, over a 2-fold range (Rea et al, 2005). This first example of individual difference in gene expression in the worm model supports the role of epigenetic variations arising during development that may ultimately represent chance variations in the assembly of the multiple proteins present in transcription complexes (Finch and

Kirkwood, 2000). In another model, cultured mammalian cells with a reporter gene did not respond synchronously or to the same level to a diffusible inducer (Zlokarnik et al, 1998).

The fly is a more complex animal with a beating heart. At 25 °C, early development takes 24 h to larval hatching. Three mobile feeding larval stages (LI-LIII) take 7 more d to pupation. During the 4-day pupal stage, without feeding or movement, the adult body is formed from the imaginal disks (metamorphosis). Adult life spans are about 40 d. Adult flies can over-winter, with extended life span from cool temperature and shorter photoperiods (Flatt et al, 2005; Finch, 1990, p.313; Schmidt et al, 2005). Unlike nematodes, the fly does not have alternate larval stages equivalent to the non-feeding dauer. Juvenile hormone (JH), a series of steroid-like molecules, influences or regulates growth of all developmental stages, particularly the timing of molts and metamorphosis, and also adult diapause (Flatt et al, 2005). JH synthesis is regulated by insulin-like peptides secreted by neurons (Section 5.4). JH also regulates stress resistance and immune responses that are like innate immunity of vertebrates.

Female egg-laying declines exponentially after a fairly stable phase, also observed in the medfly (*Ceratitis capitata*) (Novoseltsev et al, 2004). Both species have post-reproductive phases that only weakly correlated among individuals with the cessation of egg-laying. As with the worm, somatic cells are not replaced. Major damage is accumulated to the brittle exoskeleton from wear-and-tear (Finch et al, 1990). Unlike the worm, the aging fly shows some indication of neuron loss, in the mushroom body (Technau, 1984). The fat body, a key organ of energy reserves and immune function, gradually atrophies (Finch, 1990, p. 63). Apoptosis with DNA fragmentation increases in flight muscles and fat body (Zheng et al, 2005). The heart rate slows during aging and arrests more easily under the stress of electrical pacing, aging sharply (Wessells et al., 2004) (Section 5.6.3, Fig. 5.7). Insulin-signaling mutants with increased life span have delayed cardiac aging (Chapter 5). Little is known about vasculature of aging flies; other aging insects show indications of circulatory blockage (Arnold, 1961, 1964; Finch, 1990, p. 65).

1.2.5. Yeast

Yeast cells are similar to animal cells in their core biochemistry and organelles. We should not be surprised that the 6000 yeast genes include orthologues of insulin-like signaling and other genes in tissue-grade animals (Fig. 1.3A). Fungal genomes diverged from the animals about 1500 million years ago (Cai, 2006). Aging and life span in yeast are studied with two very different experimental models: *replicative life span* (Piper, 2006; Sinclair et al, 1998) and *chronological life span* (Fabrizio and Longo, 2003; Fabrizio et al., 2004).

The yeast replicative life span is defined by asexual reproduction through the formation of smaller buds on the surface of the mother cell. The intervals between budding lengthen as the replicative life span is approached, at about

20 cell divisions. Oxidatively damaged proteins are retained asymmetrically by the mother cell (Aguilaniu et al, 2003), which may be how the detached buds start the replicative clock at zero, independent of mother cell age. The replicative life span model resembles the Hayflick model in that both show limited cloning. The sterile postreplicative cells may have considerable remaining life span (V. Longo, personal comm). Mechanisms in replicative aging include a unique genomic instability in ribosomal DNA (rDNA) cistrons, through aberrant recombination that causes the accumulation of extra-chromosomal rDNA circles. The rDNA instability is modulated by chromatin condensation under the control of Sir2 (silent information regulator), a NAD-dependent histone deacetylase. Increased Sir2 inhibits the aberrant recombination and extends the replicative life span. Sirtuins and their orthologues have many other metabolic activities in animals (Chapter 3 and 5); e.g., diet restriction activates Sirt1 and modulates lipolysis in mammalian fat (Wolf, 2006).

The chronological life span is defined as the cell viability during prolonged periods with limited external nutrients. Yeast and other autotrophic fungi have evolved adaptive mechanisms in their natural habitats for surviving extended periods of starvation, pending episodes of surfeit. When switched from growth media to water, yeast cells become hypometabolic, extending their life span several fold to 15–20 days. Mutations in the kinase Sch9 increase life span by increasing stress resistance and glycogen reserves. Sch9, a functional homologue of Akt/PBK, which modulates life span in animals (Fig. 1.3A), also synergizes with Sir2 (Longo and Kennedy, 2006).

Ongoing studies point to the convergence of mechanisms in these seemingly different models, by the shared dependence of replicative and chronological life spans on Sch9, Ras/cyr/PKA, and Tor pathways (Longo and Kennedy, 2006). The formation of rDNA circles may be regarded as a 'yeast disease of aging' specific to the replicative senescence mode. Besides these single cell models, yeast can also grow as filaments (pseudohyphae) (Gognies et al, 2006), which enable the invasion of ripe fruit. Dense fungal mats can form, possibly including domains with metabolic gradients. These alternate life history modes with complex morphology have not been studied for aging processes.

1.2.6. The Biochemistry of Aging

Aging increases the load of oxidative damage in DNA, lipids, and proteins, yeast to humans (Sohal and Wendruch, 1996; Finch, 1990). Free radicals (ROS, reactive oxygen species) generated by mitochondria are a major source of oxidative 'bystander' damage. Other damage comes from extracellular ROS generated by macrophages, as is prominent in atheromas. Additionally, DNA, lipids, and proteins become glycated in an oxidizing process that is chemically driven by glucose and other sugars in tissue fluids. These advanced glycation endproducts (AGEs), while not initiated by free radicals, can generate ROS in further complex reactions and by activating macrophages (RAGE pathway, receptor of AGE), discussed below. In the following discussions of adverse effects of ROS, we must be mindful that ROS are essential in functions of the brain, heart, and many other organs that employ ROS in signaling processes. As examples from this large field, in the brain superoxide modulates synaptic plasticity (Hu et al, 2006), whereas in the heart nitric oxide modulates contractility (Massion et al, 2005).

Intracellular ROS is mainly derived from normal mitochondrial respiration (Barja, 2004; Wallace, 2005). The respiratory chain releases electrons that form the superoxide anion (O_2^-) by single electron reduction of O_2 (Fig. 1.11). Enzymes of free radical homeostasis include catalase; two types of supraoxide dismutase (SOD)—Cu/ZnSOD and MnSOD; and glutathione peroxidase. Superoxide is enzymatically converted by superoxide dismutase (SOD) into H_2O_2, which is then catalytically degraded by transition metals to the highly reactive hydroxyl radicals. These reactions are limited by the enzymatic degradation of H_2O_2 by catalase, or by glutathione peroxidase. H_2O_2 diffuses freely across cell membranes, unlike superoxide.

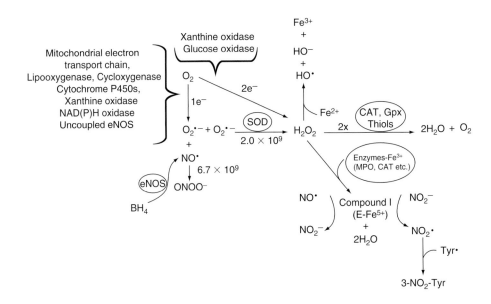

FIGURE 1.11 Free radicals and anti-oxidant homeostasis. Molecular oxygen (O_2) is reduced by loss of electrons to form superoxide (O_2^-•, 1e) or hydrogen peroxide (H_2O_2, 2e-). Superoxide spontaneously reacts with nitric oxide (NO). Most H_2O_2 forms spontaneously, or from the dismutation of O_2^-• by SOD (superoxide dismutase) and is used in cell signaling. H_2O_2 is degraded by intracellular catalase (CAT), extracellular glutathione peroxidase (Gpx) or thiols. Adapted from (Cai, 2005)

Pathways of hydrogen peroxide metabolism. Molecular oxygen (O_2) is reduced by loss of electrons to form superoxide (O_2^-, $1e^-$) or hydrogen peroxide (H_2O_2, $2e^-$). Superoxide spontaneously reacts with nitric oxide (NO) to form peroxynitrite radicals ($ONOO^-$). Most H_2O_2 forms spontaneously, or from the dismutation of O_2^- by SOD and is used in cell signaling. H_2O_2 is degraded by intracellular catalase (CAT), extracellular glutathione peroxidase (Gpx), or thiols. (Adapted from Cai, 2005.)

ROS are strongly associated with mitochondrial DNA damage (deletions, rearrangements, and point mutations). The age-related increase of damaged mitochondria DNA (Wallace, 2005; Chomyn and Attardi, 2003) has become a centerpiece in the molecular pathophysiology of aging (Brookes et al, 1998; deGrey, 2005; Harper et al, 2004; Van Remmen and Richardson, 2001). Mitochondrial dysfunctions are found in many disorders of aging, e.g., Alzheimer disease, atherosclerosis, atrial fibrillation, diabetes, deafness, muscle atrophy, retinal degeneration. However, cause and effect are not well resolved in these long-term processes of cell degeneration. Mitochondrial production of ROS increases with age in rat liver and muscle (Bevilacqua et al, 2005; Hagopian et al, 2005; Harper et al, 2004). 'Proton leak' across the inner mitochondrial membrane regulates mitochondrial ROS production with high sensitivity and increases during aging (Brookes et al, 1998; Brookes, 2004; Hagopian et al, 2005; Harper et al, 2004). Mitochondrial oxidative damage to DNA and proteins is often attributed to endogenously generated mitochondrial ROS. Because proton leak increases with oxidative damage, progressive mitochondrial impairments of various types may arise during aging through subcellular bystander damage, which propagates cell oxidative damage (Brookes et al, 1998; deGrey, 2005; Harper et al, 2004).

According to the oxidant stress theory of aging, life span should be influenced by levels of enzymes or anti-oxidants that produce or remove free radicals (ROS, NOS) (Bokov et al, 2004; Sohal and Weindruch, 1996; Stuart and Brown, 2005). The role of ROS is being tested in transgenic flies and mice by varying the levels of catalase and SOD that remove ROS (Landis and Tower, 2005; Mele et al, 2006). In flies, transgenic overexpression of mitochondrial Cu/ZnSOD increased life span by >35%, while catalase overexpression did not increase life span, reviewed by Landis and Tower (2005). Mice with partial deficits of MnSOD (heterozygote knockout, $Sod2^{+/-}$) lived slightly longer (Van Remmen et al, 2003). Although the 2.5% difference was not statistically significant, the survival curves show little overlap. This careful study also showed that SOD2 deficiency increased DNA oxidative damage (8-OH dG) and tumor incidence several-fold—e.g., lymphomas 61% versus 22%. The lack of SOD2 deficiency on skin collagen glyco-oxidation is discussed below and in Section 1.4.2.

From these results and more systematic species comparisons (Kapahi et al, 1991), I suggest that anti-oxidant mechanisms may be related to the levels of molecular turnover and repair. Flies may show these stronger effects on the life span than rodents because adult flies have no somatic cell replacement and, probably, less protein turnover, which, in mammals, removes oxidative damaged molecules. Long-lived organisms may have needed to evolve more effective repair processes (see Section 1.2.8).

Transgenic overexpression of catalase in mitochondria (mCAT) in mice increases life span by 20% (5 months) and delays important pathology (Schriner et al, 2005). This study is exemplary for its genetic design, detailed histopathology, and animal care (husbandry), even reporting the infection rate in sentinel mice. Mortality accelerations were right-shifted by increased mCAT, but without change in slope, implying that aging was delayed. Tissue changes are consistent with the Gompertz interpretation that aging is delayed. At middle age, cardiac pathology was decreased (fibrosis, calcification, arteriolosclerosis), which are common causes of congestive heart failure in human aging. In skeletal muscle, DNA oxidation (8-OHdG) and mitochondrial deletions were decreased. These findings directly link decreased mitochondrial ROS to heart pathology, which is recognized as of inflammatory origin (Query II). In a mouse model of accelerated atherosclerosis (apoE-knockout, apoE$^{-/-}$ with extreme hypercholesterolemia on standard diets), the systemic overexpression of catalase decreased aortic atherosclerosis (lesion area) by 66% and decreased F2-isoprostanes (lipid oxidation product) in plasma by 45% (Yang et al, 2004). Aortic lesion size correlated strongly with aortic isoprostane levels, again consistent with the importance of oxidized damage in inflammation. Cu/Zn-SOD had smaller effects on aortic lesions or lipid oxidation, specifically implicating hydrogen peroxide.

The hyperglycemia of diabetes is associated with another source of oxidative damage through glycation, which has not been well integrated into the free radical theory of aging. Glucose and other reducing sugars can oxidize and cross-link proteins by spontaneous and complex chemical reactions with lysine and arginine sidegroups yielding 'advanced glycation endproducts' (AGEs) that include highly reactive carbonyls (ketones and aldehydes) (Biemel et al, 2002; Monnier et al, 2005; Stadtman and Levine, 2003). Carbonyls also form by many other free radical reactions (Stadtman and Levine, 2003). Other targets of glycation are lipids (ALE, advanced lipid endproducts) (Baynes, 2003) and DNA (Bucala et al, 1984).

AGE adducts accumulate progressively during aging in extracellular matrix proteins as cross-links that reduce vascular and skin elasticity (Hamlin and Kohn, 1971; Monnier et al, 2005). Aortic stiffening causes progressive increases in systolic blood pressure (Fig. 1.6B) and pulse wave velocity (De Angelis et al, 2004) that are underway early in adult life. The formation of atheromas is superimposed on these slow arterial aging processes. Diabetes accelerates these vascular and lens changes, implying the importance of glucose and other blood sugars in damage to long-lived proteins during aging (Cerami, 1985). Conversely, AGE formation is slowed by diet restriction, which lowers blood glucose (Chapter 3). The lack of SOD2 deficiency on skin collagen glyco-oxidation (carboxymethyl lysine and pentosidine) in the study of van Remmen et al. (2003), discussed previously, points to the role of blood glucose, rather than extracellular ROS in glyco-oxidation (see below). As discussed below, AGE adducts participate in oxidative stress and inflammation.

Pentosidine was the first chemically characterized AGE cross-link identified in tissues (Sell and Monnier, 1989). Skin collagen pentosidine accumulates progressively during aging in many species, and the accumulations are accelerated by hyperglycemia and diabetes (Sell and Monnier, 1990). However, pentosidine accumulations are dwarfed by glucosepane, a recently characterized AGE that is 50-fold higher than pentosidine in skin collagen (Biemel et al, 2002; Monnier et al, 2005; Sell et al, 2005). Over the life span, glucosepane is added to about 1% of skin collagen arginine and lysine residues. This is equivalent to cross-linking of every five collagen molecules of normal individuals and every other collagen molecule in diabetics. Lens proteins accumulate far less glucosepane than skin collagen (Biemel et al, 2002). We do not yet know the specific contribution of glucosepane and diverse minor glycation products to cross-linking in skin and vascular stiffening.

Besides pentosidine and glucosepane, more than 20 other adducts derive from glucose, pentose, and ascorbate. AGEs form readily in test-tube reactions of proteins with glucose or other reducing sugars through Amadori and Maillard chemistry. The resulting brownish, autofluorescent mixtures are models for brunescent cataracts and other *in vivo* sites of AGEs (Cerami, 1985; Monnier et al, 2005). The aorta also accumulates fluorescent AGEs (Fig. 1.6D). Oxygen levels are critical to AGE chemistry and may degrade Amadori products (Ahmed, 1986). Glucosepane formation, however, forms directly from reactions that do not depend on oxygen, and is influenced by competing reactions; e.g., in the lens, the lower glucosepane may be due to high levels of methylglyoxal (Sell et al, 2005). Tissues also differ in enzymatic removal of AGEs (deglycating amidoriases) (Brown et al, 2005).

Of critical importance to inflammation, AGE adducts activate scavenger receptors 'RAGE' (receptors for AGE) on macrophages and many other cells that stimulate the production of ROS via NAD(P)H oxidases (gp91phox et al.) and electron transport (Fan and Watanabe, 2003; Schmitt et al, 2006). RAGEs are also activated by the amyloid β-peptide of Alzheimer disease and by AGEs present in cooked foods (Lin, 2003; Uribarri et al, 2003) (Chapter 2). AGEs and RAGEs appear to mediate feed-forward loops of oxidative stress and inflammation that increase bystander molecular damage in atherosclerosis, Alzheimer, and other chronic inflammatory diseases (Lu et al, 2004; Ramasamy et al, 2005) (Queries II and III).

RAGE activation also releases cytokines (e.g., IL-6) and leukocyte adhesion factors (e.g., MCP-1 and VCAM-1). Feedback loops induce RAGE by TNFα through production of ROS, mediated by NFkappaB (Mukherjee et al, 2005). RAGE signaling pathways utilize familiar workhorses in inflammation and oxidative stress, including the transcription factor NFkappaB and PI3K (Dukic-Stefanovic et al,

2003; Xu and Kyriakis, 2003). Moreover, PI3K interfaces with other signaling systems implicated in longevity (Fig. 1.3A). Lastly, RAGE activation may stimulate feed-forward 'vicious cycles' by autoinduction in the same cell (Basta et al, 2005; Feng et al, 2005; Wautier et al, 2001). RAGE-dependent processes are a major focus in atherosclerosis, particularly inflammation of arterial endothelia by AGE during diabetes (Feng et al, 2005; Naka et al, 2004; Ramasamy et al, 2005) (Section 1.5.1). RAGE-dependent processes are also implicated in Alzheimer disease and cancer. These observations are consistent with Query II that inflammation causes further bystander damage and Query III that nutrition influences bystander damage by AGE production from hyperglycemia and by AGE present in cooked food.

The molecular life span (turnover or half-life, $t_{1/2}$) is a major determinant of accumulated damage, as exemplified by AGE accumulation in arterial elastin (Fig. 1.6D). In arteries and lungs, elastin may be almost as old as the individual, as evaluated by two independent measures: D-aspartate (Powell et al, 1992; Shapiro et al, 1991), which accumulates linearly through spontaneous racemization (Fig. 1.6D) (Helfman and Bada, 1975) and by 'bomb-pulse' ^{14}C radiolabeling[1] (Shapiro et al, 1991). Human aortic elastin and cartilage collagen have $t_{1/2}$ >100 y, while skin collagen is 15 y. With lab tracer labeling, rodent elastin has $t_{1/2}$ of months to years (references in Martyn et al, 1995; Shapiro et al, 1991). Elastin progressively accumulates glyco-oxidation (AGE) (Fig. 1.6D), at the same rate as collagen, when corrected for turnover (Verzijl et al, 2000). Damage to arterial elastin and collagen contributes to the loss of elasticity and stiffening that cause the increase of blood pressure during aging (Fig. 1.6B) (Section 1.6.3, below). In Alzheimer disease, senile plaque amyloid and neurofibrillary tangles also include very long-lived proteins (also bomb-pulse ^{14}C) (Lovell et al, 2002). Other very long-lived proteins accumulate D-aspartate in tooth dentine, eye lens, and in brain white matter myelin. The accumulating oxidative damage to these life-long molecules is associated with creeping dysfunctions in arteries, skin, and eye lens; the role in myelin dysfunction is not known.

In contrast, molecules with short life spans of days to weeks have less oxidative damage. Diabetics accumulate glycated hemoglobin A1c, for example, which turns over at the erythrocyte $t_{1/2}$ of about 120 d. Erythrocyte turnover scales with body size across species ($M^{0.18}$) (Finch, 1990, p. 289). The $t_{1/2}$ of many proteins is allometrically related to body size and may be a crucial determinant of the rates of damage accumulated during aging across species. Moreover, the rates of basal metabolism correlate with molecular turnover in species comparisons of mammals. The insulin-like signaling pathways (Fig. 1.3) may mediate many of these fundamental energy relationships.

---

[1] An unplanned ^{14}C tracer labeling event occurred from atmospheric testing of nuclear weapons in the early 1960s; environmental ^{14}C has now returned to pre-1955 levels (Lovell et al, 2002).

Aging slows the turnover of many shorter-lived proteins (Finch, 1990, pp. 370–373; Goto et al, 2001)—e.g., bulk proteins in worm (Reznick and Gershor, 1979) and in mouse liver (Lavie et al, 1982; Reznick et al, 1981). The causes of slowed turnover during aging are not known and could include impaired proteasomal degradation, as in aging rodents (Goto et al, 2001). These metabolic level aging processes thus tend to accelerate the accumulation of oxidized damage. The effectiveness of diet restriction in slowing aging may be due in part to the accelerated protein turnover and decreased oxidative load (Chapter 3).

The balance of reduction:oxidation ('redox') in glutathione and other key homeostatic regulators (Fig. 1.11) is shifted to a more oxidized state (GSSG and protein-SSG) in blood, liver, and other tissues (Lang et al, 1989; Lang et al, 1990; Rebrin et al, 2003; Rebrin and Sohal, 2004), and in whole aging flies (Rebrin et al, 2004). Glutathione, the major redox couple, is at much higher levels than other redox links involving cysteine, thioredoxin, NAD, etc. (Sies, 1999). In healthy aging humans, blood GSH remains relatively stable; however, with cardiovascular disease, diabetes, or kidney disorders, blood GSH tends to drop below the normal range (Lang et al, 2000). Similar redox shifts occur during chronic infections; e.g., in HIV patients, blood GSH decreases in proportion to the viral load (Sbrana et al, 2004). Conversely, redox shifts are opposed by diet restriction (Chapter 3, Fig. 3.14). A component of the GSH shifts of aging could also be a response to low-grade infections, which would also be consistent with the increase of CRP, IL-6, and other acute phase reactants in aging populations (see below and Chapter 2). It is important to resolve the contributions to the oxidized load of aging from three sources: (I) endogenous mitochondrial free radicals and other tissue processes; (II) interactions with the commensal gut and skin flora; and (III) specific infections.

The naked mole rat (*Heterocephalus glaber*) is adding surprising findings to these debates. *H. glaber* is the most longevous rodent (at least 28 y), yet has similar body weights of lab mice (30–80 g) (Andziak et al., 2006; Andziak and Buffenstein, 2006). In comparison with lab mice (CB6F1) at 10% of the lifespan (24 m vs. 4 m), *H. glaber* had indicators of greater oxidative stress than in lab mice, e.g., 10-fold more urinary isoprostanes, 35% higher myocardial isoprostanes, and 25% lower hepatic GSH:GSSG ratios. While it might be concluded that sustained oxidative stress is not incompatable with extraordinary longevity, much remains to be learned about other aspects of metabolism in these remarkable animals. Its membrane lipids differ from other mammals by much lower levels of unsaturated fatty acids in muscle and brain, particularly docosahexaenoic acid (DHA or 22:6 n-3), which is highly susceptible to peroxidation (Hurlbert et al., 2006). The oxidizability of membranes (peroxidation index) fits well with the inverse allometry on lifespan.

These varying results across species suggest that anti-oxidant mechanisms vary within and between phyla. Besides differences in membrane composition and anti-oxidants, I suggest the importance of molecular turnover and repair. Flies may show these stronger oxidative effects on the life span than rodents because adult flies have no somatic cell replacement, except in the gut, and, probably, less protein turnover, while mammals have extensive molecular turnover, which removes oxidative damaged molecules. Long-lived organisms may have needed to evolve more effective repair processes (see Section 1.2.8).

1.2.7. Biomarkers of Aging and Mortality Risk Markers

For *populations*, the life span is expressed statistically, often as the life expectancy. However, no measurement has been found that accurately predicts the *individual* life span from the genotype, or from any 'biomarker of aging.' Clearly, the traditional aging changes of gray hair and menopause do not assess an individual's current health or future longevity. Jeanne Calment lived 70 years after menopause to achieve her longevity record of 122 years.

The N.I.A. has supported an extensive search for biomarkers that predict remaining life span (Biomarkers of Aging Program, begun in 1982) (Reff and Schneider, 1982). Biomarkers have been evaluated in biochemical, cellular, genetics, molecular, and physiological characteristics, and in behavior and cognition. Emphasis has been given to changes of 'non-pathological aging' that are distinct from disease. Two decades later, no single biomarker or combination has been found to predict longevity better than the individual age in fly, worm, rodent, or human (Finch, 1990, pp. 558–564; Warner, 2004).

Consider the limits of biomarkers in aging worms, which seem an optimal model for actuarial questions by their minimal genetic, environmental, and social heterogeneity from dominance hierarchies and social interactions (worms are self-fertilizing). Pharyngeal pumping, by which food is ingested, declines progressively during the first week and then nearly ceases a few days before death. Body movements closely parallel the pumping rates, not surprisingly because pumping provides the food needed for energy. The duration of fast pharyngeal pumping and body movements shows strong correlation with individual life spans (Huang and Kaley, 2004). When fast pumping is maintained one day longer, the odds ratio for death by, or later than, a specified date is 1.7-fold greater. The Spearman rank correlation coefficient for the duration of fast pumping and remaining life span was highly significant (r 0.49, P< 0.0001). Despite this statistic, the fraction of life span variance explained by pumping or movement was only 24%. Thus, other variables besides pumping account for about 75% of the individual differences in life span. Mutants with greater longevity have longer phases of active body movement and pharyngeal pumping. (Section 5.5.2).

Even at hatching, worms differ hugely in movements, which Kirkwood and I attributed to chance variations in cell organization and gene expression during development (Finch and Kirkwood, 2000, pp. 58–65). A concrete example is Tom Johnson's elegant study of worm-to-worm variations in expression of a stress-protective gene (hsp-16.2) in young worms, which correlated strongly with individual life spans (Rea et al, 2005). Again, the Spearman coefficient of 0.48 accounts for only 25% of the variance in life span. These sobering examples from rigorous studies suggest limits in the predictability of life spans despite strictly controlled genetics and environment. In worms, as in flies, mice, and humans, the heritability of the life span is also about 25% (Finch and Tanzi, 1997; Finch and Ruvkun, 2000) (Section 5.2).

As noted above, partial deficits of MnSOD did not alter mouse life span (Van Remmen et al, 2003). Several biomarkers of aging that respond to diet restriction were the same in $Sod2^{+/-}$ as in control aging mice (*ad libitum* fed in this study): both genotypes had identical age-related decreases of spleenocyte proliferation and increases in skin collagen of pentosidine and carboxymethyllysine. The lack of effects of MnSOD deficiency on these AGEs indicates that blood glucose was not altered. However, $Sod2^{+/-}$ mice had greater accumulations of oxidized nuclear DNA (8oxodG) in brain, heart, and liver, *and* 2-fold more lymphomas (83% vs. 41%). This study with its careful analytical chemistry and histopathology shows the uncertainty of connections between robust biomarkers of aging, tumor prevalence, and the life span.

There is reason to consider the individual disease load as more informative than tissue-level aging changes in predicting mortality risk (Karasik et al, 2005). During these same decades of the Biomarkers Program, vast clinical research has developed risk indicators of mortality for the major diseases. From the clinical perspective, disease, not aging, is the cause of mortality, as shown in the exponential increase of tissue lesions in rodent models (Fig. 1.5) and heart attack and stroke in human populations (Fig. 1.6C). Systolic blood pressure may be the most robust overall indicator of human mortality risk, with exponential age-related increases of future heart attack and stroke at all levels of systolic pressure.

The next phase of the biomarker debate may redefine the often vaguely used term 'disease.' For example, the clinical threshold of hypertension as a target for intervention is being expanded to include the 'high normal' range. A few decades ago, an informal guideline of the expected systolic pressure was "add 100 to the person's age"! Combinations of risk indicators and disease load are also being intensively studied of the inflammatory marker, C-reactive protein (CRP). In the Women's Health Study, future heart attacks occurred most frequently in those with both elevated CRP and LDL (Ridker, 2002). New models are needed to resolve the links between the diverse subtle subclinical aging changes that interact to cause circulatory failure on the background of declining organ reserves. It is shocking that 30% of diet-restricted old rats had no gross lesions at necropsy and cause of death was unknown (Shimokawa et al, 1993). Declining homeostasis of glucose and electrolytes, for example, might allow transient disturbances that would arrest a fibrotic heart, even in the absence of thrombotic blockade. The combinatorics of various mild dysfunctions gives rise to a huge number of individual pathophenotypes that may be each estimated as relative risk of mortality, but may never account for more of the variance in life span than in the worm model.

1.2.8. Evolutionary Theories of Aging

The demographics of natural populations are the basis for evolutionary theories of aging. In humans, like most other animals, the major phase of reproduction is accomplished by the young adults. Mortality from arterial and malignant diseases is low until after age 35, which approximates the life expectancy in most human populations before the 19th century (Fig. 1.1A). High levels of extrinsic mortality allow only a minority of humans to survive to older ages, until very recently. The major early causes of mortality are due to extrinsic risks, including infections, malnutrition, and trauma. A demographic pyramid with young adult ages as the largest is widely observed in natural populations. Sufficient reproduction to maintain the population can be distributed in many combinations of age groups, all governed by the level of mortality that allows a sufficient number to survive to adult ages *and* to reproduce sufficient numbers of offspring, which themselves survive to become reproductive. The reproductive schedule includes the duration of maturation, when individuals are at risk for dying before reproducing, as well as the frequency of reproduction and duration of the reproductive phase. The duration of the reproductive schedule is the prime determinant of lifespan (Hamilton, 1966; Austad, 1993, 1997; Rose, 1991, 2004).

Populations may be described by the Euler-Lotka equation, which is based on life table calculations as the net reproductive rate averaged over age classes, x (Hamilton, 1966; Rose, 1991; Stearns and Koella, 1986). The rate of population growth (r) is calculated at each age class (x) from the sum of the products of the mortality rate m(x) and the reproductive rate b(x).

$$\sum_{0}^{x} \exp(-rx)\, m(x)b(x) = 1.$$

The net population growth can not be negative for very long, or extinction results. Thus, increases in mortality m(x) must be compensated by commensurate increases in reproduction in one or another age b(x). Note that this equation is the sum of terms that are *commutative products* in each age, e.g., the number 8 is the product of (2×4) or (4×2) etc. Thus, an infinite number of different combinations of m(x) and b(x) can satisfy this equation. Because life expectancies are determined by mortality rates, we may speak naturally of the lifespans in plural that characterize a species. Lifespans are highly plastic and changeable in relation to the reproductive schedule and reproductive output. Experimental tests of these relationships are described below.

The duration of lifespans can vary widely in conjunction with the reproductive schedule. At one extreme are species that die after producing vast numbers of fertilized eggs, of which few survive to adulthood, such as in the five species of Pacific salmon (Finch, 1990, pp. 83–95). At the other extreme are species like the great apes that typically have one child at prolonged intervals, of up to ten years in orangutans (Wich et al, 2004).

Differences in extrinsic mortality between populations may lead to different reproductive schedules. In the common opossum (*Didelphis virginiana*), populations on isolated islands, which are exposed to low predation, are observed to mature more slowly and have fewer offspring per litter (Austad, 1993, 1997). Moreover, aging seems to be delayed, with slower mortality accelerations, slower collagen aging and longer lifespans than mainland opossums, which are under higher predation. These observations are consistent with the hypothesis that senescence is delayed if predation levels are lower in species comparisons (Edney and Gill, 1968), and Steve Austad's corollary that aging should also be modified commensurate with the reproductive schedule as external predation varies.

Human groups also vary in schedules of maturation and reproduction (Chapter 4, Fig. 4.5C). For example, in pre-industrial foragers, menarche occurs in the Ache by 14 y and first child at 17.7 y, while the Jo/'hoansi menarche is at 16.6 and first child at 18.8 (Walker et al, 2006). The precocious extreme is found in privileged populations with excellent health from abundant food and low loads of infections, where girls have much earlier menarche 12 years or less, closer to menarche in the great apes (Fig. 6.2). While we do not know the relative contribution of environmental factors and genetics in these populations, twin studies show that growth rates, age at menarche, and age at menopause have significant heritability (Chapter 5.2).

The force of natural selection is considered to decline during aging (Fig. 1.12A) because the majority of reproduction is achieved by the younger adults, which are the dominant age group in most natural populations due to external causes of mortality distinct from aging (Hamilton, 1966; Rose, 1991). The declining force of natural selection during aging is then considered permissive for the accumulation over time of mutations in the germ-line with delayed adverse effects emerging in adults. Examples include rare dominant familial genes for Alzheimer disease, breast cancer, or hyperlipidemia, which have little impact on young adults. Such delayed consequences of adverse mutations are not strongly selected against when effects are delayed to later ages that contribute less to reproduction. If a dominant gene caused earlier dysfunctions, its carriers would have difficulty competing for mates, and the early age phenotype would soon disappear. These concepts were introduced by J.B.S. Haldane (1941) and Peter Medawar (1952), and developed into rigorous theory by George Williams (1957) and William Hamilton (1966). In another hypothetical case, genes with adverse later effects might be selected by their benefit during development or in early ages—Williams' 'antagonistic pleiotropy' hypothesis (Williams, 1957; Williams and Nesse, 1998). Thus, the schedule of reproduction

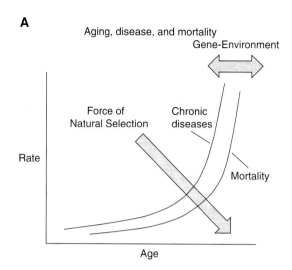

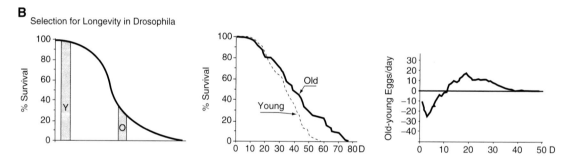

FIGURE 1.12 Evolutionary demography. A. Natural selection in aging, disease, and mortality in organisms with senescence. The force of natural selection declines during aging because most reproduction is accomplished by younger adults. With advancing age, the rate of chronic disease incidence increases exponentially (arterial events, cancer, Alzheimer disease), followed by increasing rate of mortality, as shown for rat in Fig. 1.5. Gene-environment interactions can shift these disease mortality curves, as shown for historical changes in humans (Fig. 1.1B, Fig. 2.7). Original figure (CEF). B. Using selection for reproduction at later age reproduction in flies (outbred *Drosophila melanogaster*) yielded flies that lived about 20% longer within 15 generations and had more gradual mortality acceleration; conversely, selection for early reproduction shortened life span and accelerated aging. The bottom panel shows differential in egg production between young and old selected lines. Redrawn from Rose (1984, 1991) and Luckinbill et al. (1984). Rose progressively increased the later age selected for reproduction, whereas Luckinbill maintained the selected ages.

for any species to survive (maintain Darwinian fitness) sets a lower age limit in the development of adverse phenotypes.

Many studies show the power of experimentally manipulating the reproductive schedule. In a now classic paradigm in the experimental evolution of aging, flies were selected for reproduction at later ages (Rose and Charlesworth, 1980; Rose, 1991). Within 15 generations, this selection regime yielded flies that lived about 20% longer and had more gradual mortality acceleration (Luckinbill et al, 1984; Rose, 1984; Rose et al, 2004) (Fig. 1.12B). Conversely, selection for early age reproduction shortened life span (Fig. 1.12B). These powerful effects require outbred populations and do not depend on the spontaneous emergence of new mutations and their fixation. Rather, shifts in genotype are attributed to frequency change of existing alleles, which occurs at a vastly greater rate than the mutation frequency. Moreover, the reproductive schedule and lifespan can be shifted back toward initial values in a "reverse evolution" paradigm, by switching the ages of selection (Teotonio et al, 2002; Rose et al, 2004).

These studies also show important gene-environment interactions in the density-dependence of lifespans, which were sensitive to population density in both larval and adult stages (Mueller et al, 1993; Rose et al, 2004). Density-dependent effects could involve microbial flora which grow on excreta and dead larvae. Bacteria (Hurst et al, 2000) and fungi (Rohlfs, 2005) are well known to influence larval growth and even the age of phenotype expression (Hurst et al, 2005). The microbial environment could also be important in aging fly populations that have greatly increased microbial load (Renn et al, 2007; Section 5.6.4).

However, unexpected results have come from studies of the guppy (*Poecilia reticulata*), which experimentally varied predation pressure (Reznick et al, 2001; Reznick et al, 2006). In some localities with intense predation and with high extrinsic mortality, fish mature earlier and have higher early fecundity. These different reproductive schedules show heritability that persists in the laboratory. Just as in the fly experiments, altering the extrinsic mortality from predation pressure in wild populations caused corresponding advance or delay of reproduction. When guppies were allowed to live out their days in the lab, the early maturing fish reproduce for an additional 200 days longer than the later maturing fish, contrary to the natural populations of opossums or the lab fly studies above. Moreover, the post-reproductive life spans did not differ between the early and late reproducing lines. These intriguing results challenge the evolutionary theory of senescence that was comfortably accepted for several decades.

Moreover, not all animals show reproductive senescence at advanced ages. Two species of turtles (painted, Blanding's turtles) have not shown decline in fecundity at ages over 60 y in longitudinal field studies (Congdon et al, 2003). Some older individuals continue to be successful in laying and protecting their egg clutches to hatching, as much as the average young adult. Similarly, the very long-lived rockfish (*Sebastes*) maintain seasonal cycles of *de novo* oogenesis at least up to age 80, and does not show evidence for declining fecundity (Finch, 1990, pp. 216–219; Finch, 1998; De Bruin et al., 2004).

These and many other examples support the possibility of 'negligible senescence,' or negligible decline in reproduction and other functions during the natural life span (Finch, 1990, pp. 207–247; Finch, 1998). 'Negligible senescence' as a potential life history type was considered theoretically untenable by most biogerontologists when I first proposed it, at least in part because of Hamilton's highly regarded mathematical model, which concluded ".... even under utopian conditions [of exponential fertility increase and immortality], given genetic variation....phenomena of senescence will tend to creep in" (Hamilton, 1966, p. 25). However, further theoretical developments by James Vaupel and colleagues (2004) show that the level of senescence is highly sensitive to assumptions and parameter values and that there may even be 'negative senescence' under some conditions.

Another challenge to evolutionary theory of senescence is the stable characteristics of senescence in related species, whereas evolutionary theory of the weak selection against later deleterious phenotypes should yield a great variety of different aging genes and great individual variability in aging. Indeed, there *is* great variability in life span, and specific aging phenotypes is certainly manifest between individuals. And, as well studied in twins, life span has low heritability (Section 5.2). Nonetheless, at the species and population level, some aging changes are so generally found that they may be described as canonical patterns (Table 1.1). In all well-studied human populations, arterial elasticity decreases and systolic blood pressure increases with adult age; menopause occurs by age 55 due to depletion of ovarian oocytes; reproductive tract tumors become increasingly prevalent; and bone density decreases, while the risk of disabling fractures increases. These canonical changes of human aging also characterize aging in other mammals (Finch, 1990, pp. 154–155), including details of arterial aging (Table 1.4, Section 1.5.3.3).

The basis of the canonical patterns in aging may be sought in development: Mammals share a basic body plan and program of embryonic gene regulation that determines the patterns of gene expression in differentiated cells. The human genome regulatory machinery was established at least 150 million years ago in mammalian ancestors and is apparently resistant to evolutionary change because of the densely connected transcriptional circuits required for embryonic development (regulatory kernels) (Davidson, 2006). Future studies may show the level of gene circuit regulatory lock-in that determines the replacement of molecules and cells in adults. As discussed above (Section 1.2.6), arterial elastin and other long-lived molecules inevitably accumulate molecular damage (Fig. 1.6D), whereas in circulating erythrocytes, the genomically programmed cell replacement with 120 day lifespans allows much less persistence and impact of oxidative damage. Thus, we must look to genomic regulation during development to understand the cell phenotypes that underly tissue aging processes and that may also be the basis for species differences of lifespan.

Molecular and cell repair, replacement, and organ regeneration require metabolic energy. Tom Kirkwood's 'disposable soma' theory of aging recognizes that energy resources are finite (Kirkwood and Holliday, 1979; Drenos and Kirkwood, 2005). Molecular and cell repair and regeneration require metabolic energy. At each moment, the individual organism assesses its homeostatic condition and allocates energy accordingly. Insufficient food intake attenuates immunity (Chapter 3) and growth (Chapter 4). We will examine this in the impact of diet restriction, which can attenuate immune defenses (Chapter 3), while infections attenuate growth (Section 4.6) and reproduction (Section 5.4.2). Each species has evolved within a relatively predictable balance of energy availability and energy that must be allocated for reproductive success. As one of many examples, when worker bees leave the hive to forage, a highly dangerous activity that accelerates mortality (Finch, 1990, p. 70), they decrease their immune defenses (Amdam et al, 2005). This trade-off of foraging energy against immune defenses is statistically favored because of the ultra-short life span of field bees. Theoretical modeling of trade-offs between investment in somatic maintenance and fecundity (Darwinian fitness) shows very broad curves of fitness, with optima that allow considerable variation in somatic investment (Drenos and Kirkwood, 2005). These results are consistent with observations that many biological functions do not decline appreciably and that major species differences are to be expected. A future goal of aging theory is to understand the physiological trade-offs of immunity, repair, and regeneration that define the species reaction norm of mortality rates to environmental fluctuations (Stearns and Koella, 1986).

1.3. OUTLINE OF INFLAMMATION

Inflammatory processes of innate immunity are evident participants in many tissue changes of normal aging and most of the chronic degenerative diseases of aging, as outlined in Fig. 1.2A and discussed throughout this book. Innate immune responses are the standing initial defense system against invading pathogens. The acute phase of innate immunity is mediated by secretion of systemic 'acute phase' proteins and the local activation of macrophages with rapid production of free radicals (Fig. 1.11). Acute phase responses do not depend on prior immune experience of adaptive (instructive) immunity, mediated by B- and T cells. However, exposure to new antigens during the acute phase response can activate the targeted immune responses to pathogen antigens by B- and T cells. Tissue injury from trauma or toxins can also induce inflammatory processes that go far beyond free radical production in tissue matrix remodeling and repair. Host defenses require energy, which is allocated in trade-offs, as just discussed, that determine the duration and type of inflammatory responses and the level of repair and regeneration.

The inflammatory processes at work in atherosclerosis, Alzheimer disease, diabetes, and obesity include a shared set of acute phase responses (Sections 1.5, 1.6, 1.7). Some of the same processes that macrophages employ to remove bacterial invaders are also implicated in arterial disease through the uptake of lipids by macrophages. Blood lipid responses to infections (lipid oxidation, elevated acute phase proteins, triglyceridemia) are also an atherogenic profile. Moreover, emerging evidence indicates roles for T cells in atherosclerosis (Section 1.5.3). Other tissue lesions of aging that involve chronic inflammation may also arise from an early seeding injury. Gastro-intestinal cancer, for example, is associated with local inflammation in response to *H. pylori* infections (Section 2.8.1). Remarkably, many of the acute phase genes are also upregulated in normal aging, in the absence of these specific lesions (Section 1.8). Cause and effect are unresolved in these complex, long-term processes.

1.3.1. Innate Defense Mechanisms

The acute phase of the innate immunity ('emergency line' ring-ups') include the ancient cardinal signs of inflammation in a localized injury: heat (*calor*), redness (*rubor*), swelling (*tumor*), and pain (*dolor*).[2] 'Inflammation' is now understood to include the vastly complex, multi-organ system of defense and repair, in which free radicals have major roles (Fig. 1.11) in directed cytotoxicity and in normal cell signaling.

Acute phase reactions can be stimulated by invading pathogens within one hour and, depending on the level of activation and efficacy of initial defenses, may continue for days or longer. These critical initial defenses rapidly enhance the removal of pathogens by phagocytosis, e.g., by induction and secretion of C-reactive protein (CRP), which is bacteriocidal by binding to Gram-negative bacteria and enhancing their removal by macrophages through phagocytosis. Blood clotting is enhanced by the increase of fibrinogen and other prothrombotic changes. Of major importance, energy resources are mobilized for increased cell activities and systemic responses such as fever. The liver rapidly secretes inflammatory proteins designed to neutralize invading organisms and to mobilize the needed energy. The acute phase inflammatory responses are coded by ancient genes with equivalents (orthologues) in invertebrates (Section 5.4, Fig. 5.4) as

---

[2]Cornelius Celsus (1st C. encyclopedist) in *De Medicina* described inflammation as *"rubor et tumor cum calore et dolore"* (redness and swelling with heat and pain), later expanded by Galen (2nd C. physician) " ... *et functio laesa*" (loss of function) (Plytycz and Seljelid, 2003). The inflammation in atherosclerosis and Alzheimer disease does not cause pain because the affected tissues are not innervated by pain fibers; however, joint pain from osteoarthritis is all too familiar during aging.

well as in lower vertebrates (Azumi et al., 2003) and plants (Ezekowitz and Hoffman, 2003). Transcriptional regulation is at the core of inflammatory responses, often mediated by NF-kB and PPAR.

The acute phase of inflammatory responses may be followed within days by the adaptive immune responses of lymphocyte B-cells and T-cells that recognize new antigens on an infectious invader. Antigen-stimulated immune responses involving somatic gene recombination occur in vertebrates, from bony fish to mammals, but were not evolved in worms, flies, and other invertebrates (Azumi et al, 2003; Marchalonis et al, 2002).

Inflammation in 'normal' aging involves the same cells and molecules found in the pathology of arterial atheromas and senile plaques (Table 1.3). I focus on CRP and certain interleukins (IL-1α, IL-6, IL-8, IL-10). These and other acute

TABLE 1.3 Inflammatory Components of Vascular Atheromas and Senile Plaque

	Atheroma	Senile Plaque
cells		
astrocytes	0	+ +
mononuclear cells		
macrophage	+ + + (foam cell, macrophage; CD68)	+ + (microglia, CD68)
T-cell	+ + (CD3 CD4/Th1)	0
mast cells	+ +	0
platelets	+ +	0
neovascularization	+ +	0
proteins		
amyloids		
Aβ	? (macrophages with ingested platelets)	+ +
CRP	+ +	+ (neurites)
SAP	+	+
clotting factors	+ +	0
complement C5b-9	+ (fibrinogen)	+
cytokines: IL-1, -6	+ (associated with CRP)	+
metals:	Fe	Cu, Fe, Zn

abbreviations: 0, absent; +/−, weak; +, definitive; + +, moderate; + + +, extensive. *amyloids*, Aβ: atheroma (De Meyer et al, 2002); senile plaque (Glenner and Wong, 1984; Hardy and Selkoe, 2002; Klein et al, 2001); *CRP* : atheroma (Rolph et al, 2002; Torzewski et al, 1998); senile plaque (Akiyama et al, 2000; Veerhuis et al, 1998); *SAP*: atheroma (Li et al, 1995; Meek et al, 1994); senile plaque, (Coria et al, 1988; Veerhuis et al, 2003). Aβ is detected in carotid artery plaque macrophages (De Meyer et al, 2002) and could be derived from platelets adherent to plaques, which contain the amyloid precursor protein (APP) and, when activated, release APP and Aβ-containing peptides (Jans et al, 2004); platelet APP-derived protease nexin 2 (PN-2) is an anti-coagulant (Van Nostrand, 1992). *C5b-9* (membrane attack complex); *SAA*, serum amyloid A (Akiyama et al, 2000; Finch, 2002); *B cells:* atheromas (Millonig et al, 2002); *T-cells:* atheromas (Benagiano et al, 2003; de Boer et al, 2006; Häkkinen et al, 2000; (Millonig et al, 2002); *mast cells*: atheroma (Kelley et al, 2000; Millonig et al, 2002); senile plaque *platelets*: atheroma (De Meyer et al, 2002; Nassar et al, 2003; von Hundelshausen et al, 2001); *complement*: atheroma (Torzewski et al, 1998); senile plaque (Akiyama et al, 2000; Eikelenboom and Stam, 1982; McGeer et al, 1989); *cytokines*: atheroma (Rus et al, 1996); senile plaque (Akiyama et al, 2000). *metals*: atheromas with intraplaque hemorrhages that deposit extracellular iron; also iron in macrophage from erythrocyte debris (Kolodgie et al, 2003); senile plaques accumulate metals in plaque core and periphery, and colocalized with amyloid fibrils (Lovell et al, 1998; Miller et al, 2006).

phase proteins are secreted by the liver (Bowman, 1993), but also by macrophages and other cells elsewhere. The amyloid precursor protein (APP) may also be an acute phase response in the brain (Section 1.6.2). These examples illustrate, but cannot fully represent the remarkable pleiotropies observed in the hundreds of inflammatory mediators.

When pathogens enter an organ, host defense systems respond immediately to isolate or destroy the invader and to close wounds to prevent further invasion from the skin, airways, or digestive tract. Pathogens are removed by 'professional' phagocytes, the ancient macrophage cells residing in every tissue and in the circulation. Acute phase responses are stimulated by receptors that recognize 'pathogen-associated molecular patterns' (PAMPS) of common invaders hypothesized by Janeway (Dalpe and Heeg, 2002; Medzhitov and Janeway, 2002; Netea et al, 2004). Bacterial PAMPs include their outer coat components, known as the 'endotoxins': lipopolysaccharide (LPS) of gram-negative bacteria (e.g., *Escherichia coli*) and the lipotechoic acid (LTA) of gram-positive bacteria (e.g., *Staphylococcus aureus*). LPS is recognized by specialized receptors in many cell types. In liver cells, LPS activates the Toll-4 receptors, leading to rapid secretion of CRP, IL-6, and TNFα. Bacteria are also inactivated by binding to blood lipoproteins (low- and high-density lipoproteins, LDL and HDL), which have specificities for LPS and other bacterial coat components (Khovidhunkit et al, 2004). HDL and LDL, for example, bind LPS. Some viruses are also inactivated by lipoproteins, e.g., Epstein-Barr, Herpes simplex virus. These and other pathogens are also implicated in vascular disease (Chapter 2).

Foci of chronic inflammation are broadly associated with cell proliferation. Hyperproliferation is hypothesized to be the cause of mutations arising through errors in DNA synthesis that increase cancer risk (bystander damage, Section 1.4). This hypothesis is well developed for the role of *Helicobacter pylori* in intestinal cancer (Section 2.9) and is being considered for other epithelial cancers, e.g., bladder and endometrium (Dobrovolskaia and Kozlov, 2005; Modugno et al, 2005).

Tissue fibrosis is also broadly associated with inflammation and may be considered as generalized wound healing response, which increases fibroblast proliferation and deposition of extracellular collagen and other matrix material. For example, myocarditis from Coxsackie virus infections developed focal scars with thickened collagen networks around surviving myocytes (Leslie et al, 1990). Interstitial myocardial fibrosis also arises during aging in the absence of defined infections in rodents and humans (discussed in Section 1.2.2), and is associated with increased myocardial stiffness during aging (decreased 'compliance') (Brooks and Conrad, 2000; Lakatta and Levy, 2003a,b; Meyer et al., 2006). Fibrosis is very common during mammalian aging and deeply linked, if not intrinsic, to general inflammatory processes in aging (Thomas et al, 1992). TGF-β1 signaling pathways regulate collagen synthesis and are implicated in fibrosis of liver (Lieber, 2004), lung (Chapman, 2004), and myocardium (Brooks and Conrad, 2000; Sun and Weber, 2005).

Many inflammatory mediators also have normal functions. (Gene classification systems that may be helpful in organizing data on expression should not be regarded as exclusionary of functions.) IL-6 illustrates these pleiotropies, which range from local cell effects to behaviors of the whole organism. While most circulating IL-6 is secreted by the liver, IL-6 is also made by adipocytes, neurons, and many other cells. IL-6 expression is regulated by transcription factors of convergent pathways that integrate local tissue and systemic signals (Kubaszek et al, 2003; Trevilatto et al, 2003). Moreover, IL-6 and CRP mutually stimulate transcription of the other genes (Arnaud et al, 2005). At a local site of injury, IL-6 regulates cell adhesion molecules that capture circulating neutrophils and macrophages (Kaplanski et al, 2003; Nathan, 2002). IL-6 induction can protect local cells from free-radical-induced death (Waxman et al, 2003). IL-6 is a stimulator (growth and differentiation factor) of B- and T-lymphocytes (Ishihara and Hirano, 2002; Zou and Tam, 2002). IL-6 also influences metabolism and stimulates the resting metabolic rate (BMR); the linear dose response to IL-6 increases BMR by up to 25%, as observed during fever (Tsigos et al, 1997) (Fig. 1.2B). Sustained elevations of IL-6 induce fever-related behaviors of lethargy and poor appetite. Thus, IL-6 sits in a highly integrated network sensitive to the energy state of the individual.

After the acute phase is initiated, a slower phase of adaptive immune responses may be initiated in which lymphocytes are mobilized to recognize new antigens. The differentiation and proliferation of new lymphocyte clones is regulated by IL-1, IL-6, and other interleukins (historically known as lymphokines).

The course of inflammatory responses is regulated by many checks and balances (Li et al, 2005; Nathan et al, 2002; Tracey, 2002) besides the anti-oxidant systems (Fig. 1.11). Local activation of the complement system (C-system) cascade is checked by inhibitors and short molecular life spans ('tick-over') of activated C-complexes (Morgan, 1990; Rother and Till, 1988). The complement system is integrated with inflammatory responses and is regulated by cytokines. Among many examples, TGF-ß1 represses the first component of the classical C-pathway, C1q mRNA (Morgan et al, 2000).

To counter the damage from the ongoing production of free radicals, body fluids and cells have strong anti-oxidant mechanisms. The redox recycling of glutathione in cells and in the blood is very important. Other regulators also inhibit or modulate inflammatory responses; e.g., local TNFα release may be inhibited by so-called anti-inflammatory cytokines, which include TGF-β1 and IL-10 (Elenkov and Chrousos, 2002).

Free radicals generated by inflammation also induce DNA repair mechanisms. For example, gastric infections of *Helicobacter pylori* cause infiltrations of immune cells that generate free radicals, in turn, increasing oxidative DNA damage and apoptosis in the gastric mucosa. Experimentally, *H. pylori* and H_2O_2 induce enzymes that repair oxidative DNA damage—e.g., the redox-sensitive transcription of APE-1/Ref-1 (apurinic/apyrimidinic endonuclease-1/redox factor-1), a multi-functional enzyme that mediates base excision repair of oxidatively damaged DNA (apurinic sites) (Ding et al, 2004; Lam et al, 2006). This adaptive response (one of many) increases cell resistance to genotoxic free radicals (Ramana et al, 1998).

The immune system is hormonally integrated. Pituitary growth hormone (GH) induces hepatic production of insulin-like growth factor (IGF), which is a mediator of immune and inflammatory functions (Denley et al, 2005; Russo et al, 2005). IGF-1 also feeds back to inhibit pituitary GH secretion. IGF-1 signaling utilizes the PI3 kinases (phosphatidylinositol 3-kinase isoforms) that are general workhorses in signaling (Fig. 1.3A, B).

Macrophages have high-affinity IGF-1 receptors and also secrete IGF-1 (Bayes-Genis et al, 2000), which may be important to both atherogenesis and Alzheimer disease (Section 1.6.4). IGF-1, but not GH, stimulates macrophage secretion of TNFα (Renier et al, 1996). Sex steroids influence immune functions response to trauma (Angele et al, 2000) and pathogens (Soucy et al, 2005). The deep associations of reproduction and immunity enable the evolutionary optimization in the face of the endless assault by infectious pathogenic organisms. Evidence that this selection is ongoing is the extensive genetic variations found in inflammatory responses.

1.3.2. Genetic Variations of Inflammatory Responses

Many genes that influence inflammatory responses may influence the risk of and course of vascular and Alzheimer disease (Chapter 5). Identical twins show extensive heritability in cytokine responses to LPS, accounting for a striking 50% or more of the variance in IL-1β, IL-6, IL-10, and TNFα (de Craen et al, 2005). The IL-6, IL-10, CRP, and apoE gene variants in regulatory and coding elements influence responses to infections (Bennermo et al, 2004; Kelberman et al, 2004).

In bacterial meningococcal meningitis, children carrying an IL-6 promoter variant with lower IL-6 production had 2-fold better survival (Balding et al, 2003). The lower production of IL-6 by the meningococcal LPS may reduce local bleeding (microvascular thromboses). Similarly, gene variants of IL-1β influence inflammatory responses to infections by *Helicobacter pylori*, a common pathogen, discussed above, which causes peptic ulcers and cancer (Chapter 2) (Blanchard et al, 2004; Rad et al, 2004). *H. pylori* will often enter discussions of chronic disease. IL-10 ('anti-inflammatory cytokine') has a promoter polymorphism that influences secretion by several-fold (Yilmaz et al, 2005) and is associated with different outcomes of hepatitis, meningitis, periodontal disease, and *H. pylori* (Chapters 2, 4, and 5).

CRP variants may interact with IL-6 variants. Four sites in the CRP gene are associated with plasma CRP levels: upstream promoter (Brull et al, 2003; Kovacs et al, 2005); exon 2 (Zee and Ridker, 2002); the intron (Szalai et al, 2002); and the 3'-untranslated region of the mRNA (3'-UTR) (Brull et al, 2003). Moreover, plasma CRP levels are influenced by alleles of IL-1 and IL-6 (Ferrari et al, 2003; Latkovskis et al, 2004) and of apoE (Section 5.7.4) (Austin et al, 2004; Rontu et al, 2006).

The apolipoprotein E allele apoE4, which is infamous for increasing the risk of heart attack and dementia (Section 5.7), also influences inflammatory responses. In some contexts, apoE4 protein is proinflammatory relative to apoE3. In cultured glia, exogenous apoE4, but not apoE3, induced IL-1 secretion (Chen et al, 2005; Guo et al, 2004). After surgery, apoE4 carriers had higher blood TNFα than the apoE3 (Drabe et al, 2001; Grunenfelder et al, 2004). Transgenic models confirm these effects. IL-6, TNFα, and nitric oxide (NO) production by transgenic apoE4 mice (targeted gene replacement) was greater than with apoE3 (Colton et al, 2004; Lynch et al, 2003). In its newest function, ApoE also mediates lipid antigen presentation to T-cells through CD1 mechanisms that are independent of the MHC system (Hava, 2005; van den Elzen et al, 2005). Other lipoproteins are also important in inflammation (Section 1.4.2.2).

The major histocompatibility complex (MHC) is a cluster of hundreds of genes that modulate instructive immunity and inflammation (Finch and Rose, 1995; Klein, 1986; Price et al, 1999). The MHC has many variant alleles in each of its genes and may be the most polymorphic complex locus in the human genome. The different combinations of alleles across the MHC gene complex (haplotypes) differ in proportion between human populations. MHC genes encode proteins used in antigen presentation, but also a wealth of acute phase and other inflammatory mediators including complement factors (Bf, C2, C4), HSP70, and TNFα (Finch and Rose, 1995). The MHC haplotypes are thought to represent selection for resistance to specific pathogens and toxins (Borghans et al, 2004; Klein, 1986; Wegner et al, 2004). Like IL-6, the MHC is physiologically integrated. MHC allelic variants influence insulin and glucose signaling (Assa-Kunik et al, 2003; Lerner and Finch, 1991; Napolitano et al, 2002; Ramalingam et al, 1997) and reproductive cycles (Lerner et al., 1998, 1992; Lerner and Finch 1991). Because of effects on life history traits that balance trade-offs of immunity, reproduction, and metabolism across the life span, the MHC may be considered a 'life history gene complex' (Finch and Rose, 1995).

The emerging genetics of inflammation may also involve haplotypes of the MHC. The MHC haplotypes involving TNF alleles show tentative associations with ischemic heart disease (Porto et al, 2005), whereas TNF isoform variants influence expression of the neighboring complement C4 gene (serum C4a levels) (Vatay et al, 2003). Besides the MHC gene cluster on chromosome 6 (Ch 6) with complement C2, C4, TNFα etc., other chromosomes include clusters of inflammatory and host defense genes: Ch 1, Regulator of Complement (RCA) cluster (C4bp, CR1 and CR2, DAF, factor H, MCP); Ch 2, interleukin-1 cluster (IL-1α, IL-1β, IL-1RN); Ch 11, apo A-I/C-III/A-IV gene cluster; Ch 16, CD11 cluster (integrins CD11a,b,c; adhesion receptors LFA-1, Mac-1, p150,95). Many other inflammatory genes for interleukins, chemokines, etc., are scattered across the chromosomes.

The many inflammatory mediators with genetic variants could contribute to the multi-factorial variability of many diseases. For example, the risk of gastric ulcer in *H. pylori* infections is associated with particular polymorphisms in both the CD11 cluster (Hellmig et al, 2005) and the IL-1 cluster

(Hellmig et al, 2005). The number of possible combinations among these gene variants is very large. Among the 10 or so recognized inflammatory risk factors of vascular disease, each has at least two genetic variants. Thus, the number of possible interactions approximates 2 raised to the 10th power, or 1024. This calculation gives an overestimate because some inflammatory genes are clustered on the same chromosome and hence not randomly assorted. The number of combinations grows faster for genes with more than two variants, as is the case for CRP and IL-6. These infrequent combinations could underlie sporadic cases of the major diseases that do not show obvious heritability. As human genome variations become mapped in populations in greater detail, it may be possible to find *inflammatory gene haplotypes* of polymorphic loci on different chromosomes that were selected by infectious disease. As a precedent, combinations of alleles in eight inflammatory genes and apoE were very recently found that discriminate Alzheimer disease risk groups (Licastro et al, 2006). Variants in inflammatory genes and insulin/IGF-1 are also implicated as regulators of longevity (Franceschi et al, 2005; van Heemst et al, 2005) (Section 5.7.2).

1.3.3. Inflammation and Energy

The acute phase response to infections rapidly mobilizes host energy needed to sustain fever and acute phase protein synthesis (Fig. 1.2B). White adipose tissue and liver have major roles in the energetics of host defenses (Khovidhunkit et al, 2004; Pond, 2003; Trayhurn and Wood, 2004). Plasma triglycerides increase within 2 h of infection from lipolysis in fat cells and by hepatic synthesis of fatty acids and triglycerides. Triglyceridemia may be sustained for a day or more. These generalized changes are induced by bacterial endotoxins and are mediated by IL-1, IL-6, and TNFα and other cytokines, which have direct metabolic effects. For example, TNFα acts directly on adipocytes to increase lipolysis and lower insulin sensitivity. IL-6 also stimulates lipolysis and in addition hepatic triglyceride synthesis.

Infections cause immediate and chronic energy deficits. The energy consumed by fever comes from 25–100% increases in basal metabolism (Lochmiller and Deerenberg, 2000; Waterlow, 1984). Protein, glycogen, and fat are mobilized; e.g., human energy debts in septic infections are 5,000 kJ/d (Plank and Hill, 2003), which approximates 50% of the normal daily food intake (10,000 kJ/d or 2392 kcal/d). In patients with active infections, white blood cell oxygen consumption increased by 50%, mostly from ATP turnover (Fig. 1.2B) (Kuhnke et al, 2003). The acute phase responses induce 'sickness behaviors' through hypothalamic mechanisms that decrease appetite and induce lethargy. T cell activation is closely coupled to the uptake of glucose and other extra-cellular nutrients (Fox et al, 2005). While energy partitioning to various physiological and cellular processes is understood in broad outline

(Buttgereit and Brand, 1995; Buttgereit et al, 2000; Rolfe et al, 1999), we do not know how much of the energy consumption associated with fever is due to activation of immune cells and the increased production of CRP and other acute phase proteins. The demands of immunity are considerable, because diet restriction attenuates the primary and secondary immune responses (Chapter 3) (Martin et al, 2007). Growth in children is also attenuated by infections which impair ingestion even if food is not limited (Chapter 4). Malnourished children with infections are in energy debts of 285 kcal per day of infection (McDade, 2003). The progressively reduced load of infections and inflammation in the 19th and 20th centuries is linked to the increased growth of children (Crimmins and Finch, 2006a) (Chapters 2 and 4).

White adipose tissue is considered an endocrine organ because of its many secreted peptides, particularly leptin and adiponectin ('adipokines'), which regulate metabolism and eating behavior (Ronti et al, 2006; Trayhurn and Wood, 2004). Leptin modulates appetite by binding to neurons in hypothalamic centers that regulate energy, body temperature, and reproduction; leptin also influences on insulin sensitivity and stimulates lipid β-oxidation in skeletal muscle. Adiponectin has some overlapping activities by stimulating muscle lipid oxidation by skeletal, and also inhibiting hepatic gluconeogenesis. Both leptin and adiponectin activate the critical AMP-activated protein kinase (AMPK) pathway that increases glucose uptake and lipid oxidation (Chapter 3, Fig. 3.11). Leptin is highly conserved in vertebrates, with homology to IL-6 and TNFα, and binds to class I cytokine receptors (Boulay et al, 2003). Moreover, leptin directly binds CRP in human serum and blocks binding to leptin receptors (Chen et al., 2006). These highly pleiotropic activities of leptin epitomize the nexus of immunity and energy regulation.

Because leptin is secreted in proportion to white fat mass, blood leptin levels are an index of energy reserves (Ronti et al, 2006; Trayhurn and Wood, 2004). Leptin is also a major immunomodulator with complex roles that are still emerging (Loffreda et al, 1998; Matarese et al, 2005; Steinman et al, 2003). Endotoxin induces a leptin surge, which may be an important coordinator of the acute and chronic phases of immune responses. In macrophages, leptin stimulates phagocytosis and increases secretion of IL-6 and TNFα. Adiponectin may have opposing actions (Kougias et al, 2005). In adaptive immunity, leptin is a co-stimulant of T-cell subsets, e.g., naive CD4+CD45RA+ T cells. Exogenous leptin can override energy decisions that attenuate immunosuppression, e.g., in starved mice infected with *Streptococcus* (Klebsiella pneumonia), leptin injection rapidly corrected the impaired phagocytosis (Mancuso et al, 2006). Reciprocally, diet (energy) restriction may be an intervention for the immunological abnormalities of obesity (Lamas et al, 2004), while fasting may benefit autoimmune disorders because of decreased leptin (Sanna et al, 2003).

Another relationship of fat to immunity is found in lymph nodes, where specialized adipocytes appear to supply follicular dendritic cells with fatty acids (Pond,

2003, 2005). Perinodal adipose tissue differs from adipocytes in other locations by a greater content of polyunsaturated fatty acids and by resistance to atrophy during starvation or hibernation. Intramuscular adipocytes may also be specialized.

Adipocytes also secrete acute phase proteins including CRP, IL-6, and TNFα; complement factors and serum amyloid A3 (SAA3); and prothrombotic factors plasminogen activator inhibitor-1 (PAI-1) (Lyon et al, 2003; Trayhurn and Wood, 2004). SAA-3 and PAH-1 are induced by endotoxin (LPS) and hyperglycemia (Lin et al, 2001; Lin et al, 2005). Moreover, white fat depots have numerous macrophages in proportion to obesity (body mass index) (Bruun et al, 2006; Trayhurn and Wood, 2004; Weisberg et al, 2003). The levels of inflammatory gene expression differ between white fat pad adipocytes and embedded macrophages: IL-6 is expressed in both, with TNFα more prevalent in these macrophages (Weisberg et al, 2003). The gene expression profile of white adipose tissue gives a good account for the association of obesity with the proinflammatory, pro-thrombotic blood profile in vascular events (Weisberg et al, 2003). Exercise and diet restriction can reduce the macrophage content and inflammatory expression profile of white fat (Bruun et al, 2006) (Chapter 3).

The brain receives information about the inflammatory status by detecting changes in blood sugar, cortisol, and other hormones, but also directly by the vagus and other nerves going from the gut to the brain stem and hypothalamus (Besedovsky and Del Rey, 1996; Black, 2002; Tracey, 2002). These neuronal inputs are part of *inflammatory reflexes*, which regulate hormonal secretions by the hypothalamus and pituitary and secretion of cytokines by cells throughout the body (Black, 2002; Tracey, 2002). Inflammation activates the hypothalamic-pituitary-adrenal axis and increased blood levels of the adrenal steroid, cortisol. Cortisol is called a 'glucocorticoid' because it stimulates the biosynthesis of glucose ('gluconeogenesis') (Riad et al, 2002), using carbon fragments derived from stored protein and fat. Cortisol elevations can attenuate induction of some cytokines (Franchimont et al, 2003; Nadeau and Rivest, 2003; Refojo et al, 2003), which is part of the basis for steroidal anti-inflammatory drugs (SAIDs) such as prednisone and dexamethasone.

Besides their key roles in disease, many inflammatory mediators also have normal physiological roles that are independent of the acute phase responses. During exercise, IL-6 is released by skeletal muscle in proportion to the intensity of muscular challenge (Helge et al, 2003). In adipocytes, IL-6 directly regulates insulin responsiveness (Bastard et al., 2002). Eating foods rich in fat, or induced hyperglycemia, increases IL-6 and TNFα by 50% within 4 hours (Esposito et al, 2002; Nappo et al, 2002). Could these proinflammatory responses to ingestion have been evolved as a protection against infectious pathogens that were very common in food, until recently? Chapter 6 discusses the dangers of eating raw meat in relation to our evolution. The dense synergies among the hormonal reg-ulatory systems of growth, metabolism, and immune functions may be critical to diseases that limit human life spans.

1.3.4. Amyloids and Inflammation

Amyloid proteins are closely associated with acute and chronic inflammation, and may be universally accumulated during aging.[3] Amyloid fibrils are aggregates of 10 nm filaments with repetitive β-sheets in parallel to the fibril axis (Kisilevsky, 2000; Pepys, 2005; Sipe and Cohen, 2000). The cross-β structure of amyloids is detected by binding Congo red, a birefringent dye ('congophilic amyloids'); however, cross-β structures are also formed by many peptides not yet associated with amyloidosis (Carulla et al, 2005). About 20 peptides encoded by separate genes can form amyloids. Extracellular amyloid fibrils accumulate in diseases of brain (Alzheimer, Creutzfeldt-Jakob) and heart (cardiomyopathy, atheromas). During aging, nearly all tissues accumulate some amyloid (Schwartz, 1970; Tan and Pepys, 1994; Walford and Sjaarda, 1964; Wright et al, 1969). Chronic inflammation often induces amyloids, some of which are acute phase proteins (CRP, SAA, SAP) with anti-microbial activities, discussed below. Bystander effects are also shown, with the accumulation of AGEs and other oxidative damage that attract macrophages and activate scavenger receptors (Section 1.4.4).

Three amyloids are notoriously associated with tissue damage: Aβ (amyloid β-peptide) of Alzheimer disease, *amylin* of diabetes, and *transthyretin* in cardiomyopathy. Amyloid deposits are usually embedded with acute phase proteins and sulfated proteoglycans (heparin). The amyloid bulk disrupts functions in the hereditary transthyretin amyloidoses, which damage the myocardium and peripheral nerves (Buxbaum and Tagoe, 2000; Morner et al, 2005). Oligomeric amyloid aggregates are also cytotoxic (Bucciantini et al, 2002; Kayed et al, 2003; Reixach et al, 2004) and important in Alzheimer disease (Section 1.6).

Other amyloidogenic proteins are acute phase responses and some have anti-microbial activities. C-reactive protein (*CRP*), serum amyloid A (*SAA*), and serum amyloid P (*SAP*) bind microbial pathogens. These ancient proteins form pentameric fibrils (pentraxins) that have orthologues throughout vertebrates and invertebrates (Finch and Marchalonis, 1996; Shrive et al, 1999; Ying et al, 1992). The case for anti-microbial functions is clearest for CRP, which enhances the phagocytosis (opsonization) by binding lipopolysaccharide (LPS) and other components of gram-negative bacteria (Bodman-Smith et al, 2002; Ng et al, 2004).

Infections can induce amyloids throughout the body, including the brain, as observed in HIV (Section 2.7.2). In a transgenic model of transthyretin, myocardial amyloid was observed in one mouse colony considered 'dirty,' but not in a specific-pathogen free (SPF) colony (Noguchi et al, 2002). Moreover, tissue

---

[3]Rudolf Virchow, founder of the cell theory, introduced 'amyloid' in 1854 to describe starchy hepatic deposits that reacted with iodine. However, this histochemistry was misleading: amyloids were soon identified as proteins (Andree and Sedivy, 2005; Picken, 2001), but the old term persists.

amyloids in DBA/2 mice were observed in earlier dirty colonies, but not in the cleaner later SPF colonies (Lipman et al., 1993). These responses to the microbial environment suggest that tissue amyloid deposits may be part of host defense innate immunity.

On the other side, some infectious bacteria and fungi have evolved cell-wall amyloid proteins to penetrate host defenses (Gebbink et al, 2005). The microcin amyloid of *Klebsiella pneumonia* forms cytotoxic pores, as well as non-toxic fibrils (Bieler et al, 2005), whereas the Tafi peptide of *Salmonella typhimurium* forms amyloid fibrils that enhance intestinal colonization (Sukupolvi et al, 1997). Endless host–pathogen "arms races" that select for specialized host responses may give rise to population-specific genetic risk factors in Alzheimer and other amyloidotic diseases.

1.4. BYSTANDER DAMAGE AND DEPENDENT VARIABLES IN SENESCENCE

Bystander damage is fundamental to aging. Inevitably, long-lived molecules accumulate damage from chemical agents in the immediate fluid environment, particularly glucose and free radicals such as reactive oxygen species (ROS) (Fig. 1.11). This chemical damage is described as 'bystander' because it is passively incurred. Bystander damage accumulates when the rate of incident damage exceeds the rate of molecular repair by enzymes or by 'rejuvenation' from new molecular synthesis with catabolism (turnover) of the old molecule. Bystander damage with time-dose relationships is recognized by epidemiology, e.g., pack-years of exposure to tobacco smoke (Chapter 2). Other biomedical fields have equivalents. Arterial disease includes bystander damage, as an 'aging process × exposure time interaction' (Lakatta and Levy, 2003a). Different types of bystander effects arise during immune clone differentiation through diffusible immunoregulators (Fletcher et al, 2005). It seems fruitful to expand bystander damage as a framework for resolving the levels of environmental effects in aging, exogenous and endogenous.

Four types of bystander damage may be considered. Type 1: Free radical damage, which is intensified by inflammation (Chapter 2) or attenuated by diet restriction (Chapter 3). Inflammation can also induce tissue amyloid deposits, which then become bystander targets. Type 2: Glyco-oxidation of proteins and DNA occurs non-enzymatically by spontaneous reaction with sugars that are omnipresent in extracellular fluids (AGE, or advanced glycation endproducts). Glyco-oxidation also stimulates local production of reactive oxygen species (ROS) and other inflammatory responses in arterial remodeling. Type 3: Chronic cell proliferation, which can be stimulated by oxidative stress and inflammation, leading to increased somatic mutational load, increased telomere erosion, and altered immune functions (depletion of naive T cells). Type 4: Mechanical trauma, which accumulates unavoidably during aging in the real world through accidents and mechanical wear and tear, but also violence from predation and social stress. At the microscopic level, mechanical forces in arterial blood flow (atheroprone flow) influence the location of atheromas through inflammatory patterns of gene expression (discussed briefly below and extensively in Section 1.5.3.2). This outline of bystander damage as a main category of molecular aging is an initial draft of concepts that cannot be comprehensive.

Bystander damage may be understood in distinction with two other types of molecular aging changes that are less dependent on the immediate environment: The spontaneous racemization of L-amino acids and the misincorporation (template errors) in DNA synthesis both occur at some irreducible rate that may be considered as 'intrinsic aging'. Amino acid racemization is an intrinsic property of molecular instability, which would also occur in pure water. The accumulation of D-aspartate may be used to estimate the age of the protein, with some caveats (Bada et al, 1974; Helfman and Bada, 1975). Mutations and other errors in DNA replication, transcription, and translation are inevitable because enzymes have intrinsic and irreducible errors in templating. In DNA polymerases, chain elongation depends on selection of the properly matched base among the four choices (AT,GC), which arrive at the site of synthesis by diffusion. Selection of the next base for chain elongation depends on Watson-Crick complementary pairing, which is entropy-driven (Petruska and Goodman, 1995). The role of entropy to telomere DNA erosion during somatic cell replication is undefined. Errors in transcription and translation may involve similar issues in mismatching, but much less is known (Finch and Kirkwood, 2000). Nonetheless, racemization and misincorporation are subject to the local environment. D-amino acids can be removed by repair enzymes (Brunauer and Clarke, 1986; DeVry et al, 1996). While DNA repair is well studied (base excision repair of oxidized bases), oxidized amino acids in proteins are also repaired. Repair mechanisms and chemical defenses against bystander damage may be fundamental in the evolution of life spans.

1.4.1. Free Radical Bystander Damage (Type 1)

Free radicals cause chemical damage with long-term consequences of increased mortality, as shown in examples discussed in the following chapters. Lungs are vulnerable to bystander damage with further progressive consequences to heart functions. Cigarette smoke causes chronic oxidative stress from activated macrophages (MacNee, 2001). Particulate aerosols from the combustion of fossil fuels (e.g., 'oil fly ash') cause oxidative damage and chronic respiratory disease (Ghio et al., 2000a,b, 2002). Fly ash inhalation stimulates invasion by leukocytes, which release superoxide; lung fluids had 2-fold higher levels of TNFα (which activates neutrophils) and higher GSSG (oxidized glutathione, reflecting oxidative stress). Lung damage is greatly attenuated by increased extra-cellular SOD in transgenic mice (Ghio et al, 2002). Increased SOD also blunts lung damage to hypoxia (Ahmed et al, 2003). Moreover, nitric oxide deficits (NOSII gene deletion) (Fakhrzadeh et al, 2002) or deficits of TNF-receptors (Cho et al, 2001) decrease lung inflammatory damage after ozone inhalation.

Systemic oxidative damage is caused by exposure to other inflammogens and infections. Rodents injected with the endotoxin LPS to cause sterile inflammation had rapid 5-fold increases of plasma LDL hydroperoxides (Memon et al, 2000). Lipoprotein oxidation during infections has important impact on atherogenesis, discussed below. Because oxidatively damaged molecules are recognized by macrophages through scavenger receptors, the induction of inflammatory genes during aging (Section 1.8) could be downstream to these host defenses. The uptake of oxidized LDL by vascular macrophages is a 'molecular Trojan horse' that induces inflammatory processes at the core of atherogenesis (Hajjar and Haberland, 1997) (Section 1.6). Thus, many aspects of aging could result from cell and molecular damage from extra-cellular free radicals produced during chronic, low-grade inflammation (Query II).

Chronic infections also cause chronic inflammatory bystander damage through ROS and other free radicals. Among many examples, infections by the enter-obacter *Helicobacter pylori* cause local inflammatory responses that increase DNA oxidation, cell proliferation, and the mutational load, and are a major cause of gut cancer (Section 2.8.1). Another classic example is tuberculosis (TB), which causes organ damage by host defense mechanisms that induce local fibrous connective tissue to wall off the bacillus and local amyloid deposits (Nathan et al, 2002). Pulmonary TB typically causes loss of lung tissue and 'vital capacity,' which is a major risk factor of mortality during aging (Section 1.2.2). TB also increases systemic oxidation, with higher lipid peroxidation in serum proteins and erythrocytes (Vijayamalini and Manoharan, 2004).

Amyloids (Section 1.3.4) are a crucial interface of inflammation and oxidative bystander damage through local oxidative stress (Ando et al, 1997; Butterfield et al, 2002; Miyata et al, 2000; Wong et al, 2001). The AA-amyloid fibrils in tuberculosis (TB) and rheumatoid arthritis (RA) and in a mouse model of SAA accumulate advanced glycation endproducts (AGEs): carboxymethyllysine (CML), and 4-hydroxynonenal (4-HNE, lipid peroxidation adduct) (Kamalvand and Ali-Khan, 2004). In Alzheimer brains (Girones et al, 2004; Reddy et al, 2002; Wong et al, 2001) and in a transgenic model (Munch et al, 2003), fibrilar Aβ amyloid also accumulates glyco-oxidation and lipid peroxidation adducts. In the glia surrounding brain Aβ deposits (Fig. 1.10B), AGEs are colocalized with iNOS (Wong et al, 2001) and may activate microglia through RAGE receptors (Section 1.2.6).

Metals may have a particular role in senile plaque amyloid, which has copper, iron, and zinc at concentrations 2- to 5-fold above healthy brain neuropil (Lovell et al, 1998). Aß and metal interactions are implicated in oxidative damage (Bush and Tanzi, 2002). The Aß peptide directly binds iron, which increases cytotoxic H_2O_2 production (Boyd-Kimball, 2004). Moreover, Aß binds heme to form complexes with peroxidase activity (Atamna and Tanzi, 2006). Furthermore, trace metals promote Aß aggregation (Huang et al, 2004c). There is little doubt that accumulated adducts in amyloids are proinflammatory, but their contribution to cell death is not defined.

Age-related increases of mitochondrial production of ROS through proton leak in rat liver and muscle causes bystander damage (Section 1.2.6). Diet restriction attenuates mitochondrial ROS production and DNA damage (Chapter 3). These benefits of diet restriction may be due to lower insulin and glucose, because mitochondrial ROS production is sensitive to insulin (Lambert et al, 2004). Conversely, maturity onset diabetes is associated with increased mitochondrial DNA damage and impaired energetics (Wallace, 2005).

1.4.2. Glyco-oxidation (Type 2)

Oxidative damage to DNA, lipids, and proteins is the result of unavoidable exposure to blood glucose that chemically generates AGEs (Section 1.2.6). The production of AGEs is increased by hyperglycemia and decreased by diet restriction (Chapter 3). Moreover, cooked food is an important source of AGEs, which can induce systemic inflammatory responses (Section 2.4.2). These experiments imply a large role for inflammation-induced ROS damage, which has been neglected in discussions of oxidative damage during aging because of the major focus on mitochondrial ROS. Because AGEs inevitably accumulate from the constant exposure of long-lived molecules to omnipresent glucose, bystander damage seems applicable to early stages of these general aging processes. The conceptualization of AGE formation as bystander damage is my own and open to discussion.

1.4.3. Chronic Proliferation (Type 3)

Adaptive immunity changes profoundly during aging as memory T cells increase at the expense of naive T cells. The depletion of naive T cells by chronic infections (Section 2.8) could be included in bystander effects. As noted in the overview of immune aging (Section 1.2.2), chronic infections by the ubiquitous virus CMV are associated with the 'immune risk phenotype' of impairments in the elderly, which increases mortality risk (Akbar and Fletcher, 2005; Pawelec et al, 2005). Unexpectedly, these studies also associated CMV seropositivity with greater differentiation of CD4[+] T cells specific for other antigens than in CMV-seronegative elderly (Fletcher et al, 2005). Other CD4[+] T cell specificities included varicella zoster virus (VZV) and Epstein-Barr virus (EBV). The greater T cell differentiation was characterized by shorter telomeres and loss of CD27 and CD28 costimulatory proteins. It was hypothesized that IFN-α and TNFα are secreted during activation of CMV-specific T cells and diffuse to accelerate other T-cell differentiation 'in a bystander fashion.' This concept was validated with CMV-activated T cells and T cells of other specificities, in which the inhibition of telomerase was shown to depend on IFN-α. Further evidence is the acceleration of T-cell differentiation by IFN-α therapy for hepatitis-C virus, which increased the proportion of CD28[−] T cells (Manfras et al, 2004).

In a different human population, (Khan et al, 2004) showed that CMV infection reduced immunity to EBV. Thus, chronic immune activation by CMV and possibly other common antigens can cause bystander effects by accelerating the differentiation of other T cells through secretion of IFN-α and other cytokines. The increased secretion of proinflammatory cytokines and the extreme T-cell differentiation during CMV infections may be an important link to the 'immune risk phenotype.'

Telomere erosion can be affected by bystander damage through oxidative stress. For example, telomere shortening is accelerated by oxidative stress in vascular endothelial cells (HUVECS) (Kurz et al, 2004). In diploid fibroblasts, telomere loss was attenuated by overexpressing extracellular SOD (EC isoform), which also lowered intracellular peroxides that can cause oxidative damage; the increased SOD also increased the cell replicative potential (Serra et al, 2003). SOD may decrease single-strand DNA breaks induced by oxidative stress, which enhances replicative telomere DNA loss (Sitte et al, 1998). Telomere erosion is pertinent to arterial disease because the replicative senescence of endothelial progenitor cells may be accelerated by elevated antiotensin in hypertension, or attenuated by antioxidants and statins (Section 1.5.3).

Yet other conditions shorten telomeres without primary causes of single-strand DNA breaks or other DNA damage by oxidative stress. Local secretions of cytokines during differentiation of T cells may cause other bystander effects by influencing the differentiation of neighboring immune cells (Fletcher et al, 2005) (Section 2.5.1). Inhibition of the glutathione-dependent antioxidant system that disposes of peroxides also accelerated telomere shortening and shortened the replicative potential in endothelial cultures (Kurz et al, 2004).

Telomere length may represent cumulative stress as bystander exposure (von Zglinicki and Martin-Ruiz, 2005). In different tissues of the same elderly individuals, telomere length correlated strongly in fibroblasts and blood monocytes (Friedrich et al, 2000; von Zglinicki et al, 2000). The absolute lengths of telomeric DNA differed widely, but individuals with long telomeres in monocytes had long telomeres in their fibroblasts. The cell correlations in different tissues within an individual imply systemic influences on cell proliferation, with consequent impact on telomere DNA in multiple cell types. The cumulative exposure to infections (Section 2.5.1) and stress during the lifetime (Section 2.5.2) may determine the overall levels of telomere erosion in lymphocyte clones. Systemic inflammatory responses can influence metabolic hormones, some of which regulate telomerase activity—e.g., IGF-1 (Bayne and Liu, 2005).

1.4.4. Mechanical Bystander Effects (Type 4)

Blood pulses transmit mechanical forces to the arterial endothelium that causes local molecular and cell responses as bystanders in this most vital function. Atheromas tend to form at arterial branches and curves, where the physics of blood flow alters shear forces. Growing plaques are increasingly exposed stresses that may cause fissures and fractures. Thus, the direct impact of blood flow may cause plaque instability through mechanical forces as bystander effects. Moreover, arterial flow variations 'atheroprone' and 'athero-protective' induce inflammatory gene expression in the vascular endothelia (Dai et al, 2004)—e.g., IL-1 and complement C3—but decreased expression of IL-10, an anti-inflammatory cytokine. The redox-sensitive transcription factor NF-κB is 4-fold higher in atheroprone regions. However, normal flow represses arterial inflammatory gene expression.

These examples of bystander damage suggest a casual framework for considering aging as a system of interactions, exogenous and endogenous, rather than autogenous. Recognizing that bystander damage is a major outcome of aging leads to a broader issue, about *time* as an independent variable in 'age-related' changes of senescence. Aging and time in this sense are operationally the 'duration of exposure.' In essence, most aging changes are *event-dependent*, rather than time-dependent. Event-dependence helps focus on the proximal causes of changes during 'aging' (Finch, 1988; Finch, 1990, p. 6). This recognition is explicit in epidemiological models, for example, of the cancer risks of smoking, which consider pack-years, rather than age-years of smoking. Dose-duration relationships are also understood as fundamental in arterial disease (area of artery involved, Fig. 1.6A); in colo-rectal cancer (area of intestine inflamed, Section 2.9.1); and growth attenuation by enteric infections (diarrhea days, Chapter 4.6.1). Each system of bystander damage may have boundary values in the commutative product of dose × duration, because of threshold effects and excluded values.

PART II

The second part of Chapter 1 considers in more detail the workings of inflammatory processes at work in arterial disease and Alzheimer disease, and their overlap with aging change in the absence of diseases. Shared inflammatory processes may mediate effects of diet, drugs, and lifestyle (Chapters 2 and 3); may have been the basis for the recent increases of life span in human populations (Chapter 2); may be in the developmental origins of arterial disease and diabetes (Chapter 4); may be influenced by genetic variants in aging and life span; and may have been the basis for the evolution of the longer human life span from great ape ancestors (Chapter 6). The slow degenerative changes involve complex remodeling processes in arteries and brain that extend beyond simple oxidative damage.

1.5. ARTERIAL AGING AND ATHEROSCLEROSIS

The primacy of arterial degeneration in human aging and the importance of inflammatory processes are not modern concepts. A century ago, William Osler asserted the importance of arterial degeneration in human aging: "Arterio-sclerosis is an accompaniment of old age, and is the expression of the natural wear and tear to which the tubes are subjected. Longevity is a vascular question, which has been well expressed in the axiom 'a man is only as old as his arteries'" (Osler, 1892, p. 664). Even in 1858, Rudolph Virchow considered inflammation as a primary cause of arterial disease: "I have . . . no hesitation in siding with the old view . . . in admitting an inflammation of the arterial coat to be the starting point of . . . athero-matous degeneration. . . . we have here an active process which really produces new tissues, but then hurries on to destruction in consequence of its own devel-opment," translated and cited by (Langheinrich and Bohle, 2005). After one million more scientific reports on vascular disease, these early insights are well validated: Arterial aging is fundamentally an inflammatory process from its beginnings before birth over the life span (Ross, 1995, 1999).

1.5.1. Overview and Ontogeny

The main seats of vascular aging and atherogenesis are in the arterial endothelia and the elastic lamina, which interact with multifarious inflammatory influences from the internal and external environment (Fig. 1.2A). The aorta and other cen-tral arteries are elastic reservoirs for the blood volume expelled at each heart-beat; the elasticity declines progressively during aging. The subsidiary arterioles have relatively more smooth muscle, which modulates blood pressure by adjusting the diameter (lumen), contracting in response to adrenaline, or relax-ing in response to nitric oxide, among other signals. Two distinct, but interre-lated, processes operate upon arteries throughout life[4] (D'Armiento et al, 2001; Najjar et al, 2005; Wang et al, 2006). (I) *Arterial aging* is a generalized thicken-ing and stiffening of arterial walls that slowly increase blood pressure and may lead to hypertension. (II) *Atherogenesis* is a local (patchy) growth of cells and accumulation of lipids within the arterial wall consisting of a progression from microscopic foci, to fatty streaks, to raised plaques that become fibrous and cal-cified.[5] Vascular pathologists refer to 'plaques' in reference to developed vascu-lar lesions, described in eight types or grades (Fig. 1.13). Atheromas arise focally as 'responses to injury,' in Ross's concept (1999). Large atheromas may cause stenosis by intruding into the lumen and decreasing blood flow. Clots can form on the atheroma surface, or circulating clots can be trapped, leading to

---

[4]My main sources of information and insights on vascular aging are Edward Lakatta, Claudio Napoli, and Wulf Palinski, discussions and papers.

[5]Atherosclerosis refers to pathological thickening of the inner arterial wall, while the older term arteriosclerosis ('hardening of the arteries') includes generalized arterial aging changes (loss of elasticity and intima-media wall thickening, Table 1.4) that may not be immediately associated with pathology. Arteriolosclerosis refers to aging changes in smaller arteries. Arterial plaques should not be confused with brain senile plaques in Alzheimer disease, although both arterial and Alzheimer plaques share many inflammatory processes (Table 1.3).

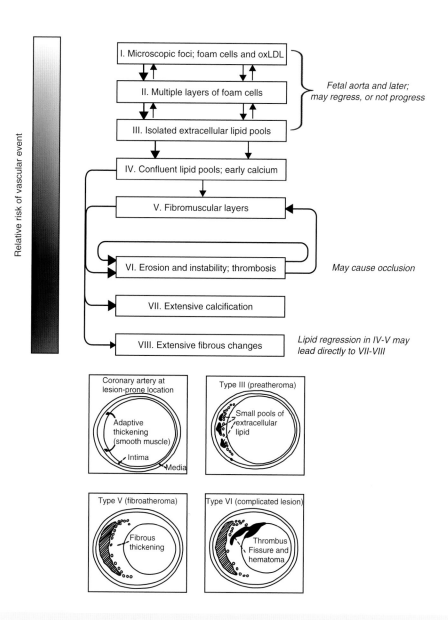

FIGURE 1.13 Natural history of atheromas from fatty streak to advanced lesions, rupture, calcification, and regression. American Heart Association grades, adapted from (Stary, 2000) and (Strauss et al, 2004): A simplified schematic of atherogenesis, beginning as microscopic foci in the embryo and growing progressively during childhood into adult life. This diagram depicts cycles of endothelial injury, lipid deposits, macrophage influx, and quiescence. I, isolated macrophage foam cells; II, multiple foam layers, but arterial structure not disrupted; III to IV, addition of expanding extracellular lipid pools and cholesterol crystals ('atheromas'); V, addition of fibromuscular layers ('fibroatheromas'); VI, fissured and thrombotic fibrous plaques; VII, calcification; VIII, fibrotic lesions without lipid cores. Advanced plaques may rupture, attracting platelets and forming a thrombus. Ruptured plaques may be clinically silent and then heal, some remaining innocuous for years.

thromboses, which block arterial blood flow, in turn, causing tissue oxygen deficits (ischemia) and tissue damage (necrosis).

The arterial system has a complex biochemistry, cell biology, and physiology evolved to serve tissue needs across a huge range of challenges in the demand for blood nutrients and oxygen, and the urgencies of hemostasis during penetrating injury. Arterial walls consist of concentric layers of cells and extracellular matrix ('connective tissue'). The innermost layer, the *intima,* consists of endothelial cells exposed directly to the blood, which are covered by a glycocalyx, as thin mesh of glycoproteins and proteoglycans (HSPGs). The endothelial lumen surface contains mechanotransducers that are sensitive to sheer stress and regulate inflammatory genes in the endothelia (Section 1.5.3.2).

The other endothelial face attaches to the *elastic lamina,* which is also a physical barrier to the pressure-driven diffusion of blood lipids and proteins. Next inside is the *media,* the thickest layer, with smooth muscle cells and matrix. The outermost layer is the *adventitia,* a sheath of matrix proteins, nerves, and capillaries. The extracellular matrix consists of elastin (its main component), collagen, fibronectin, and mucopolysaccharides; these extracellular materials account for 50% of mass in large arteries and are targets of modification during aging.

During development, arterial collagen is enzymatically cross-linked by lysyl oxidase. After puberty, further cross-links are chemically added. Arterial wall thickness is measured as the intima-media thickness (IMT) by ultrasonography. Carotid artery IMT increases universally during aging, by 2–3-fold across the life span in community studies (Fig. 1.14A) (Najjar and Lakatta, 2006; O'Leary et al, 1999). The arterial wall thickening and stiffening during aging are not benign over long life spans and predict individual risk of heart attacks, stroke, and hypertension. The top quintile of carotid IMT has 3-fold higher risk of myocardial infarcts (Cardiovascular Health Study) (O'Leary et al, 1999) (Fig. 1.14B). Combined, the wall thickening, elastin fragmentation, and cross-linking are the main *causes* of the universal increases of systolic pressure during aging. Low carotid elasticity (top quartile) was associated with 3-fold higher risk of future hypertension (ARIC Study) (Liao et al, 1999). Arterial aging rates strongly indicate future vascular health (Safar, 2005; Sagie et al, 1993).

Arterial wall thickening is due to active remodeling from endothelial cell growth and fibrosis with matrix deposition of collagen and proteoglycans (Fornieri et al, 1992; Sims et al, 2001; Sims et al, 2002; Wang et al, 2003) (Fig. 1.15A). Matrix metaloproteases (extra-cellular endoproteases, e.g., MMP-2 and -9) increase several-fold across adult ages in humans, primates, and rodents (D'Armiento et al, 2001; Lakatta and Levy, 2003a; Wang et al, 2003a). In the human thoracic aorta, collagen increases by 50% from 20 to 80 y, whereas elastin declines by 35% (Faber and Moller-House, 1952). Of major importance, elastin fibers become irreversibly fragmented with aging. The aging rat aorta intimal layer also thickens 5-fold, with increased matrix (Li et al, 1999). These processes are independent of atheromas. Wall thickening during aging is comparable in human populations with relatively little atherosclerosis and in arteries

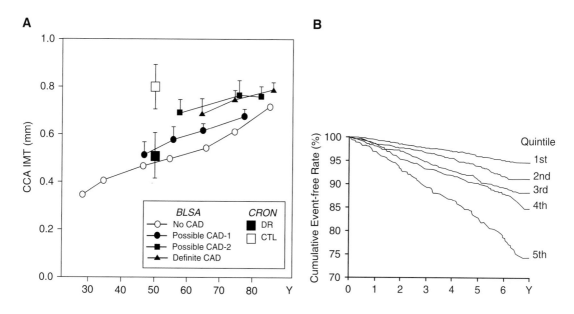

FIGURE 1.14 Carotid artery thickening during aging; risk of myocardial infarction and stroke.
A. Thickness of the common carotid artery (CCA) wall increases progressively with age (IMT, common carotid intima-media thickness). BLSA (o, Baltimore Longitudinal Study of Aging; 507 Ss, ages 42.7–85.3) (Nagai et al, 1998). BLSA subjects are mostly from upper socioeconomic strata; cardiovascular status is assessed by electrocardiographic (ECG) response to maximum treadmill exercise; all Ss reached >85% heart rate maxima for healthy age norm; none had stenosis >50% or local plaque near carotid bifurcation. No CAD (coronary artery disease) was the largest subgroup (80%). CAD-2 had silent myocardial ischemia, with IMT overlapping Definite CAD. These benchmark data suggest benefits from diet restriction (DR) in humans: CRON study (squares, Caloric Restriction Society; 18 Ss, mean age 50) who have maintained DR >3 y; controls (CTL), conventional diet matched for age and SES (Fontana et al, 2004) (Section 3.2.3). Each 0.1-mm IMT increases CAD risk by 1.91 (Fig. 1.6C). The DR CRON study IMT are slightly above the No CAD-BLSA. B. Carotid thickening as a risk indicator of myocardial infarction and stroke by quintiles of intimal plus medial layers thickness. Note the 5-fold difference in risk between the highest (25%) and lowest quintiles (5%) of IMT thickness. (Adapted from O'Leary et al, 1999.)

of aging rodents that do not develop atheromas during aging without major lipid perturbation (Najjar et al, 2005). However, generalized arterial aging changes may predispose to atherogenesis.

Arterial rigidity and loss of elasticity may be attributed to several distinct processes consistent with bystander damage I and II. The fragmentation of elastic fibers may be the largest factor in loss of elasticity. Elastin is a very long-lived

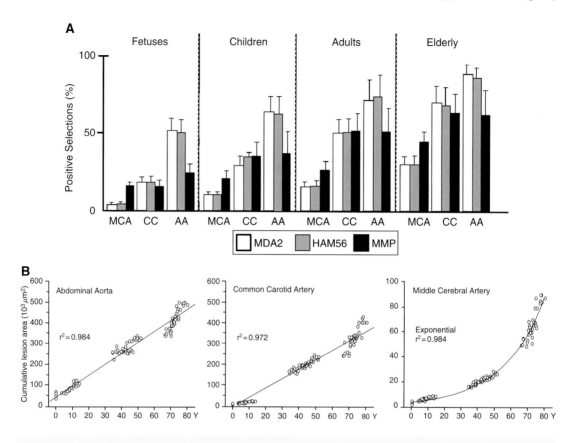

FIGURE 1.15 Atherogenesis in the large arteries across the life span. Redrawn from (D'Armiento, 2001): abdominal aorta (AA), middle cerebral artery (MCA), common carotid artery (CCA). A. Serial arterial sections were immunostained for macrophages (HAM-56), oxidized LDL (malondi-aldehyde, MDA2), and matrix metaloproteinase-9 (MMP). B. Lipid-rich area on arterial surfaces increase progressively with age, with suggestions of exponential increase in the middle cerebral artery and basilar artery (not shown here).

protein (Fig. 1.6D). Mature elastin fibrils may not ever be regenerated in adult central arteries. Elastin fragmentation is associated with foci of increased extra-cellular protease activities: MMP-2 activity was higher near breaks in the elastic lamina of aging rat aortas (Li et al, 1999). As noted above, MMP-2 generally increases during arterial aging. Elastin fragments are thought to activate elastin-laminin receptors on endothelial and smooth muscle cells, leading to the observed increased secretion of proteolytic enzymes and enhanced local cell proliferation (Duca et al, 2004; Najjar et al, 2005; Robert, 1996). A plausible sequence is that elevated TNFα induces MMP-2, which degrades elastin. Elastin receptor activation also inhibits synthesis of nitric oxide (NO), a key vascular regulator, as noted above. Elastin fragmentation may also be promoted by hemodynamic forces (O'Rourke hypothesis) (Section 1.5.3.2)

Aging arteries have increased infiltration by blood cells, lipids, and proteins. Human coronary arteries show increased staining for gamma globulin in the intimal layer, with infiltrating lymphocytes, especially around atheromas (Sims et al, 2001). In rat aorta, the permeability coefficient for albumin nearly doubled, 10 to 30 m (Belmin et al, 1993). Inflammatory gene expression increases by endothelial and smooth muscle cells during aging; e.g., cytokines in 2-year-old rats were ≥3-fold higher IL-1, -6, -17, and TNFα (Csiszar et al, 2003). Cell death markers increase, e.g., 5-fold more apoptosis in endothelial cells together with increased caspases −3 and −9 (Csiszar et al, 2004; Ungvari et al, 2004). Aging increases MMP-2 induction in response to IL-1α and TNFα (Li et al, 1999). The chemotactic protein MCP-1 (monocyte chemoattractant protein-1) and its receptor CCR2 increased in aging rat aorta smooth muscle cells (Spinetti et al, 2004). CCR2 gene variants influenced risk of myocardial infarction in association with serum MCP-1 levels (Framingham Heart Study) (McDermott et al, 2005). An MCP-1 promoter variant was associated with 5-fold greater susceptibility to tuberculosis (Flores-Villanueva et al, 2005) and may influence the impact of infections on vascular disease (Chapter 2). Other gene sets indicate a regular sequence of changes in gene expression during arterial aging (Karra et al, 2005).

Decreased availability of the free radical nitric oxide (NO) is important to declining arterial function. Endothelial NO is a key vasodilator and inhibits local platelet aggregation. Moreover, NO inhibits endothelial cell apoptosis in response to oxidized LDL and hyperglycemia. The age-related decrease in NO bioavailability is progressive (McCarty, 2004; Ungvari et al, 2004). The superoxide anion, with opposing actions as a vasoconstrictor, increases in aging rat arteries (Csiszar et al, 2002; Hamilton et al, 2001), which reduces NO bioavailability (Fig. 1.11) and may account for increased oxidative stress (3-nitrotyrosine) in arterial walls during aging. NO deficits are accelerated by hypertension (Hamilton et al, 2001; Taddei et al, 2001).

Atheromas arise as progressive focal accumulations of inflammatory cells, lipids, and other debris. Atherogenesis and vascular occlusion occur in several stages that progress from fatty streaks to fibrous plaques to more complex raised lesions with calcification (Fig. 1.13) (Strong et al, 1999). Other pathways to rigidity involve cross-linking and calcification. Collagen and other matrix materials secreted by endothelia become cross-linked by non-enzymatic glycation (AGE) (Section 1.2.6). Calcification may become universal after midlife (Blumenthal et al, 1944), in association with the mineralization of elastic fibers ('elastocalcinosis') and increased pulse wave velocity (Dao et al, 2005). Overall wall thickening by cell growth and matrix deposits should also increase rigidity.

Atheromas may be associated with gaps in the inner (subendothelial) elastic lamina, where there is observed infiltration of macrophages, lipids, and other blood substances. Gaps of the inner lamina increase with age, particularly in human coronary arteries (Sims et al, 2001; Sims et al, 2002). Patchy loss of endothelial cells also occurs in coronary arteries (Davies et al, 1988; Sims et al, 2002). As atheromatous plaques advance, LDL cholesterol accumulates in characteristic 'foam cells,' which derive from vascular smooth muscle cells and from invading macrophages. Extracellular proteases facilitate cell migrations from the blood into atheromas and of medial cells into the intima (Garcia-Touchard et al, 2005). Cell adhesion molecules (CAMs) on the endothelia increase binding of macrophages and platelets. Advanced plaques have large deposits of lipids, cholesterol crystals, and necrotic debris in the atheroma core (Fig. 1.13).

Atheromas are not randomly located, but are most frequent at arterial branches and along inner curves, where the vascular geometry disturbs laminar and slows blood flow (Blumenthal et al, 1954). The localization of atheromas by the physics of blood flow to zones of low shear stress has been elegantly developed (Dai et al, 2004; Moore et al, 1994; Traub and Berk, 1998; Wootton and Ku, 1999). A striking example is the carotid arteries, where atheromas arise only in small zone within the carotid sinus. Levels of sheer stress regulate patterns of gene expression in vascular cells that are 'atheroprone' and proinflammatory, as described below. These localized inflammatory responses are considered as 'responses to injury' (Ross, 1995, 1999), consistent with bystander process that are both physical (sheer stress) and biochemical (oxidant stress, inflammation).

Slow plaque growth gradually narrows the lumen of medium to large arteries (Fig. 1.13). Plaques with fibrous caps and smooth muscle cell proliferation are more stable and less prone to thrombosis (Fuster et al, 2005; Moore et al, 1994; Ross, 1995; Virmani et al, 2003; Wierzbicki et al, 2003). Plaque growth induces remodeling changes in the arterial wall, which is considered adaptive. In response to local blood flow changes, the arterial volume expands locally to alleviate local constriction. New collateral vessels are often formed (*vasa vasorum*) (Epstein et al, 2004). These compensations may serve remarkably well for the progressive stenosis, up to some critical point.

However, plaques may become unstable and rupture, attracting platelets and triggering clotting or atherothrombosis (Fig. 1.13) (Fuster et al, 2005). Blood flow shear stress caused by protrusion of the plaque into the lumen may precipitate plaque instability on the plaque wall (bystander damage type 4, Section 1.4.4) (Slager et al, 2005). Unstable (vulnerable) plaques have thin caps and necrotic cores with macrophages and lipid deposits. The higher levels of apoptosis (induction of caspase-3) in vascular endothelia may enhance thrombus formation (Durand et al, 2004). Caps may be weakened by matrix metaloproteinases and other extracellular proteases that degrade collagen, elastin, and fibronectin and that are secreted by endothelia and by infiltrating macrophages, mast cells, and neutrophils (Lindstedt and Kovanen, 2004). Increased MMP-9 is associated with plaque instability (Loftus et al, 2000). Adaptive immunity with B- and T-cells may have a major role in plaque degeneration (Section 1.5.3.1).

Clots (thromboses) tend to form on uneven surfaces of atheromas, which may not be symptomatic ('silent ischemia') until there are demands for increased blood flow. Thrombus formation may not immediately cause critical ischemia and can induce further local changes (Henriques de Gouveia et al, 2002). Far worse, clots may release fragments into the circulation that can completely block blood flow in smaller arteries and arterioles (thromboses), causing heart attacks or strokes (Libby, 2003). About 50% of infarcts are attributed to clots from small atheromas. Elevated blood fibrinogen, another inflammatory response, favors clotting. Plasma CRP elevations may be markers of unstable plaques (Schwartz et al, 2003). Ultrasonography is approaching cellular levels of resolution to detect plaque stability (Fuster et al, 2005; Langheinrich and Bonle, 2005; Tuzcu et al, 2001).

Aneurysms are another inflammation-related lesion. These outpocketings of the outer wall are filled with blood under pressure and may burst with fatal effects. The abdominal aorta is the most common locus, affecting 5% or more by age 65 (Palinski, 2004; Wanhainen et al, 2005). Aneurysms involve the medial layer, with smooth muscle cell atrophy and inflammatory changes extending to the outer adventitial layer (Palinski, 2004; Zhao et al, 2004). Adventitial changes include increased 5-lipooxygenase (macrophages, mast cells), which produces proinflammatory leukotrienes from arachidonic acid; and MMPs, which may weaken the medial layer. Little is known about mechanisms that may favor atheroma stenosis versus aneurysms. Th1/Th2 cytokine balance is implicated in transplant studies with aortic allografts (Shimizu et al, 2006), whereas hyperlipidemia increases aneurysms in humans (Wanhainen et al, 2005) and in a mouse model (Zhao et al, 2004).

Of great importance, arterial aging begins before birth in 'prodromal lesions' (Davies, 1990; Hirsch, 1941; Hirvonen et al, 1985; Leistikow, 1998; Napoli et al, 1999; Palinski and Napoli, 2002; Stary, 2000). Fetal arteries have microscopic cell clusters of macrophages and oxidized LDL that may be seeds of adult plaques (D'Armiento et al, 2001; Napoli et al, 1999; Sims, 2000). The mass of oxidized LDL, macrophages, and MMP-9 increases linearly in the aorta and common carotid, but may accelerate exponentially in intra-cerebral arteries (Fig. 1.15B).

Between age 10 and 20 y, intimal layer macrophage density increased progressively in coronary arteries (Sims et al, 2002). By early adult life, advanced arterial lesions are common. An early glimpse of this came from autopsies of soldiers killed during the Korean and Vietnam Wars. Many of these healthy young men had coronary artery degeneration, nearly one-third had >50% narrowing (Joseph et al, 1993; McNamara et al, 1971). These findings are confirmed by large multi-ethnic autopsy samples: PDAY Study (Pathobiological Determinants of Atherosclerosis in Youth) (Strong et al, 1999) and Bogalusa Heart Study (Berenson, 2004; Li et al, 2003). By age 30, about 50% of men and 35% of women have raised coronary lesions (Strong et al, 1999).

Lipids accumulate faster in children exposed to maternal hypercholesterolemia during pregnancy (FELIC Study, Fate of Early Lesions in Children) (Napoli et al, 1999) (Section 4.8). The variability of lesion size increased during later childhood, implying influences include diet and exercise (Chapter 3). Obesity may accelerate coronary atherosclerosis in young men more than in women (McGill et al, 2002) (Chapter 3). The greater arterial degeneration in men corresponds to the strong sex biases in cardiac disease and mortality (Tuzcu et al, 2001) (Section 2.10.4).

The fate of the prodromal fatty streaks is not fixed. Fatty streaks, while 'clinically silent,' may regress or develop further into advanced plaques that are associated with occlusive vascular disease. The transience of fatty deposits in neonatal aortas is well known (Hirsch, 1941). Thus, the level of atherogenesis in early life may not predict advanced lesions later in life (Madsen et al, 2003; Stary et al, 1994). In adults, advanced atheromas may regress during stain treatment (Petronio et al, 2005) (Chapter 2) or certain wasting conditions (Eilersen and Faber, 1960) (Chapter 3).

1.5.2. Hazards of Hypertension

The central arteries develop as highly elastic reservoirs for the blood volume expelled at each heartbeat. In children, the aorta literally balloons at each heartbeat in response to the force of the pulse wave. By puberty, arterial thickening and stiffening begin to increase the pulse wave velocity and blood pressure into the adult range, >100 mm systolic pressure measured on the arm ('cuff,' or brachial pressure) (Fig. 1.6B). Progressive increases of systolic pressure after age 30, about 0.7 mm systolic pressure/year, soon enough depart increasingly from the clinical goal of <120 mm Hg systolic and <80 mm diastolic[6] (O'Rourke and Nichols, 2005). These age findings were established by the Framingham Study, a pioneering community-based study, and are generalized to aging populations worldwide. By age 80, average pulse wave velocity has doubled and the systolic pressure has crept up to about 140 mm; this degree of elevation was formerly considered 'border-line hypertension,' but is now considered risky and warranting intervention. Worse, pulse pressure in the aorta increases with aging are greater than the brachial systolic pressure, up to 4-fold (O'Rourke et al, 2004; O'Rourke and Nichols, 2005; Safar, 2005).

---

[6]*The Sixth Report of the National Committee on Detection, Evaluation, and Treatment of High Blood Pressure* (Anonymous, 1997a). Systolic pressure (brachial, or cuff) is accepted as a stronger risk indicator of vascular complications than diastolic pressure; shown by Framingham and confirmed by meta-analysis of two huge data assemblages (Black, 2004). Pressure wave reflections ('augmentation index') of the central pulse wave form give more information about vascular disease than cuff pressure. Brain and kidney arteries are more exposed to this higher pressure than other tissues (O'Rourke and Nichols, 2005).

Uncontrolled systolic hypertension increases the risk of stroke, heart attack, congestive heart failure, and kidney failure. These hazards operate even in the supposedly normal range of systolic blood pressures. Vascular mortality risks from ischemic heart disease and stroke increase exponentially with blood pressures above 115/75 mm Hg; the curves are strongly age stratified. The Framingham Study concluded "cutoff points to define …hypertension are arbitrary" (Sagie et al, 1993). The reality of these hazards is confirmed by the benefits of drug treatments, which lowered cardiovascular events, congestive heart failure, and stroke by about 30% during 4.5 y (SHEP, Systolic Hypertension in the Elderly Program) (Perry et al, 2000). Stroke incidence was decreased by about 1% for every 1 mm of lowered systolic pressure. However, at any systolic pressure, age increases mortality risks, by about 50-fold from 40–89 years (meta-analysis, 61 prospective studies) (Lewington et al, 2002) (Fig. 1.6C).

Even modest increases of systolic pressure increase the risk of subsequently developing clinical hypertension. Systolic pressures of >160 mm increase to a prevalence of about 30% by age 60 y in most populations. The risk of hypertension is predicted by basal elevation years before. Even those with mild elevations (131 mm average) had a 50% higher risk of hypertension (Franklin, 2005; Franklin et al, 2005). Hypertension has the malignant feature of causing further arterial wall thickening.

Hypertension can synergize with hyperlipidemias, particularly elevated LDL cholesterol. Carotid IMT increased with blood pressure, except when LDL cholesterol was low (Los Angeles Atherosclerosis Study) (Sun et al, 2000). Thus, elevated systolic blood pressure, which increases in prevalence with age (Fig. 1.6A), appears to increase arterial susceptibility to damage from LDL cholesterol. Synergies of hypertension and hyperlipidemias are shown in animal models (below, 1.6.4). Hyperlipidemias and inflammatory factors are discussed in 1.6.4. Other blood indicators are discussed in 1.5.4.

1.5.3. Mechanisms

Arterial aging changes and atherogenesis appear to share inflammatory process that are, at least in part, driven by the physics of blood flow. Flow characteristics operate on arteries in two modes: in signal transduction through flow sensitive membrane links to the cytoskeleton and by direct force on the rigid body of atheromas. Inflammatory processes that participate in both modes may also interface with external infections and inflammogens (Chapter 2).

1.5.3.1. Inflammation

For nearly two centuries, inflammation has been a suspected cause of vascular disease, from Virchow to Ross, who emphasized that processes in atherogenesis are shared with other major chronic inflammatory diseases, including pulmonary fibrosis, rheumatoid arthritis, and renal glomerulosclerosis. Synergies of hyperlipidemia and hypertension illustrate Ross's hypothesis that atherosclerosis is an inflammatory 'response to injury.' True to Celsus's classic signs of inflammation (*calor*, or heat), atheromas are hotter than flanking vascular tissues, e.g., by 1°C in a rabbit model (Verheye et al, 2002). Currently, inflammation can be both cause *and* effect in arterial disease (Tracy, 2002). As described below, hemodynamics has a major role in both the arterial thickening of usual aging and atheroma formation, with fundamental involvement of inflammatory processes.

Inflammatory processes of innate immunity are at the core of atherogenesis. Lipid accumulation by macrophages, particularly oxidized LDL, is mediated by scavenger receptors (SR-A, CD-36) (Ricci et al, 2004; Shashkin et al, 2005), leading to the characteristic 'foam cells' of atheromas. Foam cells secrete cytokines and chemoattractants that activate smooth muscle cells. Cell growth factors (MCSF) and cell adhesion factors (VCAM1) mediate attachment of macrophages and platelets (Cunningham and Gottlieb, 2005; Dai et al, 2004; Passerini et al, 2004). Toll-family receptors (TLRs) mediate cytokine secretion, including TLR 4, which also binds LPS endotoxin (Miller et al, 2005).

During atherogenesis, many inflammatory proteins are produced by endothelial cells, smooth muscle cells, and macrophages (Table 1.3). The growing list includes cytokines (IL-1, IL-6, IL-8, TNFα) and complement (C) factors (C1q, C1r, C3, C5). Many of these genes are regulated by NF-κB family transcription factors, which are redox sensitive and mediate gene regulation during inflammation and oxidative stress (Li et al, 2002; Li et al, 2005b; Monaco and Paleolog, 2004). NF-κB increases in smooth muscle cells of atheromas relative to adjacent normal arterial areas (Bourcier et al, 1997; Hajra, 2000).

Many complement proteins are activated in atheromas, but fewer complement inhibitors are found (Yasojima et al, 2001a,b). Cell death in arterial plaques is closely associated with the terminal complement membrane attack complex, C5b-9 (Niculescu et al, 2004). The anaphylactic peptide C5a is also produced during complement activation and is a potent chemoattractant and activator of macrophages, causing release of TNFα and reactive oxygen species that cause further oxidative damage (Query I and II). Plasma elevations of C5a may be a risk factor in cardiovascular events (Speidl et al, 2005) together with CRP (Fig. 1.16). CRP can also activate the complement system (Pepys and Hirschfield, 2003). Both CRP and complement factors are produced by plaque smooth muscle and macrophages, more than in normal arteries (Jabs et al, 2003; Yasojima et al, 2001a,b).

CRP at acute phase levels can increase LDL uptake by macrophages (Fu and Borensztajn, 2002; Zwaka et al, 2001) through inducing the receptor for oxidized LDL (LOX-1) (Li et al, 2004). PTX3, an anti-microbial pentraxin related to CRP can be made by macrophages and vascular smooth muscle cells, and is increased by oxidized LDL (Klouche et al, 2004; Rolph et al, 2002). Systemic CRP and fibrinogen enhance macrophage accumulation in plaques. Moreover, CRP elevations may influence T cell responses of adaptive immunity, through inhibiting dendritic cell differentiation (Zhang et al, 2006). Subsets of the inflammatory proteins of atheromas also occur in senile plaques of Alzheimer disease (discussed below).

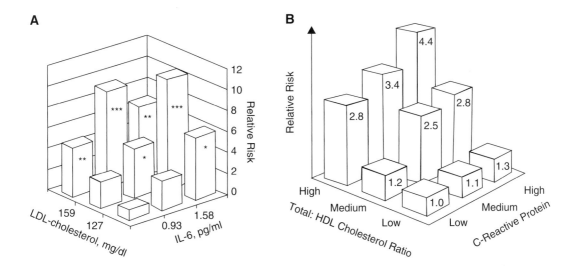

FIGURE 1.16 Additivity of blood inflammatory and lipid risk markers for cardiovascular events.
A. IL-6 and LDL cholesterol in the PRIME study (Prospective Epidemiological Study of Myocardial Infarction; population based sample of 10,600 men, 50 to 59 y from France and Ireland. IL-6 also correlated with CRP and fibrinogen. (Redrawn from Luc et al, 2003.) B. C-reactive protein, HDL, and risk of first myocardial infarction (MI) in the Physicians' Health Study of apparently healthy men (randomized study of 22,071 middle-aged U.S. male physicians, 95% Caucasian without prior MI, stroke, TIA, or cancer at the start. (Redrawn from Ridker et al, 1998.)

Arterial amyloid accumulations may be universal by middle age (Schwartz, 1970) and can include a variety of proteins (Buxbaum, 2004; Kawamura et al, 1995). SAA (serum amyloid A) and SAP, both acute phase proteins,[7] are common in atheromas (Li et al, 1995; O'Brien et al, 2006; Yamada et al, 1996). Elevated plasma SAA is a coronary risk factor (Yamada et al, 1996) and is a source of the SAA in aging arteries. By binding to HDL during the acute phase response, SAA impairs HDL's antioxidative protection to LDL and becomes 'proinflammatory'; SAA/LDL complexes are more oxidized than native LDL and are coronary risk factors (Chait et al, 2005; Ogasawara et al, 2004; Van Lenten et al, 1995). Another amyloid protein, medin-amyloid, is common by age 60 in the aorta (Peng et al, 2002; Peng et al, 2005a,b). Medin, a peptide fragment of lactadherin, is made by smooth muscle cells and is

---

[7]SAP is an acute phase reactant in mice, but not humans, whereas SAA is an acute phase reactant in both species.

deposited on the elastic lamina, where it may facilitate macrophage binding; lactadherin inhibits rotavirus infections and participates in angiogenesis.

Atheromas accumulate advanced glycation end products (AGEs), which are hypothesized to accelerate lipid oxidation, as is observed in diabetics (Reaven et al, 1997) (bystander damage, type 1 and 2, Section 1.4.1). Blockade of the receptor for AGE (RAGE) by a soluble truncated protein (sRAGE ligand) suppressed atherosclerosis in a mouse model with a 10-fold dose response (Naka et al, 2004). Conversely, endothelial RAGE overexpression enhanced diabetic damage to retina and kidney (Yonekura et al, 2005).

Increased formation of superoxide (O_2^-) is characteristic of endothelial dysfunctions in arterial disease and is attributable to increased NAD(P)H oxidase activity (Guzik et al, 2006). The NAD (P)H oxidase subunit p22phox is 50% higher in diseased than healthy coronary arteries, in correlation with inflammatory cell content. Consequences include quenching of nitric oxide (NO) and activation of redox pathways that promote remodeling. The importance of superoxide to arterial disease is indicated by benefits to endothelial functions in rodent models of increased superoxide dismutase by gene transfer (Longo et al, 2000).

Iron accumulates as a bystander process of oxidative damage, as well as causes bystander damage (Section 1.4.1). Oxidized LDL cholesterol (oxysterols) is associated with depots of intracellular ferritin in macrophages and foam cells (Li et al, 2005d; Stadler et al, 2004). Superoxide also releases iron from aconitase (Fe-S complex) (Longo et al, 2000). Iron (Fe^{2+}), in turn, causes oxidative injury from the hydroxy radical (Fenton/Haber-Weiss reaction) (Fig. 1.11) leading to cell death. Necrosis in the plaque core increases risk of plaque rupture. Iron chelators decreased caspase induction and apoptosis in animals (Li et al, 2005d). Frequent human blood donors had about 40% fewer cardiovascular events (Meyers et al, 2002), consistent with hypotheses that lower body iron is protective by decreased oxidation of low-density lipoprotein cholesterol (Meyers et al, 2002) and lowered intracellular soluble iron (Li et al, 2005d).

A further outcome is the calcification of atheromas (Fig. 1.13, stage VII), a focal calcification differing from the more universal and diffuse arterial elastocalcinosis (Dao et al, 2005). Calcification is associated with cell death (apoptosis) of vascular smooth muscle and accumulations of monocytes, distinct from foam cells, mast cells, and oxidized lipids (Jeziorska et al, 1998; Tintut et al, 2002). Medial layer cells can differentiate as osteoblasts to form calcium phosphate crystals resembling bone mineral (Abedin et al, 2004). Neovascularization also stimulates ectopic calcification (Collett and Carfield, 2005). Calcification is an independent risk factor in vascular mortality (Doherty et al, 2003; Sangiorgi et al, 1998).

Lastly, and of possible major importance, B and T lymphocytes are common in atheromas. A recent study showed 10-fold increases of T cells in unstable atheromas with increased INFγ and IL-4 (De Palma et al, 2006). T cell spectratyping showed oligoclonal expansions, suggesting antigen-driven recruitment, differing between plaques of individuals, which could be critical to atheroma instability and cell lysis. The elevated plasma CRP that predicts vascular events may sensitize endothelial cells to T cell cytotoxicity. (Nakajima et al, 2002). Ubiquitous CMV infections, which are implicated in the increase of highly differentiated T cells during immunosenescence (Section 1.2, Sections 2.2 and 2.7) could increase autoimmune interactions leading to plaque instability.

1.5.3.2. Hemodynamics

As noted above, atheromas tend to form at arterial branches and along inner curves, where the vascular geometry slows blood flow and produces low shear forces (Moore et al, 1994; Traub and Berk, 1998; Wootton and Ku, 1999). Later, as plaques protrude into the lumen, they are increasingly exposed to increased tensile stress on the plaque wall, which may cause fissures and fractures (Slageret et al, 2005a,b). Thus, normal blood flow may cause plaque instability through mechanical forces.

Signal transduction is the other major mode of hemodynamic influences on arterial functions. Blood flow directly regulates inflammatory responses through mechanosensors in endothelia (Li, 2005). The role of blood flow in the progression of plaques is shown in elegant studies that combine hemodynamic models and molecular biology (Cunningham and Gotlieb, 2005; Dai et al, 2004; Pfister et al, 2005). Flow force transduction is thought to be mediated by endothelial cell cytoskeleton through links, which include G proteins, ion channels, integrins, PDFG-receptors, etc. Downstream mechanisms include activation of machinery shared with inflammatory responses including NF-κB transcription factors and Akt kinases (Kakisis et al, 2005; Li, 2005).

Another inflammation-related mechanism is the sphingomyelinase in caveola of endothelial cells, which is flow-activated and produces transients of ceramide (Czarny and Schnitzer, 2004), a long-chain fatty acid. Ceramide mimicked the flow-activation of eNOS, which produces NO, a key vasodilator and endothelial cell regulator that is at lower levels in atheromas than healthy endothelia (Cunningham and Gotlieb, 2005; Wilcox et al, 1997). Furthermore, sphingolipid and eicosinoid pathways have multiple synergies in inflammatory responses (Pettus et al, 2005) that may mediate the increased production of prostaglandins by macrophages during aging (Wu, 2004).

Distinct arterial waveforms, 'atheroprone' and 'athero-protective,' cause different patterns of gene expression in the vascular endothelia (Dai et al, 2004). Atheroprone flow induced a number of proinflammatory genes (IL-1, IL-6, IL-8; tumor necrosis factor receptor superfamily, member 21 [TNFRSF21]; complement C1r and C3; and PTX3), but decreased expression of IL-10, an anti-inflammatory cytokine (Dai et al, 2004; Passerini et al, 2004). NF-κB was 4-fold higher in endothelial cells of atheroprone regions, consistent with activation of inflammatory genes (Hajra et al, 2000). In contrast, normal arterial flow represses arterial inflammatory gene expression, e.g., VCAM1, which mediates cell adhesion, via a TNF-dependent pathway (Yamawaki et al, 2003; Yamawaki et al, 2005).

Atheromas accumulate replicatively senescent endothelial cells above normal aging arteries (Minamino et al, 2004). Telomere DNA loss in vascular endothelial cells correlates with the grade of atheroma (Edo and Andres, 2005; Okuda et al, 2000). Replicatively senescent endothelial cells have lower eNOS, a key regulation of vasodilation noted above (McCarty, 2004). A loss of NO production would decrease the protection of endothelial cells from apoptosis in response to oxidized LDL and hyperglycemia. The declining production of NO during cell senescence is blocked by maintaining telomere length by transfection with hTERT, the catalytic unit of telomerase (Minamino et al, 2002). Moreover, telomerase in endothelial progenitor cells is inhibited by angiotensin II (Ang II), which induces oxygen-derived free radicals through gp91phox and other subunits of the various NAD(P)H oxidase complexes. The inhibition of telomerase by Ang II was blocked by SOD, or by an angiotensin receptor (AT1) antagonists (Imanishi et al, 2005). These findings epitomize the multiple interactions of oxidative damage and inflammation across multiple levels of molecular, cellular, and physiological organization in atherogenesis.

I suggest that endothelial cell senescence represents bystander damage from proliferation stimulated by blood pulsation and inflammation (bystander types 3 and 4, Section 1.4). The weaker correlations of telomere loss with age than grade of atheroma (Okuda et al, 2000) support bystander mechanisms in the inflammatory milieu of the atheroma. Moreover, shortened telomeres in circulating white blood cells of hypertensives were correlated with carotid artery plaque load, possibly reflecting systemic inflammation (Benetos et al, 2004).

Endothelial cell senescence is linked to the insulin/IGF-1 pathways implicated in vascular disease and in longevity (Fig. 1.3). During serial endothelial culture leading to replicative senescence, Akt kinase levels increased 4-fold, which is consistent with the arrest of growth in early passage by activation of Akt (Miyauchi et al, 2004). Akt activation inhibits FOXO3, a transcription factor orthologue of DAF-16 in worms that controls transcription of MnSOD and other anti-oxidant genes (Fig. 1.3A). Thus, Akt activation in atheromas could increase oxidant stress by diminishing the capacity to remove reactive oxygen species. The IGF-1 pathway is a target of drug development for vascular disease (de Nigris et al, 2006).

Besides their sensitivity to flow-induced inflammatory gene expression, atheroprone arterial regions show greater sensitivity to LPS, the endotoxin of common infections: In a mouse model, LPS caused greater induction of the NFkappaB in atheroprone than in resistant regions (Hajra et al, 2000). Moreover, the atheroprone regions had greater induction of VCAM and E-selectin, proatherogenic genes that use NF-κB. Inflammation in atherogenesis is greater after priming by LPS and possibly during infections (Chapter 2).

Blood flow regulates nitric oxide (NO), a key vasodilator that may be protective in atherosclerosis by inhibiting apoptosis, platelet aggregation, smooth muscle proliferation, and white blood cell adhesion apoptosis (Tai et al, 2005). Free NO from endothelial nitric oxide synthase (eNOS) reacts with superoxide to form peroxynitrite and other reactive oxygen species (ROS) (Fig. 1.11), which can cause molecular damage (Cai, 2005; Heck et al, 2005). The increased levels of protein nitration in atheromas and in aging arteries independently of atheromas (e.g., >2-fold) are attributed to NO-derived oxidants (van der Loo et al, 2000). The increased production of superoxide in aging arterial walls and atheromas is hypothesized as an important source of oxidative damage.

Hypertension is strongly associated with increased arterial wall thickening, atherosclerosis, and vascular mortality in humans (see above). Animal models document these associations (Lerman et al, 2005). A transgenic hypertensive rat with increased angiotensin II had thicker aortic walls with more smooth muscle cells and collagen (Rossi et al, 2002). However, hypertension-induced changes may not progress to atherosclerotic plaques without hyperlipidemia. Moreover, hypertension interacts with hyperlipidemia. In the hyperlipidemic Watanabe rabbit model, 3 months of induced hypertension caused a 4-fold greater increase of aortic lesions (Chobanian et al, 1989). Increased synthesis of collagen and tropoelasin are implicated in the aortic compensatory responses to tensile stress from hypertension (Xu et al, 2000; Xu et al, 2002). Synergies in the age-related increase of hypertension and hyperlipidemia could accelerate mortality from vascular causes (see Section 1.5.3.3).

Lastly, the loss of arterial elasticity during arterial aging could also be hemo-dynamically driven. According to O'Rourke's hypothesis (O'Rourke and Nichols, 2005), elastin fibers fragment from fatigue during repeated stress cycles. So far, elastin has not been characterized for fatigue and fracture characteristics. Using natural rubber as a model and assuming 10% stretch per cycle, as in the thoracic aorta, elastin fractures might emerge by 800 million cycles (heartbeats) in the third decade (O'Rourke, 1976), which is at the onset of stiffening and elevations of systolic pressure (Fig. 1.6A). Alternatively, I suggest that elastin degradation is enzymatically caused by endoproteinases (MMP-2) as were localized to sites of elastic lamina fragmentation in aging rat aortas (Li et al, 1999). Elastin fiber fatigue might increase protease susceptibility. Both mechanisms are consistent with accelerated loss of elasticity in hypertension.

1.5.3.3. Aging

The vascular aging changes in arterial wall thickening and atherogenesis are very slow, indolent processes that typically take decades before adverse impact. Edward Lakatta and colleagues propose that 'aging' is a key parameter in the progression of arterial disease (Lakatta, 2003; Lakatta and Levy 2003a,b; Wang and Lakatta, 2006). "[Vascular aging changes] . . . create a metabolically and enzymatically active milieu . . . conducive for superimposed atherosclerosis. An important corollary is that age should no longer be viewed as an immutable cardiovascular risk factor." (Najjar et al, 2005, p. 460). The consideration of vascular disease in terms of '(aging process) × (exposure time)' (Lakatta, 2003) joins the discussion of bystander/event-related aging (Section 1.4). A shift in thinking is underway which challenges the assumption that aging is an immutable process. In an emerging view, the rate of arterial aging processes is dependent on multiple interactions in the internal and external milieu of the individual.

TABLE 1.4 Comparisons of Arterial Aging Changes in Humans and Mammalian Models with Atherosclerosis and Hypertension

Arterial Parameter	Human	Monkey	Rat	Rabbit	Atherosclerosis	Hypertension
Diffuse intimal thickening	+	+	+	+	+	+
Lipid deposits	−	−	−	−	+	+/−
Macrophages	+	−	−	−	+	+
T cells	+	−	−	+	+	+
Matrix ↑	0	+	+	+	+	+
Ang II-ACE ↑	+	+	+	+	+	+
Endothelial dysfunction	+	+	+	+	+	+
Extra cell. Matrix	+	+	+	?	+	+
ICAM ↑	?	?	+	?	+	+
MCP-1/CCR2 ↑	+	+	+	+	+	+
NADPH oxidase ↑	?	?	+	?	+	+
TGF-β1	?	+	+	?	+	+
VEGF ↑	+	?	?	+	+	+
Lumenal dilation	+	+	+	+	?	+/−
Wall stiffness ↑	+	+	+	+	?	+
Collagen ↑	+	+	+	+	?	+/−
Elastin degeneration	+	+	+	+	0	0
Telomere shortening	+	+	+	?	+	?

Adapted from Lakatta (2003), Lakatta and Levy (2003a,b), Wang and Lakatta (2006), Najjar et al (2005).

There is extensive overlap between arterial age changes and the cell processes in atherogenesis. Arterial aging processes are broadly shared in rodents, rabbits, monkeys, and humans (Table 1.4). Thus, vascular aging processes join brain amyloid accumulation and ovarian oocyte loss in the mammalian canon of aging. Species vary in the extent of particular changes and in the proclivity to atherogenesis in response to diet and stress. Wall thickening and atheroma formation both share many molecular and cellular changes that are broadly considered inflammatory processes (D'Armiento et al, 2001; Najjar et al, 2005). Both have subclinical phases beginning early in life: Prodromal atheromas appear to begin even before birth in the form of minute cell foci that may develop later into life-threatening atheromas. Vascular aging and atherogenesis involve local cell proliferation, invasion of macrophages, and excess production of collagen. Aging increases the permeability to albumin and other blood proteins (Section 1.6.3). As also noted, aging arteries have elevated cytokines (TNFα) and genes associated with apoptosis (caspases), chemotaxis (MCP-1), and matrix remodeling (MMP-2). Senescence of endothelial progenitor cells (section above) impaired proliferation and migration (Heiss et al, 2005). In old rat arteries, smooth muscle cells secrete more proinflammatory cytokines, whereas old endothelial cells secrete more of the prothrombotic PAI-1 (plasminogen activator inhibitor-1); production of vasodilators (NO, prostacyclin) decreases, whereas vasoconstrictors increase (angiotensin II and endothelin) (Najjar et al, 2005). Moreover, the interactions of hypertension, which increases sharply during aging, could synergize with hyperlipidemia (Chobanian et al, 1989; Sun et al, 2000; Xu et al, 2000; Xu et al, 2002) (Section 1.6.3) in the accelerating vascular mortality.

Primary cultures of vascular cells also show major donor age effects consistent with increased atherogenesis. Human vascular smooth muscle cell cultures showed progressive decline in proliferation and migration from donors across adult ages (Ruiz-Torres et al, 2003). Stimulation of proliferation by insulin and IGF-1 declines with donor age (Ruiz-Torres et al, 1999; Ruiz-Torres et al, 2005). Endothelial lines derived from two donors aged 36 and 90 years (hmEC36 and hmEC90, respectively) differed in the capacity for new blood vessel formation on collagen-gels (Koike et al, 2003): the younger hmEC36 supported much more angiogenesis. Proteases critical for angiogenesis differed correspondingly: Active MMP-2 was produced only by hmEC36, whereas hmEC90 produced much more protease inhibitor (TIMP-2). Cultured human vascular endothelial cells also progressively lose telomere DNA (Chang and Harley, 1995).

Rodent models show cell aging changes. Smooth muscle cells from old rats secrete more proinflammatory cytokines, whereas old endothelia secrete more of the prothrombotic PAI-1 (plasminogen activator inhibitor-1); production of vasodilators (NO, prostacyclin) decreases, whereas production of vasoconstrictors increases (angiotensin II and endothelin) (Najjar et al, 2005). Smooth muscle cells from 2-year-old rats had greater induction of MMP-2 production in response to IL-1α and TNFα (Li et al, 1999), which could enhance elastin degradation, as noted above. Aging may increase endothelial responses to mechanical injury: Older rats had much greater myo-intimal proliferation in response to 'de-endothelialization' by wire scrape than young adults (Hariri, 1986). This elegant study showed that the age effect persisted when old aortic segments were transplanted to young aortas. No generalizations are at hand, because other experimental models present different age changes in vascular proliferative responses (Torella et al, 2004). These finding suggest that aging arteries are more sensitive to atherogenic stimuli or injury. Clearly, multiple processes are at work in vascular aging and atherogenesis across the life span.

These and many other arterial changes address Query I of bystander oxidative damage promoting inflammation and Query II of inflammation causing further bystander damage. The co-occurrence of macrophages and oxidized lipids in fetal arteries exemplifies the fetal origins of adult arterial disease (Chapter 4) and points to specific and fundamental roles of oxidant damage and inflammation in arterial aging. These hypothesized interactions of oxidized lipids and inflammation are directly tested by transgenic over-expression catalase in mice (Section 1.2.6), which attenuated arteriolosclerosis and myocardial calcification and fibrosis in ad lib feeding (Schriner et al, 2005) and in a hyperlipidemic model of accelerated atherosclerosis attenuated the size of arterial lesions and plasma and arterial lipid peroxidation (Yang, 2004a). Thus, the pathogenic interactions in Fig. 1.2A,B are ongoing processes throughout the life history. We must also recognize effects of the progressive increase in systolic pressure during aging on endothelial changes, which are expected to be compounded by inflammation and obesity (Chapters 2 and 3). We may anticipate a detailed theory that accounts for accelerating mortality during aging from hemodynamics, which incorporates microscopic and macroscopic vascular changes to predict population mortality risks.

1.5.3.4. *Endothelial Progenitor Cells*

Circulating endothelial progenitor cells (EPCs) are increasingly implicated in vascular disease by roles in plaque repair (endothelialization) and neovascularization of ischemic tissue (Dong et al, 2005; Urbich and Dimmeler, 2005). Adults maintain circulating EPCs (CD34[+], CD133[+]) that are derived from the bone marrow. EPCs may 'home' to sites of ischemia and enhance in vascular repair and angiogenesis. EPC numbers varied inversely with total cholesterol and LDL cholesterol (Chen et al, 2004) and other clinical atherosclerotic risk factors (Vasa et al, 2001; Steiner et al, 2005), and were 40% lower in a sample of coronary patients (Vasa et al, 2001). Although EPC numbers did not show age declines, there may be age decreases in proliferation and migration (Heiss et al, 2005). These deficits correlated with brachial flow-mediated dilation, a measure of endothelial dysfunction.

Rodent models also showed EPC deficits in hypercholesterolemia and the benefits of supplemental EPCs. In hypercholesterolemic mice (apoE−/−), arterial fatty deposits were diminished by infusion of EPCs from normal mice, whereas fewer EPCs were obtained from 6-month-old apoE−/− with advancing atherosclerosis (Rauscher et al, 2003). The old-derived EPC induced patterns of arterial wall gene expression that resembled gene expression in advanced lesions in mice and in humans (Karra et al, 2005). Thus may bone marrow aging contribute to atherogenesis. Moreover, EPCs can transdifferentiate into myocardial lineage cells that contribute to myocardial regeneration (Murasawa et al, 2005). The EPC capacity for neovascularization of ischemic tissue may depend on their unusual resistance to oxidant stress through elevated MnSOD (He et al, 2004). Endothelial cell replicative senescence may decrease the pool of EPCs that repair vascular damage and increase risk of atheroma rupture. Statins may also modulate EPC cell senescence by suppressing Chk2, a DNA damage checkpoint kinase that is induced by telomere dysfunction (Spyridopoulos et al, 2004).

Inflammation and smoking also inhibit EPC functions (Section 2.5.2). To anticipate this subsequent discussion, a specific inflammatory class of endothelial cells (IEPs) was recently described. (Holmen et al, 2005). Circulating IEPs have higher expression of inflammatory markers, which inhibits their functions. Blood levels of IEC correlated with serum CRP in vasculitis patients.

1.5.4. Blood Risk Factors for Vascular Disease and Overlap with Acute Phase Responses

The blood indicators of vascular disease include several acute phase reactants in response to infections, e.g., IL-1, IL-6, and CRP elevations (Section 1.3). Moreover, the combination of elevated triglycerides and LDL- and low HDL-cholesterol that are risk indicators of vascular events (Braunwald, 1997; Castelli, 1996) is also observed during infections.

In this brief review of a huge field, vascular event predictions improve by including other markers, particularly of inflammatory proteins, in addition to LDL or HDL cholesterol (Fig. 1.16). Plasma elevations of CRP and IL-6 are separately and together considered as risk indicators for a first-ever or recurrent vascular event. Even modest elevations of CRP (top two tertiles) increase risks of the first or recurrent heart attacks. The strongest predictor of vascular events was elevated CRP in combination with lower cholesterol: HDL cholesterol ratio [Physicians Health Study (Libby and Ridker, 2004) and Women's Health Study (Ridker et al, 2000). Even after adjusting for cholesterol, high CRP predicts stroke (Rost et al, 2001)]. However, IL-6 associations may be as strong as CRP. In the PRIME Study (Prospective Epidemiological Study of Myocardial Infarction) of healthy middle age, IL-6 was the strongest predictor (Luc et al, 2003): The highest tertile of CRP, fibrinogen, IL-6, and LDL cholesterol were each associated with 2–3-fold higher risk; however, the best predictor was IL-6 in combination with LDL cholesterol. Other vascular risk markers include fibrinogen, homocysteine, Lp(a), plasminogen activator inhibitor (PAI-1), and TNFα. For a balanced view of the complex contending statistical arguments on CRP and other risk factors, see Davey Smith et al. (2006).

A substantial portion of sporadic events occur within the normal range of lipid risk factors, e.g., 35% of heart attacks in the original Framingham sample (Castelli, 1996). High CRP predicted stroke, after adjustment for total and HDL cholesterol (Rea et al, 2005). Infections may be unidentified risk factors lurking in these large population studies, because acute infections induce many of the same dyslipidemias and other acute phase changes shared with vascular risk factors (Esteve et al, 2005; Khovidhunkit et al, 2004; Ohsuzu, 2004). Blood triglycerides increase during acute infections, as energy is mobilized by lipolysis. Concurrently, infections decrease HDL and the 'reversed cholesterol transport'.[8] Both shifts are vascular risk factors. The same changes are induced by bacterial endotoxins, which cause similar remodeling of HDL and LDL particles. Acute infections also increase the oxidation of blood LDL and VLDL, the uptake of oxidized lipids by macrophages, and the inhibition of reversed cholesterol transport, which removes cellular cholesterol to the liver for recycling.

During the acute phase, HDL is remodeled into the proinflammatory 'acute phase HDL' in complex and incompletely understood mechanisms (Ansell et al, 2003; Khovidhunkit et al, 2004; Van Lenten et al, 2006). Normal HDL particles have anti-oxidant activities that protect LDL from oxidation (Getz and Reardon, 2004; Kontush et al, 2003) and that inhibit LDL-induced monocyte chemotactic responses (Ansell et al, 2003). Normal HDL also blocks some proinflammatory activities of CRP (Wadham et al, 2004).

---

[8]Total cholesterol and LDL differ in response to infections by species with increases in rodents and rabbits, but decreases in humans and primates.

Many infections impair the protective effects of HDL. The 'acute phase HDL' has fewer anti-oxidant activities, due to the loss of antioxidant proteins, transferrin, and the paraoxinases (PON-1, PON-3), which hydrolyze oxidized lipids in LDL (Van Lenten et al, 2006). The acute phase remodeling involves binding of LPS to the LPS-binding protein (LBP) and the phospholipid transfer protein (PLTP), which normally regulates the transfer of phospholipids from cell membranes to HDL (Levels et al, 2005). LPB and PLTP are acute phase responses and may be directly bacteriocidal because of their structural similarities to lipid transfer proteins that increase bacterial permeability (Kirschning et al, 1997). Acute phase elevations of serum amyloid A (SAA) displace the apoA-I on HDL, which impairs reversed cholesterol transport (Miida et al, 2006). SAA also enhances cholesterol uptake by macrophages.

The Toll-receptor pathways that mediate responses to infections are also implicated in atherogenesis (Bjorkbacka et al, 2004). Cholesterol efflux from macrophages is mediated by cross-talk between Toll-like receptors on macrophages and LXR receptors (the nuclear receptor liver X receptor) (Castrillo et al, 2003). Toll-activation by infections thus could contribute to atherogenesis by favoring the accumulation of cholesterol in arterial macrophages. The LXR pathway is emerging as a key nexus of innate immunity in protection of macrophage apoptosis (Valledor, 2005) The macrophage scavenger receptor (MSR-A), which binds viral and bacterial pathogens, also mediates the uptake of oxidized lipoproteins (Gordon, 2003; Suzuki et al, 1997).

Two other inflammatory changes could enhance lipoprotein uptake by vascular macrophages: Infections tend to oxidize lipoproteins and release ceramide and sphingomyelin (Auge et al, 2002; Hajjar, 2000) and the increased CRP, as noted above (Fu and Borensztajn, 2002; Zwaka et al, 2001). Hajjar and Haberland (1997) describe the uptake of oxidized LDL by vascular macrophages as a 'molecular Trojan horse' by inducing inflammatory processes that contribute to atherogenesis. The increased ceramide and sphingomyelin from lipoprotein oxidation during infections also stimulate proliferation of vascular smooth muscle cells (Auge et al, 2002). Infections in vascular disease are discussed in Chapter 2.

This brief review of a huge literature shows the profound involvement of inflammation in arterial aging. Modulations of arterial aging by systemic inflammation and pathogens (Chapter 2) and by diet (Chapter 3) will draw on the elements discussed above. Many of these same factors are also central to Alzheimer disease.

1.6. ALZHEIMER DISEASE AND VASCULAR-RELATED DEMENTIAS

Unlike heart attacks, Alzheimer disease and vascular-related dementias are rare (<1%) before age 65. Alzheimer disease prevalence accelerates with a doubling of risk every 5 y (Fig. 1.10A). The pathologic markers of Alzheimer disease are senile plaques (extracellular 'neuritic plaques'), neurofibrillary tangles (intra-neuronal 'tangles') (Fig. 1.10B), and selective neuron loss. Tangles and plaques arise in the brain at least 30 years after the fatty streaks of fetal arteries (Finch, 2005). The prevalence of dementia after age 80 ranges widely from 10% or lower to more than 50%, depending on the population (Fig. 1.10A). These individual outcomes in aging may derive from the same gene-environment interactions that influence vascular aging and pathology, discussed in later chapters.

1.6.1. Neuropathology of Alzheimer Disease

Brain amyloid generates inflammation that interacts with neuronal regression. During 'normal aging,' nearly all humans accumulate some form of solid brain Aβ (Delaere et al, 1993; Mizutani and Shimada, 1992; Morris and Price, 2001), which is a focus of local inflammatory reactions. Senile plaques are extracellular aggregates of amyloids and inflammatory proteins, best known for the β-amyloid peptide 'Aβ' of 42 amino acids ($A\beta_{1-42}$), which is proteolytically derived from the amyloid precursor protein (APP). However, the molar proportion of Aβ and the many plaque components is not known.

Senile plaque fibrillar $A\beta_{1-42}$ is stained by the dye Congo red ('congophilic'). Aβ deposits are very heterogeneous in morphology and degree of fibrils, ranging from the classic senile plaques with fibrillar amyloid to diffuse amyloid deposits that are not congophilic. The classic Alzheimer 'neuritic plaque' has abnormal neurites along with congophilic Aß fibrils, reactive glia, and inflammatory proteins (Fig. 1.10B). The curving dendrites near plaques are predicted to have slowed neurotransmission (Knowles et al, 1999). Synaptic density (dendritic spines) drops sharply in neurons passing near neuritic plaques in transgenic mice (Spires et al, 2005). The inhibition of neurite outgrowth by aging glia (Fig. 1.9) may be a model for the glial contribution to abnormal neurites in senile plaques.

Brain amyloid pools are very dynamic. Aβ is transported in both directions from the periphery across the blood-brain barrier. Slight increases in production of the Aβ peptide from extra gene copies (Down syndrome, transgenic mice) could enable slow plaque accumulation. Conversely, brain amyloid can be removed by circulating antibodies in the transgenic mice and, possibly, in Alzheimer patients. Insulin and IGF-1 may also influence brain Aβ peptide pools (Section 1.6.5, below).

Although amyloid accumulations are universal or nearly so during later aging, neuritic plaques are not found in all nondemented elderly (Braak and Braak, 1991; Price and Morris, 1999). Diffuse amyloid deposits are not fibrillar and have fewer inflammatory components (Braak and Braak, 1991; Price and Morris, 1999). Although diffuse plaques are not associated with cognitive deficits, nearby neurons show subtle changes (D'Amore et al, 2003).

Various vascular abnormalities (microangiopathies) arise during aging and Alzheimer disease. Microvessels proliferate, with greater density and cork-screw-like tortuosity in later Alzheimer disease (Perlmutter et al, 1990). Angiogenesis is associated with senile plaques (Perlmutter et al, 1990; Wegiel et al, 2003) and in the basilar arterioles of Alzheimer brains and transgenic mice (Beckmann et al, 2003; Burgermeister et al, 2000; Calhoun et al, 1999; Krucker et al, 2004; Van Dorpe et al, 2000). Plaques are next to, or penetrated by, one or more cerebral microvessels in human dementia (Ishii, 1958; Kawai et al, 1990; Wegiel et al, 2003). New plaques may arise from the budding of large plaques close to the perivascular zone (Wegiel et al, 2003). These findings suggest a role for the angiogenic inflammatory factors that increase in senile plaque genesis (see below).

Vascular tortuosities during aging may be increased by hypertension (Akima et al, 1986; Hiroki et al, 2002; Moody et al, 1997). Transgenic Alzheimer mouse models also show a lower vascular density preceding the deposits of brain amyloid and vascular amyloid (Krucker et al, 2004). Blood flow slows, even before amyloid deposits (Niwa et al, 2002). We must also consider the 30–50% age-related decrease of microvasculature, shown in two rat strains (Sonntag et al, 1997; Sonntag et al, 2000), which may overlap with the vascular changes in transgenic Alzheimer mice. Growth hormone and IGF-1 contribute to these changes in aging rats (see below).

Neurofibrillary tangles are the other Alzheimer hallmark as reported in Alzheimer's original case of pre-senile dementia (Alzheimer, 1911). These intra-neuronal bodies are abnormally configured microtubule proteins (normally part of the cytoskeleton). Neurofibrillary tangles are paired filaments of polymerized hyperphosphorylated tau, an accessory microtubule protein, and do not contain the Aβ peptide. Besides their prominence in Alzheimer brains, tangles also accumulate sporadically during 'normal' aging absent Alzheimer disease (Mizutani and Shimada, 1992; Morris and Price, 2001). All nondemented centenarians examined had some tangled neurons (Silver et al, 2002).

Of major importance to the evolution of human longevity (Chapter 6), aging great apes have very modest Aβ accumulations (Gearing et al, 1997), in contrast to their abundance in aging rhesus monkeys (Finch and Sapolsky, 1999; Finch and Stanford, 2004). Alzheimer-like changes also arise to some extent in other mammals. The accumulation of brain Aβ aggregates may be common in vertebrates during aging, because the Aβ peptide is highly conserved (Section 1.2.2, Fig. 6.2).

Despite its importance for postmortem diagnosis, the amount of fibrillar Aβ is weakly correlated with the degree of neurodegeneration and cognitive deficits (Klein et al, 2001; Terry et al, 1991). Longitudinal clinical assessments by the Clinical Disease Rating (CDR) scale CDR 1-5 also recognize CDR 0.5 as a pre-clinical stage with subtle cognitive changes (Morris, 1999; Morris and Price, 2001). CDR 0.5 also overlaps with another classification of 'mild cognitive impairment' (MCI) (Petersen, 2004). CDR 0.5 brains show extensive neuron death, senile plaques, and neurofibrillary degeneration (Price and Morris, 1999; Price et al, 2001), corresponding to Braak neuropathology stages III to V (Fig. 1.17) (John Morris, pers. comm.). Cognitive dysfunctions correlate 4-fold better with synapse loss than amyloid load. Synapse loss represents both neuron loss and neuron atrophy (Section 1.2.2).

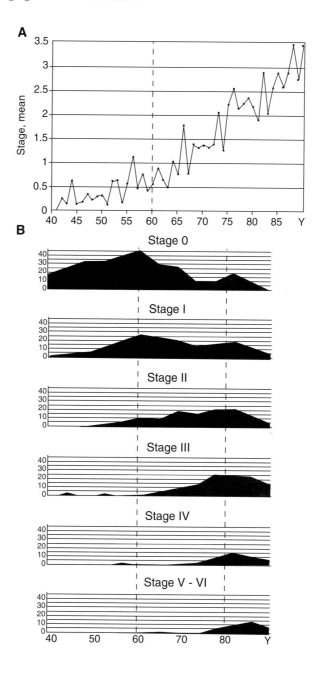

FIGURE 1.17 For legend see page 90.

Excess Aβ in the brain is widely believed the major, if not the primary cause, of Alzheimer disease (Selkoe, 2000; Yankner, 2000). The gaps between evidence that Aβ initiates Alzheimer disease and the weaker correlation of cognitive changes with the amyloid load are known as the 'amyloid conundrum' (Klein et al, 2001). Strong evidence comes from overproduction of APP and Aβ. Down syndrome (trisomy 21) gave important early support for the amyloid hypothesis because the trisomy 21, with its extra copy of the APP gene, increases Aβ production. By age 50, all Down brains have neuronal tangles, neuronal Aβ, and various extracellular Aβ including the classic amyloid plaques (Lott, 2005; Nixon, 2005; Sparks, 1996). In a rare case of partial trisomy of chromosome 21 that did not include the APP locus, this individual lived to age 78 without Alzheimer changes (Prasher et al, 1998). A mouse model of Down syndrome (trisomy chromosome 16) shows similar effects from deleting the extra APP gene (Gardiner, 2005). Transgenic mice overexpressing normal or mutant human APP develop early onset deposits of Aβ. Although several transgenic AD mice have synaptic deficits and impaired memory, neurofibrillary degeneration and neuron death are lacking (Holcomb et al, 1998; Jankowsky et al, 2004; Jankowsky et al, 2005; Mucke et al, 2000). The full package of amyloid and neurofibrillary degeneration occurs in a triple transgenic mouse with mutant APP and tau (LaFerla and Oddo, 2005; Oddo et al, 2003a,b).

Fibrillar $A\beta_{1-42}$ was the initial candidate for neurotoxicity in Alzheimer disease research (Yankner et al, 1989; Yankner, 2000), while others argued that fibrillar $A\beta_{1-42}$ is neuroprotective (Lee et al, 2005). However, $A\beta_{1-42}$ oligomers show more neurotoxicity than the classical fibrils. A subclass of particularly toxic oligomers is designated ADDLs (amyloid-derived diffusible ligands).[9] Oligomeric $A\beta_{1-42}$ has

FIGURE 1.17 Age-increase in Braak stages of Alzheimer disease, based on the density of neurofibrillary tangles (NFT) in the temporal lobe, including the hippocampus. Postmortem brains (887 Ss, 20–104 y, 47% men and 53% women) from Mainz and Frankfurt University hospital autopsies. Exclusions included brain tumors, bleeding, and inflammation; prior cognitive status is unknown (Braak and Braak, 1991; Braak et al, 1998). (Redrawn from Ohm et al, 1995.) A. Average Braak Stage score by age. Stage 0, absence of NFT; Stages 1-2, NFT confined to entorhinal and transentorhinal cortex; Stages 3-4, spread to other limbic areas; Stages 5-6, extensive NFT at Khachaturian criteria (Khachaturian, 1985) for Alzheimer diagnosis. B. Distribution of Braak stages by age. Estimated times between stages: I to II, 16+ y; II to III, 14 y; III to IV, 13 y, IV to V, 5 y. The duration of Alzheimer pathogenesis may be 50 y from the first NFT into end clinical stages.

---

[9]Readers note my commercial interests in Alzheimer disease as a cofounder of Acumen Pharmaceuticals, Inc., with William Klein (Northwestern University) and Grant Krafft (Acumen).

greater neurotoxicity than fibrillar Aβ (Klein et al, 2001; Oda et al, 1995) and is elevated >50-fold in Alzheimer brains (Gong et al, 2003). In rodent models, ADDLs impair memory and long-term potentiation (LTP) (Cleary et al, 2005; Klein et al, 2001; Lesne et al, 2006; Walsh et al, 2005), possibly by binding to synapses (Lacor et al, 2004).

Given the adverse activities of the $Aβ_{1-42}$ peptide, what might be its normal functions? The near invariance of $Aβ_{1-42}$ sequence across vertebrates from fish to birds to primates implies some long-standing function. APP is axonally transported to the presynaptic terminals (Buxbaum et al, 1998; Lazarov et al, 2005) by direct binding to the anterograde motor, kinesin (Kamal et al, 2000). Neuronal activity modulated Aβ secretion in the hippocampal slice model, which caused reversible synaptic depression (Kamenetz et al, 2003). Synaptically released Aβ appears to accumulate as plaques in transgenic mice (Lazarov et al, 2002; Sheng et al, 2002). Moreover, APP, Aβ, and the APP-like proteins (APPL1 and APPL2) may have roles in neuronal differentiation during development (Kimberly et al, 2005; Millet et al, 2005; Roncarati et al, 2002; Teo et al, 2005; Torroja et al, 1999). APP and Aβ may also participate in proinflammatory stress responses that overlap with the acute phase (Tuppo and Arias, 2005). Alzheimer transgenic mice given chronic LPS systemically (12 weekly i.p. injections) had high neuronal levels of APP and Aβ (Sheng et al, 2003). These responses to LPS are consistent with the inflammatory processes in Alzheimer disease (see below) and the acceleration of Aβ deposits by HIV infections and LPS (Chapter 2).

1.6.2. Inflammation in Alzheimer Disease

Senile plaques include many inflammatory proteins also found in atheromas (Table 1.3), some of which can stimulate free radical production, e.g., cytokines (IL-6, TNFα) and complement factors. C1q, the initiator of the classic complement cascade, is directly activated by Aβ aggregates (Fan and Tenner, 2004; Rogers et al, 1992; Webster et al, 2000). Further C-system enzymes yield the peptides C3a, C4a, and C5a; these 'anaphylactic peptides' can induce microglia/monocytes to produce free radicals. Anaphylactic peptides early in Alzheimer disease are indicated by the C3c and C4d fragments present in the pre-clinical stage CDR 0.5 (Zanjani et al, 2005). The classic senile plaques of advanced Alzheimer disease have numerous reactive microglia (macrophages). Microglia are of bone marrow origin and express CD68 and other monocyte-lineage epitopes also found in atheromas. However, in contrast to atheromas (see above), B- or T cells are rare in senile plaques. Reactive astrocytes around plaques may phagocytose Aβ (Thal et al, 2000; Wyss-Coray et al, 2003), whereas in Alzheimer transgenic mice, microglia near plaques did not (Stalder et al, 2001).

Early in the modern era of Alzheimer research, it was suspected that brain inflammatory proteins were artifacts of blood-brain barrier breakdown before death. However, we (Johnson et al, 1992a,b; May et al, 1990; Oda et al, 1994;

Pasinetti et al, 1992) and others (Akiyama et al, 2000; Walker and McGeer, 1992) showed that C-system genes are expressed in normal brain astrocytes, microglia, and neurons, and are further induced during neurodegeneration.

Many inflammatory proteins found in plaques also increase during aging in the brain (Table 1.5) in the absence of Alzheimer disease, as well as in other tissues (Section 1.8). Complement activation products C3c and C4d are found in diffuse Aβ deposits of clinically healthy elderly without indications of Alzheimer disease or gross neurodegeneration (Fig. 1.18) (Zanjani et al, 2005). Rodents also increase C1q and other inflammatory gene expression during brain aging (Pasinetti et al, 1999; Prolla and Mattson, 2001; Weindruch et al, 2002). Because rodent brains do not accumulate amyloid during aging, we can infer that in human brains there is a subset of inflammatory changes during normal aging that is independent of brain amyloid deposits.

Corpora amylacea are another inflammatory aggregate accumulated during aging and further in Alzheimer brains (Cavanagh, 1999; Singhrao et al, 1995). In these microscopic extracellular bodies (3–15μ), complement proteins surround a polyglucosan core. Angiogenic-inflammatory factors also increase. VEGF and TGF-β1 are 5-fold higher in cerebrospinal fluid in both Alzheimer and vascular dementia (Tarkowski et al, 2002; Vagnucci and Li, 2003). As noted above, new microvessels arise near plaques.

The interactions of oxidation and inflammation in amyloid plaques are less resolved than in atheromas. Plaques may represent feed-forward inflammatory processes. In 1982, Eikelenboom and Stam (1982) detected complement factors in senile plaques and postulated roles in neurodegeneration. A few years later, IL-1 production was identified with microglia (Giulian et al, 1986). In 1989, Griffin and colleagues (Griffin et al, 1989) proposed that microglial activation and IL-1 induction early in Alzheimer stimulate excess production of the amyloid precursor protein (APP) (Griffin, 2005). IL-1 also induces secretion of several complement factors by microglia (Veerhuis et al, 1999). Insulin and IGF-1 are also

TABLE 1.5 Inflammatory Changes in Alzheimer Senile Plaques and Normal Aging Brain. Adapted from Finch (2005)

	Senile Plaque	Aging Human	Aging Rodent
glial activation: GFAP, astrocytes; MHCII, microglia	+ +	+	+
α$_1$-antichymotrypsin α$_2$-macroglobulin	+		
apoE, apoJ, CRP, HOX-1, RAGE	+ +	+	+[a]
Complement C1q, C3	+ +	corpora amylacea	+ C1q mRNA
Cytokines: IL-1, IL-6, TNFα	+ +	+	+

CRP is not expressed in rodent brains.

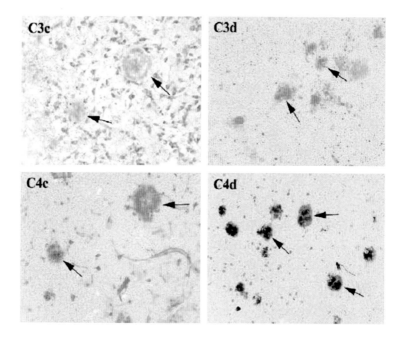

FIGURE 1.18 Increased complement deposits (C3c, C3d, C4c, C4d) on diffuse amyloid Aβ deposits in normal aging human brain (Clinical Disease Rating, CDR = 0). From collaboration with Joel Price and John Morris (Washington University) (Zanjani et al, 2005).

implicated in amyloid deposition and clearance (see below). The hypothesis that Aβ overproduction is linked to inflammatory processes is being tested by drugs and diet. As discussed in Chapters 2 and 3, non-steroidal anti-inflammatory drugs (NSAID ibuprofen) and diet restriction attenuate amyloid deposits in transgenic mice.

Other proinflammatory cascades may be driven by glyco-oxidation (Section 1.2.6 and 1.4.2; Query II). Plaques accumulate glycated proteins and oxidized lipids in Alzheimer disease (Girones et al, 2004; Reddy et al, 2002; Wong et al, 2001) and in transgenic Alzheimer mice (Munch et al, 2003). AGE adducts (Smith et al, 1994) colocalized with iNOS (Wong et al, 2001), a source of free radicals (Fig. 1.11). In Alzheimer transgenic mice, intracellular AGE colocalized with IL-1β and TNFα in astrocytes associated with amyloid deposits (Munch et al, 2003). Glycated proteins can induce oxidative stress and inflammatory responses (Section 1.2.7). The glycation of Aβ increased microglial inflammatory responses (Gasic-Milenkovic et al, 2003). Neurofibrillary tangles also become glycated, with subsequent generation of oxidative stress (Yan et al, 1995). Cause and effect are not resolved, because degenerating or stressed cells often attract macrophages and cause further inflammatory responses.

Lastly, systemic inflammatory factors that increase the risk of vascular events (Fig. 1.16) were also associated with risk of cognitive decline and Alzheimer disease in two prospective studies. In the Honolulu-Asian Aging Study (Schmidt et al, 2002) and the Health, Aging, and Body Composition Study (Yaffe et al, 2004), serum CRP elevations were associated with subsequent dementia (Section 2.6, Fig. 2.8). Neuronal CRP also increases during Alzheimer disease (Yasojima et al, 2000). There may be links of inflammatory processes of aging to the accelerating incidence of Alzheimer disease (Section 2.7).

1.6.3. Prodromal Stages of Alzheimer Disease

The onset of Alzheimer neurodegeneration is not as well defined as for vascular disease. The most detailed analysis comes from the Heiko and Eva Braak's huge autopsy series (Fig. 1.17). Neurofibrillary tangles, neuritic plaques, and various other Aβ deposits accumulate to some degree in almost all brains during aging (Fig. 1.10B). The six Braak stages, however, are based only on the neurofibrillary load (Fig. 1.17). Tangles (and plaques) appear to spread from subregions of the frontal cortex to the underlying hippocampus. Stage 0 represents brains without any tangles. Stage I, with a few localized tangles, is rare before 40 y. Later Braque stages increase after 65 y, consistent with other cognitive assessments and association with neuropathology (Kawas and Katzman, 1999; Khachaturian, 1985). Stage VI is the end stage of senile dementia. This prolonged sequence may span 50 years from initial neurofibrillary changes until definitive dementia (Ohm et al, 1995).

Neuronal endosomes show early (prodromal) changes. Endosomes mediate vesicle recycling and process the amyloid precursor protein (APP) (Nixon, 2005). Preclinical stages (Braak stages I and II of elderly brains) had enlarged endosomes and higher soluble Aβ, but no extracellular fibrillar amyloid (Cataldo et al, 2004). Late stages have extensive endosomal enlargement in neurons (up to 30-fold) (Nixon, 2005). Nixon and colleagues hypothesize that neuronal endocytic abnormalities are an early step in pathogenesis that increases the production of soluble Aβ. Other evidence comes from Down syndrome. Preceding the universal, early adult onset Alzheimer pathology, fetal Down brains have enlarged neuronal endosomes, with further deposition of extracellular Aβ deposits (Cataldo et al, 1997; Nixon, 2005). In intraneuronal $Aβ_{1-43}$ was detected in young Downs (neonate to 28 y), which had no extracellular Aβ (Hirayama et al, 2003). A trisomic mouse model of Downs also showed early endosomal pathology (Galdzicki and Siarey, 2003; Nixon, 2005).

ApoE alleles influence these changes (details in Section 5.7). The apoE4 allele, relative to apoE3, accelerates neurodegeneration in familial Alzheimer disease and in Down syndrome (Del Bo et al, 1997; Isacson et al, 2002). ApoE4 has clear effects before age 50. In Braak Stage I brains aged 22–46 y, apoE4 was 2-fold overrepresented relative to non-carriers (Ghebremedhin et al, 1998). Moreover, apoE allele associations are linked to combinations of eight other inflammatory genes in Alzheimer risk (Licastro et al, 2006).

Functional effects emerge early in E4 carriers. By PET imaging, asymptomatic E4 carriers have lower cerebral glucose metabolism in the frontal cortex even in their 30s (Reiman et al, 2004; Small et al, 2000). Further decreases of metabolism ensue at clinical stages (Alexander et al, 2002; Small et al, 2000). These metabolic impairments imply cell changes decades before clinical disease, consistent with the 30-year duration of Braak stages II to IV. Other cognitive declines are also influenced by apoE4. ApoE4 also predicted faster cognitive decline in the MacArthur Studies in Successful Aging (Bretsky et al, 2003). However, associations of later cognitive loss with midlife hypertension with apoE4 in the Honolulu Asia Aging Study (HAAS) (Peila et al, 2001) were not found by other studies (Qiu and Fratiglioni, 2005). A new concern is that apoE4 may influence brain development. In mice carrying human apoE genes, cortical neurons have less dendritic complexity in huE4/E4 mice than in huE3/E3 mice (Wang et al, 2005a).

1.6.4. Overlap of Alzheimer and Cerebrovascular Changes

Readers may have noticed a deviation from convention. Designating these senile brain diseases collectively as 'Alzheimer disease and vascular-related dementias' diverges from the convention that carefully discriminates these conditions. Alzheimer plaques and tangles and cerebrovascular lesions often co-occur in the elderly demented. Alzheimer disease and vascular dementia share many of the same risk factors (Chapter 3) and may benefit from many of the same diets and drugs (Chapter 2). This evidence, taken with the inflammatory proteins of senile plaques, suggests that Alzheimer and vascular dementia share key inflammatory processes.

Alzheimer plaques and tangles can arise in the absence of cerebrovascular lesions (Kemper, 1984; Kidd, 1964; Wisniewski and Terry, 1973). These distinctions were established in 1970 by the pioneering Newcastle Study (U.K.) (Tomlinson et al, 1968; Tomlinson et al, 1970). The conclusion that cerebrovascular and Alzheimer pathology can arise independently during aging remains valid today (Chui, 2005; Reed et al, 2004a; Terry et al, 1999). However, the combination of Alzheimer pathology and microinfarcts is commonly observed in dementia cases (Tomlinson et al, 1970; Petrovich et al, 2002).

The traditional term *cerebrovascular disease* now includes multiple types of changes in the cerebral vasculature that are hard to summarize because of their diversity: These range from focal infarcts due to a single thrombosis that causes local neuron death to more distributed hyaline degeneration of arterioles (arteriolosclerosis) that remain patent but cause chronic hypoperfusion. Helena Chui suggests the broader term *cerebrovascular-related brain injury* (Chui, 2005). The best recognized lesions of cerebrovascular aging are infarcts (Jagust, 2001; Langa et al, 2004;

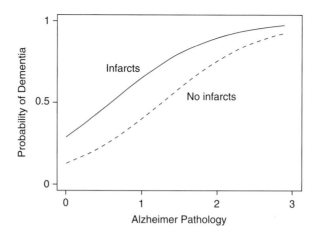

FIGURE 1.19 Clinical dementia risk increases with cerebrovascular damage and the level of Alzheimer disease characteristic neuropathology in early stages of AD. The probability of dementia diagnosis before death versus AD pathology with cerebral infarction (solid line) and without infarctions (dashed line). From The Religious Orders Study (both sexes; mean age, 84 y; 153 Ss; 44% were demented; postmortem, 99% of brains had NFT; 79%, neuritic plaques, 84%, diffuse amyloid; 35%, macroscopic infarcts; 29%, microscopic infarcts.) Macroscopic infarcts contributed progressively less to dementia with higher levels of AD neuropathology. (Text and figure adapted from Schneider et al, 2004.)

Reed et al, 2004a; Roman et al, 2004). Infarcts may be additive with the density Alzheimer plaques and tangles in predicting the level of dementia (Fig. 1.19) (Schneider et al, 2004). Depending on their location, infarcts may not cause cognitive impairments. White matter damage is also associated with vascular lesions and may contribute to dementia by slowing the neuronal conduction, which is crucial for high-speed transmission between cortical centers. Glial inflammatory changes of aging are implicated (see below).

Current cognitive tests do not resolve vascular versus pure Alzheimer contributions to dementia (Chui, 2005; Reed et al, 2004a). *First*, all studies so far are samples of convenience or of special groups that may not represent *populations*. *Second*, no 'simple metric' identifies vascular dementia. While large infarcts (>50 mL volume) are strongly associated with dementia, small infarcts in key locations also cause dementia. *Third*, no study has fully characterized premortem cerebral metabolism with postmortem cerebrovascular local blood flow, cerebrovascular amyloid, and both macroscopic and microscopic infarcts. Vascular amyloid Aβ also accumulates ('congophilic angiopathy') in association with white matter damage (Kalback et al, 2004) and increased risk of aneurysms (Van Dorpe et al, 2000). It is not known how vascular amyloid or aneurysms are related to 'prodromal' lipid accumulations in cerebral arteries (Fig. 1.15B), or to arterial 'fibrohyaline thickening,' which typically emerges by age 40 (Section 1.5.1). The vascular contribution to dementia may be stronger in the future as longevity continues to increase (Roman et al, 2002). The boundaries between 'usual aging' and Alzheimer disease are less clear at later ages.

Fourth, populations differ in the proportions of dementias. Vascular dementia may be 50% more prevalent in Japan than in U.S. Caucasians (Fujishima and Kiyohara, 2002; Jorm, 1987). Hawaiian Japanese who adopted Western diets may have less vascular dementia than on 'oriental' diets (Ross, 1999). However, a prospective study did not find associations of blood cholesterol with Alzheimer risk; as expected, apoE4 increased Alzheimer risk (Li et al, 2005). Two African-American samples had up to 2-fold more dementia than Caucasians (Demirovic et al, 2003; Mayeux, 2003a,b). Moreover, Nigerian Yorubans in Ibadan showed 50% less dementia than African Americans in Indianapolis (Hendrie et al, 2001). Indian elderly may also have less dementia (Indo-U.S. Study) (Chandra et al, 2001). These ethnodemographic differences in dementia have not been examined for neuropathology. A precedent is population differences in cancer. Breast cancer in Japan in the 1980s was 50% less at all ages than in Japanese born in the United States or U.S. Caucasians; these differences have since decreased in association with increased body fat (Pike et al, 1983; Probst-Hensch et al, 2000; Ursin et al, 1994).

Changes in cerebral blood flow and metabolism during aging may overlap with dementia. As noted above, ApoE4 carriers who are asymptomatic during middle age already have slightly depressed frontal cortex metabolism (Reiman et al, 2004; Small et al, 2000). Older patients with dementia or asymptomatic atherosclerosis typically have 10% or greater reductions in blood flow than healthy elderly (Meyer and Shaw, 1984; Schaller et al, 2005). However, cerebral blood flow also declines during normal aging by 15% from 30 to 65 y (Amano et al, 1982; Melamed et al, 1980; Plaschke, 2005) (Fig. 1.20A).

These observations on healthy subjects without risk factors for vascular pathology confirm the pioneering observations of Seymour Kety (Kety, 1956), which were initially discounted because of presumed confounds by asymptomatic atherosclerosis (Meyer and Shaw, 1984). Moreover, aging rats have progressive decrease in arteriolar density to about 35% across the adult life span, with similar changes in cerebral blood flow (Sonntag et al, 1997; Sonntag et al, 2000) (Fig. 1.20B legend). These striking changes hold for two rat genotypes that do not show occlusive cerebral atherosclerosis and are consistent with the cerebral blood flow decrease in normal human aging.

It is time to revisit Kety's hypothesis that the age decline in blood flow is due to reduced cerebral metabolism (Kety, 1956) (see above). Other studies show

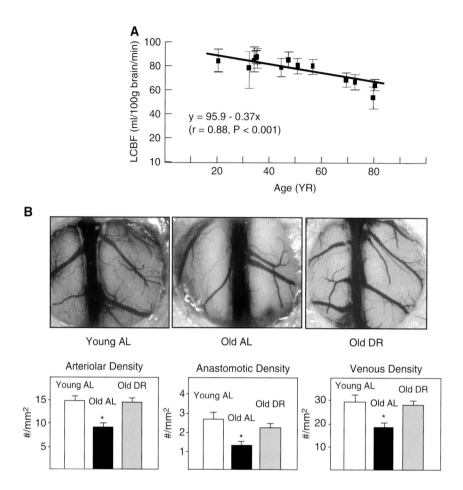

FIGURE 1.20 Brain vasculature and aging. A. Cerebral cortex gray matter blood flow declines progressively during normal human aging by 25%, 20–80 y, or about 0.4%/y (my calculation). (Redrawn from Amano et al, 1982). Cerebral blood flow (BF) was measured by the stable xenon flow CT technique on 13 healthy volunteers without vascular risk factors or diabetes, and normal cognition on the WAIS; the mean and range are shown for each subject; r of means = 0.88 (P<0.001). Cortical white matter also declined in BF with a shallower age gradient, but the age gradients were similar in gray matter cortex, basal ganglia, and thalamus. These data confirm (Melamed et al, 1980) and (Kety, 1956). B. Cerebral vasculature loss in aging rat. Cortical surface arterioles and venules in 13- and 29-m-old Brown Norway (BN) male rats. The progressive decrease in arterioles per surface area relative to age 5 m to 13 m, 1–5%; and 5 m to 29 m, −40%. Arteriolar anastamoses also decreased, by ca. 10%. Cerebral blood flow changed about 30% over the life span, close to human aging changes. The F344/BN hybrid changed similarly. Growth hormone injections for 35 d partly reversed the arteriolar loss in rats aged 30 m, but did not alter the young. (From Sonntag et al, 1997.)

more or less concurrent synaptic atrophy in normal humans and rodents during middle age (Masliah et al, 1993; Morgan et al, 1987; Morgan et al, 1990; Rozovsky et al, 2005). Moreover, apoE4 carriers show reduced cerebral metabolism during middle age, as noted above (Reiman et al, 2004) (Section 5.7.4). We are evaluating whether glial activation from inflammation and/or oxidative stress is a primary factor in synaptic atrophy, which secondarily causes the reduction of cerebral blood flow (Fig. 1.7E).

Blood pressure is another shared risk factor with vascular events and dementia. The large ARIC Study and eight others found that middle age hypertensions increased risk of later cognitive declines (Qiu et al, 2005). Vascular tortuosities during aging may be increased by hypertension (Akima et al, 1986; Hiroki et al, 2002; Moody et al, 1997). Antihypertensive drugs may decrease the risk of vascular and Alzheimer dementia (Qiu et al, 2005). Possible pathways include hypoperfusion from cerebral atherosclerosis. In rodent models, chronic hypoperfusion caused large-scale activation of microglia, as in Alzheimer brains (Farkas et al, 2004). Obesity as a risk factor is discussed below.

1.6.5. Insulin and IGF-1 in Vascular Disease and Alzheimer Disease

The inter-relations of obesity, diabetes, and glucose dysregulation are among the huge frontiers in medicine with great importance to vascular disease and possibly also to Alzheimer disease independent of the cerebrovasculature. The metabolic hormones insulin and IGF-1 are increasingly implicated in atherosclerosis and Alzheimer disease and could be critical links to the longevity pathways identified in mutant mice, flies, worms, and yeast (Fig. 1.3A, B) (Chapter 5). However, IGF-1 deficiencies show opposite effects by increasing the risk of cardiovascular disease and congestive heart failure in clinical studies and experimental models. These hormonal effects of insulin pathways are relatively new mechanisms and were first considered about 1985 for vascular disease in diabetics (Koschinsky et al, 1985) and a decade later for Alzheimer disease (Finch and Cohen, 1997).

Low serum IGF-1 is associated with vascular disease (Conti et al, 2004). Elderly in the Framingham Heart Study with the lowest IGF (serum IGF-1 <75 µg/L; lowest decile) had a 2.6-fold higher risk of congestive heart failure; during a 5-year follow-up, the hazard decreased by 27% for every standard deviation increment (Vasan et al, 2003). Low serum IGF-1 may be an independent risk factor, because the associations with vascular event did not depend on cholesterol, age, and other risk factors (Conti et al, 2004), nor on serum IL-6, which is commonly elevated in elderly and in vascular disease and that can lower IGF-1 (De Benedetti et al, 2002). Another association is with arterial plaque instability, which may be increased by low IGF-1 and low PAPPA-A, a protease which cleaves IGF-1 binding protein to release IGF-1 (Beaudeux et al, 2003).

Insulin/IGF-1 signaling is implicated in many aspects of vascular biology (Bayes-Genis et al, 2000; Frost et al, 1997; Gonzalez et al, 2001). Figure 1.3B shows the basic machinery in processes that can be cardioprotective or proatherogenic (Conti et al, 2004). Activation of IGF-1 receptors, in turn, activates PI3-kinases, serine/threonine kinase Akt, which then phosphorylates the constitutive NOS (nitric acid synthase) in the vascular endothelia. The increased nitric oxide (NO) production has multiple cardioprotective actions, which include vasodilation, platelet inhibition, and free radical scavenging. Angiotensin II inhibits this pathway, while TNFα, which is increased in atherosclerotic plaques, can inhibit IGF-1 expression (Anwar et al, 2002). IGF-1 may also be pro-atherogenic by stimulating the proliferation of vascular smooth muscle cells. Attempts to pharmacologically manipulate IGF-1, e.g., by manipulating growth hormone (GH) secretion with the somatostatin analogue angiopeptin, have not been effective (Conti et al, 2004). Leptin signaling may also converge with insulin/IGF-1 pathways in regulating cell proliferation (Tapia, 2005). Leptin in obese patients shows modest correlation with telomere loss (Valdes et al, 2005), which will be considered further below in relation to fat as a source of inflammatory factors.

The decline of IGF-1 and GH with normal aging is receiving attention as a major cause of insulin resistance during aging. GH secretion by the pituitary gradually declines during aging at the rate of 10–15%/decade of adult life (Conti et al, 2004; Obermayr et al, 2005; Rudman et al, 1981). GH is a major regulator of IGF-1 expression and secretion by liver, kidney, and vascular smooth muscle cells. Hepatic secretion may account for the bulk of serum IGF-1 decline. Age changes in GH and IGF-1 were partly reversed by donepezil, a cholinesterase inhibitor (Obermayr et al, 2005). Healthy centenarians may have higher IGF-1 (Paolisso et al, 1997; Paolisso et al, 1999; Franceschi et al, 2005) (Fig. 5.11).

Insulin/IGF-1 functions are also implicated in brain vascular aging (Sonntag et al, 1997; Sonntag et al, 2000). As noted above, rat brain shows striking decrease of vascular density. These major declines were partly reversed by injections of GH for 35 d, which increased plasma IGF-1 (Fig. 1.20 legend). Cerebral blood flow was also restored. Although these striking age changes and responses to GH have not led to clinical trials, there is reason to consider that the reduced cerebral blood flow during 'normal' aging (see above) may be also linked to the decrease of GH and IGF-1.

Another emerging possibility is the role of IGF-1/insulin in Alzheimer disease from epidemiological and clinical associations with hyperinsulinemia and maturity-onset diabetes (Carro and Torres-Aleman, 2004; Craft and Watson, 2004; Finch and Cohen, 1997; Gasparini and Xu, 2003; Steen et al, 2005). Blood insulin and IGF-1 are actively transported across the blood-brain barrier, which expresses relevant receptors (Steen et al, 2005). The importance of insulin transport was demonstrated by a recent study with healthy volunteers (Fishel et al, 2005). Induced hyperinsulinemia rapidly increased cerebrospinal fluid (csf) cytokines (IL-1α, β, IL-6, TNFα), $A\beta_{1-42}$, and F2-isoprostane, a marker of oxidative stress. Serum and csf cytokines were uncorrelated, implying that the insulin effects are not due to peripheral transport. However, plasma $A\beta_{1-42}$ was increased in association with elevations of csf transthyretin, a transporter for $A\beta_{1-42}$ from the

CNS to the peripheral blood. In a mouse model, serum IGF-1 also enhanced Aβ transport from the brain to peripheral blood by the amyloidogenic transthyretin (Carro and Torres-Aleman, 2004). Plasma IGF may be lower in sporadic and familial Alzheimer disease (Swedish APP670/671) (Mustafa et al, 1999).

Within the brain, the degradation of $A\beta_{1-42}$ may compete with insulin for IDE (insulin-degrading enzyme), which is also a candidate gene for Alzheimer disease (Gasparini and Xu, 2003; Farris et al, 2004; Leissring et al 2003; Bertram et al, 2007). Moreover, IGF-1 can be neuroprotective against Aβ (Aguado-Llera et al, 2005; Dore and Quirion, 1997) via Akt kinase (Zheng et al, 2000). Both insulin and IGF-1 and their receptors may be synthesized by brain neurons (Steen et al, 2005). Despite the major gaps, the present evidence strongly connects brain aging to the vascular and longevity pathways in insulin/IGF signaling. These metabolic associations are supported by dietary influences on Alzheimer disease (Chapter 3). The genetics of these relationships is discussed in Chapter 5.

1.6.6. Blood Inflammatory Proteins: Biomarkers for Disease or Aging, or Both?

Elevated acute phase proteins imply current or future health impairments. Serum CRP and IL-6 increases on the average after middle age in most populations (Cesari et al, 2004; Ershler and Keller, 2000; Ferrucci et al, 2005; Wilson et al, 2002). For example, a large random sample in Tuscany, Italy (InCHIANTI) showed progressive increases of CRP, fibrinogen, and IL-6 (Fig. 1.21) (Cesari et al, 2004). No age changes were seen in IL-1, TNF-, and TGF-β1. Cardiovascular disease is a major factor in these increases. Age alone, separated statistically from disease, predicted increased CRP and IL-18 in women only. Other studies also show uneven distributions of acute phase proteins, possibly subpopulations with elevated vascular risk factors including obesity (see below) or periodontal disease (Bruunsgaard et al, 1999a; D'Aiuto et al, 2005; Deliargyris et al, 2004) (Section 2.3.1).

Old age IL-6 elevations strongly associate with disability and mortality (Ferrucci et al, 1999; Harris et al, 1999; Ishihara and Hirano, 2002; McCarty, 1997). High CRP and IL-6 doubled the mortality risk in the healthy, non-disabled of the Iowa 65+ Rural Health Study (Harris et al, 1999) (Fig. 1.22). InCHIANTI associated high CRP and IL-6 with poor physical condition and hand-grip strength (Cesari et al, 2004), while the MacArthur Study of Successful Aging associated high CRP with reduced recreational (voluntary) activity and social integration (Loucks et al, 2006).

Genetic influences, while expected, have not been found. In the Women's Health and Aging cohorts, IL-6 variants did not associate with plasma levels of serum IL-6 or frailty (Reuben et al, 2003). Again, no association was found between IL-1, IL-6, and TNF alleles and mortality in Finnish nonagenarians (Wang et al, 2001). Larger population samples may be needed (Section 1.4.3).

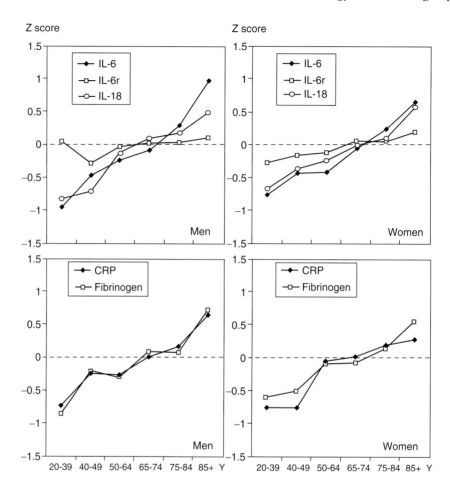

FIGURE 1.21 Blood acute phase proteins and aging graphed as z-plots in units of standard deviation (SD) from the mean. InCHIANTI Study, 1998 sample; random sample from Tuscany, Italy populations; 30 men and 30 women from each decade, 20–69 y. (Redrawn from Ferrucci et al, 2005.)

A provisional conclusion is that the *average* increases of CRP and IL-6 at later ages represent the increase of clinical sub-groups with various diseases and conditions that elevated acute phase responses. It is interesting to compare the age trends of blood proteins with the acute phase response in young adults, which are similar, with the possible exception of IGF-1 (Table 1.5). An open question is the role of infections (Chapter 2).

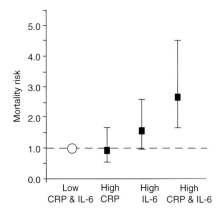

FIGURE 1.22 High levels of blood IL-6 and CRP double mortality risk in healthy, nondisabled elderly. From the Iowa 65+ Rural Health Study (1,293 Ss followed 4.6 y). High: CRP 2.78 mg/L, IL-6 >3.19 pg/mL. (Redrawn from Harris et al, 1999.)

1.7. INFLAMMATION IN OBESITY

Obesity is associated with chronic low-grade inflammation that synergizes to increase the risk of Alzheimer disease, vascular events, and other adverse outcomes of aging, according to the body mass index (BMI),[10] which is widely used to estimate obesity. For example, Alzheimer risk varied progressively with BMI in an 18-year prospective study (Gustafson et al, 2003): For each BMI unit increase at age 70 y, Alzheimer risk in women was increased by 36%; men, however, did not show these associations. There may be a female bias in mid-life obesity and later Alzheimer risk, of 2-fold in one study (Tabet, 2005). Those younger than 76 y showed a 'U-shaped' relationship between BMI and dementia, whereas at later ages, low BMI from weight loss may 'mask' these associations (Luchsinger et al, 2006). Mid-life obesity in combination with high cholesterol and systolic pressure increased Alzheimer risk additively by 6.2-fold (Kivipelto et al, 2005).

---

[10]The body mass index (BMI) is a crude but widely used measure of body fat, calculated as: height (m)/mass^2 (kg). Underweight is BMI <18.5; normal weight, 18.5–24.9; overweight, 25–29.9; obesity >30. The height-weight curves differ for men and women, and for children and adolescents. The BMI does not discriminate the type or location of fat, e.g., abdominal fat has a different physiology and pathology than subcutaneous fat (Chapter 3).

In current thinking about these complex pathologies, obesity is considered as a component of the 'Metabolic Syndrome' (Table 1.6), which is defined by three or more of the five traits that increase the risk of diabetes, cardiovascular disease, and chronic kidney disease. These traits overlap with 'syndrome X' or the 'insulin-resistance syndrome,' a cluster of metabolic dysfunctions (Kim et al, 2004; Reisin and Alpert, 2005; Reynolds and He, 2005). In some current populations, nearly 50% of adults meet 'syndrome' criteria. In a major prospective study of elderly, the combination of elevated CRP and IL-6 together with the 'Syndrome' increased the risk of cognitive impairment by 1.66-fold during the next 4.5 y (community living, 70–79 y; Health, Aging, and Body Composition Study) (Yaffe et al, 2004). In NHANES II, those with the 'Syndrome' had 2-fold higher mortality risk from coronary heart disease during 13 years of follow-up. Among those with both the 'Metabolic Syndrome' and coronary disease at entry, mortality was 4-fold higher (Malik et al, 2004). Chronic kidney disease risk is increased up to 5-fold in proportion to the number of 'Syndrome' criteria.

The relationship of obesity to inflammation is fundamental because adipocytes release IL-6, TNFα, and other proinflammatory cytokines (Hukshorn et al, 2004; Lee et al, 2005; Toni et al, 2004). Blood inflammatory cytokines tend to increase with obesity (Table 1.7). There is also a striking correlation between blood CRP elevations and leptin (Fig. 1.23), which is secreted by adipocytes; CRP induction in hepatocytes may be mediated by IL-6 or TNFα (Shamsuzzaman et al, 2004). Abdominal visceral fat is correlated with plasma OxLDL and CRP (Couillard et al, 2005). Lipid peroxides are elevated 2-fold in obese humans (plasma, MDA assay) (Yesilbursa et al, 2005) and obese rats (urinary isoprostanes) (Dobrian et al, 2004). Leptin, besides regulating food intake (Chapter 3), is proinflammatory by enhancing phagocytosis and inducing cytokines (Section 1.3.1).

The inflammatory profile of obesity implies increased oxidative stress. Free radical production (ROS) is increased in adipocytes of obese mice (Furukawa et al, 2004). Among many examples, the Framingham Study correlated BMI with plasma F2-isoprostanes, which are directly linked to lipid oxidation (8-epi-PGF$_{2\alpha}$, a stable by-product of arachadonic oxidation) (Keaney et al, 2003).

TABLE 1.6 The Metabolic Syndrome

	Women	Men
waist circumference	> 88 cm	102 cm
serum triglycerides	≥ 150 mg/dL (1.7 mM)	Same
HDL-cholesterol	< 50 mg/dL (1.3 mM)	< 40 mg/DL (<1.03 mM)
fasting blood glucose	≥ 110 mg/dl (6.2mM)	Same
blood pressure (systolic/diastolic)	>130/85 mg Hg	Same

National Cholesterol Education Program's Adult Treatment Panel (Anonymous, 2001). The choice 3 of 5 traits represents the uncertainties of definition. Gender and ethnicity also modify these five criteria. The clinical community broadly recognizes their value in describing the epidemic of obesity and diabetes.

Obesity also intensifies osteoarthritis and accelerates its onset (Bray and Bellanger, 2006; Rubenstein, 2005). Osteoarthritis is an age-related inflammation caused by mechanical stress, rather than by simple 'wear-and-tear' as once thought. Osteoarthritis may be unavoidable during aging and is more intense in joints that bear the most weight. Osteoarthritis has traditionally been considered 'non-inflammatory,' in contrast to the severe inflammation of rheumatoid arthritis. Mechanical pressures that are increased by obesity activate catabolic responses of the articular chondrocytes to cause matrix loss and accumulation of AGEs (Loeser, 2004). Acute phase proteins (CRP, IL-1) and other inflammatory molecular responses arise early in osteoarthritis (Benito et al, 2005; Bonnet and Walsh, 2005; Igarashi et al, 2004; Loeser et al, 2004). Pain in osteoarthritis is linked to inflammation. The grinding of adjacent bones as cartilage erodes often causes pain. Other pain may come from osteophytes, spurs of new bone formed in arthritic joints, which press upon nerves; their genesis appears to depend on synovial macrophages (Blom et al, 2004). Anti-inflammatory drugs may reduce pain by inhibiting cyclooxygenase-2 (COX-2) and 5-lipoxygenase (5-LOX), which produce prostaglandins and leukotrienes (Bonnet and Walsh, 2005; Hinz and Brune, 2004) (Chapter 2.9.3).

TABLE 1.7 Inflammatory Changes in Alzheimer Senile Plaques and Normal Aging Brain Acute Phase Responses and Aging Trends (bold shows differences)

	Acute Phase in Adults	Normal Aging Trends	Diabetes-Obesity
blood amyloids			
serum amyloid A	modest-large increase		
CRP			
blood complement C3	modest-large increase		
blood cytokines:			
CRP	modest-large increase	modest increase	modest increase
IL-1β			
IL-6			
TNFα			
blood coagulation (fibrinogen)	modest-large increase	modest	
blood lipids			
HDL	decrease	decrease	decrease
LDL	increase	increase	increase
oxLDL	increase	increase	increase
triglycerides	increase	increase	increase
Cortisol	modest-large increase	modest increase	modest increase
Insulin			
insulin	resistance	resistance	
IGF-1	decrease	increase	

Acute phase in adults (Wright et al, 2000). IGF-1 in aging, Fig. 5.11 and (Bonafe et al, 2003).

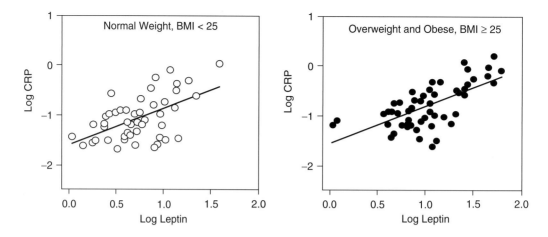

FIGURE 1.23 Blood C-reactive protein (CRP) and leptin correlations, graphed separately for BMI < 25 and > 25 (see footnote 10 for definition of BMI). CRP is elevations are strongly correlated with blood leptin, secreted by adipocytes; CRP may be regulated by IL-6 or TNFα, also secreted by adipocytes. (Redrawn from Shamsuzzaman et al, 2004.)

Lastly, I briefly mention that obesity is associated with modestly higher risks of some cancers, e.g., 10–20% higher risk of pancreatic cancer (Patel et al., 2005b; Berrington de Gonzalez et al, 2003) and advanced prostate cancer (Macinnis and English, 2006). Many factors are involved besides metabolic hormones or acute phase proteins. For example, the higher levels of endometrial cancer in post-menopausal obesity are associated with the production of estrone by fat depots, which drive endometrial cell proliferation. But again, exercise is a counterbalancing factor, possibly through improved insulin sensitivity (Kaaks et al, 2002) (Section 3.4).

1.8. PROCESSES OF NORMAL AGING IN THE ABSENCE OF SPECIFIC DISEASES

The shared inflammatory processes in the major chronic diseases discussed above also arise in tissues in the absence of these specific diseases. We have seen this already in arterial changes (Table 1.4). Some of the following examples address Query I: that bystander damage from oxidative stress stimulates chronic inflammation.

1.8.1. Brain

Microglia (macrophage/monocytic cells) show definitive activation during normal aging in rodent, monkey, and human. Overall, the increase of activated microglia during aging is 25–75% less than in Alzheimer brains (Finch et al, 2002). In rat cerebral cortex (Vaughan and Peters, 1974) and spinal cord (Stuesse et al, 2000), microglial activation progresses from maturity into old age (Fig. 1.8A) and is associated with increased production of IL-6 and TNFα (Xie et al, 2003). Humans have similar increases in activated microglia in the hippocampus during normal aging without neuropathology (DiPatre and Gelman, 1997). These cell changes are consistent with MRI imaging findings showing that white matter disorganization begins during middle age (Fig. 1.8B). White matter inflammatory changes may be important to the usual slowing of information processing.

Many of the same inflammatory proteins found in senile plaques also increase modestly in the brains of many mammals during normal aging in the absence of Alzheimer, e.g., cytokines and complement factors (Table 1.5). Complement proteins are found on the diffuse amyloid deposits of normal aging (Zanjani et al, 2005) (Fig. 1.18) and in corpora amylacea, discussed previously regarding Alzheimer disease, which accumulate modestly in non-pathological brain aging (Singhrao et al, 1995). Because aging rodent brains lack amyloid Aβ, yet show comparable microglial activation to that in humans (see above), it may concluded that microglial activation during aging *can* be initiated independently of amyloid deposits. This is a major point in interpreting the human aging changes, because tissue amyloids can activate microglia. For example, brain amyloid deposits increased the influx of blood-born monocytes, which are precursor cells of microglia (Fiala et al, 1998). Similarly, in hemodialysis patients, intestinal amyloid formed from β2-microglobulin are associated with activated macrophages (Miyata et al, 1994), which is a completely distinct protein from brain Aβ.

1.8.2. Generalized Inflammatory Changes in Normal Tissue Aging

Other tissues besides the brain show increased inflammation during aging. The variability of tissue proteases (cathepsins) between studies (Finch, 1972a) is a clue to the importance of inflammation in aging: Because these enzymes are associated with macrophages, the variability between studies could reflect variations of infiltrating macrophages, which are prominent in liver histology from aging rats in one early colony (Andrew et al, 1943). Data from rodent colonies before 1970 may be confounded by infections that have dwindled (Section 2.2.2). Nonetheless, in modern specific-pathogen free (SPF) colonies of aging rodents, lymphocytic infiltration is common and not considered pathological (Turturro et al, 2002). Fibrosis is also common in aging myocardium (Schriner et al, 2005) (Section 2.2) and other visceral organs.

Gene expression profiling by microarray chips has given further examples of inflammatory processes during aging. Microarray profiling consistently increases in many tissues during normal aging. Table 1.8 summarizes the consistent increase of inflammatory gene expression during aging in brain regions, liver, heart, and skeletal muscle. Inflammation-related genes may be the single largest category of change during aging (Table 1.9).

Several complement (C) factor mRNAs increase in brain, liver, and myocardium of aging rodents. C1q is the initiating complex of the classical C-cascade. We showed the increase of C1q in the brain during normal aging, in the striatum (Pasinetti et al, 1999), as confirmed by microarray (Table 1.8). C-system genes also have greater expression in aging human frontal cortex (Erraji-Benchekroun et al, 2005; Lu et al, 2004; Pavlidis et al, 2004). Increased expression of the complement system during aging may contribute to C-factors in the corpora amylacea and in the deposits of C3 and C4 on diffuse brain amyloid in nonpathological cases (Fig. 1.18). The 'anaphylactic peptides' (C3a, C4a, C5a) can stimulate macrophage-monocyte cells in brain and elsewhere to produce ROS that cause oxidative damage. IL-6 expression also increases in aging brain and blood vessels, consistent with blood IL-6 (see above). Most genes increased during aging are also rapidly induced in young mice by LPS (Terao et al, 2002).

These indications of similar inflammatory changes in multiple tissues during aging imply a coordinated pattern, which may involve a small number of transcription factors. The NF-κB transcription factors form multimeric complexes with one or more of the five Rel family proteins. These proteins are activated by cell oxidative stress (redox) and regulate hundreds of genes important to Alzheimer disease, cancer, and vascular disease by influencing inflammation and cell death (apoptosis) (Li, 2005; Mattson and Camanadola, 2001; Monaco and Paleog, 2004; Vater et al, 1992). For example, oxidized LDL has biphasic effects on NF-κB in vascular endothelia, which, in turn, influence expression of genes encoding adhesion molecules and scavenger receptors (Robbesyn et al, 2004). NF-κB and other redox sensitive transcription factors could be fundamental to inflammatory cascades of aging.

The progressive activation of inflammatory genes during normal aging may have a direct role in impairing gene expression for neuronal functions (Blalock et al, 2003; Blalock et al, 2004; Lu et al, 2004b). In human brain during normal aging, DNA damage was found in the promoters of certain genes with decreased activity during aging (Lu et al, 2004b). Because the DNA is extracted from whole brain regions, we do not yet know the cell types involved that might inform on the source of the oxidant damage. Because other DNA damage is attenuated by diet restriction (Section 3.2), it is plausible that inflammatory processes are involved at some level.

Inflammatory gene expression in aging is also found in the fly model, with major induction of genes encoding 20 anti-microbial peptides and other factors of innate immunity (Landis et al, 2004) (Fig. 1.24). The microbial load increases in aging flies (Section 5.6). Moreover, oxygen exposure of young flies induces subsets of the aging changes in gene expression. Thus, we see a remarkable generality in the convergence of inflammation, oxidative stress, and aging

TABLE 1.8 Inflammatory Gene Expression in Aging: Fold-increase During Aging in Rodents

Gene	Brain			Coronary Artery	Liver	Gastrocnemius Muscle	Myocardium
	Neocortex	Cerebellum	Hippocampus				
apolipoprotein E							4-13[i]
complement (C)	2[a]	3[a]	2[c]		2[g]		
C[1q] a, b, or c		4[a]	1.3[b]–2[c,d]				
C3			>10[d]				
C4	5[a]	4[a]	1.5[b]–2[c]				
cathepsin S	1.5[a]	4[a]	2[c]			2[h]	
CD68 (macrophage marker)	2[a]	4[a]				1.5[a]	
lysozyme P	2[a]	6[a]			2[g]		
serum amyloid A (SAA)				3[e]			
serum amyloid P (SAP)				3[e]	2[g]	3[h]	
Interleukin-1 (IL-1)				3[e]			
Interleukin-6 (IL-6)	1.3[j]	1.3[j]	1.3[j]				
tumor necrosis factor (TNFα)							

numbers >1.5 are rounded to the next integer; same GenBank number as the adjacent leftward entry; a. Mouse, C57BL/6NNia, m; 5, 30 m; Affymetrix (Lee et al, 2000); b. Mouse, C57BL/6 NNia, m; 2, 15 m; Affymetrix (Verbitsky et al, 2004);c. Mouse, C57BL/6 NNia, m; 3,12,18,24 m; Affymetrix (Terao et al, 2002); d. Rat, F344, m; 4,14, 24 m; Affymetrix (Blalock et al, 2003); e. Rat, F344,m; 3,26 m; GEArray , PCR (Csiszar, 2004); g. Mouse, C3B10F1, f; 7,27 m; Affymetrix (Cao et al, 2001); h. Mouse, C57BL/6NNia, m; 5, 30 m; Affymetrix (Lee, 1999); i. Mouse, 'sedentary', m; 20, 35 m; Affymetrix (Bronikowski et al, 2003); j. Mouse, BALB/c, m; 3–6,24 m; PCR, ELISA (Ye et al, 1999; Godbout et al, 2004).

TABLE 1.9 Functional Categories of Aging Changes in Gene Expression from Microarray Profiling

	Brain[a]		Liver[b]		Gastrocnemius[c]		Myocardium[d]	
	Higher	Lower	Higher	Lower	Higher	Lower	Higher	Lower
inflammation-immune	25%	5	40				15	1
stress response	17%		25		16%		8	1
energy	0–5					13		
apotosis, proliferation			15	25				
macromolecular biosynthesis and turnover		9						

a. mouse (Lee et al, 2000); b. mouse (Cao et al, 2001); c. mouse (Lee et al, 1999); d. mouse sedentary (Bronikowski et al, 2003).

(Queries I and II, Section 1.1) that appears independently in at least one invertebrate and in representative mammals. Shared gene regulatory systems may be sought that will identify ancient "kernels' of genetic machinery that modulate outcomes of aging in aerobic organisms. Chapter 2 considers the possibility that deterioration of the gut allows leakage of endogenous pathogens as a cause of systemic inflammation.

Lastly, these microarray data bring closure to a major long-standing controversy about gene function during aging. In past decades, many presumed that gene functions degenerated globally during aging (Cutler, 1975; Strehler, 1977). However, all the evidence points to high selectivity in the direction and degree of changes in gene expression during aging. Microarray profiling shows that relatively few RNAs are altered during aging: <5% of the RNAs detected changed up or down by >2-fold (Table 1.8). These results confirm our earlier work, in which RNA-driven hybridization showed that brain polyribosomal mRNA had the same 'sequence complexity' (estimate of numbers of active genes) in young and old rats, within a margin of 5% (Colman et al, 1980). Protein patterns also show the specificity of aging changes. Enzyme activity changes are highly selective (no changes in 80% of enzymes in liver and 88% in kidney) (Finch, 1969; Finch, 1972a). Another approach evaluated rates of protein synthesis in tissues of young and old mice that were injected with differently radiolabelled leucine: [^{3}H]-young, [^{14}C]-old (Gordon and Finch, 1974). After co-electrophoresis of soluble proteins from both ages, the gels were sliced. The ratios of ^{3}H: ^{14}C on 1 mm gel slices showed selective age changes in liver and brain regions (hippocampus, striatum, hypothalamus). Each tissue had a few peaks of radioactivity down the electrophoretic lane that differed by age, indicating selective shifts in protein synthesis consistent with selective shifts in mRNAs.

Although most somatic cells retain their characteristic phenotypes at the microscopic level in tissues, exacting analysis of individual cells by Jan Vijg and

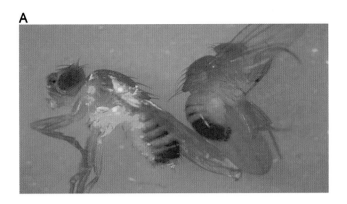

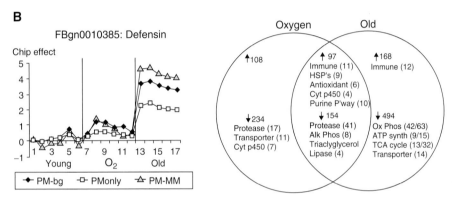

FIGURE 1.24 Aging and anti-microbial gene induction in the fly Drosophila melanogaster. A. 5-fold to 100-fold induction of anti-microbial genes, e.g., attacin (anti-Gram-negative bacteria) and drosomycin (anti-fungal). (From Landis et al, 2004.) B. Overlap of genes increased during aging and gene induced in young flies exposed to oxidative stress. (Redrawn from Landis *op. cit.*)

colleagues is pointing to increasing somatic cell diversity through quantitative variations in specific mRNA content and DNA rearrangements. For example, analysis of mRNA in single cardiomyocytes showed that aging increased cell heterogeneity in expression levels, e.g., the myosin gene (myl2) mRNA, in contrast to relative invariant expression of the mitochondrial cox-1 (Bahar et al, 2006). Aging myocytes differed by showing both increases and decreases in myl2 mRNA. The role of selective DNA damage may be suspected here, as shown for promoter DNA damage in association with decreased certain mRNAs in the aging brain discussed above (Lu et al, 2004). Moreover, chromosomal DNA rearrangements increase with aging in myocardium and liver (Suh and Vijg, 2006). While these changes are described as stochastic at the cell level, they may still be driven by systemic physiological shifts (e.g., muscle mitochondrial DNA deletions during aging are increased by hyperglycemia (Liang, 1997) and decreased by diet restriction) (Aspnes, 1997) (Section 3.3.2). Thus aging tissues become an increasing mosaic of diverse genomic alterations with a still-to-be-defined impact on cell physiology.

1.9. SUMMARY

In most chronic diseases of aging, oxidative stress and inflammation are prominent. Moreover, many tissues without specific pathology show modest inflammatory changes during aging share major subsets of those in chronic diseases of aging. The strong trends for increased blood inflammatory markers (CRP, IL-6) in many studies of aging may be mainly driven by vascular disease. Evidence for the role of insulin/IGF-1 pathways in many pathological processes (vascular disease, obesity, Alzheimer disease) seems broadly consistent with the mutations that increase longevity in experimental models (Fig. 1.3A). Major questions are the role of the age-accumulated bystander damage to proteins and lipids in the inflammatory processes (Query I) and the role of inflammation in further bystander damage (Query II). The case may be strongest for vascular disease that is attenuated by drugs with anti-inflammatory activities considered in Chapter 2. Environmental influences through infections and inflammogens (Chapter 2) and diet (Chapter 3) will evaluate Query III: that diet and environmental pathogens influence diseases with inflammatory components through bystander damage. Alzheimer disease may prove to be as multi-factorial as vascular disease.

Infections, Inflammogens, and Drugs

2.1. INTRODUCTION

Chapter 1 emphasized the role of inflammatory processes in vascular disease, from early beginnings before birth. Alzheimer disease shares many of the same inflammatory changes, although cause and effect are less clear. This chapter follows the pathways of Fig. 1.2 further by examining the role of infections and inflammatory agents in vascular disease and Alzheimer disease and selected cancers. Pharmacologic interventions through NSAIDs and anti-coagulant drugs further establish the inflammatory mechanisms in vascular disease and may extend to Alzheimer disease. These examples are discussed in relation to Query II (Section 1.1) that inflammation causes bystander damage and Query III that environmental pathogens and inflammogens influence chronic diseases with inflammatory processes through bystander damage (Section 1.4).

The environmental role in these diverse, slowly developing diseases remains counter-current to traditional thinking, because in general, Alzheimer disease, cancer, and vascular disease are not 'infectious,' by Koch's postulates. That is, with few exceptions for these diseases, infectious agents cannot be isolated, and the disease cannot be transferred and propagated to a test animal.

2.2. VASCULAR DISEASE

2.2.1. Historical Associations of Infections and Vascular Mortality

The traditional risk factors for vascular disease (hypertension, obesity, elevated LDL cholesterol, smoking) do not explain about 35% of cases (Section 1.5.3.2). From epidemiologic and pathologic studies, chronic infections may be primary causes or co-factors of inflammation in vascular disease. This controversial concept has been discussed for a century or more (Frothingham, 1911). The hypothesis of inflammation as a co-factor is strongest in human arterial disease, because prodromal microscopic foci of oxidized lipids and activated macrophages are present before birth (Section 1.5.3.1). The evidence for the role of infections in arterial disease, while considerable and supported by animal models, is still largely circumstantial for humans.

Rheumatic heart disease is a classic example of infection-caused heart disease, but with a different etiology than most cardiovascular cases. Until about 1950, rheumatic fever from 'strep' infections was still an important cause of damage to heart valves. In particular, streptococcal A substrains cause high incidence of endocarditis and mitral valve scarring (Bispo, 2000; Stollerman, 1997; Wilson, 1940). Rheumatic fever with mitral damage is life-shortening (Jones, 1956). In the 1930s, for example, few survivors of childhood infections lived to age 40, and most died within 15 years of infection (Wilson, 1940, p. 272). Rheumatic heart disease has become rarer in developed countries from public health improvements and, then after 1950, the availability of antibiotics. However, heart valves without rheumatic disease often harbor a diverse bacterial flora (see below).

Eileen Crimmins and I hypothesize that historical and modern levels of early infection are major determinants of adult vascular disease (Crimmins and Finch, 2006a,b; Finch and Crimmins, 2004, 2005). More generally, historical and modern populations also show associations of infections with later mortality. In some rural parishes of 17th century Sweden, high early infectious mortality was followed by high late life mortality among survivors (Bengtsson and Lindstrom, 2000; Bengtsson and Lindstrom, 2003). Among U.S. Civil War veterans, infectious disease in early adulthood has been associated with heart and respiratory problems after age 50 (Costa, 2000). Cardiovascular disease was twice as prevalent among older Army veterans born before 1845 compared to veterans born in the early 20th century (Fogel and Costa 1997; Fogel, 2004). In Norway 1896–1925, infant mortality, which is a proxy for exposure to infections, correlated strongly with arteriosclerotic deaths 40–69 years later (Forsdahl, 1977) (Fig. 2.1).

In the United States 1961–1971, adult cardiovascular disease is also associated with birth cohort levels of infant diarrhea and enteritis (Buck and Simpson, 1982). Other examples are discussed in Crimmins and Finch (2006a). Considered over most of the 20th century, the associations of prior infections on later mortality may explain up to nearly 25% of the decline of both morbid and mortal conditions at later ages (Costa, 2000). Relationships of early and later age mortality in birth cohorts are developed further below.

2.2.2. Modern Serologic Associations

Stepping forward, we have access to individual histories of infections through persistent antibodies. Serologic associations with cardiovascular disease were first noted in 1987 for cytomegalovirus (CMV) (Adam et al, 1987), soon followed by *Chlamydia*[1] *pneumoniae* in 1988 (Saikku et al, 1988). Other associations

---

[1]Chlamidophila is the official genus name.

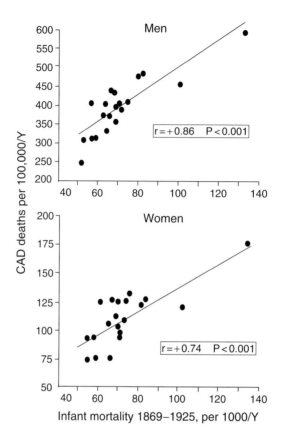

FIGURE 2.1 Past infections and cardiovascular disease in historical Norway. Infant mortality, a proxy for exposure to infections (Finch and Crimmins, 2004, 2005; Crimmins and Finch, 2006a, b), correlated strongly with arteriosclerotic deaths 40–69 years later in Norway 1869–1925. These correlations were slightly stronger for men than women. (Redrawn from Forsdahl, 1977.)

include the ubiquitous *Helicobacter pylori* and *Mycoplasma pneumoniae*; and cytomegalovirus (CMV), hepatitis virus A and -C viruses (HAV, HCV), and herpes simplex virus (HSV-1 and -2) (Belland et al, 2004; Campbell and Kou, 2004; Stassen et al, 2006; Vassalle et al, 2004). Cerebrovascular disease is also associated with *C. pneumoniae* and *H. pylori* (CagA strains) (Lindsberg and Grau, 2003). Carotid thickness correlates with antibodies to *E. coli* endotoxin (LPS) (Xu, 2000), while anti-LPS antibodies correlate with antibodies to oxidized LDL (Mayr et al, 2006). The list grows.

In the AtheroGene Study (Mainz and Paris), cardiovascular mortality and coronary stenosis were 2–3-fold higher in patients seropositive for ≥ 4 pathogens, relative to those with 0 to 3 seropositivities, with the highest odds ratios for *C. pneumoniae* and *M. pneumoniae* (Espinola-Klein et al, 2002a, b; Georges, 2003) (Fig. 2.2A, B). Carotid and femoral artery thickening (IMT) are greater in individuals with chronic infections who also carry proinflammatory alleles of IL-6, IL-1 receptors, and the endotoxin receptor CD-14 (Bruneck Study, northern Italy) (Markus et al, 2006). Blood levels of C-reactive protein (CRP), an inflammatory protein and strong risk indicator of coronary artery disease (Section 1.5, Fig. 1.16B), may also correlate with the number of different seropositivities (Georges et al, 2003; Zhu et al, 2000) (Fig. 2.2C). However, others did not find these serological associations with CRP elevations (Epstein et al, 2000; Lindsberg and Grau, 2003). This is not surprising, because seropositivity often persists long after an infection has subsided and transient elevations of CRP have subsided. Over the life span, the majority of adults become seropositive for *C. pneumoniae* and CMV (Almanzar et al, 2005; Miyashita et al, 2002).

Epidemiological associations of infections and vascular disease are increasingly supported by clinical studies and animal models (Campbell and Kuo, 2003; Coughlin and Camerer, 2003; Libby, 2003; Liuba et al, 2003). *C. pneumoniae* illustrates several key issues. This gram-negative bacterial pathogen grows only as an intracellular parasite. Infections typically begin in lungs and may propagate systemically to the vasculature by circulating macrophages. Infections are ubiquitous and reinfections very common (Belland et al, 2004; Campbell and Kuo, 2004; Grayston, 2000). *C. pneumoniae* is notorious for its broad cell targets, including endothelia, macrophages, and smooth muscle cells of atheromas. It resists antibiotics, which can suppress normal replication without eradicating its effects. Dead *C. pneumoniae* still activate the transcription factor NF-κB in endothelial cells, which could promote atherogenesis without active infection (Baer et al, 2003). *C. pneumoniae* are detected in the majority of atheromas by immunological, genomic, or ultrastructural criteria, but not in healthy arteries (Muhlestein et al, 1996; Shor et al, 1998; Shor, 2001). Heart valves tend to have more *C. pneumoniae* and other pathogens, in diseased than normal hearts (Juvonen et al, 1998; Nilsson et al, 2005; Nystrom-Rosander et al, 2003). Live *C. pneumoniae* was cultured from vascular tissues from some cardiac patients (Belland et al, 2004; Campbell and Kuo, 2004). T cells cultured from atherosclerotic carotids were immunopositive in 40% of 17 patients (Mosorin, 2000). These individual variations may arise from successful elimination of the pathogen by the host. The suppression of pathogen growth by antibiotics or cell stress may also add to these variations (Belland et al, 2004; Campbell and Kuo, 2004). However, assay criteria for *C. pneumoniae* are not well standardized and detectability varies from 0–100% (Kalayoglu et al, 2002; Peeling et al, 2000). The high genetic diversity of *C. pneumoniae* (Belland et al, 2004) may also contribute to variability. Some argue that *C. pneumoniae* and *H. pylori* in vascular lesions are an epiphenomenon because damaged or necrotic tissues, such as found in vascular plaques, are vulnerable to superinfections (Black, 2003). It is hard to prove the causal role of infections in atherogenesis because of their earthly ubiquity—everyone experiences infections (Belland et al, 2004; Campbell and Kou, 2004).

Peripheral arteries also show effects of infections. Children with acute respiratory infections had impaired regulation of the brachial artery endothelium, by the flow-mediated vasodilation test (Avon Longitudinal Study of Parents and Children, or ALSPAC Study, Fig. 2.3). The effects of infection may have persisted for a year in some individuals (the statistical significance was $P<0.06$) (Charakida et al, 2005). Longitudinal follow-up continues. Studies of children are valuable because seropositivities are less frequent than in adults.

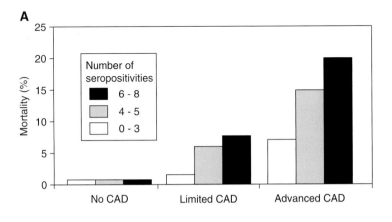

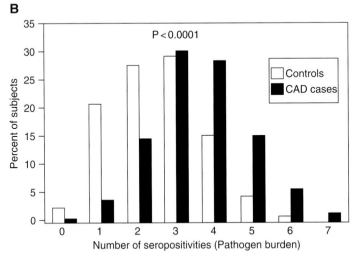

FIGURE 2.2 For legend see page 119.

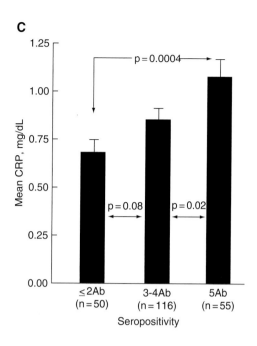

FIGURE 2.2 Past infections and cardiovascular disease. A. Cardiovascular mortality was 2–3-fold higher in patients seropositive for ≥4 pathogens, relative to those with 0 to 3 seropositivities. Pathogens with seropositive record of past or latent infection detected included *C. pneumoniae*, CMV, EBV, *H. influenzae*, *H. pylori*, and HSV-1, -2. University Clinic Mainz; 1168 Ss. (Redrawn from Espinola-Klein et al, 2002.) B. CAD cases have a higher number of seropositivities: *C. pneumoniae*, CMV, *H. pylori*, HSV-1. (Redrawn from Georges et al, 2003.) C. Plasma C-reactive protein (CRP) varies in proportion to the number of different seropositivities. (Redrawn from Zhu et al, 2000).

Antibiotics give another test of the infection hypothesis. The large WIZARD trial [weekly intervention with zithromax (azithromycin) for atherosclerosis and its related disorders] is so far inconclusive (Dunne, 2000). Experimental design is difficult, because the treatments may be most effective early during infections (de Kruif et al, 2005). Other long-term studies include the Azithromycin and Coronary Events (ACES) (Belland et al, 2004) and the Pravastatin or Atorvastatin Evaluation and Infection Therapy (PROVE-IT) (Campbell and Kuo, 2004). The first placebo-controlled, double-blind, randomized clinical trial of antibiotics on *C. pneumoniae* in vascular tissue was inconclusive (Berg et al, 2005). Although 81% of cardiac bypass patients were seropositive, *C. pneumoniae* DNA was not present in plaques of patients with advanced CAD; antibiotic treatment did not alter seropositivity.

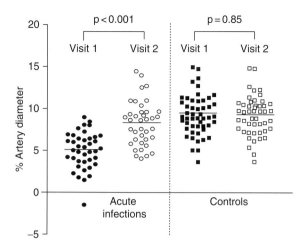

FIGURE 2.3 Childhood infections alter arterial endothelial responsiveness. Avon Longitudinal Study of Parents and Children (ALSPAC; population-based study, Bristol UK region) evaluates environmental and genetic influences on health and development. Vascular endothelial function was evaluated sonographically by flow-mediated constriction (FMD) of the brachial artery diameter. Six hundred Ss aged 10 years were assessed for health; exclusions asthma and chronic infections, or use of antibiotics or anti-inflammatory drugs; acute infections (AI) were 93% upper respiratory. About 1 year later, there was a reassessment of 50 controls without infection; of 40, prior with acute infection, but without infection since first visit. The AI group FMD response was slightly lower on the second visit (P < 0.06), suggesting a subgroup with persistent endothelial damage. (Redrawn from Charakida et al, 2005.)

Animal models show that infections may have greater synergy with arterial disease when lipids are elevated, as is common during infections (Section 1.4). In rodents, rabbits, and pigs, *C. pneumoniae* accelerated atherogenesis, but only when the models were made hyperlipidemic (Belland et al, 2004, de Kruif et al, 2005; Liuba et al, 2003a,b,c). Chronic endotoxin also required hyperlipidemia to accelerate atherogenesis (Engelmann et al, 2006). The apoE-knockout (−/−) mouse is an important model, with greatly elevated cholesterol on non-atherogenic diets that promote progressive arterial lesions not found in normal mice. ApoE knockouts develop aortic plaques by 4 months, followed by vascular rigidity and aneurysms (Wang, 2005, Wouters et al, 2005). Moreover, the lipidemia-induced lesions depend on pathogen-signaling pathways via Toll-like receptors (TLRs) linked to MyD88, an adaptor that activates kinases (Laberge et al, 2005) (Chapter 5, Fig. 5.4). The double apoE and MyD88 knockout mouse had much small aortic lesions, with fewer macrophages and lower chemokines In apoE knockouts,

C. pneumoniae caused rapid vascular endothelial damage (aortic contractility, 2–6 weeks after infection) (Liuba et al, 2000). Subsequently, the arterial wall thickens with increased ROS production. The convergence of hyperlipidemia in infection and arterial disease through pathogen-activated pathways suggests that atherogenesis is bystander outcome of the indispensable host defense mechanisms.

Future case control studies with longitudinal follow-up may be more conclusive. We may learn how to quantify effects of infections on vascular damage by the intensity and duration. There could be a threshold for acute infections of sufficient brevity that do not cause enduring damage. We may anticipate some dose-duration relationships in chronic subclinical infections and arterial disease that are like the 'pack-years of smoking' in relation to carotid thickening, as discussed below (Fig. 2.6) and lung cancer. The pathogen burden is indicated by the scaling of vascular event risk to the number of seropositivities, discussed above (Espinola-Klein, 2002; Georges et al, 2003; Zhu et al, 2000). Both research groups use similar terminology, 'pathologic burden' (Zhu et al, 2000) and 'infectious burden' (Espinola-Klein, 2002), to represent seropositivities, which does not inform on whether infections are active. I suggest the alternative term *inflammatory burden* to more comprehensively represent these long-term inflammatory influences. Besides infections, the inflammatory burden includes non-infectious inflammogens such as smoke and other aerosols and dietary AGEs produced during cooking (see below). These complexities are well expressed by Stephen Epstein and colleagues:

> Given that atherosclerosis is a multifactorial disease, Koch's postulates to establish causality will never be satisfied. These postulates . . . assume a single pathogen, require that all patients with the disease must have evidence of being infected with the casual agent and that all the infected develop the disease. In contrast . . . infectious agents are . . . neither necessary nor sufficient for [vascular] disease development . . . proof of causality can be achieved only in terms of probability rather than as certainty. (Epstein et al, 1999, p. e26).

2.3. INFECTIONS FROM THE CENTRAL TUBE: METCHNIKOFF REVISITED

A century ago, Metchnikoff suggested that autointoxication by microbial toxins in the intestinal flora causes chronic poisoning of body cells and premature death (Metchnikoff, 1901, Podolsky, 1998). Recent evidence implicates bacterial leakage from periodontal disease in vascular disease. Moreover, I suggest the lower gut should also be considered in bacterial leakage, which could be a factor in elevated circulating acute phase proteins during aging.

2.3.1. Humans: Leakage from Periodontal Disease and Possibly the Lower Intestine

The mouth normally harbors several hundred bacterial species, mostly as very high density biofilms on teeth. About 10 species of gram-negative anaerobes may be the main pathogens in vascular disease, particularly *Porphyromonas gingivalis* and *Actinobacillus actinomycetemcomitans* (Asikainen and Alaluusua, 1993). Their subgingival location is less accessible to antibiotics. We are unavoidably exposed to this high-density flora: Even tooth brushing and flossing can cause transient bacteremia (Carroll and Sebor, 1980, Slots, 2003).

The evidence for oral-vascular disease relationships is controversial. In the Atherosclerosis Risk in Communities Study (ARIC Study), severe periodontal disease was associated with thick carotid walls (Fig. 2.4); the effect was greater in men than women (Odds ratio, OR 1.46, range 1.18–1.81) (Beck et al, 2001, 2005; Beck and Offenbacher, 2001). In ARIC (Slade et al, 2003) and other studies, serum CRP, fibrinogen, and IL-6 tended to be elevated in individuals with periodontitis who were otherwise healthy (Chun et al, 2005; D'Aiuto et al, 2004; Schwahn et al, 2004). In atheromas from vascular surgery, nearly half contained DNA from at least one periodontal pathogen (Haraszthy et al, 2000).

The periodontitis-vascular association is experimentally supported. In rabbits, periodontitis induced by *P. gingivalis* increased aortic lipid deposits in proportion to the severity of periodontitis (Jain et al, 2003). *P. gingivalis* generally forms biofilms beneath the gingiva and can invade oral epithelia and vascular endothelial cells. Activation of Toll receptors by *P. gingivalis is associated with increased* IL-1, TNFα, prostaglandin E$_2$, and leukocyte adhesion molecules (ICAM-1, VCAM-1) (Choi et al, 2005a; Chun et al, 2005; Hajishengallis et al, 2004).

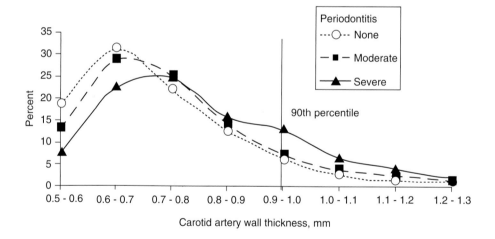

FIGURE 2.4 Severe periodontal disease is associated with increased carotid artery wall thickness. Atherosclerosis Risk in Communities Study (ARIC Study, Visit 4, 6017 subjects). Means of wall thickness: no disease, 0.74 mm; moderate, 0.77 mm; severe, 0.82 mm; most of the statistical difference was in the subgroup with thickness >1mm. (Beck et al, 2001).

The associations with vascular disease are considered circumstantial (see the analysis of 14 studies) (Kolltveit and Eriksen, 2001), because few studies measured infections by serology or bioassay (Danesh et al, 1999); smoking adds other confounds (Hujoel et al, 2000). In ARIC, 68% were seropositive for one or more of 17 bacterial species associated with periodontal disease (Beck et al, 2005). High antibody titers to ≥1 oral pathogen were associated with higher prevalence of cardiovascular disease, particularly in never-smokers. However, there were no associations of periodontal disease with prevalent cardiovascular disease after adjusting for covariates. Prospective studies should include the individual histories of oral health, smoking, and other lifestyle covariates; multiple time samples of serology for the spectrum of major pathogens; and screening for genetic polymorphisms in IL-1α and IL-1β, which are associated with risk of periodontal disease (Lopez et al, 2005).

Diverse microbial 'communities' reside in the mouth and lower intestine. The intermediate gut is normally quite sterile, stomach through jejunum (Lin, 2004). The gut epithelial cells in the crypts of Lieberkuhn have tight junctions (zona occludens) that maintain characteristic epithelial cell polarity as part of the barrier to the body cavity and prevent leakage of gut contents (Mullin et al, 2005). Cholera and other pathogenic bacteria alter this vital tight junction barrier. In aging rats, tight junctions become leakier, as assayed by transcolonic epithelial permeability; these aging effects were greater on high fat diets (Mullin et al, 2002) (Fig. 2.5A). The aging gut may have increased leakage, allowing entry of endotoxins into the circulation. As a precedent, CRP elevations are common in inflammatory bowel disease (Poullis et al, 2002). At some threshold, leakage of endotoxins could cause elevations of blood CRP and other acute phase proteins (Section 1.7).

The increase of colonic permeability with aging may be due to aberrant crypts (Mullin et al, 2002). Aberrant crypts and villi with cellular dysplasia and loss of epithelial cell polarity increase during aging in the gut of rodents (Mullin et al, 2002) (Fig. 2.5B) and humans (Finch and Kirkwood, 2000, pp. 132–137; Shpitz et al, 1998; Takayama et al, 1998). Stem cell depletion may contribute to these aging changes. Epithelial cells in the crypts of Lieberkuhn proliferate throughout life and are extruded at the tips of the intestinal villi. The crypt stem cells (Potten et al, 2001; Potten et al, 2003) apparently become stochastically depleted during aging (Finch and Kirkwood, 2000, pp. 132–137; Martin, 1998). Radiation and some carcinogens accelerate the loss of stem cells and increase the incidence of abnormal crypts (Magnuson et al, 2000; Martin, 1998). Alternately, TNFα can alter tight-junction permeability via NF-κB activation, as implicated in Crohn's disease and other chronic intestinal inflammations. Mucosal layer breakdown is not necessary for inflammatory transients to cause gut leakage of potential significance to arterial disease (Lin, 2004).

Obesity and diabetes predispose to chronic low-grade infections, which are discussed with effects of diet restriction in Section 3.2.4. The burden of infections (HSV-1 and -2, enteroviruses) shows correlations with insulin resistance particularly in those with *C. pneumoniae* seropositivity. Thus, metabolic adaptive responses to low-grade infections could be atherogenic by altering insulin sensitivity

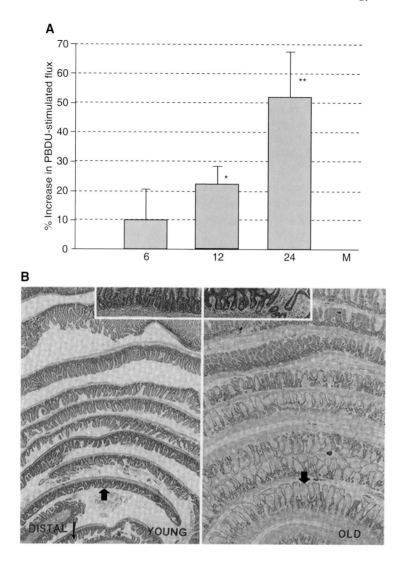

FIGURE 2.5 Changes in the aging gut. A. Aging increases colonic permeability in male F344 rats. Transepithelial flux of mannitol was induced by phorbol ester (PBDU) in the distal colon *in vitro*. (Redrawn from Mullin et al, 2002) B. Aberrant intestinal villi in aging mouse: male C57/BL; 5 vs. 30 m. Crypts of Lieberkuhn are 20% decreased; villi are enlarged, with cell loss in the lamina propria. These changes emerge after 12 m and progress further with aging. Directly from (Martin and Kirkwood, 1998).

(Continues)

C   Young   Old

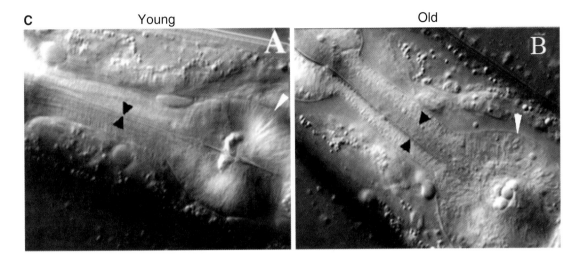

FIGURE 2.5 (continued) C. Gut abnormalities in old worms (*C. elegans*).The width of the pharynx increases from packed wads of bacteria (black arrowheads), which shows cellular deterioration (white arrowheads). (Directly from Garigan et al, 2002.)

(Fernandez-Real, 2006). Moreover, the sensitivity to low-grade infections may be associated with inflammatory gene variants.

2.3.2. Worms and Flies as Models for Human Intestinal Microbial Intrusion

In the worm model of aging, bacterial autotoxicity may be a proximal cause of death during aging (Garigan et al, 2002; Gems and Riddle, 2000; Lithgow, 2003; Mallo et al, 2002) (also discussed in Section 5.2). Wads of bacteria pack the pharynx in aging worms and there is bacterial overgrowth in the pharynx and intestine (Garigan et al, 2002) (Fig. 2.5C)—". . . the final coup de grace is bacterial invasion" (Lithgow, 2003, p. 16). The constipation of aging worms may model aspects of human inflammatory bowel syndrome, in which bacterial overgrowth into the normally sterile small intestine causes chronic inflammation (Lin, 2004; Pimentel et al, 2000). Several long-lived worm mutant resist pathogenic bacteria (Garsin et al, 2003) (Section 5.5.2).

In the standard culture conditions, worms are fed on live *E. coli* strain OP50 (Brenner, 1974). However *E. coli* OP50 may not be the optimum food because life spans may be longer and constipation lessened on diets of some species of yeast (Mylonakis et al, 2002a) or diets of the soil bacterium *Bacillus subtilis*, which may be more natural foods (Garsin et al, 2003). The concern that live *E. coli*

OP50 is mildly pathogenic is now 40 years old (Croll and Yarwood, 1977; De Cuyper and Vanfleteren, 1982; Hansen et al, 1964): "The longer life span in the absence of bacteria suggests a possible toxicity of bacterial products in the monoxenic cultures" (Hansen and Yarwood, 1964, p. 629).

Elimination of live bacteria from the diet increases life spans. A diet of UV-killed bacteria delayed the pharyngeal pack-up of bacteria (Garigan et al, 2002) and increased life spans up to 55%, without loss of fecundity (Gems and Riddle, 2000). Moreover, axenic growth on sterile media supplemented with nutrients doubled the life span (Croll et al, 1977; De Cuyper and Vanfleteren, 1982; Houthoofd et al, 2002; Houthoofd et al, 2004). The axenic cultures maintained the rate of pharyngeal pumping to later ages and increased stress resistance, but at the expense of lower fecundity (Croll et al, 1977; Houthoofd et al, 2002). Switching from axenic to bacterial media after larval maturation eliminated the longevity benefit; conversely, raising larvae on bacteria followed by brief antibiotic treatment before transfer to axenic media increased longevity almost as much as growth on sterile media throughout life (De Cuyper and Vanfleteren, 1982). However, these benefits are due not only to the elimination of bacterial toxicity, because this axenic medium was deficient in ubiquinone, a micronutrient obtained from the bacterial diet (Jonassen et al, 2003; Larsen et al, 2002).

These findings raise uncomfortable questions about artifacts from standard lab conditions that are widespread in lab models. I argue that *all* of our experimental models adapted to the lab should be scrutinized for atypical outcomes of aging. Lab husbandry has eliminated most infections and provides a uniform quality *ad lib* diet rarely found over the life span in nature. Moreover, our highly inbred lab models were initially selected for early reproduction and high fecundity that may be atypical of the evolutionary background. These concerns will be discussed further in the next chapter in interpreting the obesity common in lab rodents.

Flies also show the importance of enteric microbes to aging. In *Drosophila melanogaster* antibiotics given later in life increased life span by 30% (Brummel et al, 2004). Cell changes in the aging fly gut are consistent with the leakage of gut bacteria later in life. Aging intestinal epithelial cells accumulate virus-like particles (Anton-Erxleben et al, 1983). In the aging housefly (*Musca domestica*), intestinal cells accumulate concretions (Sohal et al, 1977) and lipid inclusions (Sohal, 1981). Bacteria are seen in sick-looking flies (the insect body cavity is usually sterile) (Flyg et al, 1988). Recent data document the increased bacterial and fungal load of aging flies (Section 5.6.4). The extensive increase of antimicrobial genes during aging in flies (Section 1.8) is consistent with the increased pathogen load of aging flies, possibly from breakdown of the barriers from the gut and exoskeleton. Chapter 5 discusses these and other genetic influences on longevity through inflammation and stress resistance.

2.4. AEROSOLS AND DIETARY INFLAMMOGENS

Chronic inflammation is stimulated by intake of non-infectious inflammogens by inhalation and ingestion. These sources have received less attention than infectious pathogens in relation to arterial disease. Airborne inflammogens may be of looming importance to future life expectancy with the accelerating global increases of air particulates (Section 6.4).

2.4.1. Aerosols

Aerosols are characterized by size (*PM10,* <10 μ particle diameter) and composition (mineral, hydrocarbon, sulfur, endotoxin, etc.) and whether the aerosols carry infectious agents (viable vs. non-viable aerosols). Inflammatory responses independently of infectious agents are induced by airborne inflammogens: Among many examples are smoke from tobacco, fossil fuel, and biomass combustion; dust from agriculture; and endotoxins from feces in the many urban locations with poor sanitation and in livestock and poultry. These sources are pertinent to current aging and to historical improvements in public health (Fig. 1.1A).

Smoke is well recognized as a non-infectious ('non-viable') aerosol with major consequences to vascular health. Cigarette smoke strongly increases the risk of heart attacks. In the United States in 1990, 20% of deaths from cardiovascular disease are attributable to smoking (Centers for Disease Control and Prevention, 1993). Second-hand smoke is also strongly associated with coronary disease (Zhang and Smith, 2003; Zhu et al, 1997) and lung cancer (Section 2.4.2). Smoking increases the carotid wall thickness in men with dose-dependency (number of pack-years as an estimate of lifetime exposure) (Gariepy et al, 2000) (Fig. 2.6). The mechanisms include proatherogenic increases of oxidized LDL and acute phase proteins. In NHANES III, smokers were twice as likely than non-smokers to have very high CRP (>10 mg/L), with dose responses to the intensity and history of smoking (Bazzano et al, 2003). Second-hand smoke also increased serum CRP into the range of primary smokers and coronary risk in the ATTICA Study (Barnoya and Glantz, 2004; Panagiotakos et al, 2004). Men incur more adverse effects of smoking than women (Fig. 2.6) (Gariepy et al, 2000).

Other types of smoke cause chronic lung damage and inflammatory responses consistent with vascular diseases. Common sources of smoke are open combustion in fireplaces, furnaces, and factories, which diffuse into the breathing environment with adverse effects on the lungs (Singh and Davis, 2002). Until the mid-20th century, exposure to wood and coal smoke was almost unavoidable, and still is in many countries (Zhu et al, 1997). 'Hut lung,' or domestically acquired particulate lung disease, is associated with inhaled smoke particulates from burning coal, wood, or other fuels and wastes (Gold et al, 2000). Cardiovascular admissions to hospitals were associated with recent exposure to black smoke PM(10) in some studies, e.g., Edinburgh (Prescott et al, 1998).

Particulate air pollutants induce vascular endothelial damage (Sandhu et al, 2005; Schulz et al, 2005). Mortality gradients in vascular diseases followed indexes of ambient air pollution in residential zones; not surprisingly, higher income zones had the least exposure to pollution (Finkelstein et al, 2005). Animal models support this epidemiology. Particulate inhalants cause chronic lung damage with lung alveolar macrophage hyperplasia, fibrosis, and accelerated atherosclerosis,

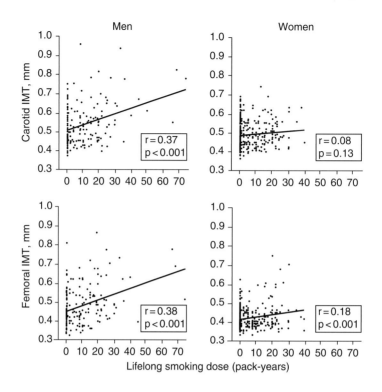

FIGURE 2.6 Smoking increases artery wall thickness in men more than women. Regressions of carotid and femoral intima-media thickness (IMT) on 'pack-years' (cumulative smoking dose). (Redrawn from Gariepy et al, 2000.)

e.g., rats exposed to wood smoke (Tesfaigzi et al, 2002) or to fly ash (Schreider et al, 1985). In hypercholesterolemic Watanabe rabbits, exposure to particulate aerosol increased the size of coronary atheromas in proportion to the number of lung macrophages that had phagocytosed particles (Suwa et al, 2002).

Dust from corn and grain also induces inflammatory responses (Buchan et al, 2002; Jagielo et al, 1996). Even lab animal bedding materials can contain appreciable bacterial endotoxin and (1– >3)-β-D-glucan from bacteria, molds, and plants. When inhaled, these common aerobiosols induce chronic inflammation (Ewaldsson et al, 2002). Humans also experience varying exposures to bioaerosols according to occupation and income, which can be a factor in the strong socio-demographic gradients in longevity. Bioaerosols are now a major concern of industrial safety (Burrell, 1994; Menetrez et al, 2001), but are still a hazard of agricultural workers. Workers in sewage plants and garbage collectors also suffer from inhalants that cause chronic systemic inflammation and elevated CRP (Rylander, 1977). Farm workers entering a swine confinement building had rapid elevations of blood complement C3 peaking at 1 h, followed by peak CRP at 2 h (Hoffmann et al, 2003). The smokers in this group had greater responses. Besides airborne live bacteria and fungi, non-viable bioaerosols may contain endotoxins of fecal origin. A specific role of LPS inhalation was shown by the induction of plasma CRP and other inflammatory responses with well-defined dose responses (Michel et al, 1997; Thorn, 2001).

The aerosol-vascular disease association is relevant to the historical increase of human longevity during the developments of public sanitation (Section 2.5) and to earlier phases of human evolution as population density increased and encountered increasing exposure to infections, inflammogens, and especially to domestic smoke for cooking and heating (Section 6.2). Genetic risk factors for resistance to domestic smoke and other types of air pollution may have evolved during this time. Curiously, European populations have a high prevalence of a null allele (GSTM1*0) of glutathione-S-transferase M1. GST makes the key anti-oxidant glutathione (Fig. 1.11) and belongs to a superfamily of xenobiotic detox-ifying enzymes with potential importance to human evolution (Section 6.4.2). The M1*0 homozygotes (equivalent to GSTM1 knockout) have impaired lung functions as children and a higher risk of asthma (Peden, 2005).

2.4.2. Food

Cooked foods have inflammogens produced by the chemistry of glyco-oxida-tion (Sandu et al, 2005). As discussed in Section 1.4.2, advanced glycation endproducts (AGE) and advanced lipid oxidation endproducts (ALEs) are produced endogenously from chemical reactions of glucose and other reduc-ing sugars with peptide lysine and arginine, which are proinflammatory, atherogenic, and carcinogenic (Kikugawa, 2004; Skog et al, 1998; Vlassara et al, 2002). This saga began in 1912 with Louis Maillard's discovery of chemical reactions between amino acids and glucose that lead to the loss of lysine and the formation of brownish condensation products (Finot, 2005; Maillard, 1912; Nursten, 2005). These reactions are the basis for browning of foods by broil-ing, or frying, which can increase AGE content 3- to 5-fold (Table 2.1) (Goldberg et al, 2004). AGEs and ALEs are also formed during food processing and storage. AGEs ingested from cooked foods are detected by immunoreac-tivity for the glycation adduct CML (N-carboxymethyl-lysine) (Table 2.1). In healthy adults, plasma CML strongly correlated with the dietary intake of AGE over a 3-fold range (Urribari et al, 2005).

The proinflammatory effects of dietary AGEs were directly shown in diet cross-over studies of diabetics (Vlassara et al, 2002). Nutritionally equivalent diets

TABLE 2.1 Advanced Glycation Endproduct (AGE) Content of Common Foods and Effects of Cooking

Food	CML, kU/g food
beef, boiled 1 hr	22
broiled, 15 min	60
tofu, raw	8
broiled	41
milk (pasteurized)	0.05
butter	265

CML (N-carboxymethyl-lysine, an AGE formed by heating); radioimmunoassay (Goldberg et al, 2004).

were prepared by different degrees of heating that yielded 5-fold differences in CML. Six weeks on the high AGE diet elevated inflammatory markers, serum C-reactive protein by 35%, and TNFα by 85% in association with 30% higher CML. Similarly, ingested dietary AGEs correlated with serum CML in renal failure patients (Uribarri et al, 2003).

Rodents show adverse effects of dietary AGEs. In a mouse model of both atherosclerosis and diabetes (apoE−/− genotype, with STZ-induced diabetes), the high-AGE diet increased aortic lesions, whereas a low-AGE diet decreased lesions below the level in the standard chow diet (Lin et al, 2003). The lesions of the high-AGE diet group had more arterial foam cells and receptors for AGE (RAGE). In another mouse model, 6 months on a high-AGE/high-fat diet induced type-2 diabetes, with impaired glucose regulation and insulin insensitivity (Sandu et al, 2005). The low-AGE/high-fat controls had normal glucose regulation despite similar adiposity. Plasma 8-isoprostane, a marker of lipid oxidation, was increased by the high-AGE diet. As a further scary example, a caramel component used for coloring beverages (2-acetyl-4-tetrahydroxybutylimidazole, THI) inhibits lymphocyte egress from the thymus by inhibiting the sphingosine 1-phosphate receptor (Schwab et al, 2005). Dietary AGE content may have unrecognized influences on rodent studies, because lab chows are typically heated during preparation.[2]

---

[2]Lab chows are typically heated for sterilization and pelleting; however, the details of temperature and duration are not easily known. One 'low-AGE' diet had 90% fewer AGEs than the 'high-AGE' diet, but this level still could be bioactive (Sandu et al, 2005). Casein, a widely used protein in chows, yields AGEs during industrial preparation (Gilani et al, 2005) (Jing and Kitts, 2002). Speculatively, low-grade, slow AGE side effects may lurk in diets containing casein and other milk-derived products as protein sources. The common nephropathy of aging F344 rats was greatly reduced by feeding on chows containing soy protein versus casein or lactalbumin (Shimokawa et al, 1993b), and median life span was 15% longer (Iwasaki et al, 1988).

These findings point to an expanding role of dietary AGEs in atherosclerosis and diabetes, and support their designation as glycotoxins' (Koschinsky et al, 1997; Vlassara, 2005). Vlassara hypothesizes that dietary AGEs, possibly synergizing with tobacco and other environmental inflammogens, sustain oxidative stress and chronic inflammation. The AGE receptors (RAGEs) that activate signaling pathways with PI3K (Section 1.3.3) may link dietary glycotoxins to longevity pathways that involve insulin/IGF-1 signaling (Fig. 1.3A) and that are also implicated in vascular disease (Fig 1.3B).

Besides their color, some Maillard products have definitive tastes and aromas (Schieberle, 2005). Caramel coloring and flavorings have been added to commercial foods and beverages for more than a century (Chappel and Howell, 1992; Nursten, 2005). These preferences may have been important in the development of cooking during the last half million years when early humans learned to control fire (Section 6.2). Cooking could have enhanced health by killing parasites and infectious organisms in animal tissues. Moreover, cooking increases the usability of many plants as foods by increasing digestibility and by inactivating toxins that are widely found, e.g., cassava and potatoes. (De Bry, 1994) suggests that early humans used Maillard products as olfactory cues to indicate when tubers with heat-sensitive toxins were sufficiently cooked. Nonetheless, evolution of the omnivorous human diet would have greatly increased exposure to toxins, implying the importance of detoxification mechanisms to enable these new foraging strategies (Sections 3.7 and 6.2.3).

Future increases of human longevity may come from better knowledge of these interactions and the mechanisms that remove ingested and endogenously produced AGEs. Dietary changes during human evolution may also have selected for genes that detoxified dietary AGEs, e.g., the recently discovered amadoriases ('AGE-breakers') (Monnier and Sell, 2006). Our ancestors ate meat increasingly by a million or more years ago, a major departure from the plant-based diets of the great apes, and, it is presumed, that of the shared human-chimpanzee ancestor (Section 6.2) (Finch and Stanford, 2004). The more recent use of fire for broiling or roasting meat would have increased AGE ingestion and selected for meat-adaptive genes.

2.5. INFECTIONS, INFLAMMATION, AND LIFE SPAN

2.5.1. Historical Human Populations

The recent longevity increases (Fig. 1.1A) also implicate the relationship of infection and inflammation to arterial disease (Finch and Crimmins, 2004, 2005; Crimmins and Finch, 2006a,b). Anonymous reviewers of these papers questioned the importance of vascular disease in deaths before the modern era. However, all evidence points to vascular disease as ancient and ubiquitous ". . . its pattern has always been the same regardless of race, diet, and the stresses of survival" (Magee, 1998, p. 663). The 5,300 year old Tyrolean "iceman" of the Bronze Age evidenced carotid artery calcification (Murphy et al, 2003), which is common in advanced atherosclerosis (Fig. 1.13) (Section 1.5.3.1) and is an independent risk factor of vascular mortality (Doherty et al, 2003; Sangiorgi et al, 1998). Two millennia later, Egyptian mummies of the 18th dynasty preserved calcified arteries and other vascular pathology (Ruffer, 1911). Most large arteries (16/24) in this sample met criteria for atherosclerosis, with half of these specimens showing vascular calcification (9/16). By the European Middle Ages, anatomists were describing arteriosclerosis as "natural to old age" (Long, 1933). Approaching the modern era, the records, scarce as they are, also show cardiovascular disease as a major cause of death in older adult ages. In 19th and mid-20th century England and Sweden, which had low life expectancy, cardiovascular disease was one of the two most important causes of mortality at the oldest ages (Preston et al, 1972; Preston, 1976). For cohorts born after the first decade of the 1800s, the deaths recognized as due to cardiovascular diseases exceed those attributed to infectious conditions. From the earliest date in Sweden, deaths from cardiovascular disease are two times higher than from infectious conditions for those 70–74. For the U.S. Civil War, Fogel and colleagues compared doctors' reports of heart disease from Union Army veterans aged 65 and over in 1910 versus veterans of the same age in 1983. Heart disease was nearly twice as prevalent in the U.S. Civil War Veterans (76% vs. 40%, age-adjusted) (Fogel, 2004, p. 31). William Osler's statement from 1892 still holds true today, "Longevity is a vascular question, which has been well expressed in the axiom that 'a man is as old as his arteries.' To a majority of men, death comes primarily or secondarily through this portal." (Osler, 1892, p. 664).

Moreover, early human ancestors were also likely to incur vascular pathology. Chimpanzees, our closest biological relative, also show extensive hypercholesterolemia, even on non-atherogenic diets, and die from heart attacks and strokes in captivity (Finch and Stanford, 2004; Steinetz et al, 1996) (Section 6.2). Crimmins and I provisionally conclude that vascular pathology during aging has been prevalent throughout human history and, quite possibly, throughout human pre-history as well (Crimmins and Finch, 2006a).

Crimmins and I are evaluating the role of infection and inflammation on later mortality in historical cohorts (Finch and Crimmins, 2004; Crimmins and Finch, 2006a, b). According to our 'cohort morbidity hypothesis,' exposure to infections early in life causes chronic infections that, in turn, promote vascular disease, leading to earlier mortality. Tuberculosis, *Helicobacter pylori*, *Chlamydia pneumoniae*, and other gastro-intestinal pathogens noted above are among many chronic infections that have recently diminished. The human environment in rural and urban areas alike was typically filthy by modern standards, with gross continuing exposure to human and animal feces. Running water was not available for convenient washing and bathing. Conditions gradually improved with national efforts in public hygiene even before the identification of infectious pathogens and development of immunization at the end of the 19th century. Besides the infectious environment, it was difficult to keep clothes clean and free of ectoparasites, especially before the availability of cheap cotton for clothing, which is easier to wash than wool or leather. Improved nutrition was another major factor in resistance to infectious conditions, due to agricultural improvements and the development of national transport systems of canal and rail (Fogel and Costa, 1997; Fogel, 2004; McKeown, 1976).

We chose to consider birth cohorts before the 20th century when infections were very common or rampant, but before tobacco smoking became popular. Smoking is a major inflammatory stimulus, as discussed above. Complete birth and death records are available from Sweden from 1751. Sweden also pioneered a national program of inoculation against small pox, begun in 1756, which attenuated these epidemics by the 1820s, decades ahead of other European countries (Skold, 2000). We also included England (1841–1899), France (1806–1899), and Switzerland (1871–1899). These early cohorts also did not benefit from antibiotics, which were not widely available before 1950. All the old age mortality examined occurred before 1973. In many countries, dramatic declines in mortality after 1970 are explained best by lifestyle and medical factors.

Initial life expectancy was low due to high early mortality characteristic of preindustrial societies, but increased considerably by 1899 (Fig. 2.7A). The historical trends for declining childhood mortality and old age mortality were remarkably parallel in Sweden, England, and France (Fig. 2.7B). As early age mortality declined, so did later age mortality in the survivors, seven decades later. The increased life expectancy at age 70 was clear in Sweden by 1850 (Fig. 2.7C). These findings support my early estimate that the steady historical increase in the adult age when mortality reaches 1% implies a slowing of aging processes (Finch, 1969, p.12).

These associations were tested with regression models for the relationships of temporal change in mortality at ages 70–74 with four childhood stages: infancy, <1 year; early childhood, 1–4; later childhood, 5–9; and adolescence, 10–14 years (Crimmins and Finch, 2006a). Infant mortality is largely attributed to infections. A key feature of this analysis is the comparison of birth cohort, followed throughout life, with the same ages in the corresponding periods. The results are consistent across these four countries: Most of the variance in old age mortality is explained by the early mortality in that birth cohort, 87–96%. The early and later mortality association of cohorts was much stronger than for periods. At a given year, the older adults in a population were born seven decades before the children and had experienced different environments that had a stronger effect on their mortality than in the current environment. Mortality of intermediate adult ages also did not predict old age mortality. The overall mortality curves shift downward quite uniformly as early mortality improves (Fig. 2.7A). Separate analysis of males and females also showed consistent associations in cohorts between early and later mortality

(Crimmins and Finch, 2006b). Many specific mechanisms can be considered in cohort morbidity through which recurrent exposure to acute infections or continiued chronic infections accelerates atherosclerosis as well as causing direct damage to heart valves and myocardium (focal lesions and diffuse fibrosis). Extensive immune activation through hyperantigenic stimulation of T cells

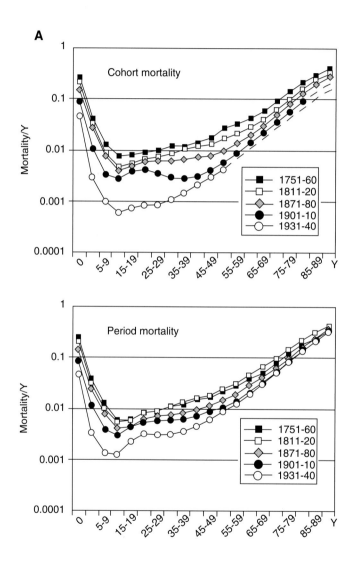

FIGURE 2.7 For legend see page 135.

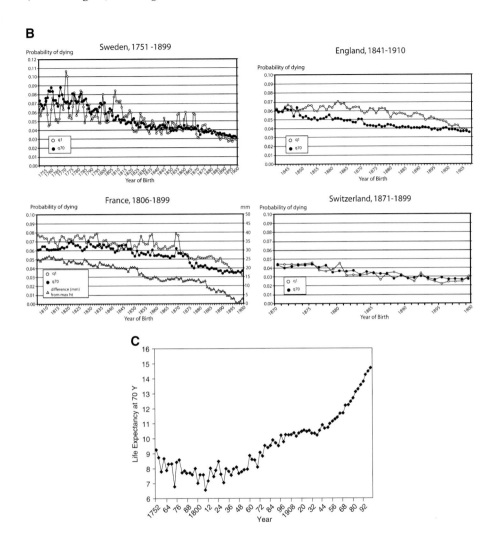

FIGURE 2.7 Swedish mortality profiles, based on national records begun in the mid-18th century. From Human Mortality Database (www.mortality.org/Public/main.html). A. Mortality across the life span by cohort and period, plotted on semi-log scale (Finch and Crimmins, 2004). B. Correlations of early and late age mortality by cohorts for Sweden (1751–1899) (*a*), France (1806–1899) (*b*), Switzerland (1871–1899) (*c*), and England (1841–1899) (*d*) with deviation from maximum cohort height at age 20–21 up to 1899 (measured in millimeters on right axis). (Crimmins and Finch, 2006a). C. Life expectancy at age 70 in Sweden (3-y moving average) showing increases by the mid-19th century, about 70 y after early age mortality had begun to decline (Finch and Crimmins, 2005).

could also have increased T cell participation in atheroma instability (Section 1.5).

Height was also examined because infections slow growth (Section 4.4). The level of early mortality strongly predicted adult height (Fig. 2.7B). In birth cohorts with high early mortality, the survivors were shorter as adults, which we attribute to the greater exposure to infections in childhood. Infections and inflammation cause the reallocation of metabolic resources and energy from growth (Fig. 1.2B), as discussed in detail in Chapter 4. There are also associations of inflammatory genes with fetal growth (TNFα-308 G/G is more prevalent in lower birthweights) (Casano-Sancho et al, 2006) (Section et al 4.10.1). These mechanisms may also account for the progressively decreasing size of adults after 50,000 years ago in human pre-history (Chapter 6, Fig. 6.7).

Our model of inflammation in the pathobiology of aging (Fig. 1.2A) also includes important links between maternal infections and inflammation to fetal and infant growth and inflammation. Influenza, malaria, and tuberculosis were common maternal inflammations until recently (Riley, 2001). Malaria and possibly other maternal infections can retard fetal growth and increase fetal cytokines (Moormann et al, 1999) (Section 4.5). Smaller babies may have lower resistance to environmental pathogens. These possibilities are not included in the Barker hypothesis of fetal origins that focused on maternal malnutrition as the main cause of the fetal retardation effect on later vascular disease (Barker, 2004), discussed at length in Chapter 4. These manifold effects of inflammation and infection on growth during childhood and on later arterial disease point to a potential unifying theory of human development and aging.

2.5.2. Longer Rodent Life Spans with Improved Husbandry

With intriguing parallels to the increasing human longevity discussed above, rodent life spans have nearly doubled in the past 50 y. Elimination of chronic infections through improved husbandry is a major factor. Additionally, arterial and myocardial disease may have been more severe in the early rodent colonies, as indicated for 19th century humans above.

Life span increases are best documented for mice of the C57BL/6J ('B6') strain, inbred since 1936 at the Jackson Laboratory (Bar Harbor, ME), a pioneering center of mouse genetics (Staats, 1985). B6 males had mean life spans of 18 m in 1948–1956 (Russell, 1966) that gradually increased to the present range of 26–30 m (Finch, 1972; Kunstyr and Leuenberger, 1975) (Fig. 2.9.A, B). Survival curves became increasingly 'rectangularized' and right-shifted: Sporadic deaths before 20 m decreased, while maximum longevity increased from 30 to 44 m (Finch, 1969; Tanaka et al, 2000; Turturro et al, 2002). These right-shifts of mortality indicate reduction of infections and match those of human populations as health improved (Fig. 1.1A). Unfortunately, the pathology of aging was not well documented for B6 mice during this transition. In modern colonies of B6 mice, the cumulative incidence of cardiomyopathy is about 40% by 24 m (Schriner et al,

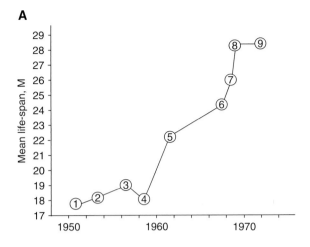

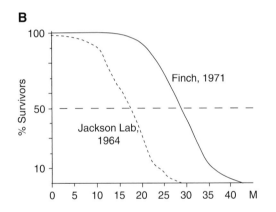

FIGURE 2.8 The life span of male C57BL/6 mice has increased progressively since 1957 as animal husbandry has improved. A. Mean life spans from sources cited by (Kunstyr and Leuenberger, 1975): (1) (Russell, 1957); (2) (Muhbock, 1959); (3) (Roderick and Storer, 1961); (4) (Storer, 1966); (5) (Russell, 1966); (6) (Grahn, 1970); (7) (Storer, 1971); (8) (Kunstyr and Leuenberger, 1975); (9) Finch, 1969 (my colony at Rockefeller University and Cornell University Medical School, NYC,1966–1971; sentinel cohort of retired male breeders). B. Survival curves of C57BL/6J male mice, from author's colony (Finch et al, 1969; Finch, 1972a) and the Jackson Laboratory (Russell, 1966).

2005; Turturro et al, 2002) (Section 1.2.2). Rat life spans also increased during the same period: In McCay's rat colony at Cornell University, where he conducted pioneering studies of nutrition and aging (Chapter 3), mean life span increased from 13 m in 1934 to 20 m in 1943 (McCay et al, 1943). Current lab rat life spans are 26–32 m.

Another striking example is the greatly improved longevity of dwarf mice with growth hormone deficiency. Thirty years ago, the Snell dwarf mouse was considered a model for accelerated aging because of short life span (< 6 m) and wizened appearance with gray hair, cataracts, and early onset tumors (Fabris et al, 1972) (Chapter 5, Table 5.3, footnote c). However, in the past decade with improved husbandry, dwarf mice have 'switched teams' to become models of slow aging, with life spans over 4 y and delayed onset of tumors. Gray hair is not common in contemporary dwarf mice and, in any case, is not a general trait of aging in B6 mice or other strains (Finch, 1973b). Husbandry improvements that enabled this remarkable transformation probably include reduced infections (see below) and better vivarium temperature control.

The general improvements in longevity across all genotypes of rodents in the past decades are not well understood. Even in the early days of laboratory rodent husbandry, some colonies were maintained well enough to achieve contemporary longevity. Slonaker's rats lived up to age 46 m (Slonaker, 1912) (Chapter 3, footnote 5), while Robertson's white mice averaged 25 m (Robertson and Ray, 1920) and the Berg-Simms colony females averaged 31 m in the 1960s (Chapter 1; footnote 3, this chapter), discussed below. I suggest that these early colonies were less inbred and closer to wild-types that were recently shown to have greater longevity (Harper et al, 2006a) (Chapter 3, Fig. 3.3).

Because the age-related pathology of aging mice at Jackson Labs before 1960 was not reported, we may look to the occasional reports on pathology from other early aging colonies.[3] This scattered literature describes conditions in aging rats that may surprise readers. In the 1960s, Wexler and colleagues documented in detail that repetitive mating can accelerate arterial degeneration in males as well as females (Wexler and Miller, 1958, 1960; Wexler and True, 1963; Wexler, 1964; Wexler, 1976). These studies employed standard rat stocks (Holtzman, Long-Evans, Sprague-Dawley, Wistar) fed on low fat (4%) diets. Lesions developed in coronary and carotid arteries in proportion to the breeding experience. Heart valve damage was common. ACTH injections

---

[3]Valuable and hard-to-find sources are *The Pathology of Laboratory Rats and Mice* (Cotchin and Roe, 1967) and *The Pathology of Laboratory Animals* (Ribelin and McCoy, 1965). Pursuit of this old literature was exasperating. Old books and journals are haphazardly discarded as useless because of their age and stored obscurely or misfiled.

or restraint stress also accelerated spontaneous atherosclerosis. Wexler and colleagues postulated that the repetitive mating caused severe stress. It is impossible to define the conditions in Wexler's colony that caused this level of stress during reproduction. Myocardial fibrosis was also associated with the severe coronary artery changes. In current clinical practice, myocardial fibrosis is associated with arrhythmias and sudden death (Siwik and Colucci, 2004; Zannad and Radauceanu, 2005).

Moreover, myocardial fibrosis with microscopic scarring was also common in several early rat colonies that may have contributed to premature death. "In older rats fibrosis may be so extensive that it is difficult to understand how the animals remain alive" (Fairweather, 1967, p. 227). Other examples include colonies with 60% prevalence of fibrosis (mild to severe fibrosis) by 20 m (Wilens and Sproul, 1938) and 100% by 20 m (Humphreys, 1957). In modern colonies, myocardial fibrosis is apparently uncommon and arises later (Bronson, 1990). Myocardial fibrosis is associated with inflammation and chronic stress (Holloszy and Smith, 1986), e.g., in rodent models, increased by TGF-β1 overexpression and decreased by TGF-β1 deficiency (Brooks et al, 2000; Siwik and Colucci, 2004). Diet-restricted humans have lower myocardial stiffness and plasma TGF-β1 (Section 3.3.2).

Arterial calcification was common in many early colonies but may be rarer today. In the Wilens-Sproul colony, calcification was noted in 46% in pulmonary arteries and 3% in coronary arteries and the aorta (Wilens and Sproul, 1938). In McCay's colony, aortic calcification occurred in 20% of *ad lib* fed, but was unexpectedly 3-fold higher (60%) with diet restriction (McCay et al, 1939). Others described 'bamboo stick aorta' with disintegration of the elastic layers and secondary calcification resembling Monckeberg's medial sclerosis (Fairweather, 1967; Mawdesley-Thomas, 1967; Wilgram, 1959). Sporadic arterial and myocardial calcification in aging rats was also reported by (Hummel, 1938; Wilgram, 1959). Moreover, calcification was associated with repetitive breeding in females (Gillman and Hathorn, 1959; Wexler, 1964). Current aging rodents have a low incidence of arterial calcification (<5%) (Bronson, 1990). Arterial calcification is associated with local nodules of *Chlamydia pneumoniae* in humans (Pierri et al, 2005) and in renal failure (Oh et al, 2002).

Coronary artery disease (CAD) was variable in the early colonies. The first report of spontaneous coronary disease on a normal (not fat-loaded) diet may have been from the Wilens-Sproul rat colony, in which 60% had some degree of coronary sclerosis by 24 m (Wilens and Sproul, 1938). Coronary artery stenosis to varying degrees was concurrent with myocardial fibrosis. In the Edinburgh colony, occlusive CAD with intimal plaques was present in 60% of rats by 17 m on a low-fat diet, causing complete blockage of a coronary vessel in some rats (Humphreys, 1957). In another colony, the incidence of coronary stenosis was about 15% (Wissler et al, 1954). CAD was particularly high in female 'retired breeders' (Wilgram and Ingle, 1959). However, in two other contemporary colonies, CAD was rare (Berg, 1967; Fairweather, 1967).

Three factors may be at work in the increased longevity of laboratory mice, ranked in reverse order of likeliness, in my opinion: genetics, diet, and infectious diseases. Improvements at the Jackson Laboratory occurred after 1959 when the Pedigreed Expansion Stock (begun in 1948) was moved to cleaner facilities (Russell, 1966). Longevity increases were not the result of intentional selection for longevity, although routine culling of sickly pups should lower overall mortality by reducing the pool of infections. The lack of correlation between life spans of parents and offspring in these early B6 colonies (Gunther Schlager, in Russell *op. cit.*) can be considered evidence against genetic drift (crosses of B6 and other strains clearly show inheritance of life span) (Jackson et al, 2002; Finch and Tanzi, 1997). Cardiomyopathies, nonetheless, may arise more frequently in aging rats maintained on diet restriction with exercise (McCarter et al, 1997) (Section 3.4.2). Dietary fat could be a factor because fatty diets can shorten life span (Chapter 3). The fats fed the first longevity group at Jackson are not known: The composition of the commercial diet was then a 'trade secret' (Elizabeth Russell, pers. comm.). In 1959, the Jackson Lab switched to Guilford Chow (11% fat, 19% protein), routinely given breeding females to enhance milk production. Chows with 4–5% fat are currently favored for aging studies (Finch et al, 1969; Turturro et al, 2002).

The major change from the 1940s to the 1970s at Jackson and elsewhere was reduction of chronic infections through improved animal and human hygiene. Some reported deaths from epidemic infections as merely 'accidental' (Robertson and Ray, 1920). Until the 1970s, laboratory colonies were often infected with microbial infections and skin parasites. Numerous pathogens were gradually minimized or eliminated, including bacteria (*Salmonella*, *Mycoplasma*); viruses [coronavirus; ectromelia (mousepox), mouse hepatitis virus, Sendai virus]; and ectoparasites (mites, pinworms) (Bell et al, 1964; Cotchin and Roe, 1967; Flynn et al, 1965; Miller and Nadon, 2000). Early colonies often had chronic respiratory disease (CRD) from endemic *Mycoplasma*[4] recognized by wheezy breathing and crusty noses. While minimizing infections and dietary fat could only increase longevity, we may never know the causes of the extensive myocardial and arterial lesions described above. The Wilens-Sproul colony rats had numerous abscesses ('suppurative lesions') in brain, ears, genitourinary tract, and lungs (Wilens and Sproul, 1938).

---

[4]Chronic respiratory disease (CRD), or catarrh (an ancient name still used), was endemic in rodent colonies up through the 1970s. CRD is characterized by extensive lymphocyte accumulations in the alveolar mucosa, increased mucus secretion and abscesses, and narrowing of the airways and their ultimate collapse (Nelson, 1940) (Nelson, 1963; 1967). I was fortunate to be tutored on CRD by John Nelson (see

(Continues)

Besides the Jackson Lab mice, another early benchmark rat colony was founded at Columbia University by Benjamin Berg and Henry Simms, which maintained advanced husbandry and exemplary documentation of age-related pathology (Fig. 1.5) (Berg, 1967; Simms and Berg, 1957; Simms and Berg, 1962). Although the Berg-Simms colony was begun in 1945, there was little respiratory disease (< 5% of rats). These rats were not selectively inbred, except to eliminate an 'eye anomaly' (Simms and Berg, 1957). Longevity in the Berg-Simms colony was in the range of modern colonies: females, median life span of 31 m and maximum of 34 m; males, median of 27 m and maximum of 29 m (Berg, 1976). Chronic lesions of aging approximated those of other rat strains in modern colonies (Bronson, 1990) and in the same age ranges: glomerulonephropathy arose before cardiomyopathy and abnormal growths (Simms and Berg, 1957; Simms and Berg, 1962), and arterial calcification was occasional. This health and longevity is remarkable for that time.

The current best practice in rodent husbandry is the 'specific-pathogen free' (SPF) colony, in which the pathogen load is regularly monitored with sentinel mice (Lindsey, 1998; Miller and Nadon, 2000). SPF status with minimal mycoplasmas and other pathogens increases fecundity and post-weaning growth and lowers spontaneous mortality (Bell et al, 1964). However, pathogen loads can fluctuate in SPF colonies with agents carried by humans and other adjacent lab animals (Taylor, 1974; Taylor and Doy, 1975). Infections are still embarrassingly common within SPF colonies at major research institutions (Jacoby and Lindsey, 1997). Although stricter barrier facilities can further reduce transmission of external infections, the expense and effort are prohibitive. Germ-free (axenic) animals lacking bacteria are problematic for aging studies: Their adaptive immunity is undeveloped, and their flaccid, grossly enlarged caecums develop fatal constrictions (volvulus) (Gordon et al, 1966).

Recent examples also show the importance of animal husbandry. Age-changes in skeletal muscle composition and function observed in 'dirty' colonies are negligible in aging rodents from SPF colonies of the same strains (Florini, 1989). Moreover, age-changes in rat liver protein oxidation (carbonyl content) disappeared in a subsequent cohort of the same strain of rats obtained 10 years later; these differences were confirmed with stored samples (Stadtman and Levine, 2003). Lastly, sporadic hippocampal neuron loss in aging may have

---

Preface). The most common agent of CRD is *Mycoplasma pulmonis*, as finally proven in 1971 with germ-free mice (Cassell, 1982; Lamb, 1975; Lindsey et al, 1985; Nelson, 1967; Slauson and Hahn, 1980). Other bacteria can cause CRD (Gay et al, 1972; Lamb, 1975). Mycoplasma are insidiously transmitted *in utero* and among cage mates; latent infections can erupt in apparently healthy SPF colonies (Lane-Petter et al, 1970), sometimes activated by Sendai virus, another sporadic scourge of aging colonies (Kay et al, 1979; Schoeb et al, 1985).

been common in early colonies (Landfield et al, 1977; Meaney et al, 1988) but is not obvious currently (Gallagher et al, 1996; Rasmussen et al, 1996). Variable stress and infections may have been involved. Moreover, early reports of neuron loss (reduced density of large neurons) could be interpreted as neuron atrophy (Fig. 1.7A). In many ways, the hygiene of lab animals parallels that of humans in modern health care: We can minimize childhood infections by immunization and hygiene, but we remain vulnerable to sporadic epidemics. *"La pest reste ici"* (J.P. Sartre, *The Plague*, 1947).

2.6. ARE INFECTIONS A CAUSE OF OBESITY?

Viral infections as causes of obesity are being discussed because of evidence that four viruses cause obesity in vertebrate models and serological associations of obesity with infections in humans with obesity and glucose intolerance. These findings should be considered provisional.

This story began with the finding that mice developed obesity when infected as weanlings with canine distemper virus (CDV, paramyxovirus closely related to measles) (Lyons et al, 1982; Lyons et al, 2002). CDV causes focal lesions of hypothalamic appetite centers with selective loss of leptin receptors, POMC and cat-echolaminergic neurons in the arcuate nucleus, and hyperplasia of adipocytes and pancreatic islets. Obesity is also induced in other animal models by infections with scrapie (prion disease), Bornavirus, the retrovirus (RAV-7), and AD-36 (human group D adenovirus) (Atkinson et al, 2005; Lyons et al, 2002). In a recent study impressive for its large subject pools, AD-36 seropositivity was 3-fold more prevalent in obese adults (30% than controls, 11%; 502 Ss); moreover, in 28 twin pairs discordant for AD-36, the seropositive individual was fatter than the co-twin (Atkinson et al, 2005). Curiously, AD-36 seropositive individuals had lower cholesterol and triglycerides. *In vitro*, AD-36 infections of adipocytes decreased increased glucose uptake and leptin secretion; these effects depend on transient expression of viral mRNA, but not viral DNA replication (Rathood et al, 2007). Unlike CDV, no hypothalamic lesions have been found in AD-36 infected mice (Dhurandhar et al, 2000). Another study of obese men who were otherwise healthy found inverse correlations between insulin sensitivity and seropositivity for common infections (HSV-1 and -2, enterovirus, and *C. pneumoniae*; AD-36 was not included in this panel) (Fernandez-Real, 2006).

If the 30% prevalence of AD-36 seropositivity in obesity is generally validated, viral infections may contribute as much to obesity as life style behaviors of eating and exercise, and moreover, may be a causal factor in these behaviors by their impact on the hypothalamus. However, responses to viral infections depend on many factors of host defense, including food intake and exercise (Chapter 3). Resolution of cause and effect in these associations is difficult because obesity and diabetes increase vulnerability to infections (Falagas and Kompoti, 2006) (Chapter 3). Nonetheless, these recent findings support the suggestion of (Lyons et al, 1982) that viral infections have roles in sporadic childhood and adult obesity. AD-36 infections that lead to obesity by causing hypothalamic lesions could be another, and milder example, of viruses that propagate by modifying behaviors, although how obesity could particularly favor AD-36 viral propagation is far from obvious.

2.7. INFLAMMATION, DEMENTIA, AND COGNITIVE DECLINE

2.7.1. Alzheimer Disease

Infections may also be causes or promoters of Alzheimer disease (AD). This new possibility is even less settled than associations of infections with vascular disease. As a first example, identical Swedish twins who are discordant for dementia may also show long-term outcomes of infections. The first twin to be affected was 3.6-fold more likely to have had periodontal disease (Gatz et al, 2006). Periodontal disease is also associated with infections that interact with arterial lesions (see above), but links of infections to AD are even more speculative.

The current (and incomplete) evidence on infections and AD centers on herpes viruses and *Chlamydia pneumoniae* (Mattson, 2004; Ringheim, 2004; Robinson et al, 2004; Wozniak et al, 2005). Causality is elusive because these infections are ubiquitous. Herpes virus infections occur widely. Postmortem, about 2/3 of all brains, normal and Alzheimer, have HSV-1 (Itzhaki, 1997). HSV-1 infections reside in some brain regions affected by AD (frontal lobe and hippocampus), as well as the trigeminal ganglion. At later ages, HSV-1 infections appear to be active by the presence of HSV-1 antibodies in the cerebrospinal fluid of about half AD and normal controls (Wozniak et al, 2005). Clearly, AD can arise in the absence of active HSV-1 infections! However, in one sample, the apoE4 allele and HSV-1 co-occurred 10-fold more frequently in AD brains than normal elderly (PCR assay). ApoE4 carriers may have a greater risk of neurode-generation from the activation of HSV-1 (Itzhaki et al, 1997). HSV-1 activation in the trigeminal ganglion causes shingles, which afflicts many elderly. A much rarer condition is herpes simplex encephalitis; survivors often have life-long cognitive impairments, possibly from neuronal apoptosis from HSV-1 (Aurelian, 2005). Other candidates are human herpes virus 6 (HHV6) seropositivity in Alzheimer (22% AD vs. 0% controls) (Wozniak et al, 2005) and CMV in vascular dementia (93% VascD vs. 34% controls) (Lin et al, 2001).

Some evidence suggests that vaccination against common infections may be protective. In the Canadian Study of Health and Aging, the risk of developing dementia during 5 years was lowered by vaccination for influenza (OR, 0.75), poliomyelitis (OR, 0.6), or diphtheria (OR, 0.41) (4392 Ss, aged $\geq$ 65) (Verreault et al, 2001). None of these infections is otherwise implicated in dementia. The protective effects of vaccination could be indirect by reduced vulnerability to other infections.

The case for *C. pneumoniae* as a casual factor in AD is less developed than for arterial disease. On one hand, *C. pneumoniae* persistently infects macrophages and can enter the brain, as in HIV (Stratton and Sriram, 2003). In a culture model, *C. pneumoniae* promoted monocyte migration across brain endothelia (MacIntyre et al, 2003). Infections of cultured human cerebral microvascular endothelial cells altered the levels of proteins associated with entry of this pathogen into the brain (increased β-catenin, N cadherin; decreased occludin) (MacIntyre et al, 2002). However, the evidence is mixed for the postmortem detection of infections. One study detected *C. pneumoniae* in cerebral vessels and glia in more Alzheimer brains than controls (Balin et al, 1998; MacIntyre et al, 2003). However, subsequent studies could not detect *C. pneumoniae* DNAs even in these same brains (Gieffers et al, 2000; Nochlin et al, 1999; Ring and Lyons, 2000). Vascular dementia studies were also mixed: positive association (Yamamoto et al, 2005) versus no association (Chan Carusone et al, 2004; Wozniak et al, 2003). Antibiotic treatment of AD patients with doxycycline and rifampin did not alter seropositivity for *C. pneumoniae* but, unexpectedly, slowed early cognitive declines (Loeb, 2004).

C. pneumoniae isolated from AD brains caused rapid formation of amyloid plaques in a normal mouse (BALB/c) (Little et al, 2004), which, like other 'wild-type' mice, never develops plaques during normal aging. Aβ1-42 containing plaques increased during the three months after infection, and a subset of plaques had fibrillar amyloid. Activated astrocytes around the plaques and distant from plaques suggest general inflammatory responses. Neuronal perikarya also had increased Aβ1-42, an early Alzheimer change (Section 1.6.3). The formation of fibrillar Aβ is puzzling because the mouse Aβ1-42 protein differs from the human in three substitutions that reduce aggregation (Section 1.6.). Nonetheless, mice overexpressing TGF-β1 (an inflammatory factor upregulated in Alzheimer brains) slowly developed fibrillar Aβ deposits around cortical microvessels; these deposits were preceded by thickening of the basement membrane. These changes are absent during aging in wild-type mice (Wyss-Coray et al, 2000).

Transgenic AD mice also show acceleration by systemic inflammation from i.p. injections of the endotoxin LPS (Godbout et al, 2005; Konsman et al, 2004; Scott et al, 2004). In the triple transgenic mouse model of AD, which has both amyloid plaques and neurofibrillary degeneration (Section 1.6), LPS caused earlier hyperphosphorylation of neuronal tau but, contrary to expectations, did not alter amyloid deposits (Kitazawa et al, 2005). In other AD transgenics, LPS induces APP and Aβ in neurons of the cerebral cortex and hippocampus, which are AD brain regions (Sheng et al, 2003). Microglial activation correlated strongly with neuronal APP and Aβ.

Aging mice had greater inflammatory responses and more prolonged 'sickness behaviors' in response to LPS (Godbout et al, 2005). The effects of aging on responses to LPS were not examined by these transgenic studies, which used relatively young mice. In stroke models, LPS pretreatment increases subsequent brain damage from cerebral artery blockade (Becker et al, 2005). Moreover, blood CRP is also elevated by LPS (Section 1.2) and elevated peripheral CRP increased damage from stroke in rats (Gill et al, 2004). Thus, in populations with high levels of infection and inflammation, stroke may cause greater brain damage and higher mortality. It is unclear if systemic endotoxins cross the blood-brain barrier. In rodents, systemic LPS binds to Toll-like receptors (TLRs) (Section 1.2 and Section 2.2.2 above) on cerebrovascular endothelia, which may increase vascular permeability to some sugars (Singh and Jiana, 2004).

Do environmental inflammogens promote AD? Smoking, while a strong risk factor in vascular disease (above), is not a clear risk factor for AD. While some case control studies indicate that smokers had lower risk of AD, recent cohort studies showed higher risk (Letenneur et al, 2004; Luchsinger and Mayeux, 2004; Sabbagh et al, 2005). Occupation and education are confounding variables. Smokers with AD may be younger at death but had the expected neuropathology (Sabbagh et al, 2005). Lastly, obesity and the metabolic syndrome are associated with chronic, low-grade inflammation (Section 1.7). As discussed in the next chapter, obesity and diabetes increase the risk of infections, while obese mice also have greater neuroinflammatory responses to LPS (Scott et al, 2004).

2.7.2. HIV, Dementia, and Amyloid

Dementia with memory loss is common in HIV sufferers with AIDS (acute immunodeficiency syndrome) (Selnes, 2005). The HIV virus enters the brain through macrophages but does not infect neurons with the production of further infectious virions. Diffuse damage and inflammation are found throughout the brain. Cases are often complex because of infections by other pathogens that cause diverse damage, e.g., demyelination (multifocal leukoencephalopathy) from the neurotropic JC virus (Del Valle and Pina-Oviedo, 2006).

Recently, diffuse amyloid Aβ deposits were found in the brains of AIDS patients (Green et al, 2005; Rempel and Pulliam, 2005) in proportion to the duration of infection (Fig. 2.10). The average age at death was 43 years, which is two decades before amyloid deposits become generally common. Nearly 50% of 150 brains from AIDS victims had diffuse Aβ deposits in the frontal cortex, most frequently near arteries (Green et al, 2005). Neuronal Aβ was also common, an early change in Alzheimer disease (Section 1.6.3). So far, AIDS brains have not shown two hallmarks of Alzheimer disease: compact neuritic plaques (Rempel and Pulliam, 2005) or neurofibrillary tangles (Green et al, 2005). These findings with well-characterized monoclonal antibodies confirm smaller studies of AIDS brains, which also included younger ages (Esiri et al, 1998; Izycka-Swieszewska et al, 2000; Rempel and Pulliam, 2005). Two mechanisms are noteworthy because of possible synergy: (I) induction of the amyloid precursor protein (APP) in neurons as an acute phase response during the brain inflammation of AIDS (Section 1.6.4) and (II) decreased degradation of Aβ by neprolysin, an endopeptidase enzymatically inhibited by Tat peptides from the HIV-encoded protein (Daily et al, 2006; Rempel and Pulliam, 2005). Both mechanisms should increase the production of oligomeric and solid Aβ. More information may be anticipated from HIV carriers who did not develop AIDS because of successful anti-viral therapy.

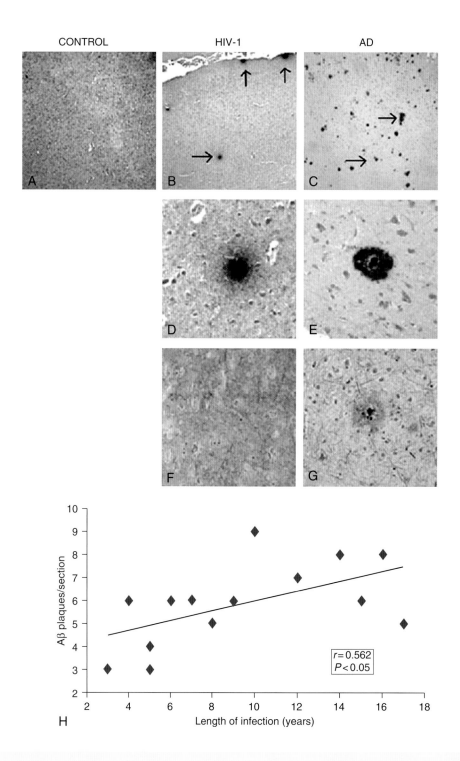

FIGURE 2.9 For legend see page 147.

2.7.3. Peripheral Amyloids

Tissue amyloid deposits (amyloidosis) are associated with chronic infections, e.g., tuberculosis (de Beer et al, 1984, Sipe, 1994, Urban et al, 1993). Peripheral tissue amyloid accumulations are also increased by endemic bacterial flora and common endemic pathogens in mice. Specific-pathogen free mice of several genotypes had no tissue amyloids (thioflavin-binding, not otherwise characterized) up through 28 m (mean life span), whereas 'conventional' (dirtier) colonies had amyloid deposits (Lipman et al, 1993). In mice transgenic for mutant human transthyretin (TTR), the amyloid deposits of the gut and the penetrance of the mutant TTR-induced peripheral neuropathy (polyneuropathy) were strongly influenced by the microbial flora (Noguchi et al, 2002). TTR amyloidosis was increased by exposure to enterobacteria and yeast, and decreased by anaerobic cocci. Social stress or social deprivation may also influence amyloidosis, e.g., more amyloid accumulated during aging when mice were housed in groups versus solitary (Lipman et al, 1993).

2.7.4. Inflammation and Cognitive Decline During 'Usual' Aging

Elevations of CRP and other acute phase proteins are common at later ages in populations (Fig. 1.23) and may be modest risk factors of cognitive declines. The MacArthur Study of Successful Aging followed high performing elderly for 7 years in a carefully controlled analysis (Weaver et al, 2002). Elderly in the highest IL-6 tertile had twice the risk of cognitive decline (Fig. 2.10A). This subgroup may be < 25% of all elderly with elevated IL-6.

Other studies show similar risks. In the Health, Aging, and Body Composition Study of well-functioning elderly (African American and Caucasian) (Yaffe et al, 2003), during 2 years, the top tertile of inflammatory markers showed a risk of cognitive declines in association with levels of CRP (OR 1.41) and IL-6 (OR, 1.34), but not for TNFα. During 5 years of observation, 23% had significant cognitive decline. Subgroups with both the metabolic syndrome (Chapter 1) and high inflammatory markers had 1.66-fold higher risk of cognitive impairment (Yaffe et al, 2004). In the Helsinki Aging Study over 5 years, the risk of cognitive decline increased with CRP > 5 mg/L (OR, 2.32) and diabetes (OR 2.18) (Tilvis et al, 2004).

FIGURE 2.9 AIDS induces Aβ-containing 'diffuse plaques' in frontal cortex sections with increasing frequency during the disease (Rempel and Pulliam, 2005). Average age 43 y (33–58). Immunostained with monoclonal 6E10, panels (a–e). Panel (a) HIV-1 seronegative control, age 46 y; (b, d, f) HIV-1 seropositive, 48 y; (c, e, g) Alzheimer disease, 84 y. Arrows, Aβ plaques in (b) and (c). Panels (d) and (e), Bielschowsky silver staining for neuritic plaques, negative for plaques from HIV-1 (f) and positive for plaques from Alzheimer (g). (h) Correlation of Aβ load versus duration of HIV-1 infection (r, 0.56, P <0.05).

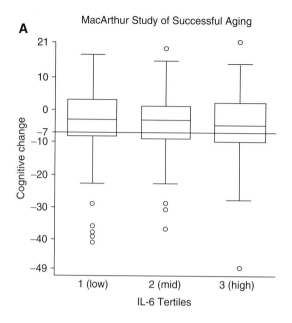

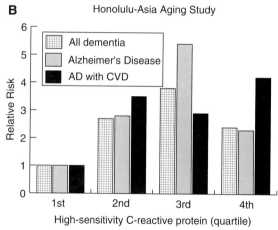

FIGURE 2.10 Elevations of acute phase proteins predict cognitive decline during aging. A. Plasma IL-6 elevations are modest predictors of cognitive decline in healthy elderly during observation over 7 y. (Redrawn from Weaver et al, 2002.) From the MacArthur Study of Successful Aging; 1,189 Ss, selected as a high-functioning sample of NHANES, age 70–79 y; assessed by 'Portable Mental Status Questionnaire' of delayed recall and the MacArthur Battery in the home for cognitive and physical evaluation. In the initial sample, IL-6 varied inversely with cognitive scores. In the 7-y follow-up,

(Continues)

However, the Longitudinal Aging Study (Amsterdam) found mixed associations: Cognitive decline was associated with elevated α_1-antichymotrypsin (ACT), but not with elevations of CRP or IL-6 (Dik et al, 2005). In the Maastricht Aging Study (MAAS) for those over 50 during 6 years, elevated CRP was associated with decline in only one cognitive test (word learning) (Teunissen et al, 2003). The InCHIANTI study of aging in Tuscan communities documents the age-related increase of IL-6 and other acute phase proteins (Cesari et al, 2004) (Fig. 1.21) and may soon report on cognition. Overall, the associations of acute phase elevations and cognitive declines are modest and may not generalize between populations. Some divergences may be due to different tests used. But, a larger question lurks.

Do the cognitive declines in "normal aging" represent incipient dementia from Alzheimer or cerebrovascular disease? Although these studies of normal aging excluded individuals with signs of dementia at entry, none was designed to identify the early, preclinical stages (CDR 0.5 or mild cognitive impairment) (Section 1.6.3). However, the Honolulu-Asia Aging Study of men clearly shows associations of blood CRP at middle age with Alzheimer and vascular dementia 25 years later (Schmidt et al, 2002). Relative to the lowest quartile, the top three quartiles showed 3-fold higher risk of Alzheimer and vascular dementias 25 years later (Fig. 2.10B). The risks did not scale smoothly with CRP levels, but are highly significant for each of the top three quartiles: for Alzheimer, for vascular dementia, and for mixed cases. These associations were independent of cardiovascular disease in this sample, which may represent selective mortality. However, InCHIANTI attributed most of the elevations of CRP and other acute phase proteins to cardiovascular disease (Cesari et al, 2004). Seropositivity to *C. pneumoniae* was prevalent among the elderly and correlated with IL-6 and TNFα (Blanc et al, 2004). As noted in Section 1.5.4, vascular and Alzheimer disease share many risk factors including elevated acute phase proteins, elevated cholesterol, and hypertension.

FIGURE 2.10 (continued) cognitive scores decreased in 33.6%. The change in cognitive score (vertical axis) over 7 y grouped by tertiles of initial IL-6, left to right in ascending order (tertiles 1,2,3). The Box plots show ± bars' of the 1.5 interquartile range; o, outliers. The horizontal line is the cut-off of significant decline. B. Plasma C-reactive protein (CRP) in the Honolulu-Asia Aging Study (males only) in 1975 showed associations of blood CRP at middle age with Alzheimer and vascular dementia 25 y later. CRP values were stratified as quartiles. OR is odds ratio of dementia risk, adjusted for possible confounders. (Redrawn from Schmidt et al, 2002.)

2.8. IMMUNOSENESCENCE AND STEM CELLS

Immune system aging is very complex: Innate immunity tends to increase, exemplified by arterial macrophages and local inflammation, whereas adaptive immunity tends to develop restriction of repertoire from oligoclonality and depletion of T cells (Sections 1.2 and 1.5.1). Inflammatory processes may interact with aging in instructive immunity and stem cell generation.

2.8.1. Immunosenescence and Cumulative Exposure

The thymus is highly sensitive to atrophic changes during acute infections, which alter the critical micro-environment and impair thymocyte proliferation (Savino, 2006). During the life span, humans and other mammals show major shifts from naive T cells to memory T cells with progressively restricted repertoire (oligoclonality) (Sections 1.2.2 and 1.4.3). This aspect of immunosenescence can be accelerated by greater exposure to antigens. The 'hyperstimulation hypothesis' of naive T cell depletion is most strongly developed for the very common infections by cytomegalovirus (CMV). Deficits of memory cells and the presence of highly differentiated T cells with CMV-specificity are strongly linked to CMV seropositivity. These changes characterize an 'immune risk phenotype' with higher mortality in the elderly, observed in two European populations (Akbar and Fletcher, 2005; Huppert et al, 2003; Pawelec et al, 2005; Wikby et al, 2005). Continued antigenic stimulation is hypothesized to drive clonal expansions of memory T cells and is predicted to eventually clonally deplete cells with the highest antigenic affinity. Moreover, the hyperstimulation by one antigen can have bystander effects that activate other T cell specificities due to local secretion of IFNα and TNFα (Fletcher et al, 2005) (Section 1.4.3).

Although CMV is a ubiquitous infection, in 60–100% of adults depending on the population, nonetheless, some individuals reach old age without becoming seropositive. By comparison with CMV-seronegative individuals aged 22–91, healthy CMV-seropositive individuals with latent infections at all ages had 25–50% fewer naive T-cells and an increase of differentiated memory T cells (CD8$^+$ CD28$^-$ effector cytotoxic) in all age groups, particularly the older (Almanzar et al, 2005). Moreover, IFNγ expression is higher in CD8$^+$ T cells with CMV-seropositivity, which would increase the body load of this powerful cytokine and possibly synergize with inflammatory processes throughout the body.

The hyperstimulation hypothesis of immunosenescence predicts that populations with chronic infectious disease should show premature T cell senescence. HIV is being examined from this perspective. Young HIV carriers have impaired T-cell responses to vacci-nation for preventing childhood infections; e.g., measles, polio, and influenza antigens induce weaker responses (Rubinstein et al, 2000; Setse et al, 2006). HIV-specific T cells have lower proliferation and cytotoxicity, both as found in immunosenescence of the elderly (van Baarle et al, 2005). Moreover, HIV patients show immune impairments to other antigens.

Multiple immunizations with a T cell-dependent neoantigen (ϕ174, non-infectious bacteriophage) caused progressively smaller responses, unlike healthy controls, presumably because of the already limited pool of naive T cells; booster immunizations with ϕ174 also increased plasma HIV viremia (Rubinstein et al, 2000). These findings support the hyperstimulation hypothesis of immunosenescence.

These effects extend to antigenic stimulation by intestinal nematodes (helminth parasites). In Ethiopians infected with HIV and nematodes, the plasma HIV load was correlated with the helminth load; successful de-worming treatment also decreased HIV viremia in 8/11 patients (Wolday et al, 2002). Ethiopian immigrants to Israel have given unique opportunities to study the reversibility of age-like immunological changes after leaving a highly infectious environment (van Baarle et al, 2005). About 60,000 Ethiopians of all ages arrived in two waves, 1984–1985 and 1991. Immigrants were often infected with worms, but not with HIV, malaria, or TB. The immigrants were characterized by abnormally low proportions of naive CD4$^+$ T cells and excess T memory cells ('broad T cell activation') (Borkow et al, 2000; Kalinkovich et al, 1998; Kalinkovich et al, 2001). Nearly half had inverted CD4:CD8 ratios <1, not found in control groups that resemble the 'immune risk phenotype' of elderly northern Europeans (Section 1.2). T cell impairments included decreased activation of ERK2 kinases, β-chemokine secretion, and delayed type hypersensitivity (DTH, memory T cell dependent). Effective de-worming restored the DTH (Borkow et al, 2000), normalized the ratios of CD4:CD8 T cells, and almost normalized the T cell activation profile (Kalinkovich et al, 1998). Evidently, elimination of the nematode antigen load partly regenerated a naive T cell pool, as occurs in HIV infections. Even when not infected with HIV or worms, by the age of 5, Ethiopians have abnormally high proportions of memory T cells, indicative of antigenic hyperstimulation (Tsegaye et al, 2003). Nonetheless, their neonatal T cell proportions were normal, suggesting effective placental barriers to maternal infections (see Section 4.6.4). Their short life expectancy (about 40 y, like other pre-industrial populations, Fig. 1.1 legend) and high memory T cell profile suggest that some Ethiopians are exposed to conditions prevailing in 18th century Europe where life span was also about 40 y (Section 2.4). These continuing studies promise unique insights on the rate of reversibility of immunosenescence after the transition to a 21st century environment with greatly improved health care, hygiene, and nutrition.

Another population in transition is the Tsimane of the Bolivian Amazon basin. These forager-horticulturalists have had limited access to modern medicine and manifest a high incidence of parasites and other infections (Gerven et al, 2007; McDade et al, 2005). Their short life expectancy (43 y, about the same as the Ethiopian immigrants above) and age-specific mortality profile resemble mid-19th century Sweden (Fig. 1.1B, Fig. 2.7A). Blood CRP elevations are consistent with their high pathogen load: By age 40, the Tsimane have had as many years with high CRP as those in the United States by age 60. Immune cells have not been characterized. Other populations of interest for accelerated immunosenescence are Gambians, who have seasonal cycles of infections that alter T cell functions (Section 4.6.2) (Moore et al, 2006), and rural Guatemalans, who received nutritional supplements and health care in controlled studies (INCAP, Section 4.2) (Scrimshaw, 2003).

Mice also accumulate memory T cell clonal expansions in response to chronic antigenic stimulation, e.g., by HSV-1, which induces a strong cytotoxic lymphocyte response (Messaoudi et al, 2006). Unexpectedly, these memory T cells were not antigen specific and were induced just as effectively by the immune adjuvant, suggesting important by-stander effects that increase T cell clonal expansion (Section 1.4.3). Moreover, normal intestinal flora also influence memory T cell clonal expansions, as shown with germ-free mice (Kieper et al, 2005). We may conclude that the individual profile of aging in instructive immunity is closely linked to the cumulative antigenic experience that certainly begins at birth with the first full encounter to the germy world and may well begin earlier in the undocumented levels of prenatal infections. Internal sources of antigens also extend far beyond enteric and oral fauna to auto-antigens, possibly including AGEs accumulated on long-lived proteins. Lastly, the trends for increased levels of proinflammatory cytokines may also influence adaptive immunity, because IL-1, IL-6, IL-18, etc., modulate many aspects of immune progenitor cell differentiation, including stem cells.

2.8.2. Immunosenescence and Telomere Loss

Chronic inflammation without infections can cause telomere shortening. Chronic smokers, for example, have shorter telomeres in peripheral blood lymphocytes (Valdes et al, 2005) and less telomerase (hTERT) (Getliffe et al, 2005). The pathway linking smoking to peripheral lymphocytes may be direct because smoke components rapidly activate blood monocytes by redox-dependent pathways (Walters et al, 2005). Chronic skin inflammation is also associated with telomere shortening. Children with atopic dermatitis have activated skin T cells; when cultured, skin T cell cultures had 25% shorter telomeres than normal blood lymphocytes (Bang, 2001). In psoriasis, blood T cells also have shorter telomeres (Wu et al, 2000).

Chronic psychological stress was correlated with telomere shortening in peripheral lymphocytes in women (Epel et al, 2004). Although these premenopausal women were considered 'healthy,' this study did not report on recent infections, which would be expected with histories of stress and which could have caused immune cell proliferation independently of perceived psychological stress. Stress is well known to increase the incidence of infections in humans (Marsland et al, 2002) and animals (Sheridan et al, 2000).

Short telomeres may predict greater mortality and shorter longevity. As noted above, CMV-seropositive individuals had shorter telomeres. Although CMV is considered a benign infection in those with healthy immune systems CMV-seropositivity is associated with higher mortality in the elderly (Pawelec et al, 2005). Again, short telomere length in blood lymphocytes was associated with increased mortality at all ages by 2-fold, with 8.5-fold more infections and 3.2-fold more heart disease (Utah blood donors) (Cawthon et al, 2003). Among stroke survivors, those with short telomeres in blood lymphocytes were more likely to develop dementia and die sooner (von Zglinicki and Martin-Ruiz, 2005). The generality of these findings is unclear.

2.8.3. Inflammation and Stem Cells

Inflammation may prove to impair stem cell generation and survival. For example, in the adult rodent brain, neuron stem cell formation (*de novo* neurogenesis) was strongly inhibited by LPS endotoxin (direct i.c.v. infusion) (Ekdahl et al, 2003). Neurogenesis was inversely correlated with the density of local microglia. Neurogenesis was restored by minocycline, an antibiotic that passes the blood-brain barrier and suppresses microglial reactions in neurodegenerative disease models. These findings give a rationale for evaluating the role of inflammation in neurogenesis during Alzheimer and Parkinson disease, which have chronic local inflammatory responses, as well as in the milder inflammation of normal brain aging (Chapter 1).

Circulating C-reactive protein (CRP) may inhibit generation of vascular endothelial progenitor cells (EPCs), which are implicated in adult vascular repair and regeneration (Section 1.5.3.4). *In vitro*, clinical levels of exogenous CRP inhibited EPC migration and adhesion; moreover, high CRP also inhibited formation of capillary tubules (angiogenesis) and the expression of proangiogenic factors (VEGF, IL-8; eNOS) (Verma et al, 2004; Suh et al, 2004). Other factors are anticipated besides elevated CRP because angina patients showed very modest correlations of CRP and circulating EPCs ($r^2 = 0.09$) (George et al, 2004).

Responses to bacterial pneumonia imply further roles of EPC. Elderly patients with bacterial pneumonia, but without clinical cardiovascular disease, had several-fold more circulating EPCs during the acute phase, relative to post-treatment (Yamada et al, 2005). Those with low EPCs before treatment had persistent lung fibrosis, which suggests that EPCs contribute to lung repair. Moreover, EPC and total lymphocyte counts were strongly correlated, consistent with the poor prognosis of lymphocytopenic pneumonia patients. This association implies the co-regulation of EPCs with other marrow stem cell populations.

In summary, these observations suggest that chronic exposure to infection and inflammogens may drive increased mortality during aging from three causes. (I) The diminished pool of naive memory T-cells truncates the primary immune response to new infections, whereas the highly differentiated state of memory cells limits the strength of the secondary responses. (II) The cytokine shift to increased IFNγ production by differentiated T cells may interact with the proinflammatory trend during aging. (III) Atherogenesis may interact with these processes at many levels, from local reactions of CMV-specific T cells in unstable atheromas to reduced generation of stem cells that may be critical in repair of vascular, lung, and neural tissues.

2.9. CANCER, INFECTION, AND INFLAMMATION

Some infections that cause chronic local inflammation also increase the risk of cancer and other abnormal growths. About 15% of all cancers are attributed to infections, directly or indirectly (Herrera et al, 2005). Links between aging, cancer, and endogenous inflammation are also hypothesized (Sarkar and Fisher, 2005). Many cancers and abnormal growths are associated with local inflammatory cell responses that stimulate cell proliferation. In the mutational theory of oncogenesis, the mutagenic progression to malignancy begins with DNA damage. Mutations accumulate during DNA replication, which may be stimulated endogenously, e.g., by sex steroids in reproductive tissues or exogenously, e.g., ultraviolet damage, carcinogens, viruses. Inflammatory processes after initiation are illustrated by the ras pathway. Ras protooncogenes (H-ras, K-ras, N-ras) are often activated by mutations; e.g., 50% of colon cancers have mutations in ras (Bos, 1989). Activated ras protein, in turn, induces IL-1 and IL-8 and other proinflammatory cytokines (Sparmann and Bar-Sagi, 2004; Liu et al, 2004). IL-8 induction involves ERK-MAPK and PI3K pathways, which also influence longevity (Fig. 1.3). IL-8 mediates the recruitment of macrophages and other inflammatory cells that promote tumor vascularization (angiogenesis). Local inflammatory responses may also produce ROS that induce further mutations on the pathway to malignancy. Several examples are discussed in more detail that represent inflammation from infections (next) and from smoking (following section) and that further illustrate the importance of bystander damage during inflammation (Chapter 1.4).

2.9.1. Helicobacter Pylori and Hepatitis B Virus

H. pylori is conclusively linked to inflammatory bowl disease and gastro-intestinal cancers, which rank second among malignancies as cause of death (Herrera et al, 2005; Parkin et al, 2005; Sugiyama and Asaka, 2004). These links are much stronger than associations of *H. pylori* with vascular disease (Section 2.2). Most humans have submucosal infections of *H. pylori*: 76% in developing countries, 58% in developed countries (Parkin et al, 2005). Infections are usually acquired early in life, and the risk is several-fold higher if parents are infected (Webb et al, 1994; Rothenbacher et al, 2002). Fortunately, most carriers (85%) are asymptomatic. However, about 15% of carriers develop peptic ulcers, with 1% proceeding to gastro-intestinal cancers. As hygiene and public health improve, the prevalence of infections decreases. In successive birth cohorts of the Bristol Helicobacter project, cancer incidence has decreased correspondingly with *H. pylori* infections (Harvey et al, 2002; Lane et al, 2002). This progression supports the general relationships of the early-life infectious load to later mortality in successive cohorts (Fig. 2.8) and is a benchmark example of by-stander effects in infections (Queries 1 and 2, Section 1.1).

The oncogenicity of *H. pylori* arises from chronic localized inflammatory responses around the mucosa to which it attaches extracellularly (Penta et al, 2005).

Mucosal cell proliferation is stimulated. Infiltrating macrophages and neutrophils produce promutagenic ROS that damage epithelial cells, in association with increased oxidative DNA damage, as assayed by intestinal 8-OHdG (Farinati et al, 2003). As further proof of the inflammation-oxidative damage link, treatments that eradicated *H. pylori* also decreased tissue level of 8-OHdG (Farinati et al, 2004). As expected from the increased intestinal proliferation, intestinal telomere DNA is also shortened in *H. pylori* infections, even without local metaplasia (Kuniyasu et al, 2003). There are instructive genetic interactions of host cytokine alleles with virulence factors of *H. pylori*. For example, cancer risk was 10-fold higher by the combined presence of a high-risk *H. pylori* virulence factor and high-risk IL-1 allele than in the opposite low-risk combination (Figueiredo et al, 2002). Anti-inflammatory NSAIDs, which inhibit COX-2, are protective in *H. pylori* infections (more on this in the next section). *H. pylori* infections are strong examples of inflammation-induced oxidative damage (Query II).

Inflammatory bowl disease is among the top three main risk conditions for colorectal cancer. After 7 y of exposure to inflammatory bowl disease, the incidence of colorectal cancer increases by 0.5–1%/y (Itzkowitz and Yio, 2004). The area of the colon surface involved in inflammation also increases the risk of colorectal cancer, giving an example of bystander damage with dose effects from time and target area (Section 1.4). Oxidant stress from inflammation is a leading mechanism in colorectal cancer. Chromosomal instability, mutational loss of function in the *APC* and *p53* genes, and induction of COX-2 and NO synthase are typical. Consistent with the inflammation hypothesis, aspirin and NSAIDs reduce the risk of colorectal cancer (Section 2.10.2).

Virus-induced inflammation is also linked to liver cancer, which ranks sixth in the world and third in the U.S. as causes of death (Parkin et al, 2005). Most liver cancers, 75% worldwide, are caused by hepatitis B and C viruses (HBV, HBC). Each infection increases the risk about 20-fold, while co-infection may increase the risk >100-fold (Donato et al, 1998). A substantial minority (5–20%) of HBV infections progresses from cirrhosis, within 5 y of diagnosis, to hepatocellular carcinoma (Imperial, 1999; Marcellin et al, 2005). HBV-induced cancer is associated with increased inflammatory expression: Although the acute phase responses during HBV were not reported in detail, IL-6 elevation correlates with the clinical severity (Tangkijvanich et al, 2000). Tumorigenesis depends on Hepatitis-Bx (HBx), a virally encoded signaling peptide that stimulates hepatocyte proliferation by activating NF-κB after viral integration. Hbx also facilitates metastasis by inducing matrix remodeling through matrix metalloproteinases and COX-2 (Lara-Pezzi et al, 2002). These latter inflammatory responses are all-too-familiar in atheromas (Section 1.5.3.1). COX-2 inhibitors suppress cell invasion in experimental models (Lara-Pezzi et al, 2002), but their efficacy has not been reported for HBV or HBC. These examples of *H. pylori* and hepatitis virus in inflammation and cancer merely scratch the surface of a growing literature that links chronic inflammation to cancer and that shows promise for anti-inflammatory drugs (see below).

2.9.2. Smoking and Lung Cancer

Smoking is the most robust example of an external inflammogen (bioaerosol) that is not infectious and that causes acceleration of mortality and premature mortality from multiple causes. Lung cancer was extremely rare before the advent of popular smoking beginning in the early 20th century. In Richard Doll's classic longitudinal study of British physicians since 1951, smokers have a risk that increases in proportion to the numbers of 'pack-years.' In contrast, those avoiding contact with cigarette smoke have negligible risk (Fig. 2.11) (Doll et al, 2004; Doll et al, 2005; Peto R et al, 2000; Vineis et al, 2004). For lifetime use, the risk of death from lung cancer is 5% in men and 10% in women. Smokers who quit retain the same risk for lung cancer indefinitely; e.g., men quitting at 60 had stabilized 10% during the remainder of their lives.

These powerful dose-response relationships in smoking and cancer define a paradigm for environmental exposures that may extend to environmental factors in cancers in general. Besides the lung, smoking also increases the risk of cancer elsewhere in the larynx, stomach, liver, pancreas, and bladder. However, prostate cancer is only weakly, if at all, related to smoking (Vineis et al, 2004). Cancer

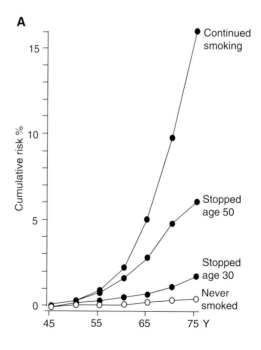

FIGURE 2.11 For legend see page 157.

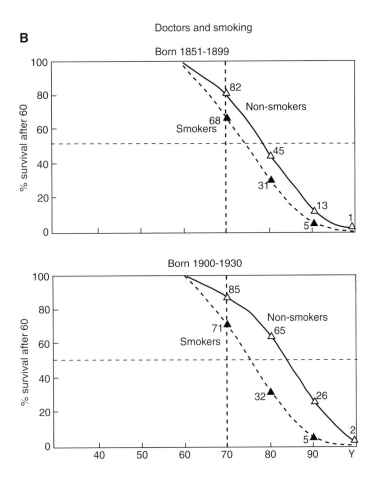

FIGURE 2.11 Smoking. A. Cumulative risk of death from lung cancer in the UK by age of smoking cessation since 1950. From national data combined with two case control studies. (Redrawn from Peto R et al, 2000.) B. Survival and smoking in British doctors. The smaller impact in doctors born before 1900 may reflect few pack-years. Note the greater life expectancy and percent surviving to age 90 in non-smokers born after 1900. (Redrawn from Doll et al, 2005.)

risk in smokers may be subject to genetic variations in detoxifying enzymes, DNA repair (Wu X. et al, 2004), and apoE4 (Fig. 5.18).

Smoking also increases the risk of vascular disease events, but the dose-response to pack-years is less clear. It is not known how tobacco smoke promotes, directly or indirectly, carcinogenesis in enteric organs that are not in direct contact with the airways.

2.10. PHARMACOPLEIOTROPIES IN VASCULAR DISEASE, DEMENTIA, AND CANCER

I suggest the term 'pharmacopleiotropy' to represent multiple domains of drug effects with overlapping specificities. Many drugs influence biochemical and cell systems far beyond the original targets. Negative or adverse effects of drugs are well recognized, as in gastric bleeding from aspirin. However, unexpected positive pharmacopleiotropies are emerging for drugs that protect against heart disease which may also reduce the risk of cancer and of AD (Table 2.2). These cross-over effects are consistent with shared anti-inflammatory effects of diverse drugs in heart disease and with evidence for the pervasiveness of inflammatory processes in "normal" aging and in Alzheimer and vascular disease. Moreover, pharmacopleiotropies are consistent with genetic pleiotropies of apoE4 as a shared risk factor in Alzheimer and vascular disease and with the shared risk factors from the environment and lifestyle (Section 5.7).

2.10.1. Anti-inflammatory and Anti-coagulant Drugs

The remarkable possibility can be considered that a cluster of major degenerative diseases is attenuated by the widely used drugs that were developed for heart disease. Meta-analyses agree in the shared efficacy of quite different drugs in reducing the risk of vascular events, certain cancers, and possibly Alzheimer disease, with effects in the broad range of 10–60% (Table 2.2). No single study can suffice, and there are many divergences between indications of efficacy from animal models and clinical effects. It is hard to interpret the drug literature on vascular disease and dementia (Baron, 2003): Clinical end-points differ between studies, as do drug doses and durations. There is great heterogeneity in age, health status, ethnicity, socioeconomics, and education. Those taking aspirin and other drugs often modify their lifestyles, which reduces their risks independently of the drug candidate. Thus, the 'possible benefits' of the drugs in Table 2.2 should be considered a moving target of continuing critical evaluation for complex drug interactions to identify subgroups by risk and benefit for remaining life expectancy.

The pharmacology of anti-inflammatory drugs distinguishes two broad groups: steroidal anti-inflammatory drugs (SAIDs) and non-steroidal anti-inflammatory drugs (NSAIDs) (Hardman and Limbird, 2001; Vane and Botting, 2003). NSAIDs alter production of prostaglandins and thromboxanes, 'isoprenoids' that have diverse and broad roles in normal physiology and in disease, e.g. the thromboxane TXA_2 enhances local platelet aggregation, while blockers of TXA_2 can be protective against thrombosis. The ubiquitous isoprenoids are also referred to as 'autocoids' because they are produced from local membrane lipids. Arachidonic acid is an autocoid substrate of the cyclooxygenase enzymes, COX-1, -2, and -3. COX-1 products mediate normal functions of gastric mucosa and kidney, as well as coagulation: COX-2 is induced during inflammatory reactions,

TABLE 2.2 Possible Benefits of Adult-Onset Degenerative Diseases by Aspirin, NSAIDs, and Statins

	Aspirin	NSAIDs	Statins
cancer			
colorectal & esophageal	+2	+2	+/−
bladder, breast, ovary, prostate	+/−	+/−	+/−
non-Hodgkin lymphoma	−1	−1	
neurodegenerative diseases			
Alzheimer disease	+	+	+/−
Parkinson	+	+	
vascular disease events			
myocardial infarct	+2	−2	+2
stroke	+/−	−1	+2

+2, consistent benefit across many studies; +1, possible benefits according to initial observations; +/−, possible benefits, but not consistent; −1, possible adverse effects; −2, definite adverse effects. Other references in Section 2.1.

cancer:
aspirin and NSAIDs (Baron, 2003; Bosetti et al, 2002; Herendeen and Lindley, 2003; Perron et al, 2003; Meric et al, 2006); non-Hodgkin lymphoma (Cerhan, 2003).
statin benefits to cancer are in Phase II trials with various tumors and are being considered for adjunct chemotherapy and chemopreventives (Chan et al, 2003; Etminan et al, 2003).

neurodegenerative diseases:
Alzheimer (Breitner, 2003; Etminan et al, 2003)
Parkinson (Chen et al, 2003)

vascular disease events:

myocardial infarct:
aspirin (Antithrombotic Trialists' Collaboration, 2002; Eidelman et al, 2003; Bartolucci and Haward, 2006)
statins (Fonarow and Watson, 2003; Heart Protection Collaborative Group, 2002; Law et al, 2003; Mostaghel and Waters, 2003; Wald and Law, 2003)

stroke:
aspirin (Bartolucci and Howard, 2006)
NSAIDs (Kearney et al, 2006)
statins (Amarenco et al, 2006; Endres and Laufs, 2006).

e.g., by LPS and other endotoxins. COX-1 and COX-2 are coded by distinct genes, whereas COX-3 is a new splicing variant of COX-1 with overlapping functions (Botting, 2003; Vane et al, 2003). PI3-K, of the 'insulin/IGF-1 metabolic longevity' pathways (Fig. 1.3), mediates many NSAIDs' actions. For example, PI3-K is required for induction of COX-2 by endotoxin (LPS) in mesangial cells (Sheu et al, 2005).

Steroidal anti-inflammatory drugs, such as dexamethasone and prednisolone (synthetic glucocorticoids), act via specific receptors to modulate subcellular pathways that are in part distinct from those regulated directly by NSAIDs. Glucocorticoids have metabolic effects during chronic treatments that differ from NSAIDs. However, there are notable convergences; e.g., the COX-2 gene promoter has glucocorticoid response elements (GRE), which enable repression by cortisol and synthetic glucocorticoids (Kramer, 2004; Santini et al, 2001).

Of the NSAIDs, aspirin (acetylsalicylic acid) has been long known as an analgesic and antipyretic at low doses and is the mostly widely taken drug worldwide (Vane et al, 2003). Aspirin has anti-coagulant activities that reduce the risk of vascular events. At 160 mg/d, aspirin doubles the clotting time by irreversibly inhibiting platelet COX-1, which makes TXA_2 from arachidonic acid, an omega-6 polyunsaturated fatty acid (PUFA). Aspirin effects on clotting last up to 10 days, the life span ($t_{1/2}$) of blood platelets. Higher doses of aspirin are used for rheumatic inflammatory diseases, but often cause gastric bleeding due to blockade of COX-1 in the gastric mucosa. However, even after its acetylation by aspirin, COX-2 activity persists for certain PUFA ω-3 and ω-6 substrates, some of which are anti-inflammatory, e.g., 15 epi-lipoxin A_4 (Arita et al, 2005). Ibuprofen and naproxen are non-selective for COX-1 and-2 (Cryer and Feldman, 1998). Other NSAIDs were developed to target COX-2 without inhibiting COX-1, effectively reducing inflammatory responses with fewer gastric side effects, e.g., celecoxib, naproxen, and rofecoxib. COX-2 and prostaglandin production are also inhibited by synthetic glucocorticoids, as noted above.

The NSAIDs field is in turmoil because of conclusive evidence for increased risk of vascular events (Hippisley-Cox and Coupland, 2005; Juni et al, 2004; Levesque et al, 2005). For example, a population-based case-control study in Finland showed that NSAIDs users had 40% higher risk of a myocardial infarct (OR, 1.40, 95% CI, 1.33–1.48) (Helin-Salmivaara et al, 2006). The various types of COX-2 inhibitors had similar effects. An underlying mechanism may be that inhibiting COX-2 may induce both *proinflammatory and prothrombotic* homeostatic compensatory responses (Doux et al, 2005). Homeostatic responses would be expected because of the importance of COX-2 to many normal cellular functions, e.g., celecoxib induced COX-2 in rat spinal cord (Hsueh et al, 2004). Moreover, due to their short half-lives in circulation (e.g., $t_{1/2}$ 11 h, celecoxob), there could be prothrombotic transients in prostaglandin conversion in the declining phase before another dose is taken. Withdrawal from chronic aspirin in stable cardiac patients, for example, may increase the incidence of thromboses (Senior, 2003). These early observations merit full study.

Statin drugs were designed to lower blood cholesterol by blocking a rate-limiting enzyme of cholesterol synthesis (HGM-CoA reductase). In addition, statins have many effects on inflammation (Balk et al, 2003; Halcox and Deanfield, 2004l; Kwak et al, 2003; Schonbeck and Libby, 2004; Stuve et al, 2003), which may account for vascular benefits not directly linked to blood lipids. Cholesterol-independent pleiotropic effects of statins include the lowering of blood CRP (Albert et al, 2001), inflammatory cell infiltration and cell death (Wierzbicki et al, 2003), and impairing of lymphocyte proliferation (Palinski and Tsimikas, 2002b). Some statin effects result directly from the decrease of mevalonate from the inhibition of HMG CoA reductase. Intracellular mevalonate is a precursor to the isoprenoids (farnesyl pyrophosphate, geranylgeranyl) that modulate enzymes with links to inflammation and vascular smooth muscle cell proliferation, e.g., the Ras and Rho kinases (Endres and Laufs, 2006; Kamiyama et al, 2003). PI3K/Akt is also involved in the induction of nitric oxide synthase by statins (Walter et al, 2004). Statins also increase circulating endothelial progenitor cells (EPCs) (Urbich and Dimmeler, 2005; Vasa et al, 2001a,b), which are implicated in vascular repair (Sections 1.5.3.4 and 2.5.2) and may modulate EPC cell senescence by suppressing Chk2, a DNA damage checkpoint kinase induced by telomere dysfunction (Spyridopoulos et al, 2004). Cardioprotective effects of NSAIDs and statins involve neovascularization (Vagnucci and Li, 2003), which may be important to both AD neuritic plaques and in vascular atheromas (Chapter 1, Table 1.3).

2.10.2. Aspirin and Other NSAIDs

Aspirin and NSAIDs have well established benefits to risks of heart attack and probably to stroke. In the huge Anti-thrombotic Trialists' Collaboration, aspirin and antiplatelet drugs collectively reduced vascular events: 25% risk reduction for myocardial infarction (primary or recurrent) and 11% reduction of stroke; aspirin at a low dose (75–150 mg/day) reduced risk by 32% (Antithrombotic Trialists' Collaboration, 2002). Low dose aspirin in other studies reduced stroke by 13–16%. This net figure represents a greater reduction in thrombotic strokes than the increase of hemorrhagic stroke in aspirin users (van Gijn and Algra, 2002; Wald and Law, 2003).

Some cancer risks may benefit from aspirin and NSAIDs (Baron, 2003; Meric et al, 2006). Colorectal cancer is the best case, in which aspirin lowered risk by 20–30% in case control and cohort studies (Morgan, 2004; Slattery et al, 2004). Gastric cancer shows similar benefits of aspirin and NSAIDs (Wang et al, 2003b). As discussed above, gastric cancer is strongly associated with *Helicobacter pylori* infections, which elevate mucosal prostaglandins (Laine et al, 1995). In one mechanism, aspirin directly inhibits *H. pylori* growth (Wang et al, 2003c). Breast cancer may also benefit by aspirin and NSAIDs (Zhang et al, 2005), particularly for cancers that have both estrogen and progesterone receptors (Terry et al, 2004). The optimum dose of aspirin for cancer prevention may be higher than for coronary disease (Chan et al, 2004). These effects are controversial and may not hold for low-dose aspirin (Cook et al, 2005).

Alzheimer disease risk may also benefit from aspirin and NSAIDs, another controversial possibility that has been considered for nearly two decades. An early indication came from informal clinical observations that rheumatoid arthritis patients seemed to show less Alzheimer disease (Jenkinson et al, 1989); although this study could not fully document the drug use profile, rheumatoid patients are typically heavy users of anti-inflammatory drugs. Another indication came from identical twins discordant for use of anti-inflammatory drugs (all classes): The twin taking anti-inflammatories had about 75% lower relative risk (Breitner et al, 1994). Recall from Section 2.7 that periodontal disease increased the risk of dementia in twins (Gatz et al, 2006).

Larger post hoc studies indicate improvements of 13% for aspirin and 28% for NSAIDs (Akiyama et al, 2000; Breitner, 2003; Etminan et al, 2003; McGeer et al, 1996; Nilsson et al, 2003). In recent longitudinal observational studies, two groups reported less Alzheimer's in users of NSAIDs, but not aspirin (in t' Veld et al, 2001; Cornelius et al, 2004). However, others observed less Alzheimer's and loss of cognition in normal individuals with 75 mg or more aspirin; NSAIDs showed similar trends (not statistically significant) (Nilsson et al, 2003).

Interventional studies of NSAIDs and Alzheimer's are in an early stage (Akiyama et al, 2000; Davey Smith and Ebrahim, 2002; Etminan et al, 2003). In Joseph Rogers's pioneering pilot study, Alzheimer patients with mild to moderate impairments had slower decline after 6 months of indomethacin, an inhibitor of both COX-1 and -2 (Rogers et al, 1993). However, subsequent trials with the selective COX-2 inhibitor Rofecoxib (alternate names: Refecoxib or Vioxx) did not show benefit in two large randomized trials lasting 1 y (Aisen et al, 2003; Reines et al, 2004).

Experimental studies give some insights into these divergent results (Imbimbo, 2004). In cell cultures, indomethacin decreases the production of Aβ42 (Fig. 2.12), as does ibuprofen (Weggen et al, 2003; Kukar et al, 2005). These effects are well documented in transgenic Alzheimer mice, in which chronic ibuprofen at clinical levels slowed brain amyloid accumulation (solid and soluble), IL-1β increase, and behavioral changes (Lim et al, 2001b; Morihara et al, 2005).

However, contrary to the consistent effects of ibuprofen, targeted COX-2 inhibitors did not give the expected benefits. Rofecoxib *increased* Aβ42 production in cells (Fig. 2.12) and in the brain (Kukar et al, 2005). Celecoxib (Celebrex) was similar. Contrary to assumptions, these activities do not require COX-1 inhibition and appear to modify amyloid production through direct allosteric effects on γ-secretase, the enzyme complex that cleaves Aβ42 from the amyloid-precursor protein. As noted above, COX-2 drugs are associated with increased risk of myocardial infarctions. Possibly, their withdrawal from general long-term use may also benefit the risk of dementia on two grounds: the shared prothrombotic risk factor of myocardial and cerebrovascular events and the increased production of Aβ42 by these drugs.

In considering further large-scale trials of NSAIDs as preventives for Alzheimer disease, we need more preclinical understanding of the pharmacopleiotropies of these powerful drugs. Genotype may also be important, e.g., apoE4 carriers taking aspirin had a *higher* incidence of Alzheimer disease (Cornelius et al, 2004). Other inflammatory gene variants could influence drug responses, particularly those associated with vascular disease (Chapter 4). Meanwhile, we may learn more about the benefits of aspirin to Alzheimer and vascular dementia, because aspirin continues to be widely advised and used.

2.10.3. Statins

2.10.3.1. Vascular Disease

Statins are considered separately because of their multiple effects on cholesterol and on inflammation. In a meta-analysis, statins reduced the risk of coronary

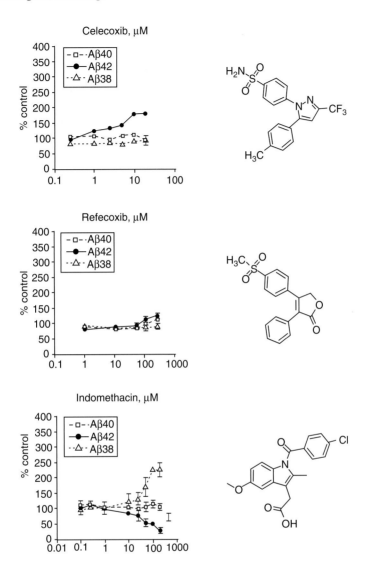

FIGURE 2.12 Production of amyloid peptide Aβ is differentially sensitive to NSAIDs drugs. Redrawn from (Kukar et al, 2005). Aβ peptides secreted by cells transfected with APPswe. Note the increased Aβ42 with celecoxib and the decreased Aβ42 with indomethacin.

events by about 60% and stroke by 17%, in association with lower LDL cholesterol (Law et al, 2003). Among secondary prevention medications for cardiovascular disease, statins reduced cardiac mortality by 24% to 42%, i.e., at least as much as aspirin and blood pressure medications (β-adrenergic blockers, and ACE inhibitors) (Fonarow and Watson, 2003; Grobbee and Bots, 2003). Statins also lowered cardiovascular mortality in patients with normal cholesterol in two major studies: the Scandinavian Simvastatin Survival Study ('4S') and the Long-Term Intervention with Prevastatin in Ischaemic Disease (LIPID) trial (Fonarow and Watson, 2003).

Statins influence vascular plaque size by mechanisms that may be independent of effects of statins on blood cholesterol levels (Wierzbicki et al, 2003). The FATS trial showed 75% decrease of cardiovascular events, despite the small improvement in stenosis (<1%) (Brown et al, 1993). These authors suggested that statins selectively depleted unstable fatty plaques with large lipid cores (Fig. 1.13, type IV), thereby stabilizing the lesions and reducing thrombosis. Plaque shrinkage during statin use is documented by sonography (Sato et al, 2003) and magnetic imaging (Vigen et al, 2005).

These unexpected benefits of statins point to broad anti-inflammatory actions, possibly through the reduction of isoprenoids from blocking HMG-coA reductase, which modifies many receptor functions in inflammatory pathways. Stain therapy is being considered for a wide range of inflammatory conditions, including multiple sclerosis, rheumatoid arthritis, and sepsis.

2.10.3.2. *Dementia*

Lower risk of Alzheimer disease was observed in statin users in epidemiological studies (Crisby et al, 2002; Jick et al, 2000; Vagnucci and Li, 2003; Wolozin et al, 2000). Evidence seems definitive that statins lower the risk of a first stroke (Amarenco, 2005; Endres and Laufs, 2006) or recurrent stroke (Amarenco et al, 2006), which should also lower dementia risks (Section 1.6). The slow turnover of brain cholesterol (about 6 months) (Casserly and Topol, 2004) implies that prolonged treatment with statins may be needed.

Animal models raise caveats for statins, as for NSAIDs. On the positive side, in cell culture models, lowering of cell cholesterol by statins decreased Aβ42 production, apparently by directing APP cleavage to the non-amyloidogenic α-secretase pathway of APP cleavage (Cole et al, 2005b). However, the lower levels of isoprenoids had opposing effects by *increasing* production of APP and Aβ42, which would be pro-amyloidogenic. This may be why lovastatin *increased* brain amyloid in a transgenic Alzheimer mouse (Tg2676), despite lower plasma cholesterol (Park et al, 2003). Rebound effects are also observed in discontinuation of statins, which are associated with increased risk of stroke and mortality (Endres and Laufs, 2006). Statin clearance after sustained administration suddenly activates rho and Rac-1, leading to oxidative bursts and decreased NO availability. Rebound transients could also arise with the statins that are rapidly cleared from plasma, noted above for NSAIDs.

2.10.4. Sex Steroid Replacement (Hormone Therapy)

Estrogen replacement therapy to compensate for age-related deficits is a possible intervention for vascular and brain dysfunctions and diseases that interact with inflammation at many levels. Major ongoing studies address benefits and risks of hormone therapy.[5] Animal models are largely supportive, but clinical findings are mixed. Besides their direct effects on many brain cell and vascular cell functions, sex steroids also modulate adaptive immune and inflammatory functions. My summary of these complex and controversial topics begins with a demographic perspective.

Cardiovascular disease, cerebrovascular disease, and Alzheimer disease show an accelerating incidence during mid-life into later ages. Sex differences in mortality are present throughout life with greater overall male vulnerability (Section 5.2): In developed countries during recent decades, age-specific death rates of adult women lag behind those of men and approximate those of adult men who are 5 y or more younger (Fig. 5.2). After middle age, cardiovascular disease becomes the first or second main cause of death in most populations (Section 1.2.2, Fig. 1.4). Mortality rate accelerations tend to be slightly faster for women than men, for both total and cardiovascular mortality (Horiuchi, 1997), but within the population average-age mortality rate doubling times of about 7–10 y (Section 1.2.1). The mortality accelerations are concurrent with menopause, which implies a role for the sharp decrease of ovarian steroid levels. However, behavioral and environmental risk factors vary widely between populations, making it is hard to resolve the contributions of age-changes in sex hormones to health and mortality after middle age.

Dementia risks accelerate exponentially after age 60, with a doubling time of about 5 y (Fig. 1.10A) (Kawas and Katzman, 1999; Mayeux, 2003). Sex differences in dementia are variable and, in a meta-analysis of 23 studies, were not statistically significant (Jorm and Jolley, 1998). The age-specific prevalence was also similar in men and women in three studies [Rotterdam Study (Ott et al, 1998), Cardiovascular Health Study (Fitzpatrick et al, 2004), and AHEAD (Assets and Health Dynamics of the Oldest Old, a survey of community living U.S. elderly) (Suthers et al, 2003)]. Nonetheless, relatively more women are demented at later ages, when calculated as a fraction of the surviving population. In developed countries at 55, the female:male ratio is about 1:1; at 85, about 2:1, and climbing

---

[5]Estrogen therapy is administered in two main modes: *conjugated equine estrogens* (CEE) taken orally and *estradiol-17β* (pill or skin patch). Transdermal estradiol differs from CEE in effect on inflammatory markers (see footnote 6). Equine estrogens (Premarin, from *pregnant mare's urine*; Wyeth-Ayerst) have been widely used since 1942, because of their availability from an abundant natural source that preceded industrial estrogen synthesis. The equine estrogens in Premarin include equilin and other compounds not made by human ovaries whose estrogenic activities are not well defined (Bhavnani, 1998; Dey et al, 2000; Rozovsky et al, 2002a). Estradiol is a minority component of Premarin and varies widely between preparations over a 3-fold range, 4.5–12% (Bhavnani, 1998).

(Section 5.2. Fig. 5.2). In populations where women have a greater life expectancy (Section 5.2), women are exposed to a proportionately greater lifetime risk of dementia (the 'demographic hypothesis of dementia prevalence') of Suthers, Kim, and Crimmins (2003). As examples, at age 55, Rotterdam women had a 2-fold higher risk of dementia in the remaining life span: women, 0.33; and men, 0.16 (Ott et al, 1998). In the AHEAD sample at age 85, the remaining life expectancy without cognitive impairment was 15% longer for women.

The greater mortality risk of males in cardiovascular deaths has been interpreted as due to protection from cardiovascular disease by ovarian steroids, principally by estrogens, which decrease >90% after menopause. Until recently, estrogen was the most widely prescribed medication in the United States and remains popular because of its effectiveness in suppressing menopausal hot flushes (Hickey et al, 2005). Estrogen therapy is supported by experimental and clinical studies. Many observational studies concluded that estrogen replacement lowered cardiovascular events by 40–60% (Barrett-Connor et al, 2005; Grady et al, 1992). For example, the Nurse's Health Study recruited women who reported no cardiovascular disease (Grodstein et al, 1997) at entry ages 30–55 in 1976: 18 years later, current hormone users had a lower mortality risk (0.63); those who acquired coronary risk factors since entry had the greatest benefit (relative risk, 0.51); the risk of death from coronary disease was 0.47. In EPAT (Estrogen in the Prevention of Atherosclerosis Trial), estradiol replacement (oral, micronized) of healthy postmenopausal women for 24 months slowed (actually decreased) carotid artery thickening (Hodis et al, 2001; Karim, 2005), a major marker of atherosclerosis (Section 1.5). In the Women's Health Initiative (WHI)-estrogen (E) Trial, coronary disease outcomes were decreased by about 35% in women who began CEE before 60. Estrogen plus progestin (CEE + medroxyprogesterone) had similar benefits (Women's Health Initiative Steering Committee, 2004; reviewed in Hodis and Mack, 2007a,b). These findings are supported by other studies and meta-analyses, which also show benefits of estrogen therapy are reduced or reversed if begun after age 60.

Hormone therapy (estrogen replacement) 'should be' protective because of consistent improvements in vascular risk markers for (lowering of LDL cholesterol and IL-6, etc.), as shown by several hundred studies (Godsland, 2001). A complication is that oral estrogen may have proinflammatory effects.[6]

---

[6]CEE and other oral estrogens elevate the inflammatory marker serum CRP by 50–100%, whereas transdermal estrogens (patch) do not (Frohlich et al, 2003; Hu et al, 2005; Lacut et al, 2003). This potentially important effect arises because the portal circulation carries, on the first circulatory pass, the estrogens absorbed from the gut directly to the liver, which is the source of most systemic CRP. Transdermal estrogens, however, are diluted by the venous circulation before reaching the liver. Fortunately, IL-6, fibrinogen, and other inflammatory risk factors in cardiovascular disease are not induced by oral estrogens. In a case control study of 492 older women within the Study of Osteoporotic Fractures, the cardiovascular risk in the top quartile of CRP was independent of estrogen usage (Tice et al, 2003).

Experimentally, estrogen attenuates the systemic and local inflammatory responses (Amantea et al, 2005; Carlsten, 2005; Thomas et al, 2003) and can attenuate apoptosis, e.g., in endothelial cells by Akt-dependent mechanisms (Koga et al, 2004).

Estrogens also have anti-oxidant effects (Behl et al, 1997; Sugishita et al, 2003). In clinical studies, estradiol decreased plasma antibodies to oxidized LDL (Hoogerbrugge et al, 1998) and the susceptibility of LDL to oxidation (Sack et al, 1994). In vascular smooth muscle cultures, estradiol decreased the production of ROS from hydrogen peroxide or CMV infections; estradiol also inhibited the CMV infection (Speir et al, 2000).

Moreover, estrogen enhances endothelial progenitor cell (EPC) production and inhibits EPC senescence (Sections 1.6.2 and 2.5.2). Young women receiving estradiol in a fertility clinic had 3-fold more circulating EPCs, probably due to increased bone marrow production, as was shown in mice (Strehlow et al, 2003). Estrogen attenuates EPC cell senescence, at least in part, by augmenting telomerase (hTERT) through PI3kinase/Akt-dependent mechanisms (Imanishi et al, 2005).

Bone density is another key benefit of estrogen therapy. The consensus holds that estrogen therapy attenuates osteoporosis and spontaneous osteoporotic fractures that are an important cause of mortality in older women (Barrett-Connor et al, 2005; Col et al, 2005; Raisz et al, 2005). Some of the same inflammatory factors that are risk factors in cardiovascular disease and that are improved by estrogen are also regulators of osteoclasts (Chapter 1) (Ginaldi et al, 2005); e.g., estrogen suppressed IL-6 in bone marrow cells and formation of new osteoclasts (Jilka et al, 1992).

But adverse side effects of estrogen are also widely recognized, particularly for endometrial cancer (Amant et al, 2005; Finch and Flurkey, 1977). The continued stimulation of cell proliferation in the endometrium by sex steroids inevitably leads to the accumulation of mutations from errors during DNA replication (bystander effect, type 3, Section 1.4.3). Moreover, breast cancer risk was increased 20% by estrogen plus progestin in the WHI Trial and Heart and Estrogen/Progestin Replacement Study (HERS) (reviewed in Hodis and Mack, 2007a,b). Although venous thromboembolism is also increased by most forms of hormone therapy (Cosman et al, 2005), the effects diminish after the first year of treatment (Hodis and Mack, 2007a). The risk of stroke in WHI-E and WHI-EP was higher for women beginning therapy after 60, while much rarer for those beginning within 5 y of menopause (<1 per 1000).

Similar reversals have occurred for dementia. Just as for cardiovascular disease, hormone therapy has shown benefits to dementia and cognitive aging in many experimental and clinical studies (Birge et al, 2001; Sherwin, 2005). In animal models, estrogen favors neuronal growth and memory, and increases resistance to amyloid and other neurotoxins (Brinton, 2004; Pike, 1999; Quintanilla et al, 2005; Rozovsky et al, 2005; Simpkins et al, 2005). Estrogen also decreases neuronal damage in stroke models (Wise et al, 2005). However, the

Women's Health Initiative Memory Study (WHIMS), an ancillary study of WHI, found that estrogen increased risk of cognitive decline by 1.38-fold for either 'mild cognitive impairment, MCI' or 'probable dementia' (Shumaker et al, 2004). Adverse effects on cognition were greater among women with lower scores at entry (Espeland et al, 2004).

These recent findings are devastating to millions of women and their physicians (Barrett-Connor et al, 2005), but strong conclusions are premature (Schneider, 2004; Morrison et al, 2006; Hodis and Mack, 2007a,b). The timing of replacement may be particularly important (Clarkson, 2002). In WHI and several other trials, estrogen therapy was initiated at 10 or more years after menopause (age at entry averaged 63 y). This delay is important because early menopause accelerates 'subclinical' atherosclerosis, as does surgical ovariectomy (Stampfer et al, 1990). The duration of estrogen deficits also influences carotid artery thickness in correlation with the time since menopause (surgical and natural) (Mack et al, 2004): thickness increased by 0.0032 mm/y after menopause (age-adjusted), which is about 50% of the overall age trend of 0.006 mm/y (author's calculation).[7] In monkeys, estrogen replacement was most effective in suppressing arterial plaque growth if begun at ovariectomy; estrogen replacement was ineffective if delayed 2 y (equivalent human age 52) (Clarkson, 2002).

Consistent with these findings, estradiol replacement did not benefit existing coronary stenosis in women about 10 y after menopause (Hodis et al, 2003a,b; Hodis and Mack, 2007a,b). The timing of estrogen replacement is the focus of ELITE (Early versus Late Intervention Trial) (Howard Hodis, University of Southern California). The use of estradiol rather than conjugated equine estrogens (CEE) may improve trial reproducibility because of variations in equine estrogen components (footnote 5).

Lastly, I return to influences of sex steroids on immune functions, as implied by the anti-inflammatory effects of estrogens. In general, females have higher serum Ig and antibody responses to diverse antigens and incur more autoimmune disease than males (Min et al, 2005; Olsen et al, 1996). During aging, lymphopoiesis differs between immune cell subclasses (Min et al, 2005). Estrogen deficits may derepress regulatory T-cell functions (CD4[+]) that control self-tolerance and responses to microbial antigens (Sakaguchi, 2004). Benefits of estrogen replacement to osteoporosis depend on T-cell subsets that support bone-resorption by osteoclasts via TNFα and TGF-β1 (Gao et al, 2004; Roggia et al, 2001). These mechanisms may extend to endothelial progenitor cells (EPC) of bone marrow origin that mediate vascular repair. As noted above, estrogen enhances EPC functions and suppresses osteoclasts, which mediate osteoporosis. The importance

---

[7]CEF calculated the slope of carotid thickness versus age curve for men without cardiovascular disease from the Baltimore Longitudinal Study (Nagai et al, 1998) (Fig.1.14A). However, both sexes had similar slopes of carotid thickening ages 20 to 90 y.

of EPCs in vascular repair (Section 1.5.3.4) and in attenuating inflammation is a rationale for optimizing hormone therapy for both osteoporosis and EPC production and functioning.

2.10.5. Plant-derived Micronutrients and Neutriceuticals

The powerful benefits of aspirin and other drugs with anti-inflammatory and anti-coagulant activities may be mimics of plant-derived biochemicals present in human diets to varying amounts: polyunsaturated fatty acids (PUFAs), curcumin, and salicylate. These and many other biogenic agents contribute to health through regulatory influences, rather than through their caloric value, and may be broadly considered as micronutrients.

PUFAs are 'essential' micronutrients required for normal brain development and adult health (DeMar et al, 2006) and are ultimately derived from plant foods (Crawford et al, 2004; Holub and Holub, 2004; Zamaria, 2004). PUFAs may have been important in human brain evolution, during the transitions to meat-rich diets (Section 6.2.2).

PUFAs bind to PPAR, SREBP, and other transcription factors that directly modulate the genetic control of fat and carbohydrate metabolism in brain, fat, and liver cells (Sampath and Ntambi, 2004).

α-linolenic acid (18:3ω3) is an essential 'omega-3' fatty acid that must be obtained from the diet[8]. The closely related linoleic acid (18:23ω6) is an 'omega-6' PUFA. After ingestion, the 'parental' PUFAs are enzymatically elongated and desaturated to yield eicosinoids, which have certain opposing activities. Eicosapentanoic acid (20:5ω3) ('EPA') and docosahexanoic acid (22:6ω3) ('DHA') have anti-inflammatory and anti-thrombotic activities, whereas arachidonic acid (20:4ω6) gives rise to ω-6 autocoids with opposite activities. Cyclooxygenases and lipoxygenases convert arachidonic acid to prostaglandins and leukotrienes (Section 2.6 above).

Fish fat and oils are rich sources of eicosapentanoic acid and docosahexanoic acid (both ω-3). Plant foods lack EPA and DHA, but may contain α-linolenic acid (ω-3). Egg yolk also contains ω-3 PUFAs (Renaud, 2001). Popular vegetable oils (corn, safflower, sunflower) are rich in linolenic acid (ω-6). Meat is rich in arachidonic acid (ω-6): pork and poultry > beef and lamb, in both the lean meat and visible fat (Li et al, 1998). Of these, pork fat was the highest (175 mg arachidonic acid/100 g) and lean beef the lowest (21 mg/100 g). Typical U.S. diets yield 1–3 g of α-linolenic acid (ω-6), but 80 mg DHA (ω-3). 'Mediterranean' diets tend

---

[8]The chemical nomenclature 18:3ω3 in α-linolenic acid specifies that the 18 carbon fatty acid has three double bonds, with three carbon atoms separating the methyl group and its nearest double bond (ω-3, or n-3). The closely related linoleic acid (18:2 3ω6) is ω-6. Other ω-3 PUFAs have $\geq$ 3 double bonds: eicosapentanoic acid (20:5ω3) has five double bonds; docosahexanoic acid (22:6ω3) has six double bonds.

to be rich in α-linolenic acid (ω-3). At high dietary ratios, the ω-6 PUFAs compete at the enzymatic level with ω-3 to diminish the yield of eicosapentanoic acid and docosahexanoic acid (ω-3); this shift is considered prothrombotic (see above). The optimum ratios and amounts of dietary PUFAs remain controversial.

Epidemiological studies link the intake of linolenic acid (ω-3) to lower cardiovascular and stroke and improved risk indicators (Crawford et al, 2004; Harris and Levine, 2005; Holub and Holub, 2004). For example, in a rural Japanese community, the carotid artery thickness (IMT) at age 63 varied inversely with ω-3 consumption (Hino et al, 2004). Their high fish consumption yielded about 2.2 g/d of ω-3 PUFAs; this level approximates the 'Mediterranean' diets and exceeds the typical U.S. consumption of about 1.3 g/d. Nonetheless, intervention trials and case control studies with fish oils have been inconclusive (Wilkinson et al, 2005).

The dietary proportions of ω-3 versus ω-6 PUFAs influence coagulation through platelet membrane composition. For example, Eskimos with diets rich in fish oils have low cardiovascular disease in association with slow coagulation in some studies (von Schacky and Dyerberg, 2001). ω-3 PUFAs decrease platelet production of the prothrombotic thromboxane TXA_2 (Section 2.10.1 above) (Adan et al, 1999; Kramer et al, 1996) and attenuate atherosclerosis in hypercholesterolemic rats (Adan et al, 1999). Dietary PUFA regulation of coagulation is attributed to the partial replacement of arachidonic acid (ω-6) by eicosapentanoic acid (ω-3) in platelet membranes, which lowers production of TXA2; e.g., 3 wk of increased fish consumption lowered TXA_2 (Mann et al, 1997). Diet composition may have had a major role in human evolution, in the transitions from the herbivory of great ape ancestors to the high meat intake favored by humans (Chapter 6).

The PUFA framework is being extended to Alzheimer disease (Calon et al, 2005; Mucke and Pitas, 2004). PUFAs are important for normal brain functions and development; e.g., synapses are enriched in docosahexanoic acid. The same transgenic Alzheimer mice that responded to NSAIDs (see above) also show strong effects of dietary PUFAs (Calon et al, 2004; Calon et al, 2005). Depletion of docosahexanoic acid (ω-3) by an ω-6 rich diet (safflower oil) caused huge deficits (>90%) in glutamatergic synapses (NR2A & -B) and in the PI3K subunit, p85α. Oxidative stress (carbonyl content) was increased and learning was impaired. Supplements of docosahexanoic acid partly blocked these deficits. Docosahexanoic acid activates the PI3K/Akt pathway and blocks caspase activation, which may link PUFA functions to insulin-like signaling pathway in longevity (Fig. 1.3A).

Human elderly have not consistently associated dietary ω-3 and supplements with cognitive functions (Maclean et al, 2005). Short-term supplements with EPA did not slow cognitive decline in Alzheimer patients, not surprisingly (Boston et al, 2004). A good model for such studies is EVA (Etude du Vielliessement Arteriel; Nantes, France), which used erythrocyte membrane lipid composition as an index of dietary PUFA (Heude et al, 2003). Over 4 years, higher erythrocyte ω-6 content was associated with higher 1.91-fold risk of cognitive decline, whereas ω-3 content reduced risk by 0.59. If the vascular studies of PUFAs are any guide, the benefits of PUFAs to Alzheimer disease will not be proven soon.

Another type of inflammatory regulator involves ω-3 PUFAs, which are oxidized by COX-2 or cytochrome P450 (*CYP* gene family) to numerous agents. Among the emerging functions are the 'resolvin' RvE1, which inhibits leukocyte infiltration (IC50 of 5 nM) (Arita et al, 2005). These aspirin-independent pathways confound analysis of dietary PUFAs in vascular disease (Arita, 2005), e.g., in self-reports, blood salicylate was detected in 14% of aspirin 'non-users' (Smith et al, 1999). This discrepancy could represent benign inaccuracy, or the more interesting possibility of unrecognized dietary salicylates (see below). Many other examples show the difficulty of assessing dietary or other lifestyle factors in health.

Two other plant-originated substances in human diets, curcumin and salicylate, are interesting candidates for benefits to shared risk factors for vascular and Alzheimer disease. Curcumin, a biphenol with a remarkable range of activities, is a major component of turmeric, a traditional Asian spice and preservative from the herb *Curcuman longa*. In Arurvedic medicine, curcumin is considered anti-inflammatory and, in fact, inhibits COX-2 in various cells (Cole et al, 2005a; Lantz et al, 2005; Sharma et al, 2005). Relevant to arthritis, curcumin synergized with celecoxib to inhibit synovial cell growth (Lev-Ari et al, 2006), which is relevant to arthritis. Curcumin induced glutathione biosynthesis and inhibited NF-kappaB activation and interleukin-8 release in alveolar epithelial cells (Belmin et al, 1993; Biswas et al, 2005; Orlandi et al, 2000; Pardio et al, 2005). Curcumin may also be anti-thrombotic. Lastly, and relevant to atherosclerosis in human endothelial cells, curcumin attenuated the repression of thrombomodulin by CRP (Nan et al, 2005). In diet-induced hypercholesterolemia, curcumin increased HDL-cholesterol by 50% and decreased LDL cholesterol by 40% (Arafa, 2005).

Curcumin fed to transgenic Alzheimer mice attenuated oxidative damage and amyloid deposits, whether introduced early before amyloid formed or at later ages (Cole et al, 2005a; Lim, 2001; Yang et al, 2005). Curcumin crosses the blood-brain barrier and binds directly to amyloid deposits. The apparently low incidence of Alzheimer disease in India (Section 1.6.4) (Chandra et al, 2001) is intriguing, in view of the heavy use of turmeric in regional cooking. Clinical trials are evaluating curcumin in Alzheimer disease, vascular disease, cancer, and osteoarthritis. Moreover, there are potential synergies of curcumin with DHA in Western diets that are typically low in DHA and polyphenolic anti-oxidants (Cole and Frautschy, 2006).

Curcumin also has antimicrobial activities; e.g., curcumin attenuated HSV-2 transmission in a mouse model (Bourne et al, 1999). Other useful drugs may be found among ancient traditional spices and food preservatives. Some spices have anti-bacterial, anti-viral, and anti-fungal activities that may have been highly adaptive ("some like it hot") before the advent of refrigeration and sterilization (Billing and Sherman, 1998; Goff and Klee, 2006).

Dietary salicylates may give some of the benefits identified with aspirin (acetylsalicylate) (Hare et al, 2003; Paterson and Lawrence, 2001; Paterson et al, 2006). Many fruits, vegetables, herbs, and spices are rich in salicylates. Vegetarians had 40% higher serum salicylate, with some overlap in non-vegetarian low dose (75 mg/d) aspirin users (Blacklock et al, 2001). The higher salicylate intake of vegetarians is consistent with dietary plant sources. How fascinating that salicylates are important to plants as host-defense mechanisms and are induced in response to attacks by insects and viruses (Shimoda et al, 2005; Ton et al, 2002; Traw et al, 2003). Fruit and vegetables grown without insecticides may have higher salicylates. The anti-inflammatory activities of salicylates work by different mechanisms than aspirin. About one-third of oral aspirin is rapidly converted by carboxyesterases in the gut and liver to salicylic acid and related dihydroxybenzoic acids (Blacklock et al, 2001). Acetylsalicylate is rapidly cleared ($t_{1/2}$ 20 min), while salicylate clears more slowly (blood $t_{1/2}$, up to 30 h) (Hare et al, 2003). In contrast to acetylsalicylate, which inhibits COX-1 and COX-2 by acetylating serine at the enzyme active site (see above), salicylate inhibits prostaglandin synthesis by repressing COX transcription (Awtry and Loscalzo, 2000; Hare et al, 2003). There is always more to aspirin.

Two other natural COX inhibitors have come to light. Olive oil contains '(−)oleocanthal', a phenolic adduct that strongly inhibits COX-1 and -2 in rank order: indomethacin > oleocanthol > ibuprofen (Beauchamp et al, 2005). Oleocanthol may be among the benefits imputed to the Mediterranean diet. Ingestion of 50 ml extra-virgin grade olive oil is estimated to yield 9 mg of (−)oleocanthol, which is 10% of the ibuprofen dose recommended for analgesia.

The overlapping risk factors for vascular disease and Alzheimer disease are tantalizing targets for simple nutritional interventions. PUFAs, curcumin, and salicylates are likely to be joined by many other dietary micronutrients in wild plants and cultivars. There may be a common biochemistry in view of the conjugated double bond systems that these three classes of compounds share. Synthetic drugs developed for vascular disease and cancer may interact with micronutrients from animal and plant foods, as indicated for curcumin and celecoxib, and alter therapeutic outcomes.

2.11. SUMMARY

Arterial disease, some cancers, and possibly Alzheimer disease are promoted or accelerated by infections and environmental inflammogens. Drugs with anti-inflammatory actions appear to show corresponding benefits. These strong bidirectional effects are consistent with the major role of inflammation in the progression of vascular disease, cancer, and Alzheimer disease. Query III (Section 1.1) is well answered with major evidence for inflammation in bystander damage in aging from infections and inflammogens in aerosols and diet. The acceleration of telomere shortening by inflammation may prove to be a major mechanism in immune dysfunctions during aging (bystander type III damage, Section 1.4.3). The molecular mechanisms may include PI3K/Akt signaling, which is on the insulin signaling pathway of many mutations that increase life span of laboratory animals (Fig. 1.3A and Chapter 5). New drugs that selectively target PI3K isoforms for cancer (Kang et al, 2005; Osaki et al, 2004) and vascular disease (Walter et al, 2004) may have broader influences on longevity. Chapter 3 considers evidence that lower caloric intake and moderate physical activity can attenuate many of these chronic diseases and aging processes, in approximate parallel with the beneficial effects of anti-inflammatory drugs. The evolution of human longevity (Chapter 6) will further consider how humans became increasingly exposed to inflammation and the role of diet-aging-disease interactions.

CHAPTER 3

Energy Balance, Inflammation, and Aging

3.1. INTRODUCTION

The preceding chapter described how infections, micronutrients, and environmental inflammogens interact with arterial and Alzheimer diseases. Many examples show the synergies of inflammation and oxidative damage. This chapter considers how diet and exercise influence outcomes of aging, with a focus on inflammation and immunity, and the role of energy balance on somatic maintenance.

Diet restriction (DR) is the best documented manipulation of aging rates. DR attenuates many diseases with inflammatory processes and, in permissive environments and genotypes, increases longevity. Laboratory rodents, adapted to confinement with excess food, may be models of modern human lifestyles that promote obesity, the metaphoric 'couch potato'. Wild mice show very different responses to DR, suggesting the plasticity of metabolic genetics and energy strategies.

Dietary manipulations also further evaluate the Queries (Section 1.1) on the role of inflammation in free radical damage (Query II) and oxidant stress during aging, and effects of nutrition (Query III). The oxidant stress theory of aging, which attributes aging outcomes to damage from normal metabolism, may also be understood in terms of energy allocation strategies. At all times, individual organisms have finite energy resources for allocation to meet basal functions and the specific needs of growth, reproduction, immunity, or somatic repair (Fig. 1.2B). The gross energy balance is (not so simply) the difference of environmental energy input (food, temperature) against the expenses of basal and specialized activities. At any moment, energy may be allocated for host defense responses to invading pathogens, to flee from predators; or, for reproduction, foraging, and tissue repair in response to traumatic injury. Severe challenges may slow growth and halt reproduction. Reproductive success depends on highly evolved homeostatic (physiological) mechanisms that use external and internal information to allocate energy for survival *and* for sufficient reproduction. These energy-demanding processes vary by the stage of life history and may vary widely between sex, species, and phyla.

The energy allocation strategy varies with the phase of life history according to optima evolved for the genotype *and* within boundary values constrained by the associated mortality risks as described by life history theory (Section 1.2.8). Many species have evolved 'time-out' alternatives to reduce energy demands and mortality risks during adverse conditions. Among familiar examples, nematodes may enter diapause during larval development (dauer stages) when food is scarce, whereas bears seasonally hibernate.

The energy allocation framework helps understand how DR can modulate aging processes and longevity. Three phenomena are considered: the slowing of aging by DR; slowing of aging by exercise; and, acceleration of aging by obesity and hyperglycemia, extending discussions from Chapter 2.

3.2. DIET RESTRICTION AND AGING

'DR' is a protocol that restricts food below *ad libitum* (*ad lib*) intake, while providing required micronutrients. Depending on the study, DR may be equivalent to 'caloric restriction' or 'energy restriction' (Mattson, 2005; McCay et al, 1935; Spindler et al, 1990; Walford et al, 2002; Weindruch and Walford, 1988). Typical DR paradigms for lab rodents that provide −30% to −40% less daily food than *ad lib* intake also sharply reduce reproduction and may be considered as 'semi-starvation.' Slightly more severe DR is rapidly fatal to small rodents.

3.2.1. Overview of Animal Models

In the 1930s, Clive McCay discovered that DR had two remarkable effects when imposed after puberty: Besides the 30% increase of adult life span, DR suppressed degenerative aging changes in many tissues (McCay et al, 1935; McCay et al, 1939a; McCay et al, 1943). While the suppression of chronic diseases by DR extended earlier work[1], the extension of longevity and the system-wide effects on aging and pathology were novel. A rarely discussed additional observation of McCay is that DR suppressed chronic lung disease (McCay et al, 1939b; Saxton et al, 1946). This once common scourge of rodent colonies was due to endemic mycoplasma infections that confounded rodent studies then and for several more decades (Section 2.5.2, footnote 4). The suppression of chronic infectious respiratory disease by DR gives insights about energy balance, immunity, and aging.

Since McKay, DR with sufficient micronutrients has been shown to increase longevity in most lab models of aging (Allison et al, 2001; Finch, 1990, pp. 512–537; Masoro, 2005; Mattson, 2005; Partridge et al, 2005; Sohal and Weindruch, 1996; Weindruch and Walford, 1988). For example in male mice, DR at 40% below *ad lib* from age 4 m increased the median life span by 20% and maximum by 15%; total body weight was 55% lower (Fig. 3.1A). DR can be imposed during middle age with shorter benefits to longevity. Alternate-day *ad lib* feeding as a DR paradigm has similar benefits to life span as a restricted ration of food per day (Goodrick et al, 1990; Masoro, 2005; Mattson, 2005; Weindruch and Walford, 1988).

---

[1]McKay extended extensive prior work showing nutritional influences on chronic diseases of aging. By 1920, undernutrition was known to slow tumor growth (Moreschi, 1909; Kritchevsky, 2003; Rous, 1914; Weindruch and Walford, 1988). Conversely, high-fat diets were known to accelerate atherogenesis (Anitschkow and Chalatow, 1913; Jukema and Simoons, 1999). Osborn and Mendel had shown that undernourished, growth-arrested rats, aged 18 m, could regain growth when diet was restored (Osborne and Mendel, 1914; Osborne et al, 1917; Osborne and Mendel, 1993; Simoni et al, 2002). 'Undernutrition' differs from DR of the modern era because of undefined deficits in vitamins and other micronutrients.

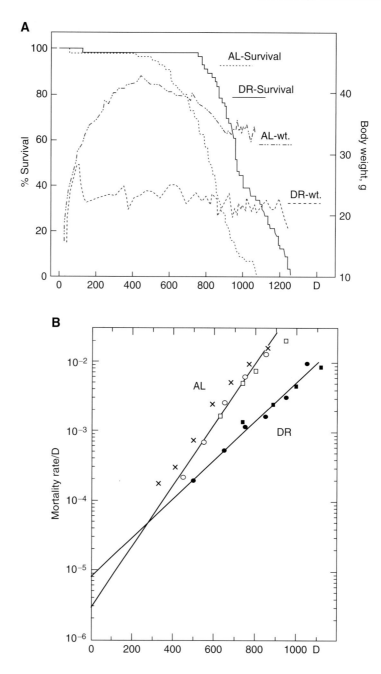

FIGURE 3.1 For legend see page 179.

(Continues)

The increase of median and maximum life span is specifically due to slowed acceleration of mortality as measured by the Gompertz slope (Fig. 3.1B) (Section 1.2.1) (Berg, 1976; Finch, 1990; Merry, 2005; Sacher, 1977). The slowed acceleration can be expressed as the mortality rate doubling time (MRDT), which DR increases by about 70%. The background mortality (initial mortality rate) is more variable between studies, and may be increased or decreased during DR (Finch, 1990, p. 508). The increased mortality before midlife in some studies (Goodrick et al, 1983; Merry, 2005; Ross, 1959) may indicate stress from fighting or stress during growth. Importantly, pre-midlife mortality variations can confound

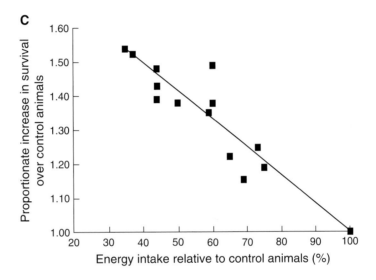

FIGURE 3.1 (continued) A. DR, longevity, and body weight in C57BL/6NNia male mice: AL, *ad lib*; DR, 40% diet restricted; S, survival; BW, body weight. Food provided as pellets of NIH-31, cereal-based open formulae with 5% fat (Turturro et al, 2002). Individual mice differ in *ad lib* food intake. Because the coefficient of variation of body weight is 2-fold larger in *ad lib* than DR groups, about 50% of the variance in body weight is attributable to individual food intake; the residual variance may represent differences in metabolic efficiency. B. DR slows mortality acceleration in rats: mortality rate slopes (Gompertz plots). From Sacher (1977, p. 616), based on data of (Berg and Simms, 1960; Ross, 1959). C. Level of DR and maximum life span. Data from 24 studies of rodents; the increase in maximum life span normalized to *ad lib* fed ($r^2 = 0.96$) (Merry, 2002).

mortality slope calculations.[2] Because the slower mortality acceleration corresponds to lower incidence of pathological lesions and many other aging changes, DR is considered to slow or delay the fundamental processes in aging (Finch, 1990, pp. 512–537; Finch et al., 2002; Merry, 2002; Weindruch et al, 2001). Over a wide range of 20–65% DR, life span increased proportionately (Fig. 3.1C). Depending on the protocol and animal model, mortality may increase above −60% DR; e.g., in a mouse model, DR at −60 % *ad lib* caused high mortality after 8d (Dagon, 2005). Thus, extreme DR may not have generalizable benefits to longevity. Notably, humans starve to death as DR approaches 50% (Section 3.2.3).

The benefit of DR to rodent life span is attributed to the limitation of energy input (caloric restriction): There is no increase of life span from selective restriction of carbohydrate, fat, or protein unless caloric intake is restricted (Masoro, 2005; Weindruch and Walford, 1988). Two general physiological responses to DR are consistent with the energy limitation hypothesis: lower fasting blood glucose and higher glucocorticoids (Han et al, 2001; Masoro et al, 1992; Sabatino et al, 1991) (Fig. 3.2). Cortisol in humans and corticosterone in rodents are gluconeogenic by inducing enzymes in the liver and other tissues that process catabolized reserves to glucose.

Despite the slower weight gain during −40% DR, rats show increases of total fat mass and number of adipocytes (Bertrand et al, 1980; Lesser et al, 1973; Yu et al, 1982). In male F344 rats, total fat accumulations were maximum after midlife in both *ad lib* and DR groups and then declined in all rats before death. The epididymal fat pad showed similar growth, with up to 2-fold increases of weight and 30% increases of adipocyte numbers. Lean body mass also increased in DR and *ad lib* groups.

Wild-derived mice (a true wild-type) showed no effect of DR on the mean life span, but a subgroup of 8% did outlive the *ad lib* group (Harper et al, 2006a) (Fig. 3.3A). Their maximum life span of 1600 d was below the lab mouse record of 1742 d (figure legend). These wild-derived mice are smaller than lab mice (Fig. 3.3B, C) and live as long as conventional lab mice on DR (Miller et al, 2002b). As in lab strains, DR caused an initial loss of weight that stabilized at 15 grams, which was 55% below the maximum weight of *ad lib* fed wild mice (Fig. 3.3B). Nonetheless, these mice did show several responses to DR as expected from lab mice: lower body weight (Fig. 3.3C), 80% fewer tumors, and elevated corticosterone and decreased testosterone (Harper et al, 2006a) (hormonal responses to DR are discussed in Section 3.2.5).

Wild mice at capture have much less fat (4%) than *ad lib* fed wild mice lab-reared (12%) or conventional lab mice (Fig. 3.3C). When purged of parasites and adjusted to lab conditions, wild-derived mice eat less *ad lib* than lab mice per gram body mass (Austad and Kristan, 2003). Lab rodents may be considered as

---

[2]Increased mortality which is common early in DR (Finch, 1990, pp. 507–509) will statistically force a lower slope on a linear regression model, even if later mortality is not reduced. In Fig. 3.2B, the early mortality was not included to avoid this bias (Sacher, 1977, p. 616), based on data of (Berg and Simms 1960; Ross, 1959).

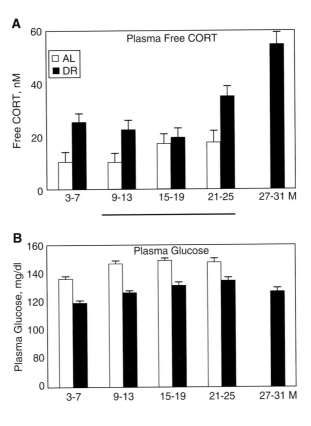

FIGURE 3.2 Diet restriction (DR) elevates blood glucocorticoids and lowers glucose. Plasma corticosterone (free CORT) (A) and glucose in male F344 rats, longitudinal sampling. Free CORT data from Table 4 of (Sabatino et al, 1991); plasma glucose from Table 1 of (Masoro et al, 1992). (Redrawn from Patel and Finch, 2002.)

models for modern human lifestyles with *ad lib* food and few physical demands (Section 3.6). In contrast, the great apes, with whom we share ancestors, spend most of their waking hours foraging over considerable distances (Chapter 6). Wild rodents also move extensively to meet energy demands and even on running wheels cover several miles a day.

More generally, the relationship of body fat to life span is far from resolved. Other studies of inbred rodents have strong associations of fat load to longevity [reviewed in (Allison et al, 2001; Weindruch and Walford, 1988)]. For example, in two studies of DR rodents total fat mass correlated with life span: F344 rats

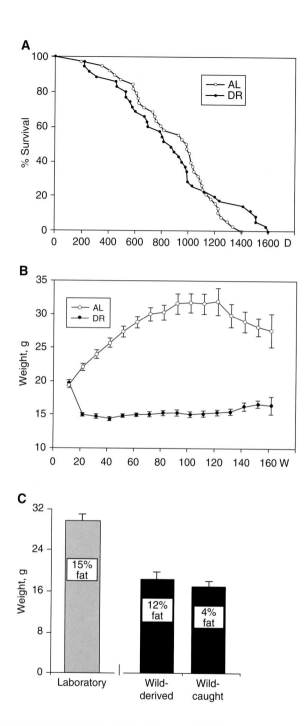

FIGURE 3.3 For legend see page 183.

(Bertrand et al, 1980; Yu et al, 1982) and C3B10F1 mice (Weindruch and Walford, 1988, p. 71). However, fat load and dietary intake may be independent variables in longevity. In a classic experiment with obese mice, DR increased life span to that of controls on DR and slowed collagen aging. Nonetheless, the obese mice still had 2-fold more fat/g body weight than the controls (Harrison et al, 1984). Thus, high fat loads do not preclude normal longevity in some conditions. Humans also show modest associations of body fat with mortality risk over a wide range (Section 3.4, below).

Because DR suppressed lung infections in MacKay's early colony, aging of germ-free mice is of interest. In early colonies, germ-free mice lived slightly longer (Gordon et al, 1966). As observed under modern conditions (Tazume et al, 1991), *ad lib* fed germ-free mice lived 20% longer than specific-pathogen free (SPF) mice and did not show senescent weight loss, suggesting effects from endogenous pathogens in the SPF mice. While DR increased life spans in both groups, the SPF mice outlived the germ-free. Frustratingly, no data were given on organ pathology. The germ-free status profoundly alters immune system functions, with unknown consequences to aging.

DR paradigms that provide a single ration of daily food may not apply simply to some invertebrate models. DR did not increase longevity in the medfly (Mediterranean fruit fly, *Ceratitis capitata*; restricted food provided once per day) (Carey et al, 2002). The lack of DR benefit to life span in this paradigm may be due to a form of starvation, because *Drosophila melanogaster* (not a true fruit fly) feeds at least once an hour (M. Piper, cited in Partridge et al, 2005). Female fly life spans show a strong inverted-U dose response of food concentration (Clancy et al, 2002) (Chapter 5, Fig. 5.6). On an alternative DR paradigm with a series of nutrient dilution, the fly feeding frequency was increased in proportion to dilution, with shortening of life span (Carvalho et al, 2005).

However, interpretation of lab DR experiments must consider nutrition in context with the reproductive schedule. The fruitfly *Anastrepha ludens* shows gradients in the interactions of nutrition, egg production, and mortality, with some

FIGURE 3.3 Wild *(Mus musculus)* mice live longer and respond differently to diet restriction (DR). Wild-caught mice (Idaho stock), males, 40% DR after 4 m (Harper et al, 2006a). A. Survival. Median life span was not altered by DR, but the longest lived mice (8% total) were DR. The longest lived DR survived to 1600 d. The credible maximum life span for lab mice may be 1742 d (F1 hybrid of B6CBA; DR until 1541 d) (Harrison and Archer, 1987). Wild mice derived from tropical islands did not live as long as the Idaho stock (Miller, 2002). B. Body weight *ad lib* (AL) or 40% DR (Harper et al, 2006a). C. Wild mouse body weight and fat content: laboratory (4-way cross, see footnote 2) and wild-derived *ad lib* fed, age 4 m; wild-caught (Austad and Kristan, 2003).

contour transects that do not alter life span (Carey et al, 2007). Thus, DR gradients on mortality should not be simply interpreted as degrees of starvation.

Moreover, DR would not be expected to increase the long life spans of social insect queens, which are fed high levels of food to support their continuing egg production. In a very different life history, ferox trout acquire greater longevity than slower growing members of their cohort when they switch their diet to larger prey fish (Finch, 1990, pp. 142–143). Modeling of ferox growth rates shows parameter domains (windows) in mortality rates and competition for prey food that favor extreme longevity (Mangel and Abrahams, 2001). The manipulations of aging by nutrition must consider the 'reproductive costs,' which will lead to understanding of the resource allocation strategies evolved in each species and sex.

3.2.2. Diet Restriction and Disease in Rodent Models

The attenuation of specific chronic diseases by DR gives an almost complete account of why DR to 30-40% below *ad lib* increases longevity in lab rodents. DR delays and attenuates most spontaneous diseases of aging (Lipman et al, 1999a; Weindruch and Walford, 1988). To a first approximation, DR right shifts (delays) the schedule of chronic pathology. The robust generalizability of these findings is remarkable given the diversity of chronic degenerative changes in the lab rodent genotypes. Instructive examples come from studies on two widely used inbred rodents: the Fisher 344 rat ('F344') and C57BL/6 mouse ('B6').

In aging male F344 rats, three conditions account for most mortality, all of which were attenuated by DR: chronic kidney disease, cardiomyopathy, and tumors (Section 1.2). DR delayed the onset age of chronic kidney disease, as well as degeneration of skeletal muscle and bone (Lipman et al, 1999a; Maeda et al, 1985; Shimokawa et al, 1993b; Weindruch and Walford, 1988). Shared pathophysiologic mechanisms in these different organs may be seated in kidney dysfunctions. Aging rats are vulnerable to progressive renal degeneration (glomerulosclerosis), with progressive inflammatory responses and glycated proteins (AGE) to major dysfunction. Human kidneys increasingly show similar changes during aging, possibly in association with high protein diets (Brenner et al, 1982; Hostetter et al, 1986). The 'renal-hyperparathyroid disease' of aging rats elevates serum parathyroid hormone and calcitonin in correspondence to the degree of glomerulosclerosis; in turn, the elevated parathyroid hormone and calcitonin mobilize calcium and cause bone loss (Armbrecht et al, 1988; Kalu et al, 1988; Maeda et al, 1985). DR attenuates all these changes and prevented the renal degeneration from reaching 'end-stage renal disease,' which is a major cause of death (Yu et al, 1982). Cardiomyopathy was closely linked to the degree of kidney disease (Maeda et al, 1985) and was also attenuated by DR (Lipman et al, 1999; Maeda et al, 1985). Most tumors in aging rats are benign, e.g., the testicular interstitial cell tumors found in nearly all aging F344 rats, which, like rarer malignant growths, are attenuated by DR (Maeda et al, 1985).

The bone, parathyroid, and myocardial pathology and systemic pathophysiology illustrate multi-organ degenerative cascades stemming from renal dysfunctions. In humans, chronic kidney disease is becoming a major problem during aging due to the increase of diabetes; other consequences include anemia and very high risk of coronary heart disease (Astor et al, 2006; Foley, 2005; Foley et al, 2005). The restriction of energy had a larger effect on kidney degeneration than protein restriction alone (Masoro, 1989). In humans, low protein diets are clinically effective in slowing chronic kidney disease (Mitch, 2005; Remuzzi et al, 2006).

In aging male B6 mice, the main degenerative diseases and causes of death are also slowed by DR (Turturro et al, 2002). The diseases overlap with F344 rats but with different proportions. Sarcomas involving spleen and liver are the major cause of death (80%), the 'reticulum cell sarcoma'(Dunn, 1954; Finch et al, 1969; Finch and Foster, 1973), whereas testicular tumors are rare (Bronson, 1990). Although delayed by DR, sarcoma incidence eventually becomes as prevalent as in *ad lib* feeding. Kidney disease, affecting 60–80% of B6 mice, was also attenuated in severity and delayed by DR (Turturro et al, 2002). Cardiomyopathy (fibrosis and myocarditis) and thrombosis, which may be less common (<50%) in aging B6 mice than in F344 rats (Bronson, 1990, Tables 4, 7, 8), were also attenuated by DR (Turturro et al, 2002). Extreme hypercholesterolemia is required to induce aortic atherosclerosis, as in apoE-knockout mice (apoE–/– on the B6 background, Section 1.2.6), which again is attenuated by DR (Guo, 2002).

Tumor suppression by DR has received great attention (Kritchevsky, 1995; Weindruch and Walford, 1988; Weindruch, 1992). Further examples of tumor suppression by DR from this century-deep literature (see footnote 1) include spontaneous and carcinogen-induced breast cancer (Dirx et al, 2003b; Kritchevsky, 1995; Thompson et al, 2004a,b); prostate cancer (TRA rMP mouse) (Suttie et al, 2005); intestinal tumors (APC mutant model) (Mai et al, 2003); leukemia, whether spontaneous (Shimokawa et al, 1993b) or radiation-induced (Yoshida et al, 1997); and transplanted astrocytomas (Mai et al, 2003). Observations by physicians on malnourished human populations suggest a lower incidence of malignancy (Keys et al., 1950, pp. 1053–1056; Murray and Murray, 1981). Even short-term DR can increase latency and incidence over the rodent lifespan (Klebanov, 2007). Conversely, many tumors attenuated by DR can be accelerated by high-fat diets. Given the diverse mechanisms in cancer, it is remarkable that DR has such broad effects across genotype-specific abnormal growths.

But the lower chronic diseases in DR do not fully account for the increased life span in rodents! Causes of death are not always single and simple. At later ages, humans and other mammals accumulate multiple degenerative changes or co-morbidities (Section 1.2; rats, Fig. 1.5). Even the inbred status does not eliminate the wide variations between individuals in the location and severity of various co-existing lesions at later ages, as well documented for genetically identical worms in the same culture dish (Section 5.2) (Finch and Kirkwood, 2000, pp. 16–18). Although the smooth acceleration of mortality (Fig. 1.1C) would indicate a simpler situation, we have yet to develop a theory of mortality and aging that accounts for the impact of diverse lesions.

The reduction of chronic aging lesions by DR adds the remarkable puzzle that about one-fourth of DR rodents at death have no organ degeneration by careful histopathology (Shimokawa et al, 1993b). Lacking definable pathology in this

ad lib subgroup, I suggest that death from cardiac arrest could be due to fluctuations of blood glucose, which might be more labile in the lower blood glucose
characteristic of DR, particularly in the fasting state before next feeding. A precedent is the sudden 'dead-in-bed syndrome' of humans. Transient hypoglycemia
is implicated in sudden death from cardiac arrest in type 1 diabetics (insulin-defi-
cient), who have 3-fold more unexpected death than healthy young (Heller,
2002). This hypothesis might be tested by detailed serial sampling of blood to
characterize variability of glucose and insulin, and examination of time of death.

3.2.3. Diet Restriction, Starvation, Vascular Disease, and Longevity in Humans

We do not know how DR applies to humans. If applicable, DR will operate in
a lower range than the $\geq 50\%$ below *ad lib* tolerated by rodents, because 50% or
more DR is fatal to humans, discussed below. Consider the current evidence for
mortality as a function of total fat, measured as body mass index (BMI),
weight/height^2 (metric) (Fig. 3.4). By convention (National Center for Health
Statistics), BMI of healthy adults is ≥ 18.5–25; BMI ≥ 25 is overweight; ≥ 30 is obesity. These criteria for overweight and underweight are being further specified
for growth stage in children, gender, and ethnicity.

All populations consistently show U- or J-shaped curves of BMI and mortality,
with increasing mortality at the extremes. Two major U.S. studies that sample
overlapping subpopulations are being intensely discussed because of differences
in the BMI mortality curves (Fig. 3.4); the legends describe the populations.
As documented in NHANES (Flegal et al, 2005), mortality risk is low over the
broad range, BMI 18.5–30, which encompasses about 70% of the adult U.S. population (Fig. 3.4A). These findings were recently extended by a prospective study
of the NIH-AARP cohort aged 50–71 (Adams et al, 2006). Both studies agree that
risks of obesity decreased with age, but controversies continue about the possibility of a 'safe' level of fat; e.g., NHANES shows negligible effect of BMI 25–30
on mortality in 70 and older. The impact of obesity is greatest in non-smokers in
the NIH-AARP sample, which showed a steep J curve for BMI > 25 in both men
and women. These studies concur with the general conclusion that obesity, particularly morbid obesity with BMI > 35, is a mortality risk factor through diabetes
(not identified here). Extreme thinness (BMI < 17.5) indicates anorexia or wasting
disease, and is hazardous because atrophy of the myocardium during extreme
weight reduction can cause sudden death (Galetta et al, 2005; Sullivan et al, 2002).

Where might our Venus of Willendorf (cover image) fit on these curves? Although
her obese profile suggests a BMI > 30, we could not estimate mortality risks for obesity in the Paleolithic even if we knew the distribution of BMIs and ages at death,
because environmental hazards were so much greater than in these modern
populations, and life expectancy was probably much lower (Fig. 1.1, legend).

Moreover, the BMI is a bulk measure of fat that does not resolve the various
types of fat depots which differ by physiology and association with diabetes.
Visceral fat in particular is strongly implicated as an independent mortality risk

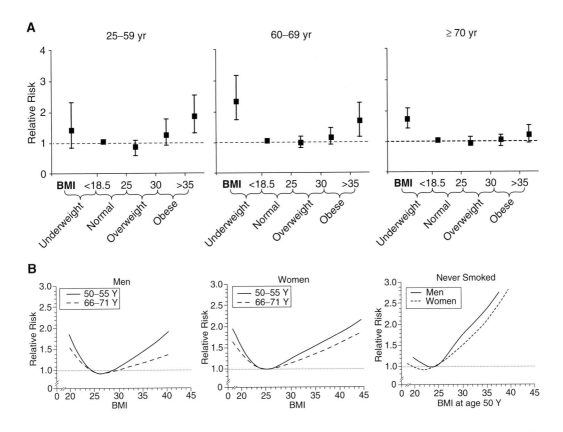

FIGURE 3.4 Body mass index (BMI) and mortality risk in U.S. population samples. Adult BMI ≥ 25 is classified as overweight and BMI ≥ 30 obese. A. The relative risk 1.0 is for BMI from 18 to < 25. From the National Health and Nutrition Examination Surveys (NHANES) through 2000. NHANES collects health data by direct interviews and medical examinations to obtain a statistically valid profile of the non-institutionalized U.S. population of all ages. (Redrawn from Flegal et al, 2005.) B. Prospective study of the NIH-AARP cohort aged 50–71 years at enrollment in 1995–1996. The respondents were 18% of AARP membership (313,047 men; 214,218 women). Non-smokers also show definitively increased mortality with BMI >25. (Redrawn from Adams et al, 2006.)

factor in mortality. The fat-mortality relationship is curvilinear, suggesting a threshold level (Kuk et al, 2006). Visceral fat is more strongly correlated with abdominal circumference than the BMI and more closely linked to the risk of diabetes (Despres, 2006; Frayn, 2000). Thus, the broad range of BMI with little apparent effect on mortality risk seen in NHANES may hide higher risk groups. Moreover, recall from Fig. 3.3B and the discussion of obese lab mice, that longevity in wild mice was independent of fat levels over a 2-fold range. These controversies aside, evidence is building that DR has many benefits to vascular risk factors.

The first controlled study of DR was the 'Minnesota Starvation Experiment,' conducted in 1945 by Ancel Keys[3] and an expert team (Keys et al, 1950; Keys, 1994). Their objective was to model 'semi-starvation and rehabilitation' as a guide to the optimum treatment of WWII starvation victims. The young male volunteers were average age 25.5 y, with initial BMI of 21.8 and in excellent health. The 50% level of diet restriction (average 1800 kcal/d, or 7531 kJ) was adjusted for the individual *ad lib* intake. Under close observation and in a congenial environment with state-of-the-art health care, most of the volunteers (32/36) managed to endure 50% DR for 24 wks. However, this regimen was unsustainable and caused progressive debilitation. Abnormal behaviors emerged by 6 wks, including confusion, depression, lassitude, loss of sex drive, and suicidal thoughts. The required exercise of walking 22 miles/wk became increasingly difficult. Most experienced severely painful lower limb edema, but all had general edema (increased extracellular fluid space) (Keys et al, 1950, p. 926). No serious infections were observed, and the incidence of colds was not increased. The study was terminated by 24 wks when the average BMI reached 16, now recognized as very hazardous. Average weight had declined by 32% and body fat by 70% (Keys et al, 1950, p. 284).

With food restored, mood and behavior slowly normalized. Initial *ad lib* food intake was up to 10,000 kcal/d, gradually normalizing to 3200–4500 kcal/d (Keys et al, 1950, p. 78). Weight recovered rapidly and overshot initial values. However, the replaced mass was mostly fat; one year later, fat was still 40% over starting values (*ibid.*, p. 70). Major directed exercise was required to regain muscle (Kalm and Semba, 2005).

Half of the group survived to age 80 or more and were recently interviewed (Kalm and Semba, 2005). These survivors thus lived at least 8 y longer than expected for men born in 1920 who were about age 24 when the study was begun (U.S. Social Security Table for 1920 cohort: 71.5 y life expectancy). Decades later, (Keys, 1994) stated that there were "no lasting effects." But no data are reported. The lifetime health profiles of those who predeceased the present survivors might give insights about causes of earlier mortality. As discussed in Section 4.7, severe famine may have remarkably little effect on the mortality of the survivors. Starvation during WWII has not altered Dutch adult mortality up

---

[3]This study was motivated by urgent need for information on how to safely restore food to the survivors of starvation during WWII. The Minnesota Starvation volunteers were 'conscientious objectors', who included Max Kampelman, later prominent in nuclear arms reduction (Kalm and Semba, 2005). Keys was an early advocate of the cardio-protective lifestyle through regular exercise and a diet with low fat and fresh fruit and vegetables. He showed that blood cholesterol varies with dietary saturated fatty acids and cholesterol, and inversely with polyunsaturates (the 'Keys equation'). Keys later added the Centenarian status to his achievements.

to age 57, nor did Finnish famine of 1866–1868 alter life spans of adult survivors. However, birth cohorts exposed to famine during pregnancy from malnourished Dutch mothers have increased adult heart disease (Section 4.7).

Few population-level studies have been made of the effects of DR on heart disease or longevity in those transiently malnourished as adults. During both world wars, vascular mortality apparently declined in association with lower caloric intake (Crawford and Blankenhorn, 1979; Keys et al, 1950; Keys, 1994; Strom and Jenson, 1951). Interviews with physicians present during the famine in Leningrad (St. Petersburg), 1941–1942 "…were positive about the relative reduction in coronary disease" (Keys et al., 1950, p. 617). However, starvation did not prevent horrible epidemics of typhus and dysentery in the German POW camps, also fostered by the execrable sanitation (Markowski, 1945). The two-volume report of Keys et al. (1950) discusses many other first hand observations of chronic and infectious disease during malnutrition. Table 3.1 summarizes these data for comparison with Biosphere and CRON studies, discussed later.

An unplanned semi-starvation 'experience' with additional emotional and physical stress absent from the Minnesota experiment occurred in 'Biosphere 2' (1991–1993) (Verdery and Walford, 1998; Walford et al, 1992; Walford et al, 2002). Eight adult men and women, ages 27–67, including Roy Walford, a leading proponent of DR (Finch, 2004b), spent two years under the Biosphere's huge glass domes in the Arizona desert, which were designed to support ecosystems that would provide all food and oxygen, but with external electrical power to maintain air conditioning and other machinery. However, the food production was overestimated, and yielded only 1750–2100 kcal/d, with sufficient micronutrients (Walford et al, 2002). This ration is marginally above the 1800 kcal/d (50% DR) in the Minnesota Starvation Experiment (Table 3.1). Because all 'biosphereans' received the same rations irrespective of body size (110 lbs to 208 lbs), it is not possible to calculate the level of DR more precisely than in a range of 20–40%

TABLE 3.1 Diet Restriction and Cardiovascular Risk Indicators in Humans

	Food Intake, kcal/d	Body Mass Index	Blood Pressure, mm Hg	Total Cholesterol, mg/dl	HDL Cholesterol, mg/dl	Tri-Glycerides	C-reactive Protein, g/ml
Minnesota 1944*	1,800	16.6 (−24%)	94.7/64.4 (−10%, sys)	151 (−10%)			
Biosphere 1991–1993**	1,750–2,200	19	90/60	125 (−30 %)	55 (+30%)	80	
CRON Study 2004+	1,112–1,958	19.6 (−18%)	101/61 (−30%, sys)	158 (−18%)	63 (+30%)	48 (−64%)	0.3 (−80%)

*Minnesota Starvation Experiment: (Keys et al, 1950, 1994). Values at termination of the experiment (% changes from beginning).
**Biosphere 2: (Walford et al., 2002); approximate mean values.
+CRON study of the Caloric Restriction Society (Fontana et al, 2004; Meyer et al, 2006).

DR. Hunger became so intense between meals that it was finally necessary to lock up the food stores (Alling and Nelson, 1993, p. 86).

An average weight loss of 17% weight stabilized in the first year at BMI of about 19 (Weyer et al, 2000). These BMI values are higher than those in the Minnesota Starvation Experiment (BMI 16) and are in the range of the current self-selected DR group (BMI, 19.5) in the CRON Study (see below). Cardiovascular risk factors improved, including 35% lower blood total cholesterol (initial average 190 mg/dl dropping to 125 mg/dl) (Verdery and Walford, 1998). Both LDL and HDL cholesterol decreased in parallel, which increased the LDL–HDL ratio. Lower fasting glucose (−21%) and insulin (−42%) are consistent with the observed lower glycated hemoglobin (HbA1$_c$, −30%), which reflects integrated exposure to blood glucose. These positive vascular changes cannot be attributed only to DR, because all engaged in intense physical activity, up to 80 h/wk in maintaining the Biosphere. However, the 'melting' fat depots released polychlorinated biphenyls (PCBs) into the blood (Walford et al, 1999), which may have had adverse cytotoxic effects (see below).

Despite the physical and social stresses and the lower white blood cell count (−31%), there were no persistent infections or serious illness (5 'off-work' days due to illness, < 0.1% total) (Walford et al, 2002). Unlike those in the Minnesota Starvation experiment, there was little depression or lethargy, and sexual activities continued at some level (discretely, Walford did not provide quantitative data). Menstrual cycles were reported to 'continue' by the four young women, despite major loss of body fat. This apparent challenge to the hypothesized critical level of fat to support ovulation (Frisch and Revelle, 1970) is discussed in Section 3.6. However, no data are available on cycle length or ovulation.

An additional confound in interpreting these data as a 'DR experiment' is the abnormalities in the gas composition that developed. The huge concrete surfaces in the Biosphere structure absorbed atmospheric oxygen (Walford et al, 1996), which caused a serious decline in oxygen levels from 21% to 14.2%, equivalent to 14,000 feet altitude. Another abnormality was that the atmospheric pCO_2 and pCO were close to sea level, an abnormal ratio which could promote CO-induced apoptosis (Tofighi et al, 2006). Symptoms of high-altitude sickness[4] were consistent with hemoglobin saturation curves (Paglia and Walford, 2005). However, none of the eight developed compensatory erythropoeisis, which would be expected at this pO_2.

---

[4]In our phone conversations, Walford's voice became flat and halting. After about 16 m, he could no longer do simple arithmetic. When supplemental oxygen was pumped in to the Biosphere, his voice and cognition soon recovered (Alling, 1993). Walford practiced and preached DR before and after the Biosphere (The 120 Year Diet, 2000). We cannot know if his terrible neuromotor disease was connected to his exotic lifestyle, which went beyond nutrition (Finch, 2004a).

There may be long-term consequences from the combinations of DR, intense physical activity, elevated blood PCBs, and abnormal atmosphere. After returning to the outside world, Walford at age 69 slowly developed 'atypical parkinsonism and motor neuron syndrome' (Lassinger et al, 2004) causing his death 10 years later. His lifespan of 79, though, was not premature for his birth cohort. The elevated blood PCBs may have been a factor in his terrible creeping neuromotor pathology, because PCB neurotoxicity is implicated in Parkinson disease (Finch, 2004b; Grandjean et al, 2001; Lee and Opanshuk, 2004; Steenland et al, 2006). Moreover, PCBs are proinflammatory and may be factors in cancer (Ruder et al, 2006; Walker et al, 2005) and vascular disease (Hennig et al, 2002, 2005). PCBs and other fat-soluble industrial pollutants released from fat during weight loss warrant consideration in campaigns to reduce body fat. The remaining Biosphereans' health status should be followed further.

Sound data on DR are coming from several ongoing studies by the CRON study of the Caloric Restriction Society and CALERIE (The Comprehensive Assessment of the Long-term Effects of Reducing Intake of Energy). Although self-selected, these individuals had blood lipid profiles and other clinical characteristics close to the median of their U.S. age group (Fontana et al, 2004a; Meyer et al, 2006b). It must be noted that these subjects are not randomized controls from a general population, such as was needed to prove the benefits of aspirin and statins to heart disease (Chapter 2), and we know little of their prior lifestyles.

In the CRON study, men and women of average age 50 have maintained DR since 2001 (Fontana et al, 2004a, 2006a). Body weights have stabilized at BMI of 19.5 kg/m^2, within the normal range, with lower risk factors for vascular disease, relative to age-matched healthy controls on more typical American diets (Fontana et al, 2004a; Meyer et al, 2006b): blood cardiovascular indicators include 75% lower cholesterol ratio of total cholesterol: HDL-C; 80% lower C-reactive protein; 50% lower TNFα and 15% lower TGF-β1 (Table 3.1). Plasma triglyceride levels were in the 5th-percentile of 20-year-olds. These blood lipid values were reached within 1 year. Serum T_3 (thyroid hormone, triiodothyronine) is 20% lower, while serum T_4 and TSH did not change. The lower serum T_3 was attributed to the DR regimen because endurance runners with similar BMI who ate a more typical Western diet did not have lower T_3 (Fontana et al, 2006a).

Arterial indicators are also improved. The carotid wall thickness was slightly higher than age group norms of those with no indication of cardiovascular disease (shown on Fig. 1.14). Diastolic blood flow velocity has improved to younger values, in association with decreased stiffness of the left ventricle (Meyer et al, 2006). The reduction in stiffness implies less myocardial fibrosis, which is implicated in arrhythmias that can cause sudden death (Zannad and Radauceanu, 2005). In rodent models (Sun et al, 2005a), myocardial fibrosis and collagen levels are increased by TGF-β1 overexpression and decreased by TGF-β1 deficiency (Brooks and Conrad, 2000; Siwik and Colucci, 2004). DR also decreases myocardial fibrosis in aging B6 mice (Turturro et al, 2002; Section 2.5.2).

In the CALERIE study, 48 volunteers were selected for good physical and mental health, with body compositions expected for their ages (BMI 27.5, range 25–30; men <50 y; women, <45 y) (Heilbronn, 2006; Larson-Meyer et al, 2006). Participants received "significant monetary compensation." Four randomized groups differed by level of DR (12.5% and 25% DR) and exercise (12.5% DR). By 6 months the DR groups had lost more than 10% initial weight. DR also lowered core temperature, fasting insulin, T_3, and leukocyte DNA fragmentation (−5%, comet assay). Visceral fat and fat cell size decreased in correspondence with improved insulin sensitivity. However, DR did not alter fasting glucose or serum protein carbonyl (measure of oxidant damage, Section 1.4.2). Energy expenditure (24 h metabolic chamber) decreased in proportion to non-fat body mass and was 6% lower than expected from the loss of metabolic mass. The lower T_3 and proportionate 24-hour energy expenditures show metabolic adaptations that also occur during obesity weight-reduction through DR and exercise.

3.2.4. Diet Restriction, Infections and Inflammation

Chronic energy deficits, with or without micronutrient defects, increase susceptibility to infections (Cunningham-Rundles et al, 2005; Felblinger, 2003; Kikafunda et al, 1998; McMahon et al, 1993; Scrimshaw, 1959, 2003; Scrimshaw et al, 1968). Without doubt, adequate nutrition enhances recovery from most systemic infections. Consider these examples from a huge field of study: Rene Dubos's classic studies showed that fasting for 30 h before infection of prepubertal mice sharply increased mortality from *Klebsiella pneumoniae*, tuberculosis, and staphylococcus (Dubos, 1955; Schaedler and Dubos, 1956; Smith and Dubos, 1956). *Ad lib* feeding for only 24 hrs restored resistance to control levels (Schaedler and Dubos, 1956). However, DR imposed during primary immunization impaired secondary immune responses, even though food was restored (Martin et al, 2007). Moreover with DR, sepsis (systemic infections) from intestinal puncture caused earlier mortality and impaired macrophage activities (Sun et al, 2001). And, there is general agreement that DR lowers the white blood cell count, by ≥ 50% in rodents (McCay et al, 1935; McCay et al, 1939a,b; McCay et al, 1943; Weindruch and Walford, 1988, p. 184) and by 20% in macaques (Roecker et al, 1996; Weindruch et al, 1997). Having recognized the larger adverse effects of DR on pathogen resistance, much may be learned from the exceptions.

McCay's finding that DR attenuated chronic bacterial lung infections (Section 3.2.1) has been extended in various rodent models (Miller, 1991; Mo et al, 2003; Pahlavani, 2000; Spaulding et al, 1997). DR also has powerful anti-inflammatory effects, which we and others have proposed are a major basis for the slowing of aging by DR (Chung, 2001; Morgan et al., 1999). These findings were also anticipated 50 years ago by Nevin Scrimshaw's benchmark review, which concluded that malnutrition reduced the severity of infections in about 20% of 484 studies, e.g., malaria parasitemia in humans and domestic animals (Scrimshaw, 1959). However, few generalizations seem possible because many pathogens have specific micronutrient requirements and because of specific interactions of host and pathogen genotypes.

In unique observations from 1973–1993, the Murrays studied large groups of African nomadics who were famine refugees (4382 Ss) (Murray et al, 1995). Adults with severe weight losses of ≥ 25% were evaluated for chest and gut diseases, including parasites. Despite the high prevalence of infectious diseases, only 22% of famine victims showed symptoms of infections. During the first 2 weeks of refeeding, latent infections rapidly emerged (Fig. 3.5), particularly malaria, brucellosis, and tuberculosis, in association with bloody diarrhea and fever. During weight gains averaging 4.2 kg, symptomatic infections increased 10-fold. Serum CRP was <10 mg/L in most (82%) before refeeding. Of those with initially low CRP, after refeeding, 32% had huge CRP elevations (49 ± 7 mg/L). The group of 68% with low CRP before and after refeeding closely matched the

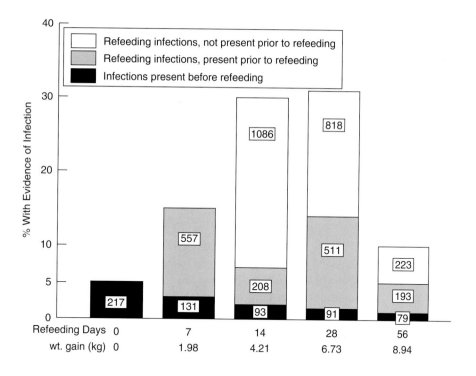

FIGURE 3.5 Infections in African famine victims, examined medically before and after refeeding. Symptomatic infections rapidly increased 10-fold, particularly falciparum malaria, brucellosis, and tuberculosis, which were initially latent. (Redrawn from Murray et al, 1995.)

78% without symptoms. Increased leptin, an immunoregulator, would also be expected from refeeding and from the resurgence of infections (Section 1.3.3). In another study of Masai pastoralists, skin lesions from herpes simplex virus and molluscum contagiosum (pox virus) were absent during famine and emerged about 6 weeks after refeeding, afflicting 50% of children (Murray et al, 1980). These field observations may not meet modern criteria (Beisel, 1982) and differ from the infections observed in starving POWs, as noted above (Markowski, 1945).

These African observations, however, led to further insights into DR effects and the important hypothesis that anorexia of the acute phase response is a host defense mechanism (Section 1.3.1) (Murray and Murray, 1979).[5] In a pioneering experiment, mice that were lethally infected with *Listeria monocytogenes* (gram-positive) were observed to cease feeding within 4 h; the mortality of infected mice was *doubled* by force-feeding to *ad lib* intake (Murray and Murray, 1979b). Moreover, starvation for 48 h enhanced clearance of *Listeria* from liver and spleen (Wing and Barczynski, 1984; Wing et al, 1986) and, again, decreased mortality (Wing and Young, 1980). These effects are due to acute energy deficits.

Anorexia is now well recognized as a behaviorally integrated acute phase response to microbial endotoxins in mammals and birds (Exton, 1997; Hart, 1990; Johnson, 1998; Owen-Ashley et al, 2006). The bacterial endotoxin LPS induces transient anorexia, mediated by IL-1 at the hypothalamic level through prostaglandins; the LPS-induced anorexia is attenuated by NSAIDs and can even be evoked as a conditioned response (Exton et al, 1995; Exton, 1997). LPS-induced sickness behaviors include sleep and reduced exploratory locomotion. Anorexia is also induced by gastro-intestinal parasites. Rats infected with a nematode (*Nippostrongylus brasielensis*) developed anorexia in proportion to the larval dose; after parasites were cleared, rats became transiently hyperphagic (Horbury et al, 1995).

Anorexia nervosa may also increase resistance to influenza infections and colds (Barbouche et al, 1993; Bowers and Eckart, 1978; Wade et al, 1985). In one of the few clinical reports, anorectics responded to influenza immunization with greater primary antibody levels (Armstrong-Esther et al, 1978). The lower fever of anorectics during bacterial infections (Birmingham et al, 2003) is expected from the smaller elevations of the fever-inducing cytokines IL-1, IL-6, and TNFα (Nagata, 1999) and may be considered as an outcome of limited energy resources (Fig. 1.2B).

The sexes differ importantly in anorectic responses to infections. The LPS-induced anorexia was greater in female than male rats (Wichmann et al, 2000):

---

[5]Hippocrates asserted in the 5th Century BCE "...in times of epidemics, the body should be kept thin and weak", echoed in the old maxim "Feed a cold and starve a fever". Other historical lore and early experiments on diet and infections are surveyed by (McCay, 1947; Murray et al, 1978a; Murray et al, 1995).

Feeding during estrus was most affected and is estrogen-dependent (Geary et al, 2004). These findings concur with women's stronger acute phase responses and survival during severe sepsis (systemic infections) (Geary et al, 2004). Their greater elevations of IL-10 ('anti-inflammatory' modulator) may be a factor in these important sex differences (Schroder et al, 1998).

Some experiments have extended the Murrays' observations that acute DR can attenuate infections, at least in a protected lab environment. In young rats, −25% DR for 3 weeks enhanced clearance of *Streptococcus* from the lung (Fig. 3.6A) and attenuated inflammation, as shown directly by the smaller macrophage production of NO and TNFα (Fig. 3.6B) (Dong et al, 1998). In a mouse model of fatal cerebral malaria, modest DR increased survival to 50% from zero in the *ad lib* fed and improved cell immunity (CD4[+] T-cells) (Hunt et al, 1993). Deaths from infection/septicemia due to infected skin ulcers in mice were decreased 3-fold by 40% DR (infections were not defined) (Perkins et al, 1998).

However, the effects of DR on responses to influenza virus in aging rodent models are opposite to these observations. Aging DR mice given influenza intranasally had *greater* mortality than *ad lib* fed mice and a much higher lung virus load (Gardner, 2005). However, DR attenuated age impairments in lectin-induced T-cell proliferation in this and in other studies (Fig. 3.7) (Effros et al, 1991; Weindruch et al, 1982). DR also delayed shifts of CD4 and CD8 memory cells (Miller, 1997) and attenuated decreases in IL-2 (Pahlavani, 2000). Thus, the impact of DR on immune responses must consider integrative systemic functions, not just specific cell responses.

Hibernation has been compared with DR because of the prolonged phases of low food intake (Walford and Spindler, 1997; Wilkinson and South, 2002). Like DR, hibernation may also attenuate certain infections. In bats (*Myotis lucifugis*), the infectivity of equine encephalomyelitis virus (EEV) was much less during hibernation (Main, 1979). Hibernating squirrels (*Citellus erythrogens*) injected with fungal spores were asymptomatic; upon the squirrels' awakening, the spores caused skin infections (Sharapov, 1984). As in DR, hibernating squirrels have fewer white blood cells, which increase after feeding (Bachman, 2003). Hibernation also lowers plasma complement activity (Maniero, 2002).

How does restricted food intake influence infections? The Murrays suggested that starvation limits microbial pathogen growth by induced deficiencies of various micronutrients, such as iron, zinc, and methionine (McMahon et al, 1993; Murray et al, 1995). Free iron, which is limiting for microbial and fungal growth, is tightly regulated and further sequestered from circulation during acute phase responses (Beisel, 1995; Bullen et al, 2005; Exton, 1997). LPS rapidly induces hepcidin, a key regulator of iron metabolism that mediates the hypoferremia of inflammation (Kemna et al, 2005). The importance of iron was directly shown in iron-deficient African nomadics: Those receiving iron supplements had 5-fold more sympto-matic infections, including activation of malaria, brucellosis, and tuberculosis (Murray, 1978; Plata-Salaman, 1996). This result suggests the importance of iron

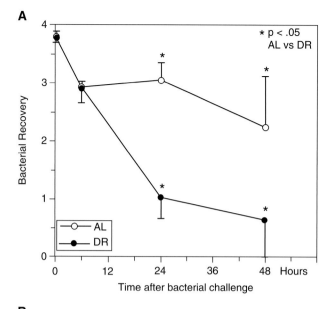

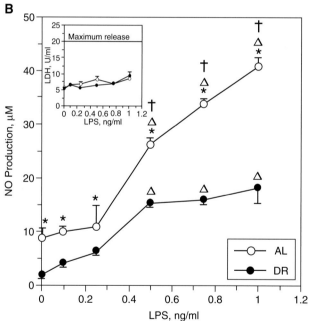

FIGURE 3.6 Diet restriction (DR) enhanced certain responses to Streptococcus infections. Young F344 male rats after 3 weeks of DR were given aerosol infection with *Streptococcus zooepidemicus* followed by ozone challenge. (Redrawn from Dong et al, 1998.) A. DR increased bacterial clearance in the lungs (CFU/ml lavage) and suppressed inflammatory responses (not shown). B. Isolated alveolar macrophages from DR rats had less LPS-induced nitric oxide.

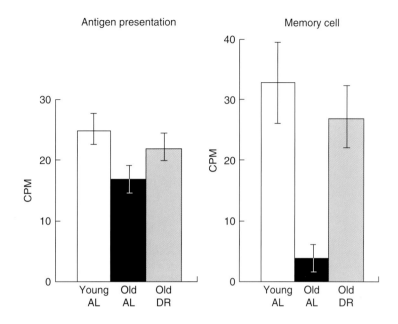

FIGURE 3.7 Diet restriction (DR) enhanced immune memory in aging mice maintained on DR as adults: Age-related loss of antigen presentation with influenza virus was not attenuated by DR, whereas memory T cell responses were almost completely maintained in old DR mice. (Redrawn from Effros et al, 1991.)

regulatory mechanisms during the human evolutionary transitions to meat-rich diets in Africa (Chapter 6).

Additionally, I suggest that lower blood glucose in fasting and in DR (Fig. 3.2B) restrict bacterial growth. Conversely, infections are more frequent in hyperglycemia and diabetes (Dubos, 1955; Savin, 1974). A well-controlled study showed 5-fold higher risk of postsurgical infections at postoperative glucose at >220 mg/dL, despite antibiotic therapy (Pomposelli et al, 1998). Glucose control in diabetic cardiac surgical patients decreased postoperative infections by 40% (Zerr et al, 1997). Hyperglycemic rodents are also more vulnerable to infections, illustrated by three of many other good studies. In fasting mice, access to 5% glucose in the drinking fluid sharply increased mortality from staphylococcal infections (Smith and Dubos, 1956). Hyperglycemic rats had higher mortality from *Candida albicans*, together with suppressed macrophage responses and deficits of IFNγ (Mencacci et al, 1993; Mosci et al, 1993). Moreover, lung influenza virus load was proportional to blood glucose at infection; this vulnerability was eliminated by insulin (Reading et al, 1998). Apparently, glucose competes with the influenza virus for binding by the SP-D protein, thereby reducing viral neutralization (Allen et al, 2004; Reading et al, 1997). SP-D (surfactant protein-D) is a soluble collectin with major importance to host defense in the lung; SP-D neutralizes many viral infections that are also enhanced by hyperglycemia.

Besides increasing resistance to certain infections, DR also attenuates acute phase responses in young rodent models. In the classic pharmacologic model of sterile edema induced by subcutaneous injection of inflammogens, James Nelson and colleagues showed that DR for 2 m shortened the duration of the local inflammatory response (Fig. 3.8) (Klebanov et al, 1995). Moreover, DR attenuated the LPS-induced transient increase of blood TNFα by 50% (Tsuchiya et al, 2005); the ozone-induced lung inflammation, which causes oxidative damage and fibrosis (fibronectin induction) (Elsayed, 2001; Kari et al, 1997); and allergic lung inflammation induced by house dust mite antigen (Dong et al, 2000). DR tends to attenuate macrophage responses to LPS; however, conclusions are tentative because of the different assays and animal models (Finch and Longo, 2001; Longo and Finch, 2003; Tsuchiya et al, 2005). Ongoing studies may resolve the role of elevated glucocorticoids (Fig. 3.2A) in attenuating inflammation (Section 3.5). Other mechanisms could include downregulation of acute phase responses. DR lowers hepatic mRNA for serum amyloid A (SAA4) and complement factors: C9, C4 binding protein, mannose binding lectin (Corton et al, 2004; Dhahbi et al, 2004).

In summary, there is no doubt that undernutrition lowers resistance to pathogenic infections in most circumstances, which could undermine the effects of DR to cardiovascular functions over the long term in our germy world. The physio-

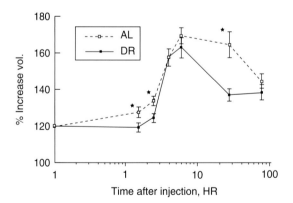

FIGURE 3.8 Diet restriction (DR) attenuated edema induced in the foot pad by local injection of carrageenan (algal extract), an inflammogen that induces a transient sterile edema. Young BALB/c mice were fed ad libitum (AL) or DR (−40%) for 2 mo. (Redrawn from Klebanov et al, 1995.)

logical domain wherein DR improves resistance to certain pathogenic infections merits further study.

3.2.5. Somatic Repair and Regeneration

Diet restriction (DR) has even less consistent effects on age impairments of somatic repair and regeneration. In a classic wound-healing paradigm, two studies agree that age impairments in cutaneous healing of full-thickness wounds were not improved by long-term DR: mice (Reed et al, 1996), rats, and monkeys (Roth et al, 1997). However, refeeding of old DR mice for 30 d restored healing rates to the young in association with increased fibroblast proliferation, synthesis of collagen-I, and serum IGF-1 and IGF-like binding protein-3 (IGFBP-3) (Reed et al, 1996). Age decreases of serum IGF-1 were not blocked by DR, which is no surprise, because DR, like fasting, lowers serum IGF-1 (Richardson et al, 2004) and insulin, while increasing growth hormone (GH) (Parker et al, 1972; Xu and Sonntag, 1996).

Turning to the clinical geriatric setting, older institutionalized patients suffer badly from impaired healing of skin wounds, chiefly bed-induced pressure ulcers. Malnutrition due to loss of appetite is among the many causes of impaired healing (Harris and Fraser, 2004). Nutritional supplements may improve ulcer healing (Lee et al, 2006; Mandal, 2006). Of course, malnutrition in geriatric patients is not equivalent to DR as discussed elsewhere in this chapter.

Liver regeneration may be enhanced by DR. In the partial hepatectomy model of rodents, removal of two-thirds of the liver stimulates rapid division of the remaining hepatocytes with complete regeneration of the liver mass within 1 week. The slower activation of hepatocyte DNA synthesis in aging rats (Bucher et al, 1964) may be ameliorated by DR (Chou et al, 1995), but has not been studied in depth. In human hepatitis C virus infections, DR improved liver function during 24 m (Iwasa et al, 2004).

In young adults, DR may impair wounding and regeneration, depending on the model. Young mice on 30 days of DR had 45% less epithelial cell proliferation (Hsieh et al, 2004). Refeeding caused a rebound of proliferation in skin, mammary, and T-cells (Hsieh et al, 2005). While these effects of DR are interpreted as anticarcinogenic, they are also consistent with energy allocation away from somatic growth and repair (Fig. 1.2B). The reduction of metabolic growth factors by DR (IGF-1 and insulin, see above) was confirmed *in vitro*: Serum from DR adult rat and monkey (not aging) supports less cell growth (FaO hepatomas), which was restored to *ad lib* serum levels by adding insulin and IGF-1 (de Cabo et al, 2003). The protective effects of DR to xenotoxins (Section 3.2.4) may also apply: In a toxicity model that depends on hepatocyte proliferation, DR raised the threshold dose for lethal thioacetamide toxicity above that in *ad lib* fed young rats and accelerated promitogenic and repair responses (EGF receptor and IL-6) (Apte et al, 2003). In a non-clinical example, feather regeneration in zebra finches (*Taeniopygia guttata*) is also impaired by DR (Wiersma and Verhulst, 2005): Adult birds on −67% DR had modest impairments in feather regrowth (4% shorter), while foraging activity was increased 5-fold, discussed below as an evolutionary strategy.

Stem cell regulation may also be sensitive to DR, depending on the tissue (Tapia, 2005). DR slowed age declines in the number of marrow hemopoietic stem cells and restored their ability to repopulate irradiated donors; stem cells from old DR mice were more vigorous than from young *ad lib* mice (Chen et al, 2003b). However, the brain may respond differently: DR did not alter the large (> 80%) early age loss in neuronal stem cell production in mouse hippocampus ages 2 to 12 m or prevent the modest further declines up to 24 m (Bondolfi, 2004).

Generalizations about DR in somatic repair and regeneration may not be possible until we understand the hierarchy of energy allocation during energy and nutrient restriction (Fig. 1.2B), which may differ widely between species according to special adaptations. We must be cautious about over-interpreting findings on DR from our inbred rodent models, which have been selected for different growth and metabolic patterns than their wild-type mice (Fig. 3.3).

3.3. ENERGY SENSING IN DIET RESTRICTION AND SATIETY

Consideration of energy-sensing systems raises important questions about how DR works. All cells process information about their ATP production, pO_2, and glucose ('biochemistry'). Tissue grade organisms have additional highly evolved energy-regulating mechanisms systems in their nervous system that integrate systemic metabolic information from the extracellular fluid and blood, with information from local cells and tissues ('physiology').

Vertebrate systemic energy is regulated by the nervous and endocrine systems, which govern energy acquisition through foraging and feeding and energy expenditure through thermogenesis, locomotion, and specialized behaviors, many of which are specifically modified by DR in proportion to energy deficits. Humoral factors in the vascular and lymphatic systems are averaged across tissues. Moreover, *local* cell information is also neuronally transmitted to the brain, with specific afferents from liver and fat, both visceral and subcutaneous; reciprocally, distinct brain neurons project to both visceral and subcutaneous fat (Kreier et al, 2005). The hypothalamus is a major recipient of metabolic signals and a major seat of metabolic regulation. Hundreds of neuronal circuits within the hypothalamus and extending to other brain regions regulate metabolism, growth, reproduction, response to infections, and response to threats by predators (Grove et al, 2005; Horvath, 2005; Simerly, 2005). Some pathways have specific transcription factors and neurotransmitter phenotypes, e.g., those inhibiting reproductive behaviors during threat stimuli (Choi, 2005). Besides regulating metabolism by pituitary and hypothalamic peptides, the autonomic output has major importance to fat, liver, pancreas, and adrenal medulla. Fat-sensing pathways are incompletely mapped, as is much of the autonomic innervation that directly mobilizes glycogen and fats. Flies and worms also have complex neuroendocrine mechanisms of energy regulation shown in the long-lived mutants with altered insulin-like signaling in neurons (Sections 5.5. and 5.6).

3.3.1. Physiology

Blood glucose and fatty acids regulate metabolism, directly through effects on liver and pancreas, and indirectly through neuroendocrine controls. Energy deficits rapidly activate the hypothalamic-pituitary-adrenocortical axis. DR rodents have 20% higher afternoon elevations of corticosterone (Fig. 3.2A), which may be due to increased hypothalamic-pituitary-adrenal cortical activity. Plasma glucocorticoids are increased during running and other 'anorectic' behaviors of DR rodents in support of gluconeogenesis (Duclos et al, 2005; Rivest and Richard, 1990). The lower blood glucose in DR is in part due to increased 'insulin sensitivity,' which enhances insulin-mediated glucose uptake by muscle cells.

Glucose and glucocorticoids cross the blood-brain barrier to act directly on hypothalamic neurons that regulate food intake and macronutrient selection (Porte et al, 2005; Tempel, 1992; Yang, 2004c). Hypothalamic neurons are exquisitely sensitive to blood glucose levels. Neuronal gene expression is also modulated by glucose independently of insulin levels, e.g., fasting induces GLUT-1, MPK-1, and other genes associated with glucose metabolism and transport (Mastaitis et al, 2005). Several peptides that control energy are also modulated by DR. Chronic 30% DR or acute fasting increased NPY-mRNA and decreased POMC mRNA (ratio 2:1) in the arcuate nucleus of the hypothalamus (Shimokawa et al, 2003; Makimura et al, 2003; Xu, 1999). The NPY and POMC neuropeptides have opposing actions on appetite: NPY elevations strongly stimulate feeding and can inhibit reproduction when energy is restricted (Gonzales et al, 2004a, b). The fasting-induction of hypothalamic NPY and decrease of POMC are blocked by adrenalectomy (Makimura et al, 2003), indicating important links to glucocorticoid increases during acute by fasting and chronic DR. Energy allocation during infection and host defense is mediated by these integrated hypothalamic systems (Broberger, 2005; Turrin and Rivest, 2004). In rats given gastro-intestinal nematode infections that induced anorexia (Section 3.2.4), the infections elevated hypothalamic NPY to the same levels as in pair-fed non-infected DR controls, indicating the sensing of energy deficits (Horbury et al, 1995).

Adiposity-related hormones including leptin and insulin activate hypothalamic and other subcortical centers that regulate energy balance. Levels of blood insulin and leptin vary in general proportion to fat mass; both act on hypothalamic centers (arcuate and ventromedial nuclei) that suppress anabolism and activate catabolism. Leptin infusion to hungry rats suppresses feeding and the associated wheel-running behavior (Exner et al, 2000). Leptin may also be thermogenic during DR (Ritz et al, 2005), which typically lowers core temperature by 1°C in mice (Koizumi et al, 1992; Rikke et al, 2003) and monkey (Lane et al, 1996). Rat genotypes that are prone to obesity on fatty diets are less sensitive to the anorectic effects of infused leptin, as measured by NPY mRNA and weight gain given *ad lib* food (Levin and Dunn-Meynell, 2002; Levin and Dunn-Meynell, 2004).

Decreased CNS leptin signaling is implicated in obesity. Old rats with 2-fold larger fat depots and 4-fold higher serum leptin than young (30 vs. 6 mo) were leptin resistant. Infused leptin inhibited food intake 70% less in the old and did not induce hypothalamic NPY mRNA, unlike the young (Scarpace et al., 2000a). Moreover, the EC50 for phosphorylation of STAT3 was 5-fold higher, with 70% less total induction of this key metabolic transcription factor (Scarpace et al., 2000b). These important findings implicate the decreased hypothalamic sensitivity to leptin with aging in obesity and in appetite despite leptin elevations.

Ghrelin, a gastro-intestinal tract peptide hormone also expressed in hypothalamic neurons, also interacts with these systems (Nørrelund, 2005). Ghrelin and NPY stimulate appetite and are among the most potent orixigens. With *ad lib* food, ghrelin rises just before anticipated feeding, whereas ghrelin decreases in obesity. Plasma ghrelin is increased by short-term DR 25% below *ad lib*, and by 24 hours fasting; these increases are blocked by leptin infusion (Barazzoni, 2003). Ghrelin may be the main cause of GH elevations during DR and fasting, through specialized receptors in the brain (GHS-R1a, GH secretogogue receptors). Fasting GH is elevated, whereas IGF-1 is decreased; fasting may be considered as a state of GH resistance, the converse of obesity.

Besides hormonal mechanisms, hepatic glucose production is directly modulated by the vagus nerve, possibly in response to fatty acids released by adipocytes during negative energy balance that act directly on hypothalamic neurons (Pocai et al, 2005). In parallel, fatty acids may also act directly on the liver ('portal hypothesis') (Kabir et al, 2005).The similarity of hypothalamic responses to short-term fasting and chronic DR suggests that the chronic DR is 'read' as an energy deficit, despite the fact that body fat slowly accumulates during DR at 40% *ad lib* (Bertrand et al, 1980) (Section 3.2.1). Although much will still be learned from studying aging changes in different cells, future studies must grapple with aging at the systems level of energy regulation. Elucidation of the 'gero-metabolome' will require analysis of multiple loci across the diurnal cycle, using the forthcoming technology of multiple reporter genes *in vivo*.

3.3.2. Biochemistry

Subcellular energy is regulated by individual enzymes and pathways with extensive overlap, including AMPK, insulin signaling, sirtuins, and TOR (Fig. 3.9). Mutations in these and related pathways influence longevity in flies, worms, and mice (Chapter 5). These energy-sensing systems are implicated in DR, but also have major roles in development.

The AMP-activated protein kinase (AMPK) pathway mediates energy balance in yeast and animals by integrating nutrient and hormonal information (Hahn-Windgassen et al, 2005; Kahn et al, 2005). AMPK activation inhibits ATP consumption and induces catabolic processes. In the pancreas, AMPK inhibits insulin secretion. Hormonal activators include adiponectin (liver) and leptin (muscle) by phosphorylation of AMPK. Hypothalamic neuronal AMPK is a key regulator of

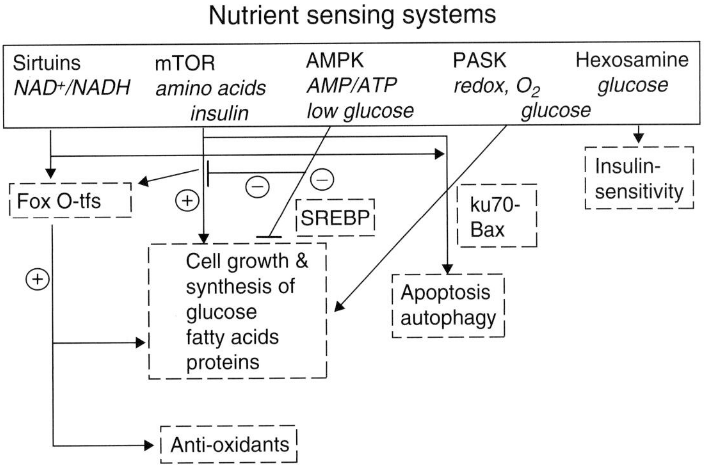

Nutrient sensing systems

FIGURE 3.9 Nutrient sensing systems in vertebrates that have many orthologues in yeast, flies, and worms. (Drawn by CE Finch from Barthel and Schmoll, 2003; Lindsley and Rutter, 2004.)

systemic energy through glucose utilization, fatty acid oxidation, and appetite (Fryer and Carling, 2005; Kahn et al, 2005). AMPK activity is exquisitely sensitive to the AMP:ATP ratio, which is closely linked to cell glucose and pO_2.

AMPK interacts with the mTOR pathway. mTOR, a key energy-sensing enzyme system, regulates cell growth and biosynthesis in response to amino acid pools: Declining free amino acids lower TOR activity, which decreases the ribosomal S6 kinase and attenuates translation; concurrently, lowered TOR stimulates protein catabolism by increasing lysosomal autophagy (Maloney and Rees, 2005; Sarbassov dos et al, 2005). Worm life span was increased by inhibiting its corresponding TOR (*let-363*) by RNAi (Vellai et al, 2003). TOR may interact with insulin-like signaling in fly and worm (Chapter 5) (Partridge et al, 2005a,b; Walker et al, 2005).

mTOR is also activated by the tumor suppressor LKB1, an AMPK kinase. Activation of PI3K/Akt may inhibit AMPK directly by phosphorylation. Although AMPK activity was 2-fold higher in aging mouse liver, it was not changed during fasting or DR (Gonzalez et al, 2004a, b; Mulligan et al, 2005). We need more understanding of AMPK activity responses to DR in other tissues, particularly hypothalamic centers.

In the liver, the increased glucocorticoids stimulate the catabolism of fatty acids for energy ('gluconeogenesis'), while decreasing the synthesis of fatty acids and cholesterol (Corton et al, 2004; Dhahbi, 1999; Dhahbi, 2002; Dhahbi et al, 2004; Sabatino et al, 1991) (Fig. 3.10). The degradation of oxidized proteins is

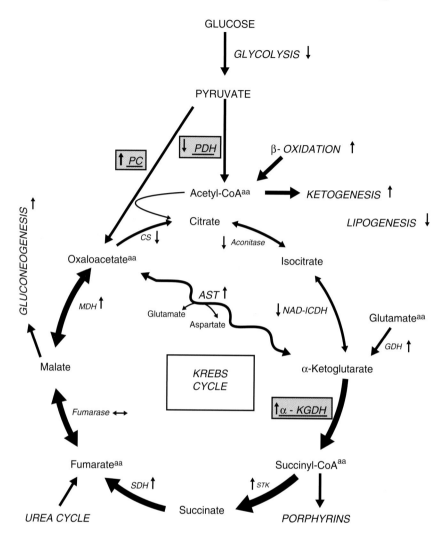

FIGURE 3.10 The Krebs cycle during diet restriction (DR) shows selective changes in rat liver, indicated by small vertical arrows. (Redrawn from Hagopian et al, 2004.) Gray shading indicates key regulatory sites. aa shows entry of amino acids into cycle. aa shows entry of amino acids into cycle. Gluconeogenesis is increased during DR by increasing pyruvate carboxylase (PC), which diverts pyruvate to oxaloacetate. Decreased glycolysis: aconitase, −25%; NAD isocitrate dehydrogenase, −30%; STK, succinyl–CoA thiokinase, +25%. Other enzymes shown include a-ketoglutarate dehydrogenase (aKGDH); malate dehydrogensase (MDH); pyruvate dehydrogenase (PDH); succinic dehydrogenase (SDH); In a different study, DR decreased PDH by −50% (Dhabi et al, 2001).

increased by DR through increased proteasome degradation in liver (Goto et al, 2001) and skeletal muscle (Selsby et al, 2005). Protein catabolism feeds carbon fragments for the increased gluconeogenesis by the liver and increases flux of nitrogen through the urea cycle

Heat shock proteins—e.g., HSP 70 and other chaperones—are decreased in rat liver and muscle during DR and rapidly induced by refeeding (Dhahbi et al., 2002, 2004). DR attenuated the age decreases in HSP-27 and HSP 72, whereas HSP 90 was increased 4-fold (Selsby et al, 2005). HSP 90, a highly abundant protein, functions in a multi-chaperone complex with various 'client proteins,' including Akt/PKB, IGF receptor, steroid receptors, RAF-1 kinase, etc. For example, the HSP/Akt complex facilitates Akt phosphorylation by PDK1 (Zhang and Burrows, 2004).

A race is on to identify transcription factors that are shared regulators in the insulin-like signaling network of genes. The effects of DR on many diseases of aging with inflammatory components give reason to look for transcription factors that modulate the overlapping inflammatory gene networks implicated in AD, cancer, diabetes, and vascular disease (Finch et al., 2002; Longo and Finch, 2003). NF-κB and other redox-sensitive transcription factors are implicated in transcriptional changes in DR (Kim et al, 2002; Merry, 2004). Models include PPARα knockout mice and drug antagonists, such as the pan-PPARα agonist 'WY-14643,' which induces sets of genes that overlap with short-term DR (Corton et al, 2004). In liver, the transcription factors PPARα, LXR, and RXR regulate many genes during DR that also have major roles in inflammation (Fig. 3.11).

The glycation of extracellular proteins is decreased by DR and starvation. According to the Cerami hypothesis (Cerami, 1985), extracellular glucose is a major driver of aging through the formation of advanced-glycation endproducts (AGEs) (Sections 1.2.7, 1.4, 1.4.2). DR may attenuate glyco-oxidation of extracellular proteins during aging processes according to the principle of mass action by lowering blood glucose. Conversely, hyperglycemia and diabetes may accelerate glyco-oxidation by mass action. At the subcellular, glyco-oxidation may be less coupled to blood glucose because of more complex biochemistry and involvement of mitochondrial ROS.

DR decreases the load of oxidatively damaged proteins, lipids, and DNA which accumulate generally during aging (Section 1.2.6). Total proteins from rodent brain, liver, and muscle of aging DR rodents have 10–30% lower carbonyl and dityrosine content than in *ad lib* controls (Forster et al, 2000; Leeuwenburgh, 1997; Selsby et al, 2005). DR also lowers tissue lipid oxidation. Even in old rats, short-term DR diminishes oxidized proteins and lipids (Radak et al, 2002), demonstrating the lability of these oxidation products when energy balance become negative. DR also attenuates oxidative DNA damage (Lee and Cerami, 1990; Thornalley, 2003), e.g., 8-oxodeoxyguanosine (8-OHdG) in rat liver mitochondria (Lockie et al, 1992; Lopez-Torres et al, 2002). DNA deletions in muscle mitochondria, a different type of DNA damage than 8-OHdG, change in parallel with protein glyco-oxidation: Both are decreased by DR (Cassano et al, 2004) and

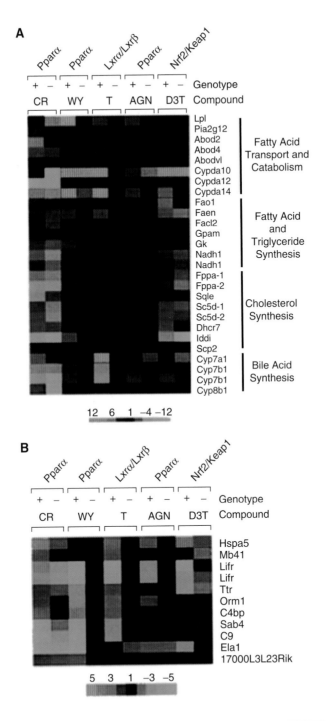

FIGURE 3.11 For legend see page 207.

conversely, are increased by chronic hyperglycemia (Cassano et al, 2004; Fukagawa et al, 1999).

Of major importance, DR decreases mitochondrial production of ROS and other free radicals, as shown in mitochondria from liver (Fig. 3.12A) (Barja, 2004; Bokov et al, 2004; Sohal and Weindruch, 1996) and muscle (Fig. 3.12B) (Bevilacqua et al, 2005). Moreover, oxidative damage to mitochondria is decreased correspondingly by DR, shown here for DNA oxidation (8-oxodG) and lipid oxidation (TBARS) each by 50%.[6] DR also increased enzymatic breakdown of free radicals (Sohal and Weindruch, 1996) and induces anti-oxidant defenses (Bokov, 2004; Merry, 2004). As noted above, DR lowered lung macrophage production of nitric oxide (Fig. 3.6B) (Dong et al, 1998).

These oxidative changes are paralleled by changes in glutathione, a major redox couple (Section 1.2.6). Levels of oxidized proteins correlate with oxidized glutathione (GSSG), which increases 2-fold in tissues of aging mice (Rebrin et al, 2003; Rebrin and Sohal, 2004) and in whole aging flies (Rebrin et al, 2004). Correspondingly, the glutathione redox potential also becomes more pro-oxidizing in most tissues (Fig. 3.13). Together with decreases of oxidized proteins in aging mice, DR decreased oxidized glutathione (GSSG and protein-SSG content) and shifted the glutathione redox potential to a lower oxidative state in liver and muscle of aging mice (Rebrin et al, 2003). The smaller responses of these redox shifts to DR in aging brain are puzzling and suggest important tissue differences in redox homeostasis.

Hyperglycemia may be considered the converse of DR by increasing glyco-oxidative damage in association with a proinflammatory state ('Brownlee hypothesis') (Brownlee, 2001). Mechanisms include increased mitochondrial

---

[6]In liver and muscle, most of the superoxide produced by mitochondrial oxidative phosphorylation is dismutated to H_2O_2. The freely diffusing H_2O_2 accounts for 20–40% of cell H_2O_2 production; steady state levels are about 10 nM varying by cell type (Jezek and Hlavata, 2005).

FIGURE 3.11 Gene expression changes during diet restriction (DR), and cardiovascular drugs are mediated by lipid-activated nuclear receptors in the liver. Signals are compared to *ad lib* (AL) control. In (A), *bolded* genes are regulated by DR Scale, -fold changes. Expression of genes in mouse liver that mediate lipid metabolism (A) and that are associated with cardiovascular disease (CVD); (B) DR and drugs that lipid-activated nuclear receptors agonists of PPAR'U, RXR, and LXR: *WY* (WY14,642; PPAR'U agonist, ChemSyn); *T* (T0901317; LXR agonist); *AGN* (AGN 194,204; RXR agonist, Allergan); *D3T* (1,2-dithiole-3-thione, anti-oxidant activator of oxidant-inducible Nrf2). WY, T, and AGN diminish CVD in AL fed mice. DR increased expression of genes mediating fat utilization and decreased that of fatty acid, triglycerides, and glycerolipid synthesis. (From Corton et al, 2004.)

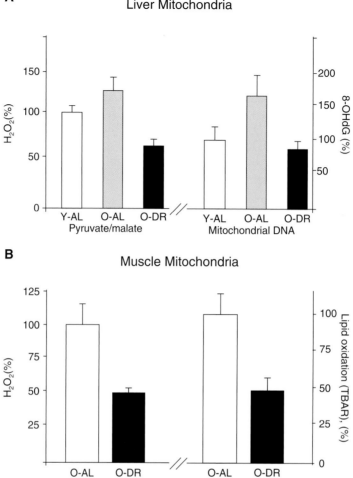

FIGURE 3.12 Mitochondrial aging: Diet restriction (DR) attenuates free radical production and oxidative damage. A. Liver mitochondria from male adult Wistar rats fed *ad lib* age 11 m (Y-AL) or 24 m (O-AL), or DR from 12–24 m (O-DR). Using mitochondrial complex I substrates (pyruvate/malate), the mitochondrial production of H_2O_2 was decreased by 47% by 12 m of DR, but did not significantly increased by age; short-term DR for 1.5 m decreased H_2O_2 production by 23%. Mitochondrial oxidative DNA damage (8-oxoDG) increased 100% with age in AL, and attenuated by DR. Liver nuclear DNA 8-oxodG was unchanged in this assay (not shown). DR did not alter mitochondrial O_2 consumption. (Redrawn from Lopez-Torres et al, 2002.) B. Skeletal muscle mitochondria from male (F344 x Brown-Norway) F_1 rats fed *ad lib* age 18 m (O-AL) or DR from 6 m and examined at 18 m (O-DR). Production of H_2O_2 increased 18% with age (12–18 m, not shown); DR attenuated the age increase. Mitochondrial lipid peroxidation (TBARS) increased 24% (18–24 m, not shown); DR attenuated the increase. This powerful study also showed that the age increase in proton leak was slowed by DR. Proton leak may account for 25% of resting energy expenditure. (Redrawn from Bevilacqua et al, 2005.)

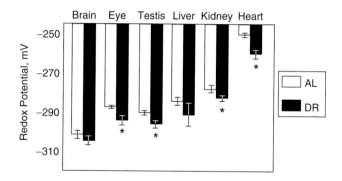

FIGURE 3.13 Glutathione redox potential, calculated by the Nernst equation, is shifted to less oxidation (more negative values) by DR in mice aged 22 m (Rebrin et al, 2003).

superoxide production (Nishikawa et al, 2000; Piconi et al, 2006) and formation of AGE on extra-cellular proteins that attracts macrophages and can stimulate free radical production (Section 1.4.2). In muscle, elevated glucose decreased glutathione levels by repressing glutamylcystein-synthetase, the rate-limiting enzyme of glutathione synthesis (Powell et al, 2001). Systemically, hyperglycemia increases IL-1 and TNFα (Ling et al, 2003). In cultured monocytes, hyperglycemia induces IL-6 and TNFα secretion (Morohoshi et al, 1996). These cytokine changes have direct importance to insulin action: TNFα inhibits insulin receptor signaling in adipocytes, hepatocytes, and skeletal muscle and is implicated in the insulin (Kirwan et al, 2001). Adipocytes from non-diabetic rats cultured with high glucose had elevated superoxide and 8-OHdG and increased inflammatory proteins, including serum amyloid A (SAA), lipocalin 24p3, and pentraxin-3. Adipocytes from the streptozotocin-diabetic rat model cultured in normal glucose also had increased superoxide production, which was blocked by transfected Mn-SOD (Lin et al, 2005).

A provisional conclusion is that DR counteracts hyperglycemic and diabetic damage by reducing the ROS production by mitochondria. However, tissue fluid glucose at any level inevitably causes oxidative damage in one of the central processes in aging. The effects of DR in attenuating inflammatory activity by macrophages would be expected to decrease bystander damage (Query I, Section 1.1). Because macrophages are activated during aging in many tissues, the original free radical theory of aging requires expanding and recasting to include bystander damage from macrophage activation and other host defense mechanisms (Queries I and II). The biochemistry of DR in aging is beginning to acknowledge the complexity of tissue differences and effects of genotype, including sex.

3.3.3. Relevance to Arterial Disease and Cancer

The decreased glyco-oxidation of proteins by DR is cogent to diabetes because DR attenuates glycation and lipoprotein oxidation, each of which accelerates atherogenesis. Arteries of human diabetics and a mouse model of diabetic-accelerated atherogenesis have increased glycation (AGE) (Reaven et al, 1997). DR decreases adhesion molecules that are implicated in atherogenesis, e.g., vascular cell adhesion molecule 1 (VCAM-1) and intercellular adhesion molecule 1 (ICAM-1) (Zou et al, 2004). We may soon know how DR alters sRAGE, the soluble receptor of advanced glycation endproducts, which is implicated in atherogenesis in humans (Falcone et al, 2005) and mouse models, both diabetic and euglycemic (Hudson et al, 2005).

Cell oxidative responses to oxidized lipids are also attenuated by DR. Aortic endothelia cultures from DR mice were less reactive to oxidized LDL, with 50% less nitric oxide and nitrotyrosine production and 30% less adherence of blood monocytes than from *ad lib* fed controls (Yang et al, 2004). (Endothelial nitrotyrosine is a measure of bystander damage from reactive oxygen species, whereas monocyte adhesion is a factor in atheroma development). In the apoE-knockout mouse model of atherogenesis, DR attenuated aortic lesions with decreased foam cells and oxidized lipids (F2-isoprostanes) (Guo et al, 2002; Yang et al, 2004). These improvements are due to lower production of H_2O_2, proven by overexpression of catalase and Cu/Zn-SOD. The overlapping anti-inflammatory roles of DR and exercise may synergize to reduce vascular events (Section 3.4).

Overproduction of superoxide induced by hyperglycemia is broadly implicated in diabetic vascular pathology (Brownlee, 2001; Nishikawa et al, 2000). In endothelial cell cultures, high glucose levels increased matrix metaloproteinases (MMP-9) and oxidation of proteins (nitrotyrosine) and DNA (8-OHdG) through mechanisms that include enhanced superoxide production (Callaghan et al, 2005; Nishikawa et al, 2000; Piconi et al, 2006; Uemura et al, 2001). Acute hyperglycemia induces Mac-1, a monocyte adhesion molecule, and β2-integrin, which is proatherogenic and interacts with lipoprotein(a) (Sampson et al, 2002; Sotiriou et al, 2006). MMP-9 induction may be important to elastin degradation in atherogenesis (Section 1.6).

DR lowers cancer incidence, either spontaneous or induced by applied carcinogens (Corton, 2004; Dhahbi, 2004; Klebanov, 2007) (footnote 1). Lower serum IGF-1 in DR may attenuate tumor growth (Kari, 1999; Sell, 2003). The increased DNA repair and catabolism of xenobiotics may contribute to the lowering of cancer incidence by DR rodents, either spontaneous or induced by applied carcinogens (Corton et al, 2004; Dhahbi et al, 2004). IGF-1 regulation is associated with systemic anti-carcinogenic mechanisms in DR (Berrigan et al, 2005; Kari et al, 1999; van Noord, 2004) that may also prove to be links to the genetics of longevity (Section 5.7.1). IGF-1 is implicated in human breast cancer because it promotes cell growth via insulin receptors and indications that high IGF-1 may interfere with chemotherapy (Boyd, 2003; Ibrahim and Yee, 2005). In mice, IGF-1 overexpression increased spontaneous mammary tumors, synergizing with the p53 oncogene (Hadsell et al, 2000). However, in carcinogen-induced mammary tumors in rats, the protective effect of DR could not be attributed to lower IGF-alone, because IGF-1 infusions of DR rats did not increase tumor incidence to that from DR and refeeding (Zhu et al., 2005). Elevated IGF-1 and insulin in obesity and diabetes are also implicated in colorectal cancer (Giovannucci, 2001; Ma et al, 2004).

More generally, DR, by improving insulin-sensitivity in obesity, diabetes, and aging, may be a long-term strategy in cancer prevention. However, adherence to protocol is a major problem. In the first randomized controlled primary prevention trial of a low-fat diet with postmenopausal women (N = 48,835), only 19% kept to the diet throughout the 8 years; the lowest fat intake group had 9% less breast cancer during 8 years, at the margin of statistical significance (Prentice et al, 2006). Colorectal cancer (Beresford et al, 2006) and cardiovascular disease (Howard et al, 2006) showed similar small benefits of low-fat diets.

Glucocorticoids are also implicated, independently of IGF-1. In various rodent models, the suppression of tumors by DR was linked to corticosterone elevations during DR. Adrenalectomy abolished the protective effects of DR on carcinogen-induced skin tumors (Pashko and Schwartz, 1992, 1996; Schwartz and Pashko, 1994). Mammary tumors also respond to the increased glucocorticoids in DR. In carcinogen-induced mammary tumors, graded DR up to −40% *ad lib* attenuated tumor growth and altered cell cycle genes in proportion to the blood corticosterone elevations; DR induced p27 and decreased cyclin D1 (Zhu, 1999). Apoptosis was also increased by DR, with induction of Bax and caspases 3- and -9 (Thompson et al, 2004a,b). Mammary cell cultures showed similar growth inhibition and induction of p27 by corticosterone, which were reversed by antisense downregulation of p27 (Jiang et al, 2002).

Suppression of cell proliferation in many tissues by DR could reduce the accumulation of errors during DNA replication, from which premalignant changes arise. DR slows normal cell turnover in the skin (Hsieh et al, 2004) and intestine (Albanes et al, 1990; Patel et al, 2004). The lowering of core temperature by torpor (Section 3.2.1) may be important because DR mice maintained at 30°C to suppress torpor did not show the anti-proliferative effect of DR, as observed at conventional room temperature (Koizumi et al, 1992). Energy balance, determined by both dietary intake and physical activity, may interact with genetic susceptibility for cancer development and progression.

3.4. EXERCISE, CARDIOVASCULAR HEALTH, AND LONGEVITY

Physical activity in the form of directed regular exercise is proving to strongly benefit health and longevity in humans through benefits to basal functions and the attenuation of diseases in the circulatory, endocrine, and nervous systems. In each system, exercise appears to influence inflammatory processes.

3.4.1. Humans

The benefits of regular modest exercise to lowering mortality (Poehlman, 2001) are most consistently shown in elite socioeconomic groups of health-rich populations. Data until recently came from observational studies of self-selected lifestyles, with a focus on 'premature' mortality from cardiovascular disease (Erlichman et al, 2002). A general caveat is the lack of information on the lifestyles and prior drug and health history of respondents in self-selected exercise categories. Thus, these studies cannot be compared with the randomized studies of aspirin and other drugs, which proved cardioprotective (Section 2.9).

In the Harvard Alumni Health Study (Lee et al, 1995; Lee et al, 2004), men who expended ≥1,000 kcal/wk in regular moderate physical activity (62% of respondents) had about one-third lower mortality risk relative to the sedentary (<500 kcal/wk; 17% of respondents) (Fig. 3. 14A). To a first approximation, walking 1 mile burns 100 kcal. The exercise 'dose-response' appears linear over some range. These benefits apply to those with the usual cardiovascular risk factors of hypercholesterolemia, hypertension, obesity, and smoking. Other surveys support these conclusions, but statistical strengths vary. In the U.S. Railroad cohort, the mortality benefit from moderate exercise was just below significance (Menotti et al, 2004). Socioeconomic status (SES), which strongly influences mortality (Section 1.2) (Bauman, 2004; Berkman, 2005), may be a factor in differences between studies ('Harvard,' mainly white collar; 'Railroad,' blue collar). The impact of SES on cardiovascular health is clearly revealed in treadmill stress tests of Cleveland Clinic outpatients (Shishehbor et al, 2006) (Fig. 3.14B). In general, lower SES status is associated with poorer health across the life span (Berkman, 2005).

Exercise may allow a higher caloric intake without penalty to cardiovascular disease. In NHANES I, those with normal weight who exercised had lower mortality from cardiovascular disease *despite* their higher caloric intake (Fang, 2003). Obesity and low physical activity were independently associated with cardiovascular mortality, whereas caloric intake was not. Physically demanding human occupations that increase food intake may also not alter body weight (Mayer, 1956).

An instructive extreme is the hugely obese sumo wrestlers. Despite BMI ≥ 35 and 25% of their body weight as fat, sumo wrestlers maintain normal blood glucose and lipids when they are in training (Karam, 1996; Matsuzawa, 1997). In prime condition, the sumo's fat is largely subcutaneous, whereas in obese sedentary Japanese of the same BMI, the fat is mostly visceral (Karam, 1996; Saito et al, 2003). After retirement, usually by age 35, sumos incur a high risk of diabetes and premature mortality, with 10 years less life expectancy than other Japanese (Saito et al, 2003). Even within this upper range obesity, sumo wrestlers with lower BMI have lower mortality (Hoshi and Inaba, 1995), consistent with U.S. data (Fig. 3.4). Thus, physical fitness can counteract obesity and diabetes, even at the BMI extremes.

The concept of 'healthy obesity' in humans is controversial in the current era of expectations for evolutionarily extreme longevity to postreproductive ages.

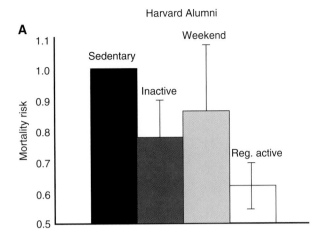

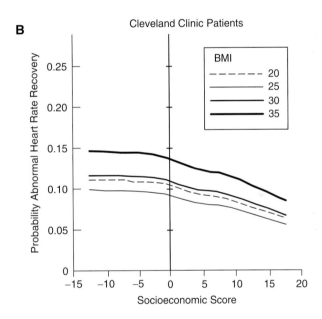

FIGURE 3.14 A. Exercise and mortality risk in the Harvard Alumni Health Study (all men) (Lee et al, 2004): *sedentary,* 500 kcal/wk walking, climbing stairs, sport/physical recreation (1453 Ss); *inactive,* expending 500–999 kcal/wk, same activities (1127); *weekend,* ≥1,000 kcal/wk in physical recreation 1–2 times/wk (580); *regularly active,* all others expending ≥1,000 kcal/wk (5621). B. Cardiac abnormalities after exercise are sensitive to socioeconomic status (SES), smoking, and body mass index (BMI) in Cleveland Clinic patients (30,043 Ss) referred for evaluation of 'known or suspected coronary artery disease.' The probability of abnormal heart rate recovery varied by SES score and BMI. Subsequent mortality correlated inversely with SES (Shishehbor et al, 2006). These findings concur with global associations of low SES with elevated cardiovascular morbidity and mortality.

In earlier eras, the ability to become fat was a sign of health and wealth, which may be the model represented in the numerous plump fertility goddess statues from the Upper Paleolithic and Neolithic periods (Section 6.2.3).

Interventions of exercise and diet are effective for those with impaired glucose tolerance and obesity (metabolic syndrome, Table 3.2A, Section 1.7, Table 1.6). Exercise reduces the incident risk of diabetes in humans by as much as 50% (Bassuk and Manson, 2005; Yamaoka and Tango, 2005). In the first large-scale randomized controlled trial (Orchard et al, 2005) (Table 3.2B), exercise and DR were twice better than placebo in eliminating the metabolic syndrome after 3 years. In those healthy at entry, the exercise-diet group had 41% less future incidence of the metabolic syndrome. Exercise and weight loss were more effective than treatment with metformin (glucose-regulating drug for type-2 diabetes),

TABLE 3.2 A Diagnosis of the Metabolic Syndrome

Three or more of the following clinical markers of diabetes and vascular disease

	Women	**Men**
waist circumference	> 88 cm	102 cm
serum triglycerides	≥ 150 mg/dL (1.7 mM)	same
HDL cholesterol	< 50 mg/dL (1.3 mM)	< 40 mg/DL (<1.03 mM)
fasting blood glucose	≥ 110 mg/dl (6.2 mM)	same
blood pressure	>130/85 mg Hg	same

National Cholesterol Education Program's Adult Treatment Panel (National Cholesterol Education Program, 2001).

TABLE 3.2 B Interventions: Absence of the Metabolic Syndrome after 3 Years

Initial Status	Intervention		
	Lifestyle: 7% Weight Loss Plus Exercise	**Metformin**	**Placebo**
glucose intolerance	38%	47%	53%
glucose intolerance **plus** metabolic syndrome	38%	23%	18%

(Diabetes Prevention Program) (Orchard et al, 2005). *Subjects*: 3234 volunteers at baseline, including both sexes of African American, Hispanic, Native American, White. Subjects randomly assigned to the three groups. *Lifestyle intervention* ('intensive'): weight loss >7% of clinical body weight achieved by low-calorie, low-fat diet and exercise of 150-min brisk walking/wk, plus placebo pill. *Metformin*, 850 mg, twice daily plus 'standard lifestyle.' *Placebo*, placebo pill plus recommended 'standard lifestyle.' *Exclusions*: Coronary heart disease or other major illness; prior diagnosis of diabetes or use of medications that impair glucose tolerance; triglycerides >600 mg/dL. *Criteria for glucose intolerance*: Fasting plasma glucose 95–125 mg/dL; 75 g glucose load causing 2-h plasma glucose 140–199 mg/dL. Lifestyle intervention was least effective for young adults (22–45 y) and more effective for men (64%) than women (37%); no significant differences between ethnic groups.

but without exercise. A smaller study of intensive exercise in elderly obese (12 weeks of treadmill/cycle, 60 min/d) improved insulin sensitivity by 35% in proportion to the reduction of visceral fat (O'Leary et al, 2006). We may anticipate that gender and genetic variation will influence the choice of lifestyle and drug interventions.

Breast cancer risk may also benefit from exercise and is about 35% lower in women who exercise than in sedentary women, across adult ages (Bernstein et al, 2005; Patel et al, 2003). These robust relationships hold across adult ages, vary in proportion to the level of exercise, and are found in White and Black women. The maintenance of 'normal body weight' is a recognized modifier of breast cancer risk. Improved insulin-sensitivity and reduction of body fat by exercise could be a shared mechanism with vascular disease.

3.4.2. Rodent Models

The associations of regular exercise with lower mortality in humans are generally consistent with the rodent studies. Rodents may also model adverse effects of exercise in individuals stressed by disease loads (SES effects in Fig. 3.14B). *Ad lib* fed lab rodents are mainly sedentary and do little 'voluntary' wheel running (Holloszy, 1992; Russell et al, 1987). Life-long voluntary wheel running has mostly positive effects on longevity in *ad lib* fed rodents. The self-selected runners may live up to 20% longer with right-shifted survival curves (Bronikowski et al, 2003; Goodrick et al, 1983; Holloszy et al, 1985; Holloszy, 1997; McCarter et al, 1997; Poehlman et al, 2001). The Gompertz slope was lower in one study (Goodrick et al, 1983), implying slowed aging. Not surprisingly, voluntary runners weigh less than the sedentary, e.g., 15% or more of the adult weight (McCarter et al, 1997) (50 g); (Goodrick et al, 1983) (100 g); (Holloszy et al, 1985) (200 g). Surprisingly, running did not increase food intake despite the lower body weights relative to the sedentary.

However, voluntary running can also increase mortality under apparently benign conditions; e.g., the combination of running and DR increased higher mortality during middle age in male Long-Evans rats (Holloszy and Schechtman, 1991). Subclinical infections were suspected because these rats ran 20–50% less than in a later study from the same lab (Holloszy, 1997). John Holloszy's choice to publish these mixed findings is an exemplar of scientific ethics. Even when rodent colonies are documented as specific-pathogen free (SPF) (Section 2.5.2), acute infections are well known to arise sporadically. Another study of *ad lib* fed F344 male rats did not find increased longevity with access to running wheels; again, the amount of running was "very little" (McCarter et al, 1997), suggesting some malaise. A provisional conclusion is that voluntary wheel running can increase life span by about 20% under favorable circumstances, but that the benefits of exercise are much smaller and less reliable than DR at −40% *ad lib* feeding in sedentary rodents.

The impact of running on diseases of aging in *ad lib* fed rodents is also unclear. Running cut kidney disease by almost half in F344 rats (McCarter et al, 1997), but not in Long-Evans rats (Holloszy et al, 1985). DR and running increased cardiomyopathy 3-fold in rats that lived longer than the DR or running groups and may have been a cause of death (McCarter et al, 1997). In some older reports reviewed by (Poehlman et al, 2001), running *shortened* the lifespan. Possibly, the chronic lung infections prevalent in the early colonies were exacerbated by exercise.[7] Early studies that did not use specific-pathogen free (SPF) animals (Section 2.5.2), despite apparent health, must be considered cautiously. Only the colonies of (Bronikowski et al, 2003; McCarter et al, 1997), and (Holloszy et al, 1985) had barrier-SPF status. Variation in pathogen load in humans might be a factor in the SES effects on exercise on longevity (Fig. 3.14B).

Ambient temperature may be another hidden variable. Temperature influences voluntary running and is often not well regulated. DR lowers core temperature in rodents by $\geq 1°C$ (see above) (Koizumi et al, 1992; Lane et al, 1996; Rikke et al, 2003), whereas running is thermogenic (Hebebrand et al, 2003; Rivest, 1989). In one of the few studies conducted at a defined thermoneutral ambient temperature, Tom Johnson's lab shows that DR did not increase wheel running (Gutierrez et al, 2002). This result should be better known because of its implications to the design and interpretation of studies of rodent exercise and aging.

3.4.3. Mechanisms in Exercise and Longevity

In great contrast to the sendentism of *ad lib* fed rodents, DR increases voluntary running (Hebebrand et al, 2003; Lane et al, 1996; Overton and Williams, 2004; Russell et al, 1987). Even modest DR at −10% below *ad lib* increased running by up to 8 k/day (Russell et al, 1987). With DR at the −30% to −40% *ad lib* used for aging-longevity studies, voluntary running is sustained during most of the life span, whereas the *ad lib* fed become progressively less active after maturation, irrespective of wheel-running opportunities (Holloszy, 1992; McCarter et al, 1997; Slonaker, 1912). Because rodents vary widely in their individual use of running wheels (Lazarov et al, 2005; Slonaker, 1912), it is hard to dissociate the self-selected behaviors of *ad lib* food intake and physical activity.

Macaques also vary widely in DR-induced locomotor activity; surprisingly, middle-aged obese monkeys were more responsive to DR-induced activity (Moscrip et al, 2000). In humans, obesity and preferences for fatty foods and sedentary activities show familial patterns that suggest heritability (Wardle

---

[7]James Slonaker (Stanford University) (Baumberger, 1954) reported the first longitudinal kymographic studies of voluntary activity of rats across the lifespan. He showed that playful activity declined after adolescence; that long-distances were run, up to 5 miles daily; that running declines during middle-age (males shut-down before females); that infections diminish running; and that individual differences in spontaneous activity persist up to the advanced old age of 45 m, also a record lifespan for those early days (Slonaker, 1912).

et al, 2001), yet identical twins can be discordant for obesity in association with sedentism (low levels of self-selected exercise) (Williams et al, 2005). Recall from Section 2.6 that obesity discordant twins differed in seropositivity for adenovirus AD-36. The low motivation of *ad lib* fed lab animals for wheel running gives clues to foraging behaviors and other adaptations in energy regulation (discussed below).

The benefits of exercise may challenge the time-honored 'rate-of-living' hypothesis. According to Rubner's (1908) statement, and already anticipated by Aristotle,[8] there is a maximum energy production over the life span, such that greater expenditures should shorten life span. However, within humans and other mammals, many examples show that energy expenditure *and* food intake can increase to meet demands, but without cost to health or longevity (Speakman, 2005). Another elegant study from John Holloszy showed that mild cold stress that increased *ad lib* food intake by 44% did not alter life span (Holloszy and Smith, 1986). Rats were made to stand in cool water 4 hours/5 days week. Although mean and maximum life spans were identical, the age-related pathology differed: cold-exposed rats had 50% fewer sarcomas, while cardiovascular lesions were increased from 65% to 100% and severe myocardial fibrosis was increased 10-fold. How puzzling that such major shifts in the proportion of lesions had no effect on average or maximum longevity!

Two major levels of function are affected by exercise: the systemic level, including cytokines, glucocorticoids, and lipoproteins; and cell responses in skeletal muscle, heart, and fat. Exercise increases pituitary growth hormone (GH) secretion, a response that decreases during aging (Weltman et al., 2006). GH, as an anabolic hormone, supports muscle cell hypertrophy during exercise (Kraemer and Ratamess, 2005; Linnamo et al, 2005). While muscle-specific IGF-1 isoforms respond to muscle stretch, intensive training is required to increase serum IGF-1 and IGFBP-3 (Elloumi et al, 2005; Koziris et al, 1999).

Exercise also reduces the oxidative load in muscle (Goto et al, 2004; Radak et al, 2002). While single bouts of exercise in sedentary animals can transiently increase the load of oxidized proteins and lipids, regular exercise increases the GSH/GSSG ratio and other anti-oxidant homeostatic responses (Radak et al, 2001; Radak et al, 2004). Young adult humans who were sedentary but not obese responded to regular aerobic exercise with 15% decrease in oxidized LDL and 28% increase in blood glutathione peroxidase by 4 m (Elosua et al, 2003). Older coronary patients given 3 months of aerobic training had 50% lower blood CRP and 2-fold higher IL-10 ('anti-inflammatory' cytokine) (Goldhammer et al, 2005).

---

[8]Aristotle, 350 BC: "A lesser flame is consumed by a greater one, for the nutriment, to wit the smoke, which the former takes a long period to expend is used up by the big flame quickly". From "On Longevity and Shortness of Life", G.R.T. Ross, translator. Aristotle also noted associations of lifespan with size in different species. Also see (Speakman, 2005; Speakman and Krol, 2005).

In rats from the above study in which running did not increase life span (McCarter et al, 1997), nonetheless the myocardial lipid peroxidation was decreased and anti-oxidant defenses were increased (Kim et al, 1996). These effects indicate overlapping anti-inflammatory roles of DR and exercise.

Exercise also decreases the systemic inflammatory profile (Bruunsgaard, 2005). Exercise consistently increases blood IL-6, a proinflammatory cardiovascular risk factor normally secreted by skeletal muscle cells (Chapter 1). IL-6 has lipolytic activity that increases energy for muscle; however, effects of IL-6 on insulin sensitivity of liver and skeletal muscle are unclear (Bruunsgaard, 2005; Pedersen et al, 2003). The resolution of this paradox may come from better understanding of IL-6 and TNFα interactions. Exercise attenuated the acute phase response to LPS with a smaller induction of serum TNFα (Starkie et al, 2003).

Other cardioprotective actions include increased insulin sensitivity and lower systolic pressure, hyperlipidemia, and fat (Bassuk and Manson, 2003; Goldhammer et al, 2005). Fat depots accumulate macrophages; plasma CRP and IL-6 are elevated; and there is higher production of reactive oxygen species and altered anti-oxidant homeostasis (Chapter 1). Fat cells also secrete mediators of insulin resistance: adiponectin, leptin, TNFα. The lower secretion from exercise may be a factor in increased glucose uptake by muscle (Coker and Kjaer, 2005; Holloszy, 2005). Glucose uptake by skeletal muscle can increase up to 20-fold, depending on intensity and duration, and increases with exercise intensity. Exercise improves the efficiency of glucose uptake by skeletal muscle by two pathways: insulin-independent and increased insulin-sensitivity to uptake of glucose. Exercise also releases glucagon and other hormones that attenuate or antagonize insulin action, including a serum factor is still unidentified (Holloszy, 2005). Exercise increases glucose production so that blood glucose in healthy subjects remains relatively constant (Coker and Kjaer, 2005; Holloszy, 2005).

In a rat model of non-insulin-dependent diabetes mellitus (OLETF rat), wheel running for 6 m attenuated obesity and lowered blood glucose, insulin, hemoglobin A_{1c} (Miyasaka et al, 2003). Human diabetics also respond to exercise in combination with DR. Besides reducing myocardial lipid peroxidation in aging mice (Kim et al, 1996), voluntary running also attenuated inflammatory expression: 70% of the mRNA increases in aging sedentary mice were attenuated by running, including TNFα, complement C1q, and apoD and apoE (Bronikowski et al, 2003). Extreme exercise, as in a marathon, however, induces CRP and other acute phase responses (Siegel et al, 2001; Weight et al, 1991).

Arterial endothelial functions relevant to arterial disease are sensitive to diet and exercise. As measured by flow-mediated dilation (FMD in the brachial artery) (Chapter 2; Fig. 2.3), NO-dependant endothelial vasodilation transiently diminishes after eating a fatty meal. The impairments peak 4 h after eating during the postprandial lipidemia (surge of triglycerides) and may last 6 h. Impairments are independent of LDL and HDL cholesterol and are linked to triglyceride-rich chylomicrons, which include ApoE. The number of impairments in FMD scale linearly with triglyceride elevations above a threshold of about 800 mm/dL

(Gaenzer et al, 2001). Regular exercise markedly diminishes the triglyceridemia (Barrett et al, 2006; Miyashita et al, 2006), e.g., treadmill running, whether experienced as a 30-min session or distributed in 10 bouts of 3 min. These and many more findings point to the suppression of postprandial lipemia by exercise in arterial health (Chandrruangphen and Collins, 2002). These findings are also consistent with the Harvard Alumni Health Study showing the benefits of regular moderate exercise to mortality (Fig. 3.14A). Transient arterial endothelial impairments may also be decreased by anti-oxidants (vitamins C and E) (Plotnick et al, 1997) or alcohol (red wine) (Cuevas et al, 2000). Postprandial lipemia shows genetic influences of lipoprotein system genes, including apoB, apoE, lipoprotein lipase (LPL), and the scavenger receptor (SR-B1); e.g., in those over 55 with the metabolic syndrome, apoE4 carriers had 40% higher postprandial triglyceridemia than apoE3 carriers (Reznik et al, 2002).

In conclusion, moderate regular exercise consistently enhances health and longevity in humans and lab animals, relative to the sedentary. In non-obese humans who exercise and who eat more because of energy demands, the increased caloric intake does not appear to cause increased mortality risk, relative to the sedentary. Obesity increases the risk of mortality and diabetes, which can be partly ameliorated by exercise and diet. The long-term benefits of diet or energy restriction in non-obese humans are not known, although all vascular risk factors are improved (Section 3.2.3). The mechanisms of exercise include improved insulin sensitivity and reductions of oxidant stress and inflammation.

Genetic influences are likely to be important. For example, the apoE4 allele, which accelerates atherosclerosis (Section 5.7.4, Fig. 5.17) increased the risk of exercise-induced silent myocardial ischemia 2.5-fold (Katzel et al, 1993). Sex differences add to the complexity. In a training program, women, but not men, showed increased HDL if they did not carry the apoE4 allele (Leon et al, 2004).

3.5. DIET, EXERCISE, AND NEURODEGENERATION

3.5.1. Alzheimer Disease

Because obesity is broadly proinflammatory (Section 1.7) and because blood inflammatory markers are associated with cognitive declines (Section 2.6), we may ask how diet and exercise influence neurodegenerative aging. Rodent experiments show effects of diet and exercise that concur with clinical associations of Alzheimer disease with high calorie intake and obesity (Grant, 2003; Luchsinger and Mayeux, 2004; Petot and Friedland, 2004).

In two Alzheimer transgenic mouse models, DR at −35% *ad lib* attenuated brain deposits of Aβ-amyloid by 50% within 3-4 months (Patel et al, 2005; Wang et al, 2005) (Fig. 3.15). The rapidity of the effects of DR show that brain Aβ deposits are metabolically dynamic. Conversely, high fat diets increased the brain Aβ load (Levin-Allerhand et al, 2002; Refolo et al, 2000; Shie et al, 2002).

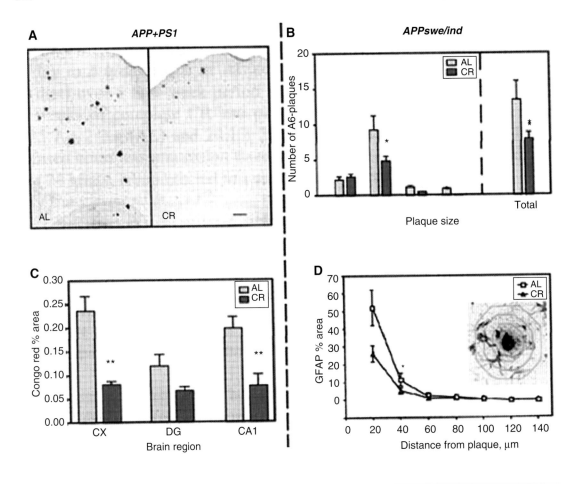

FIGURE 3.15 Diet restriction attenuates the accumulation of amyloid deposits in two transgenic mouse Alzheimer models: APP(swe/ind) (J20) and APP(swe) + PS1. Forty percent DR starting by 5 wk attenuated Aβ1-42 peptide deposits by up to 55% within 15 wk. Glial activation around the Aβ deposits was also lowered by DR. (Redrawn from Patel et al, 2005.)

Exercise also modifies amyloid deposits in mouse models. Male transgenics in enriched housing with exercise wheels and toys had 50% fewer amyloid deposits by age 5 months than with standard caging (Lazarov et al, 2005). Brain Aβ varied inversely with individual running. Several mechanisms are considered: Running increased brain neprilysin, an amyloid-degrading enzyme; running also increased EGR-1, a transcription factor expressed in microglia that regulates inflammatory gene responses to Aβ (Giri et al, 2005; Lynch et al, 2004). However, female mice of the same transgenic line responded oppositely, according to other researchers:

Running was associated with *increased* Aβ, but paradoxically, better cognitive function (Jankowsky et al, 2003; Jankowsky et al, 2005). These mouse models support associations of obesity and Alzheimer and benefits from exercise, but the findings are less consistent in humans.

An 18-year prospective study of Alzheimer risk showed that, for every 1.0 unit increase in BMI at age 70 years, risk in women was increased by 36%; men, however, did not show these associations (Gustafson et al, 2003). In normal elderly observed for 4 y, high fat intake increased risk by 2.3-fold in apoE4 carriers (CI, 1.0–4.7); the caloric intake ranged 2.5-fold between extreme quartiles (Luchsinger et al, 2002). Others also found associations of mid-life obesity and Alzheimer risk, but only in women: 2.07-fold (CI, 1.49–2.89) (Tabet, 2005). Women younger than 76 showed a 'U-shaped' relationship between BMI and dementia, whereas at later ages, low BMI from weight loss may 'mask' these associations (Luchsinger et al, 2006). Mid-life obesity in combination with high cholesterol and systolic pressure increased Alzheimer risk additively by 6.2-fold (C.I. 1.94–19.9) (Kivipelto et al, 2005). In contrast, a prospective study did not find associations of blood cholesterol with Alzheimer risk (Li et al, 2005a).

Exercise reduced the Alzheimer risk up to 50% in two prospective 5-year studies. In the Canadian Study of Health and Aging, a prospective cohort study of cognitively normal elderly, those with habitual moderate exercise (walking or its equivalent ≥ 3 times per wk) showed 50% lower Alzheimer risk (CI, 0.29–0.90) and all dementia by 67% (Laurin et al, 2001). The Cardiovascular Health Cognition Study showed 50% lower AD in the most physically active group (CI 0.33–0.79); however, apoE4 carriers did not show these benefits (Podewils et al, 2005). In a case control study, low physical activities in middle age were associated with 4-fold higher Alzheimer risk (Friedland et al, 2001). Exercise may act on the shared risk factors of vascular and Alzheimer disease (Chapter 1). These mixed findings do not allow broad conclusions! Other lifestyle choices may also be involved besides exercise.

3.5.2. Synaptic Atrophy in the Absence of Neurodegeneration

Exercise and DR attenuate some atrophic synaptic changes that arise without the dire neuron loss and degenerative changes of Alzheimer disease (Section 1.2.2; Fig. 1.7). Neuron loss is not apparent in middle age, when glial activation and synaptic atrophy are well defined (Section 1.2). The low level of neuron loss during normal aging gives an optimistic basis for reversal of synaptic atrophy of aging.

Exercise and physical fitness consistently and significantly improve cognition and other brain functions in the elderly. The pioneering study of Spirduso et al. (1978) showed that elderly who played racket sports had reaction times that were far better than sedentary elderly, and not different from younger players. In electroencephalographic (EEG) studies, aerobically fit elderly had normal-for-young speed of visual-evoked EEG potentials (P95 +N135) (Dustman et al, 1990). Physical fitness is consistently associated with higher level functioning in the executive control processes (meta-analysis, 18 studies) (Colcombe and Kramer, 2003). In brain imaging studies (fMRI), physically fit elderly have less atrophy of frontal cortex regions than the sedentary (Colcombe et al, 2004) (Fig. 3.16). The most fit also had more activation in prefrontal and parietal cortex regions that mediate executive control and that are also major sites of neurodegeneration in Alzheimer disease.

Rodent models show benefits of exercise to brain function. In young rodents, running increases the *de novo* generation of neurons (neurogenesis) in the

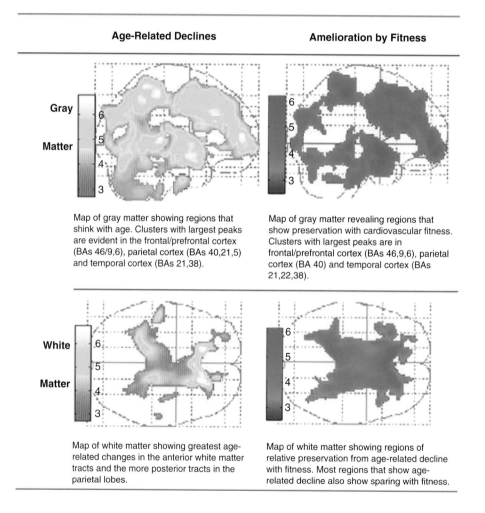

Age-Related Declines   **Amelioration by Fitness**

Gray Matter

Map of gray matter showing regions that shink with age. Clusters with largest peaks are evident in the frontal/prefrontal cortex (BAs 46/9,6), parietal cortex (BAs 40,21,5) and temporal cortex (BAs 21,38).

Map of gray matter revealing regions that show preservation with cardiovascular fitness. Clusters with largest peaks are in frontal/prefrontal cortex (BAs 46,9,6), parietal cortex (BA 40) and temporal cortex (BAs 21,22,38).

White Matter

Map of white matter showing greatest age-related changes in the anterior white matter tracts and the more posterior tracts in the parietal lobes.

Map of white matter showing regions of relative preservation from age-related decline with fitness. Most regions that show age-related decline also show sparing with fitness.

FIGURE 3.16 Cerebral cortex atrophy (fMRI) during aging is attenuated by exercise. (Directly from Colcombe et al, 2004.) Non-demented, high-functioning, community-dwelling volunteers, av. 66.5 years (55–79); fitness verified by oxygen consumption (VO_2) on a treadmill test.

hippocampus (van Praag et al, 1999) and brain levels of growth factors: BDNF (Cotman and Berchtold, 2002; Vaynman et al, 2004), which supports neurogenesis, and IGF-1, which induces BDNF and VEGF (Carro et al, 2000). Glutamate receptor functions in the cerebral cortex (NMDA binding sites and phosphorylation) (Dietrich et al, 2005) and BDNF and synapsin I in the hippocampus (Vaynman et al, 2004) were also increased by running activity. In aging rodents, running activity slowed the decline of neurogenesis (Kronenberg et al, 2005). Moreover, middle-aged (19 m) mice responded to running exercise with enhanced neurogenesis and improved learning (van Praag et al, 2005).

The importance of the reversal of growth factor deficits to neurogenesis is shown in the long-lived Snell dwarf mutant mice, which have elevated production of IGF-1 in brain cells and neurogenesis above wild-types (Sun, 2005). Brain expression of IGF-1 and GH is independent of systemic hormonal deficits in Snell dwarf mice and wild-types. Aging Snell dwarfs also maintain learning better than wild-types.

Diet restriction (DR) also slowed the age-related loss of striatal dopamine receptors (dopamine D2 receptor subtype) (Roth et al, 1984) (Fig. 3.17A). Other dopaminergic processes slowed by DR include dopamine outflow (K+-stimulated) (Diao et al, 1997) and dopamine-stimulated receptor activation (phosphoinositide hydrolysis) (Undie and Friedman, 1993). DR attenuated the age deficit in maze learning (spatial memory) (Pitsikas et al, 1990). These effects arise early in DR: In young rats short-term DR increased the sensitivity of D1 receptors by 35% (Carr et al, 2003; Haberny, 2004). Short-term effects of DR were also observed in attenuating amyloid deposits in Alzheimer transgenic mice.

The progressive synaptic atrophy of normal brain aging (Figs. 1.7A, B and 3.17A) is also concurrent with reduced cerebral blood flow and glial activation (Chapter 1, Fig. 1.7C). DR attenuates the glial activation of astrocytes and of microglia (Figs. 3.17B, C) (Morgan et al, 1999). We hypothesize that glial activation during aging from interactions of oxidant stress and inflammation is a primary cause of synaptic atrophy. The increase of astrocyte cell size during aging (Fig. 1.7C) (Finch et al, 2002; Hansen et al, 1987) is associated with increased expression of the intermediate filament GFAP (Morgan et al, 1999; Nichols et al, 1993), and these increases are attenuated by DR. The age increases of GFAP transcription (intron, mRNA) and protein per cell are attenuated by DR (Fig. 3.17B). With our 'heterochronic coculture model' (Rozovsky et al, 2005), the glial age was shown to strongly decrease support for neurite outgrowth, inversely with GFAP expression (Fig. 1.19).

We are analyzing the transcriptional controls that mediate GFAP responses to DR, which may be part of the causal chain leading to neuronal atrophy. The GFAP promoter has an extensive array of canonical inflammatory response elements, including an NF-1/NFkB sequence motif that mediates responses to IL-1β and TGF-β1 (Krohn et al, 1999) and H_2O_2 (Wei et al, 1999 and in prep). Because DR attenuates the aging increase in GFAP transcription and lowers brain levels of oxidized proteins and lipids (see above), we hypothesize that the increased GFAP transcription is in response to local oxidant stress, directly or through cytokines secreted by activated microglia.

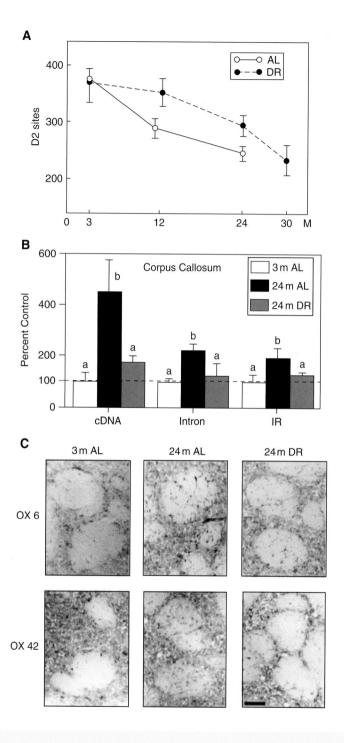

FIGURE 3.17 For legend see page 225.

(Continues)

Besides synaptic atrophy, white matter (myelin) is slowly eroded during aging (Section 1.2 and Fig. 1.9B). DR attenuates the glial inflammatory activation during aging in the myelinated corpus callosum and cortico-striatal tracts, which enable high-speed exchanges within the brain (Fig. 3.17C) (Morgan et al, 1999). Another indication of DR as myelin-protective is that DR decreases an age-related hind-limb paralysis found in some rat colonies that is associated with spinal motoneuron degeneration (radiculoneuropathy) (Berg et al, 1962; Everitt et al, 1980; Morgan et al, 2007).[9] The segmental myelination degeneration in spinal roots may be secondary to axonal atrophy (Kazui and Fujisawa, 1988; Krinke, 1983; Mitsumori et al, 1981). Hind-limb paralysis with myelin degeneration could be developed as a model for dietary interventions in diabetic neuropathy.

3.6. LABORATORY RODENTS AS MODELS FOR THE 'COUCH POTATO'

Our domesticated rodents may be models for the 'couch potato' syndrome of sedentary obesity and poor physical fitness. For several hundred generations, lab rodents have been selected for fast growth and maturation; high fecundity with the capacity to nurse large litters to weaning; rapidly succeeding litters; and docility (Blank and Desjardins, 1985; Miller et al, 2002). Moreover, this selection occurred during confinement with few physical demands, with *ad lib* food, low levels of infectious pathogens, and no macropredators besides the experimenters. I suggest that selection for rapid growth and high fecundity in this utterly unnatural environment may have altered metabolic gene regulation to phenotypes that model human lifestyles in a low infectious environment with few physical demands.

---

[9]The aging phenotype of hind-limb paralysis (radiculoneuropathy) is not known to most biogerontologists. The incidence varies widely: 67% in an SPF colony of Wistar rats (Salmon et al, 1990) to 25% in the NIA–Charles River colony (1978–1983; 9 genotypes, mean onset age 31 m). It may be even less common in aging mice (Bronson, 1990) and was never observed in my B6 aging colonies.

FIGURE 3.17 (continued) Diet restriction (DR) attenuates synaptic atrophy and glial activation in aging rat brain. A. Dopamine (D2) receptors in striatum decline more slowly during aging in rats maintained on DR (Roth et al, 1984). B. DR attenuates aging changes in expression of astrocytic GFAP (glial fibrillary acidic protein; intermediate filament protein). (Redrawn from Morgan et al, 1999.) C. Microglia in myelinated corticostriatal projections (Morgan et al, 1999). F344 male rats, DR from 3 m. OX6 represent the Mhc-2 antigen; OX 42, the complement CR-3 receptor.

Continued fat accumulation during middle age is common in rodents confined to small cages without exercise wheels and *ad lib* food. In some colonies, rodents continue to gain weight; e.g., Sprague-Dawley rats may reach 700 g by 2 y (Adelman, 1978), but this may not be universal. Although C57BL/6 mice typically have stable weights by 12 m (Adelman, 1978; Finch et al., 1969),[10] high-fat diets can also induce obesity in the 'B6' (Koza et al, 2006). High fat 'breeder chows' used to enhance milk production were once widely used for studies of aging.

Other domestic animals were similarly selected for growth and fecundity: rabbits, cattle, chickens, turkeys, etc. All tend to obesity when confined to small spaces with *ad lib* food. Primates also tend to obesity in confinement (Moscrip et al, 2000; Steinetz et al, 1996). Besides obesity, confinement is well known to alter behaviors, especially in social animals. Neuronal stem cells may also be influenced by lab confinement, as shown for the chickadee (*Parus atricapillus*), in which there was 2-fold less neurogenesis in caged captives than adult wild-caught birds (Barnea and Nottebohm, 1994). In rodents, environmental enrichment increases adult neurogenesis in association with improved learning: In young adult rats (Bruel-Jungerman et al, 2005) and in aging mice enriched from 10 to 20 m (Kempermann et al, 2002).

Insights about domestication come from studies of wild-derived mice (Austad and Kristan, 2003; Harper et al, 2006; Miller et al, 2002). Wild-derived mice differ importantly from inbred lab strains. In the Idaho-derived stock, puberty (vaginal opening) is delayed up to 3 m (Miller et al, 2002). [Vaginal opening marks the first ovulation (Bronson, 2001)]. Average life spans approximate those of lab mice on DR. Metabolic hormones are altered in the direction of the long-lived mutant dwarf mice (Chapter 5) and of lab mice on DR. Blood levels of insulin-like growth factor 1 (IGF-I) are lower by 50%; leptin, by 70%; and glycosylated hemoglobin, by 60%. The lower glycosylated hemoglobin on *ad lib* food implies lower blood glucose and high insulin efficiency, which might reduce overall oxidative molecular damage from glucose (AGE accumulation, Section 1.3) and would be consistent with the absence of DR effects on mean life span (Harper et al, 2006) (Fig. 3.4A).

These findings raise the key question: "Are wild mice calorically restricted in nature?" (Austad and Kristan, 2003), which is convincingly negated. Food intake, when corrected for body mass, was equal to or higher in wild-derived than in

---

[10]My first colony of C57BL/6J male mice was fed Purina 'Lab Chow' with 4.3% fat; their maximum weight stabilized at 29 g (Finch, 1969; Finch et al, 1990), which was about 5 g less than in John Yuhas' colony at Jackson Labs where mice were fed 'breeder chow' with 12% fat (Finch, 1969). Female B6 mice also reached stable weight of 24 g by 12 m on 4% fat Purina 'Rodent Chow' (Nelson et al, 1985). On another diet with 5% fat, B6 females weighed more than 30 g (Turturro et al, 2002), which could be due to genetic drift or differences in diet. The fat composition of rodent chows is not always available (proprietary rights).

lab mice. Although adult wild-caught mice are smaller by about 35%, their size overlaps the lower range of lab mice and the wild-derived. The *gross* food consumption of lab mice does not exceed that of wild mice under mild temperatures. By these criteria, wild mice in the field are not subject to chronic DR. Spontaneous activity also needs study. The 30% greater *gross* energy consumption of *ad lib* fed lab mice is likely a result of artificial selection for faster growth and greater fecundity.

The 3-fold higher body fat of wild mice adapted to the lab than the wild-caught (Fig. 3.3C) could represent the benefits of *ad lib* food, lower stress and physical demands, and a lower parasite load. These conditions have been enjoyed by many in the 'developed world' since 1950 when antibiotics became available. Current discussions of obesity usually emphasize lifestyle choices of higher intake of fatty foods and lower physical activity. However, the lower levels of infections and parasites may be as important. Even subclinical infections can impair growth in domestic animals and humans (Hart, 1990) (Section 4.6.5).

The very recent increase of obesity is too sudden and too general to be a result of genetic selection, as in domestic animals. Nonetheless, gene differences among the inbred strains may inform about interactions of physical activity, immune activity, appetite, and obesity. The widely used DBA/2 mouse strain has unusual responses to diet (DR shortens the life span) and other features associated with a deficit in the complement system, the important anaphylactic C5a peptide.[11] The relation of the C5a deficit to diet responses is consistent with the close integration of host defense and energy regulation. These differences are not

---

[11]In contrast to the rule, DR shortens the lifespan of DBA/2 mice, whether imposed throughout adult life, or at later ages, shown in two independent studies, versus C57BL/6 (B6) or B6D2 hybrids (Fernandes et al, 1976; Forster et al, 2003). The 2-fold greater 'open-field' exploratory activity of DBA/2 mice (Sprott and Eleftheriou, 1974) may also be a factor in these atypical responses to DR. Infections and susceptibility to amyloidosis may be causes of the shorter and more variable DBA/2 lifespans relative to B6 and other strains. DBA/2 are more vulnerabile to pneumonia and other infections, particularly during DR (Ashman et al, 2003; Fernandes et al, 1976). DBA/2 mice acquired more amyloid in the myocardium and other tissues in an early colony with chronic viral infections (Lipman et al, 1993). The general role of infections in stimulating amyloid deposits is discussed in Section 2.6.2. These vulnerabilities may be reflected in their 2-fold higher coefficient of variations in lifespan (Austad, 2006). DBA/2 mice also show unusual impairment of fertility on high fat diets (Tortoriello et al, 2004). One molecular defect is known: DBA/2 and some other widely used strains (CE/J, FVB) carry a frame-shift mutation in the complement C5 gene which blocks formation of the important anaphylactic peptide C5a (Pasinetti et al, 1996); the longer-lived B6 are 'wild-type' at this locus. The lack of C5a peptide decreases resistance to infections (Ashman et al, 2003), and increased brain responses to injury (Pasinetti et al, 1996) shown with congenic strains.

widely known to biogerontologists and should alert us all for other peculiarities of inbred lab rodents.

3.7. ENERGY BALANCE IN THE LIFE HISTORY

DR reveals trade-offs to optimize reproduction during energy shortages that may arise from the infectious load or from poor foraging opportunities in nature. In female mammals, the level of nutrients is 'read' somehow by neuroendocrine reproductive control centers, which determine whether the individual has sufficient reserves to support pregnancy and nursing. If food is restricted beyond some threshold, ovulation ceases by homeostatically suppressing the required gonadotrophin pulsatile secretions (Howland and Ibrahim, 1973; McShane and Wise, 1996; Nelson et al, 1995). The lab rodent threshold for ovulatory cycles is about −20% DR (Chapin et al, 1993; Nelson et al, 1985). In B6 mice, DR initiated after puberty suppressed ovulatory cycles in 80% within 2 months (May et al., 1992), while slowing the loss of ovarian oocytes (Fig. 3.18) (Nelson et al, 1985). The loss of hypothalamic estrogen receptors (ERα) was also diminished by DR in mice (Timiras et al, 2005). Restoration of food rapidly restores reproductive cycles (Holehan and Merry, 1985; McShane and Wise, 1996; Nelson et al, 1985; Segall and Timiras, 1976).

The slowing of reproductive senescence by DR is hypothesized to be an evolved and adaptive response to food fluctuations (Harrison and Archer, 1989; Holliday, 1989; Koochmeshgi, 2004). By slowing oocyte loss during food shortages, reproduction may be postponed to better times when foraging success may improve (Masoro and Austad, 1996). The record extension of reproduction by DR may be a successful pregnancy at age 32 m, which exceeded the oldest maternal age in *ad lib* fed rats by 6 m (Holehan and Merry, 1985).

The suppression of fertility cycles by DR is broadly consistent with the 'critical fat hypothesis' for reproduction, e.g., that puberty requires ≥ 22% fat by weight (Frisch and Revelle, 1970; Johnston et al, 1971). However, the 'critical fat level' hypothesis is challenged because the hypothalamic control of ovulation is not tightly linked to the same body fat levels in different species and experimental models (Bronson and Manning, 1991). Recall that low BMI in the Biosphere did not block menstruation (Section 3.2.3). Blood leptin levels that are closely linked to fat depots, may be permissive for ovulation, depending on other metabolic hormones or nutrients (Bronson and Manning, 1991; Dunger et al, 2005). In female rats, the delay of puberty by 30% DR was blocked by leptin infusions into the brain (i.c.v.); conversely, puberty was advanced by central leptin infusion (Zeinoaldini et al, 2006). In hamsters, the blockade of ovulation by 2 d fasting was overcome by glucose (Morin, 1986), implying roles for glucose itself, or for the expected surge of insulin. Although the 'critical fat hypothesis' is no longer considered generally valid (Bronson and Manning, 1991), no one doubts

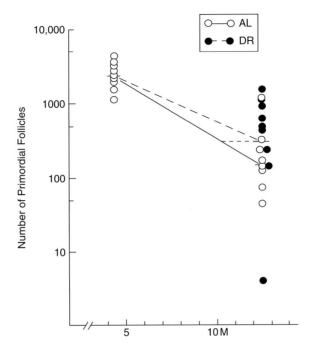

FIGURE 3.18 Diet restriction (DR) delays reproductive senescence and slows ovarian oocyte loss during aging in C57BL/6 mice. (Redrawn from Nelson et al, 1985.) 20% DR from 3.5–10.5 m suppressed ovulatory cycles. After restoration of *ad lib* feeding, all DR mice regained estrous cycles, with cycle lengths characteristic of younger *ad lib* fed mice, whereas most (80%) of the *ad lib* fed controls of the same age had ceased cycling. At the ovarian level, DR attenuated oocyte loss by about 2 m (dotted horizontal line). The scatter represents individual variations of oocyte stocks, which are not measurement errors (Finch and Kirkwood, 2000, pp. 24–28).

that endogenous energy and nutrient resources are critical regulators of maturation and reproduction.

Hypothalamic responses to energy restriction differ importantly between species. Human puberty is preceded by slowly elevating serum leptin and fat (Dunger et al, 2005). However, in mice, ovulation at puberty is concurrent with decreases of both body fat *and* leptin (Bronson and Manning, 2001). In wild-derived deer mice (*Peromyscus maniculatus*), 30% DR for 5 weeks impaired spermatogenesis and lowered testosterone, whereas male lab mice did not show these impairments (Blank and Desjardins, 1985). It will be interesting to learn if wild-derived male *Mus musculus* were also able to maintain testosterone and fertility on 30% DR, which had little effect on longevity (Fig. 3.3A).

How do energetic drains from infections influence reproduction? The extensive reallocation of energy during fever approaches the effect of 30% DR, e.g., each degree of fever increases basal metabolism by 10–15% (Fig. 1.2A legend). It is cogent to recall that until recently, chronic and acute infections were very common, if not nearly universal, in human populations. Fetal growth and viability are influenced by the maternal infectious burden (Section 4.4 and 4.5). Given the evidence that DR in lab rodents suppresses ovulatory cycles, much remains unknown about energy allocation to host defense and reproduction. In a novel approach to this major question, male birds of a species that shows declining male fertility with age (*Sula nebouxii*, the blue-footed booby) were injected with bacterial endotoxin (LPS) to evaluate the impact of immune challenge (Velando et al., 2006). LPS increased reproductive success of the old males (59% more chicks raised to fledge), whereas young adult males showed 16% fewer. It is hypothesized that the LPS increased the effectiveness of the older and frailer birds in brood care, a behavioral change that represented a reallocation strategy. Other reallocation strategies are shown in malnourished women, whose basal metabolism decreases during pregnancy, opposite to those who enter pregnancy well nourished (Section 4.4.4, Fig. 4.8).

The huge increase of voluntary running by rodents during DR (Section 3.4.3) is hypothesized to be a motivated behavior to increase the foraging range (Cabanac, 1985; Masoro and Austad, 1996; Overton and Williams, 2004). Even 10% DR increases running (Section 3.4.3) (Russell et al, 1987). Leptin treatment suppresses the DR-induced hyperactivity and exploratory activity (Buyse et al, 2001; Exner et al, 2000). With severe DR, rats do not maintain weight and may run themselves to death within a week through 'self-starvation'(Morse et al, 1995; Routtenberg and Kuznesof, 1967, 1968). Thus, expenditure of energy reserves in running may be considered as a desperate foraging strategy.

The costs of foraging were simulated by imposing bar-pressing to gain access to a large food depot (Vaughan and Rowland, 2003): As the required bar-pressing increased, feeding frequency decreased and the meal size increased, so that the total food intake was stable. Leptin-deficient obese mice had higher threshold for bar-pressing effects on feeding frequency, consistent with their slower responses to DR in accessing sugar solutions (Ramirez and Sprott, 1978). In another test of these concepts, Zebra finches were given different energy intakes by mixing seeds with chaff (Wiersma and Verhulst, 2005; Wiersma et al, 2005). With increasing chaff:seed ratios, the time spent foraging increased 5-fold; consistent with energy needs, foraging increased as temperature was lowered. These responses to DR are considered to model the hyperactivity of anorexia nervosa, which also shows associations of leptin (Holtkamp et al, 2005).

Obesity presents the converse of DR, with decreased voluntary activity (sedentarianism), tendency for hyperglycemia, and lower insulin efficiency, as observed in lab rodents, primates, and humans. Obesity increases the risk of diabetes; both are characteristic of the metabolic syndrome (Table 3.2), which is associated with accelerated mortality and aging in the arteries and eyes. As a corollary to the hyperactivity hypothesis in energy deprivation and anorexia, I suggest that sedentism is an adaptive behavior evolved with different energy set points under genetic control. When body energy reserves are ample, becoming sedentary would enhance fitness by reducing foraging or exploration, with higher risk of predation and accidents. Thus, obesity with low physical activity defines the other extreme from the increased activity during food shortages. It would not be surprising if human populations had different genetic polymorphisms that pleiotropically influence appetite, efficiency of fat storage, and voluntary activity.

DR induces stress-resistance and detoxifying enzymes, which may be adaptive during food shortages (Finch, 2004a). The increased activity and foraging range could increase exposure to toxins not present in preferred foods. In herbivores and omnivores, diet selection is optimized for maximum energy, while minimizing the ingestion of plant toxins (Duncan and Gordon, 1999). Plant foods have a remarkable diversity of toxins, produced endogenously or by associated fungi, etc., that vary widely by season and locale. An example of delayed effects of toxin ingestion during foraging is the clover disease of sheep, which causes sterility due to phytoestrogens found at some seasons in some clovers (Adams, 1976; Adams, 1990). DR increases the catabolism of toxins (Finch, 2004), described as 'xenohormesis' (Lamming et al, 2004). Starvation and DR induce various P450 cytochromes, which can accelerate toxin clearance (Bauer et al, 2004; Chou et al, 1993; Seng et al, 1996). Stress proteins (heat shock) and enzymes of DNA repair (*Rad511* induction) are also increased. The DR responses of increased locomotion and clearance of toxins are specific cases in optimum foraging theory, which recognizes multiple trade-offs that affect reproduction and somatic maintenance (Finch et al, 2004b; Yearsley, 2005).

3.8. SUMMARY

Diet restriction remains the most robust intervention to aging in lab rodents by increasing lifespan and attenuating changes at all levels, including atherosclerosis, Alzheimer disease, tumors, and other chronic degenerative diseases. Human volunteers show many positive effects of comparable DR, but effects on mortality remain to be defined. If immune responses to infections are attenuated by DR in humans, as in rodent models, then chronic DR may add hazards from infection that could counter-balance the benefits to cardiovascular functions.

The mechanisms of diet restriction (DR) and exercise in slowing aging changes and chronic diseases are poorly understood. Decreased oxidant stress, inflammatory processes, and increased life span are well documented in conventional lab rodents. DR decreases two sources of oxidative damage: Intracellular mitochondrial ROS production is decreased in muscle mitochondria in aging DR, while extracellular glyco-oxidation is decreased by the lower blood glucose. These two processes have not been integrated into a theory of oxidative damage. The close connection of inflammation and oxidative stress is implied but not directly proven by the experiments (Queries I and II, Section 1.1). However, strong evidence shows that DR attenuates both inflammation and oxidative damage, whereas obesity and high fat diets can increase both inflammation and oxidative damage (Query III).

Future studies could probe the inflammation-oxidative damage nexus with dietary manipulation of transgenic overexpressors of catalase and SOD, which increased life span (Schriner et al, 2005) and attenuated atherosclerosis (Yang et al, 2004) on *ad lib* diets (Section 1.2.6). Because wild-derived mice show very modest life span increases in response to DR, we must ask if our inbred lab rodents are misleading models for aging studies.

Despite the overwhelming evidence that obesity increases the risk of chronic disease, there is reason to consider obese and caloric intake as independent variables (Section 3.2.3, CALERIE Study and obese mice). The benefits of DR and exercise may be largest in environments that promote obesity and sedentism.

Some responses to DR can be interpreted as evolved adaptations. Suppression of ovulatory cycles and slowing of ovarian aging could enable reproduction at later ages, pending improved resources. While DR suppresses inflammation, resistance to pathogenic infections may be increased, which is a concern in lifestyles with severe diet restriction.

Exercise is an important consideration in application of DR to humans because of additional energy demands concurrent with reduced food intake. Laboratory rodents increase voluntary running activity during DR, which may be a model for the hyperactivity of anorexia. On *ad lib* feeding, regular running has a modest impact on life span, less than DR. These findings support the lowering of mortality by moderate exercise in the Harvard Alumni Health Study. Relative to sedentary and obese humans, those who exercise regularly have lower risk for cardiovascular impairments and better brain function, and better glucose regulation. Despite this impressive and growing body of evidence, it would be premature to conclude that exercise fundamentally alters human aging processes. The next chapter extends the inflammation-nutrition queries to development, where arterial aging begins and the stage may be set for vulnerability to obesity and the metabolic syndrome.

CHAPTER 4

Nutrition and Infection in the Developmental Influences on Aging

4.1. INTRODUCTION

Developmental exposure to infections and poor nutrition can profoundly influence the outcomes of aging. The 'Fetal Origins' theory of Barker and colleagues, discussed below, has focused on links of adult metabolic and vascular disease to nutrition during development. In addition, the importance of infection and inflammation during development to later outcomes of aging is argued in this chapter. Inflammatory processes are prominent in arterial disease, Alzheimer disease, cancer, diabetes and obesity, and osteoporosis (Chapter 1). The Finch-Crimmins hypothesis proposes direct links of these chronic conditions to early inflammatory exposure (Finch and Crimmins, 2004, 2005; Crimmins and Finch, 2006a,b).

Aging begins during development in three concrete ways: (I) The adult capacity for somatic repair and regeneration is set during development. The extent of molecular and cell turnover ('rejuvenation') in each organ is controlled by the gene regulatory programs installed during differentiation (Chapter 1). Cell replacement varies widely. In some systems, cells are continually replaced (erythrocytes, hepatocytes, macrophages). However, there is little to no replacement of some cells (neurons, naive T cells, oocytes) and of some cell organizations (kidney nephrons, eye lens). Molecular replacement also is set during development through cell-specific patterns of gene expression. Arterial elastin and lens crystalins accumulate progressive damage during adult life *because* these molecules are made only during development and not replaced during adult life. Because of their molecular long life spans, these molecules progressively accumulate oxidative bystander damage, e.g., aortic elastin (Fig. 1.6D). (II) Fetal arteries have microscopic foci of macrophages and oxidized LDL that are early stages of atheromas (Fig. 1.6A, Fig. 1.15). Even before birth, synergies of oxidative stress and inflammation are at work. Maternal cholesterolemia can accelerate the postnatal accumulation of arterial lipids (Section 4.8). (III) Organ development is sensitive to environmental factors acting pre- and postnatally, including nutrition, infections, inflammation, and other stressors. Each organ system has critical periods during development when environmental factors have greatest impact on cell number and homeostatic set points. This chapter addresses the complex interactions of nutrition with infections during development that can alter outcomes of aging, and extends the themes of prior chapters.

Chapter 3 discussed evidence that diet restriction during adult life improves adult health, especially in sedentary lifestyles. The efficacy of drug interventions for vascular disease may involve anti-inflammatory effects, as well as the anti-coagulant and hypocholesterolemic activities (Chapter 2). The role of infections in stimulating arteriosclerosis through inflammatory processes is plausible, though not universally accepted. Inflammatory processes may be attenuated by diet restriction, particularly in obesity. As discussed in this chapter, maternal *under*nutrition is considered a cause of small birthweight; subsequent *over*nutrition that leads to catch-up growth with earlier onset obesity increases the risk of high blood pressure and diabetes. In turn, maternal obesity increases the risk of diabetes and obesity in the subsequent generation. The current theory of fetal origins of adult disease has focused on nutritional influences.

However, infections and inflammation may also have major roles. Infections at any age can cause energy deficits equivalent to malnutrition. Early infections can profoundly influence adult mortality from infections through immune pathways and accelerated immunosenescence (Fig. 1.2A). And, resistance to infections may be diminished by undernutrition, but also by 'overnutrition' that leads to hyperglycemia (Chapters 2 and 3). Atmospheric inflammogens also need consideration, e.g., maternal smoking also decreases birthweight and, independently of birthweight, increases the risk of childhood obesity (Section 4.5.3). These complex interactions are best understood from an ecological perspective.

This chapter begins with a historical synopsis of the Fetal Origins theory but does not attempt to give full details, which are hotly debated. The broad theory that adult diseases have fetal origins (developmental influences) is widely recognized through the leadership of David Barker, Clive Osmund, and many other colleagues in the past two decades. Review of those seminal papers shows a strong role of infections that, though well documented, is not widely known. Although no one denies developmental influences on chronic diseases of aging, the early influences are diverse and extend beyond low birthweight, the current focus of many studies.

The role of birthweight and adult height in adult health and longevity is then discussed, with a focus on nutrition and infections. Twins are an important example: Despite their low birthweight, adult twins have normal adult health and life expectancy. Other factors are at work in the associations of low singleton birthweights with later growth and mortality. Revisiting the classic Barker-Osmund studies shows influences of infection on later diseases. Many other studies clearly show the impact of maternal infections and early life infections on later adult health and mortality. Immune hyperstimulation during development, as well as in adult life, appears to deplete naive T cells used in instructive immunity and limit protective responses to new infections (Sections 1.2 and 2.8). Infections may also have an unrecognized role in the effects of pre- and postnatal exposure to malnutrition in Europe during World War II ('epidemic shadows,' discussed below). The efficacy of nutritional supplements pre- and postnatally may depend on the infectious load. These examples from unhygienic environments of the 20th century help to understand the remarkable recent increase of human life spans. The old world examples are relevant guides to future changes in the infectious and inflammatory environment, which may be progressively worsening (Chapter 6).

The mechanisms are multifarious in these hugely complex developmental variations. Infections during pregnancy can affect the placenta and fetal nutrient supply. Fetal arteries are also clearly influenced by maternal cholesterol, which can alter the rate of arteriosclerosis postnatally (Section 4.8). Additionally, fetal growth interacts ($G \times E$) with alleles of TNFα and other inflammatory mediators that mediate resistance to infectious pathogens. Lastly, I consider maternal nutrition and infections in terms of fetal-maternal competition and imprinting, returning again to the critical role of the insulin/IGF system that regulates not only metabolism and aging, but also development.

4.2. SYNOPSIS OF THE FETAL ORIGINS THEORY

The concept that adult health is sensitive to environmental influences on development is not new. A good starting place is the remarkable 1934 study of Kermack, McKendrick, and McKinlay of 18th and 19th century cohorts of Britain and Sweden (Kermack et al., 1934). Survivors of early mortality in these birth cohorts retained characteristic mortality rates throughout the life span into old age. Mortality improved in successive generations, again across the life span. Another of their key insights is that these effects are transgenerational, i.e. the improved health of mothers preceded and enhanced the health and physique of their children. The reduction of virulent infections was indicated in the environmental improvements.

After the starvation in World War II, nutrition joined the discussion of environmental effects on long-term health. Many studies showed that growth can be irreversibly attenuated by caloric deficits during critical periods (Widdowson et al, 1964; Widdowson and McCance, 1975) and that puberty can be delayed, but not irreversibly, by disease and nutrition (Tanner, 1962, 1981). Infections can also attenuate postnatal growth of mice (Dubos et al, 1966). Subsequently, there seemed to be few lasting effects, with rapid rebound of health and fecundity after the Dutch Hunger Winter, 1944–1945 (Section 4.7) and in the Minnesota Starvation Experiment (Section 3.2.3).

A major effort was launched after World War II to improve maternal health and early growth by nutritional supplements in impoverished populations (Kramer, 1993; Pelletier, 1994; Ramakrishnan, 2004; Scrimshaw et al, 1968; Scrimshaw, 2003). Malnutrition and infection were recognized to synergize with effects that multiplied their individual contributions to mortality. Moreover, infections can *cause* malnutrition: by impairing ingestion and reallocating energy (Fig. 1.2B) for host defense, chronic infections or series of acute infections can slow growth. In many studies, nutritional supplements alone had limited benefit. The INCAP studies in Guatemalan villages, for example, provided either supplemental food or excellent medical care, 1959–1964. The nutritional supplement decreased respiratory and diarrheal infections by 70%, but the medical treatments had negligible benefit to preschool children (numerous reports summarized in (Scrimshaw and Guzman, 1995; Scrimshaw, 2003; Schroeder, 1995). At the end, these children's height and weight did not differ between the villages, nor was the parasitic load changed. It is generally recognized that child health improvements require a full program that fundamentally alters the local environment, including education and hygiene, in addition to vaccination and drugs. Still, the explosive population growth during the Industrial Revolution is attributed to improved food and better distribution in McKeown's *The Modern Rise of Population* (McKeown, 1976) and then Fogel and Costa's *Technophysio Revolution* (Fogel and Costa, 1997), with less importance given to public health and hygiene.

In the early 1970s, Dorner proposed that metabolic hormonal regulation (ACTH, insulin, GH, TSH) and feeding behavior are epigenetically programmed at critical phases of development, with long-term impact on adult metabolism; papers in German are summarized in (Dorner, 1974; Dorner, 1976; Plagemann, 2005). Based on the recognized effects of maternal diabetes on fetal development, Dorner hypothesized critical phases of development in the hypothalamic metabolic and appetite centers, analogous to the time window of sensitivity to fetal sex steroids during hypothalamic sexual differentiation.

A decade later, Barker hypothesized that maternal malnutrition is the main influence on adult vascular health, through growth retardation leading to small birthweight (Barker and Osmond, 1986; Barker, 2004). This analysis of birth cohorts showed strong correlations between of infant mortality and later cardiovascular disease mortality for the survivors (Fig. 4.1A). Concurrently, Brenner noted links of low birthweight to adult hypertension, which he attributed to impaired kidney development (Brenner et al, 1988). Low birthweight babies have fewer nephron tubules, which places them at greater risk of cumulative damage to these irreplaceable structures. Deficits in functional nephrons can raise blood pressure, which is associated with increased risk of heart attack and stroke (Fig. 1.6C). Then, Hales with Barker further noted the association of diabetes at later ages with lower birthweight and early rapid postnatal growth (Hales et al., 1991; Hales and Barker, 2001). The diabetes was attributed to adult onset insulin insufficiency linked to pancreatic β-cell defects acquired during development.

Further, the Barker group found associations of low birthweight with elevated adult systolic pressure (Fig. 4.1B). As observed a follow-up study of low birthweight babies from Sheffield, England, by age 50, systolic pressure was lower by 6 mm for each kg higher birthweight (Martyn et al., 1995). These findings, though controversial, were generally confirmed in a huge meta-analysis: systolic blood pressure varied inversely with birthweight in children, adolescents, and

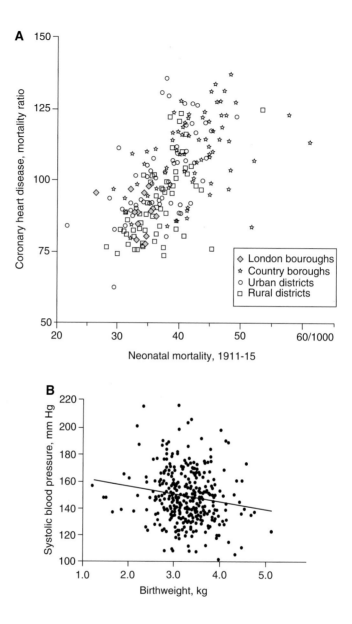

FIGURE 4.1 Early and later age correlations of mortality and birthweight. A. Mortality rates of infants (1911–1915) and adult (male) (1968–1978) from ischemic heart disease (coronary artery disease) in England and Wales (Barker and Osmond, 1986). The regression coefficients (r, 0.69) approximate those of Norwegian historical cohorts in an overlapping period, 1895–1925 (Forsdahl, 1977) (Fig. 2.1; r, 0.86). B. Systolic pressure at age 50–53 varied inversely with birthweight: Adults with low birth weights (<2497 g) had 17 mm Hg systolic pressure above the heaviest (>3859 g) (337 Ss, born 1939–1940; Sheffield, UK) (Martyn et al, 1995).

(Continues)

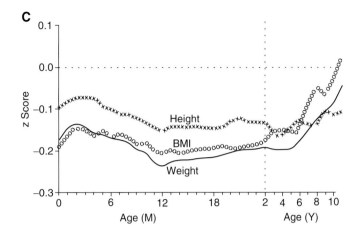

FIGURE 4.1 (continued) C. Early growth in Finnish boys who developed coronary heart disease as adults in relation to height, weight, and body mass index (BMI) from birth to age 11 y, expressed as deviations from the mean (*z-scores*, see below) (Barker et al., 2005). From the Helsinki Birth Cohort Study (Eriksson, 2005), second cohort of births 1934–1944 (4360 men), Helsinki University Central Hospital, who were exposed to food shortages before and during World War II. About 60% of the families were laborers, and some were known to be malnourished. Deviations from the mean at each age of the coronary subgroup are expressed in standard deviations (z-score). For example, the birthweight of the coronary subgroup was 0.2 SD below the mean. However, short length at birth was not a risk. The catch-up of body weight (increased BMI score) after age 2 y predicted coronary events better than BMI at any age. Low birthweight, low BMI at age 2 y, and high BMI at 11 y each were predictive. Girls had a similar pattern (not shown here).

adults, with average effect of 2 mm higher pressure per kg lower birthweight (80 studies, 440,000 Ss worldwide up to age 80) (Huxley et al., 2000). Head size (circumference) at birth, however, was even more strongly associated with adult blood pressure than birthweight. The 2 mm pressure/kg birthweight effect seems modest, relative to the effects of aging on systolic blood pressure, which approximates 5 mm/decade during adult life (Chapter 1, Fig. 1.6B). Other long-lasting effects of the fetal environment may be adaptive responses to food availability that supports catch-up growth. Diabetes at later ages is also associated with lower birthweight and postnatal growth. According to the 'thrifty gene hypothesis,' type-2 diabetes is a 'thrifty genotype rendered detrimental by progress' (Neel, 1962; Neel, 1999). Rapid secretion of insulin could be adaptive during uncertain food supply, but maladaptive in affluent times when food is reliably available and physical demands are low. Hales and Barker (2001) further considered a 'thrifty phenotype' developed by the growth retarded fetus, which was hypothesized to program glucose-insulin metabolism during development in response to maternal malnutrition. Consequent insulin resistance would increase efficiency of fat storage, leading to obesity. Catch-up growth by those small-at-birth is a major co-variate in adult risk of metabolic disorders predisposing to vascular disease (Barker et al., 2005) (Fig. 4.1C). Genetic influences on fetal growth (Section 4.10) could be adaptive.

Another important human complexity came to light in these decades: socioeconomic status. Marmot and colleagues (1978) showed strong SES associations with heart disease, attributable to differences in smoking and sugar consumption (Marmot et al, 1978)[1]. SES is now well-known for lifelong effects on health (Berkman, 2005; Marmot, 2006).

In the current model of fetal origins of adult disease, development is adjusted to enable 'predictive adaptive responses' in anticipation of the postnatal environment (Barker, 2002, 2004; Bateson, 2007; Gluckman and Hanson, 2005; Plagemann, 2005; Vickers et al, 2005; Welles, 2007). Animal models show complex dose responses, in which maternal under- and overnutrition can both predispose to adult obesity and diabetes, depending on postnatal nutrients. Additionally, adult stress responses may also be developmentally modified. This plasticity, or programmability, is restricted to particular developmental stages and is often conditional depending on multiple factors (Vickers et al, 2005). Thus was 'the Barker hypothesis' extended to include multifarious influences of the maternal environment during critical or 'plastic' phases of development on outcomes of aging (Bateson, 2004; Gluckman, 2004; Plagemann, 2005). This synopsis represents the majority view that nutritional factors are paramount influences on chronic degenerative diseases of aging, principally vascular disease, cancer, and diabetes.

However, nutritional factors do not fully explain the early mortality, which is dominated by infections, as recognized by Kermack et al. (1934) and discussed below (Fig. 4.2). Crimmins and I have proposed a 'cohort morbidity hypothesis' to link early and later health through inflammatory processes (Finch and Crimmins, 2004; Crimmins et al 2006a,b). The level of chronic inflammation and infection from early in life influences later life health by interacting with the inflammatory processes in most chronic diseases. We consider that inflammation synergizes with malnutrition in the pathogenesis of adult chronic diseases (Fig. 1.2A). Acting at many levels within the gene regulatory matrix, the infectious load causes reallocation of nutrients, in turn attenuating organ development and growth. These insults may be superimposed on, and reciprocally modify, the developmental programming as studied in 'clean' animal models. Inflammatory mechanisms in later disease have not received as much emphasis as nutrition alone in the developmental theory of aging. Their consideration from the beginning could have developed a deeper research agenda that included the synergies of infection and nutrition during development, which were well recognized by the international development community.

---

[1]Soon after, in 1980, the Thatcher government tried to suppress the politically explosive report on *The Health Divide* (Sir Douglas Black: *Inequalities in Health: Report of a Research Working Group*), initiated under the prior Labour Party government. Reprinted with comments (Townsend and Davidson, 1982).

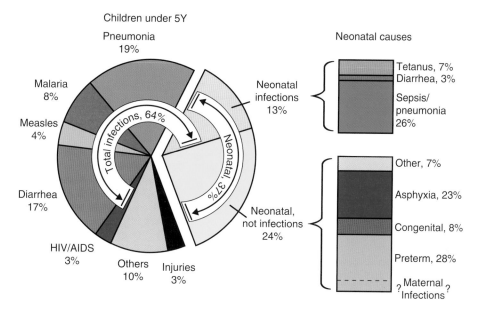

FIGURE 4.2 **Pie chart of mortality causes for children under 5, worldwide 2000–2003** (Adapted from World Health Organization, 2005b). The bar graph shows neonatal causes with my interpretation of maternal infections.

4.3. THE BARKER STUDIES OF INFECTIONS AND VASCULAR DISEASE

Barker's early papers are explicit in the importance of early infections to later age mortality. The initial Barker-Osmond report (Barker and Osmond, 1986), besides its main focus on ischemic heart disease, also analyzed mortality from respiratory infections by cohort and period. The cohort from England and Wales was born 1921–1925 and did not have access to antibiotics until adulthood. Adult deaths from rheumatic heart disease and bronchitis were as strongly associated with infant mortality[2] as cardiovascular death (Table 4.1A, reformatted from this

---

[2]Early mortality distinguishes *stillbirths* from *infant mortality,* dying after birth up to age 364 days. This interval is subdivided in two periods: (I) *neonatal mortality,* liveborn and dying 0 to <28 days and (II) *postneonatal mortality* during 28–364 days.

report). Infant mortality was attributed to two main causes of similar magnitude: infections (39%) and 'congenital causes' (41%). These figures for England-Wales of the mid-1920s approximate the current proportions of death causes worldwide before age 5 (Fig. 4.2), despite the much higher total mortality 80 years before. In the correlations of overall infant mortality with the adult cause of death in this population, adult bronchitis ranked highest, followed by adult stomach cancer, and then of equal weight, adult ischemic- and rheumatic heart disease (Table 4.1B). Most correlations are >0.5.

The infant mortality was also subdivided into deaths during the neonatal (0–27 d) and postneonatal periods (28–364 d) (not shown in Table 4.1). Adult

TABLE 4.1 Infant Mortality and Adult Death by Cause in 20th Century England and Wales

TABLE 4.1 A Causes of Infant Mortality (≤ 1 y) in England and Wales 1921–1925

Cause of Death	Infant Deaths (Total 291, 082)
congenital	41%
bronchitis & pneumonia	21%
diarrhea	11%
other infections	7%
other causes	20%
all infections 39%	

Calculated from (Barker and Osmond, 1986).

TABLE 4.1 B Correlations of All Infant Mortality with Specified Adult Causes of Death, 35–74 Years

Cause of Death	Correlation Coefficient, r
bronchitis	0.82
cancers:	
cervix	0.60
lung	0.46
stomach	0.79
ischemic heart disease	0.73
rheumatic heart disease	0.72
stroke	0.54

From (Barker and Osmond, 1986), Table 1 and text.

TABLE 4.1 C Standardized Mortality Ratios and Weight at Birth and at 1 Year

Age/Birth Weight Classes	Cause of Death (Number of Cases)		
	Ischemic Heart Disease (434)	Chronic Obstructive Lung Disease (43)	All Causes (1186)
Birth Weight			
≤5.5 lb	104	93	101
6	77	59	69
7	90	75	83
8	85	50	80
9	62	69	70
≥10	81	33	77
1-year weight			
≤18 lb	111	129	89
19–20	81	86	89
21–22	98	41	85
23–24	71	61	68
25–26	68	52	73
≥27	42	29	58

(Barker et al., 1989b), Table 1. The inverse trend of size and mortality from 'all cause' and ischemic heart disease was significant (P<0.001 and <0.002, respectively). Excluding lung and heart disease eliminated the 'all cause' significance. The lowest birth weight <5.5 lb corresponds to WHO standards <2500 g (Section 4.4.3) and comprised 4.4% of this sample.

death from ischemic heart disease was equally strongly correlated with neonatal and postneonatal deaths, with deaths from 'bronchitis and pneumonia' ranking highest over both periods (all r, 0.68–0.69). Stroke death, however, correlated better with neonatal (r, 0.66) than postneonatal (0.44) mortality. Adult deaths from bronchitis correlated more with postneonatal deaths (0.83) than neonatal deaths (0.58); deaths from 'bronchitis and pneumonia' again ranking highest (0.85), followed by diarrhea (0.74). Consistent with the major role of infections, adult death from rheumatic heart disease correlated more strongly with postneonatal deaths (0.72) than neonatal (0.55) deaths; the early causes of death were mainly from bronchitis and pneumonia (0.73).

While poor nutrition in early life has an undeniable role in mortality, these data on a pre-antibiotic cohort also show the importance of infection, to which even well-nourished infants are vulnerable. Among many examples, rheumatic heart disease is due to early streptococcal infection (Chapter 2). Another pathogenic pathway may also be considered (Fig. 1.2A) in which high infectious exposure early in life accelerates immunosenescence by depleting the pool of naive T cells (Section 2.8). The depletion of naive T cells is implicated in increased vulnerability to influenza among elderly ('immune risk phenotype') (Huppert et al, 2003; Wikby et al, 2005) (Section 1.2).

Further analysis of these 212 districts of England and Wales (Barker et al, 1989b) strengthened the role of neonatal and postneonatal influences. Adult ischemic heart deaths had independent trends with both neo- and postneonatal mortality. Bronchitis deaths trended mainly with postneonatal, whereas stroke trended mainly with neonatal mortality. Neonatal mortality was attributed to adverse intrauterine environment, which caused lower birth weights. A given example was a hospital with high maternal mortality, and neonatal mortality had average birth weights that were 289 g lower than in other hospitals with low neonatal and maternal mortality. These observations are consistent with infections causing deaths of lying-in mothers and babies, but also, I suggest, with prenatal effects of infection and nutrition on fetal retardation. The early-later age correlations in mortality with infections suggest that district differences in the infectious environment persisted for decades. As a possible mechanism, immune hyperstimulation is recognized to deplete naive T cells and is associated with oligoclonal memory T cells in unstable atheromas (Section 1.5.1) (De Palma et al, 2006).

Soon after, another paper described early body weight as a risk factor for ischemic heart disease (Barker et al, 1989b). In six districts of Hertfordshire among the above 212, the risk of ischemic heart disease in men up to age 70 was inversely correlated with weight at birth and at 365 days (Table 4.1C). Chronic obstructive lung disease, which accounts for 10% of adult deaths, had a similar relationship to birth weight. This report emphasized both pre- and postnatal growth retardation in the risk of later heart disease. Growth during the first year is very sensitive to infections (Fig. 1.2B) (Section 4.4), even with the breast-feeding that most of these men received. I suggest that postnatal growth retardation of these men reflects chronic infections that can accelerate immunosenescence with links to unstable atheromas, as noted above.

The next report linked adult height with these same diseases (Barker, 1990). The counties with taller averages had lower mortality of infectious origins from chronic bronchitis and rheumatic heart disease (caused by infections) and from ischemic heart disease and stroke (not immediately linked to infections). The relative mortality risk of men for each cause of death varied by average height in counties, given as the ratio of shortest:tallest height class: bronchitis, 1.8-fold; rheumatic heart disease, 1.4; ischemic heart disease, 1.28; stroke, 1.33. Women showed similar trends. In both sexes, reproductive tract cancers had the opposite trend, with consistently higher incidence in counties with taller average height, an association that has been verified and extended, e.g., for breast cancer.

Infections were recognized for interactions with nutrition from the beginning: " . . . frequent intercurrent infections [can lead to] impaired nutrition" (Barker and Osmond, 1986, p. 1081). In many districts of Europe before WWII, average health was close to the current developing world in infectious disease. However, the subsequent focus sharpened to nutrition, and maternal infections were not discussed in a review on fetal nutrition and cardiovascular disease (Barker et al, 1993). The malnutrition-infection synergy has not been given much attention as the fetal origins field expanded, but is well recognized in health-poor developing countries where chronic infectious disease is more prevalent than in the health-rich developed countries.

Further findings are emerging from recent Barker–Osmond collaborations with the Helsinki Birth Cohort Study, which has detailed data on parental characteristics and childhood growth (Eriksson, 2005). In the cohort born 1934–1944, birth weights <2500 g predicted threefold higher adult risk for coronary heart disease (CHD) (O.R., 3.63). Slow growth up to 2 y also increased risk of CHD (Barker et al, 2005) (Fig. 4.1C) and stroke (Osmond et al, 2007). Catch-up growth ('obesity rebound') after age 2 increased adult risk of diabetes type 2 and CHD. Malnutrition is discussed as a likely factor in growth impairments, because these children and their mothers were exposed to food shortages before and during World War II: about 60% of the families were laborers, and some were known to be malnourished (Eriksson, 2005). Moreover, preceding generations were not well nourished, the average reaching 3000 kcal/d only after 1890 (Heikkinen, 1996). Adult height of Finns increased mostly in the 20th century (Silventoinen et al, 2000), approximating the trend for increased food consumption (Heikkinen, 1996). Nutritional deficits would also have been permissive for infections, a real possibility in this pre-antibiotic cohort which has not been considered in these Helsinki analyses.

These associations of early growth impairments and later vascular disease risk have been confirmed in many studies, but certainly not by all. Major issues beyond the methodological have been raised (Elford et al, 1991; Paneth and Susser, 1995; Paneth and Susser, 1996; Huxley et al, 2000). However, it seems rash to declare losers and winners, and wiser to focus on the emerging complex links between development and aging, and their gene-environment interactions.

Human health at any age is an outcome of multiple contingencies. For example, consider smoking, which all agree is harmful. Yet, most life-long smokers (85%) do not die of lung cancer (Fig. 2.11). Moreover, Jeanne Calment, who holds the record life span of 122, regularly smoked up to age 117 (Allard et al, 1998, p. 73). There may be constitutional factors (genetic and developmental variations, Section 5.2) that protect some smokers from lung cancer or premature mortality. Let's now broaden the discussion from the focus on maternal nutrition as the main cause of fetal growth retardation to other environmental effects from infections and inflammation: gene-environmental interactions. The next sections consider interactions of infections, inflammation, nutrition, and growth to adult disease and mortality. This evidence further develops the cohort morbidity hypothesis (Finch and Crimmins, 2004; Crimmins and Finch, 2006a) and expands the domain of fetal origins into the real germy world.

4.4. SIZE, HEALTH, AND LONGEVITY

Larger-sized animal species generally live longer, whether feral or domestic. Among mammals, life span broadly scales with adult size according to allometric relationships of adult body mass and length (Calder, 1984; Finch, 1990, pp. 267–271). Yet, women are about 10% shorter than men, but live about 10%

longer in most populations. Moreover, the allometry of life span, despite its statistical power, also includes major species deviations (Finch *op. cit*; Speakman, 2005), e.g., the naked mole rat, 30–80 g, that lives at least 28 y (Section 1.2.6), or even more extreme, the 6 g Brandt's bat that lives at least 41 y (Podlutsky et al, 2005).[3] We must be mindful that the allometry of life span is not derived from any known invariant property of cells or physiology.

Human height and weight vary widely across populations, modern and historical. Little is known about the genetic basis for these variations between populations. However, in all populations, pre- and postnatal development is very sensitive to environmental factors that influence adult height and weight: nutrition and infections. The following synthesis of diverse evidence shows that the levels of nutrition and infection during development are major determinants of adult size, but are also major determinants of adult mortality from infections and vascular disease. I will argue that small size at birth, which is very common in health-poor[4] populations, is in response to energy restriction from the maternal load of infection and inflammation, in addition to nutritional deficits (Section 4.9). Responses to energy limitations include lower maternal metabolism during pregnancy and smaller food intake required by the small-sized offspring to reproduce within a shortened life expectancy. Identical twins in health-rich populations contrast starkly with pathological growth retardation: Despite the 900 g birthweight deficits, in healthy circumstances twins have 'true' catch-up growth and as adults have normal health and longevity.

4.4.1. Adult Height, Vascular Disease, and Longevity

In most modern populations, taller people live longer (Davey Smith et al, 2000; Davey Smith and Ebrahim, 2002). In the U.S. NHANES I survey (1971–1974), short height predicts mortality, with strongest effects in the range 50–75 y (Sunder, 2005). These relationships are represented in Waaler plots (Waaler, 1984; Fogel and Costa, 1997; Fogel, 2004) defined by contours (isoclines) of mortality rates as a function of height and body mass index (BMI) (Fig. 4.3A) (Sunder, 2005). The optimal BMI for minimum mortality is similar for both sexes. The asymmetry of the height-BMI contours in women indicates a subgroup with different pathophysiology.

---

[3]Wild-caught male Brandt's bat, *Myotis brandtii*. Another allometric longevity outlier may be the 2 g Kitti's hog-nosed bat, *Craseonycteris thongylongyai*. Bumble-bee sized, this is the smallest mammal and is a bit smaller than the smallest rodent, the pygmy shrew *(Sorex minutus)* at 2.5-5 g, which lives at least 18 m.

[4]When populations are well nourished and have minimum infectious disease, I suggest they be designated as 'health-rich,' as predominates in the 'developed' nations. A current ethic is to distinguish developed and developing countries. However, all countries include health-poor subpopulations that develop and live in unhealthy environments and have shorter life expectancy. Health-poor populations also tend to be lower socioeconomic status and, in some countries, are increasingly obese.

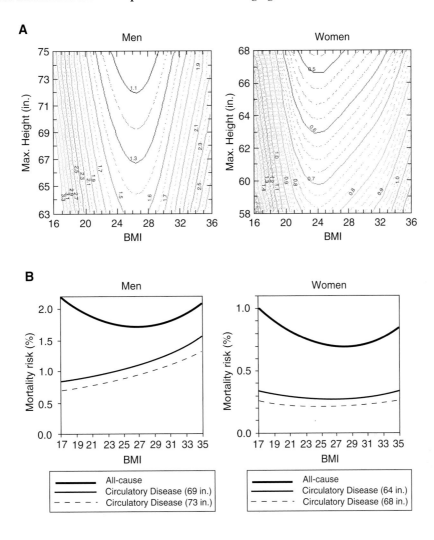

FIGURE 4.3 Adult height decreases mortality risks in NHANES I. (From Sunder 2005.) A. Contours (isoclines, Waaler plot) (Waaler, 1984) of mortality rates as a function of height and body mass index (BMI) at age 60 based on non-parametric regressions in which the BMI-height surface predicted relative mortality risk. B. Height and mortality risk from cardiovascular disease for a 60-year-old man with height of 69 inches (175 cm). An additional 4 in (10 cm) of height would decrease mortality risk 14%. BMI has a small effect on mortality risk from vascular causes, consistent with the small effect of BMI within the range 20–30 m/kg^2 on total mortality in NHANES (Fig. 3.4A, Chapter 3).

Cardiovascular mortality may be the most strongly correlated with height in men and women (Fig. 4.3B): In NHANES I, each inch of additional height reduced the risk of vascular death in men by 3.5% and in women by 5.25% (Sunder, 2005). The BMI has a small effect on mortality risk from vascular causes, consistent with overall causes of death in the NHANES for BMI of 20 to 30 (Fig. 3.4A, Chapter 3). Similarly, in the Physicians Healthy Study (United States), each inch of additional height reduced the risk of heart disease by 2–3% (Hebert et al, 1993). Most other studies concur (Langenberg et al, 2005; McCarron et al, 2002; Nwasokwa et al, 1997), including studies of twins (Silventoinen et al, 2003).

Dementia, both Alzheimer disease and vascular dementia, also varied inversely with height at midlife (Israeli Ischemic Study, 1,892 men) (Beeri et al, 2005). If replicated, these findings will further the broad overlap of risk factors and mechanisms in cardiovascular, cerebrovascular, and Alzheimer disease (Section 1.7.4).

The lower risks of being tall derive from many factors. First, relative tallness implies minimal growth retardation and better health during development. Other factors may follow from healthy development of a larger size. At birth, the diameter of coronary arteries scale in proportion to the height and weight: Larger arteries show less vulnerability to occlusions (Section 4.4.5). Additionally, glucose tolerance, a vascular risk factor in the metabolic syndrome (Chapter 1, Table 1.8), may be better in the taller (Brown et al, 1991; Leger et al, 1997). Glucose tolerance was impaired in men shorter than controls by 3.5 cm and women shorter by 3.0 cm (adjusted for BMI and age) (Brown et al, 1991). Other causes of death may have opposite relationships to height: Aortic aneurysms (McCarron et al, 2002) and cancer as noted by (Barker, 1990), among other conditions (Gunnell, 1998). Associations of height with different causes of death and life span may be expected to differ across populations because these conditions vary in prevalence.

Socioeconomic status (SES) deeply influences health throughout life, briefly mentioned in Section 4.2. In NHANES I and some other studies, low SES is linked to shortness and higher mortality, particularly from cardiovascular disease (Allebeck and Bergh, 1992; Floud et al, 1990; Marmot et al, 1978; Sunder, 2005). These interactions are broadly consistent with the Fetal Origins theory, because early age mortality and the inflammatory load are also worse in lower SES (Alley et al, 2005; Koster et al, 2006). Even in developed countries, low SES increases exposure to the same adverse influences of infection, inflammation, and poor nutrition, which once prevailed prior to the 20th century in the most developed countries of those times.

In historical cohorts from 18th and 19th century northern Europe, neonatal mortality was inversely correlated with adult height (Crimmins and Finch, 2006a) (Fig. 4.4), while both neonatal and childhood mortality correlated inversely with mortality rates at older ages (Chapter 2, Fig. 2.7B). These relationships extend the hypothesis of Kermack, McKendrick, and McKinlay (1934) (Section 4.2) that successive cohorts in England and Sweden had lower mortality throughout life because of improved health during childhood. They also noted a relationship to height ('physique') but provided no analysis. As discussed in Chapters 1 and 2, the reduction of early infections would also reduce the chronic inflammatory load,

max. height, mm

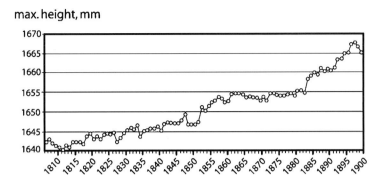

FIGURE 4.4 Adult height is predicted by neonatal mortality. Historical changes in male adult height in France (military recruits, age about 21 y, 1806–1895). Neonatal mortality correlated strongly with adult height (r^2, 0.93). Height changes in Sweden 1820–1895 are similarly correlated (r^2, 0.88). A gradually decreasing burden of infection and inflammation is hypothesized to be the common factor in these correlations of early age mortality, growth stunting, and later age mortality (Crimmins and Finch, 2006a).

thereby attenuating the inflammatory processes in vascular disease along with other causes of morbidity during aging that share many inflammatory mechanisms.

Adult height has increased progressively in most countries since the mid-18th century (Floud et al, 1990; Fogel, 2004; Tanner, 1981). Among many examples, during the past 250 years in Norway, male height increased by 21 cm from an average of 158 cm (62″) in 1761 to the current 179 cm (70.5″) (Waaler, 1984). The progressive increase of height and lowering of old age mortality in the 18th and 19th centuries was interpreted as the shared benefits of lower metabolic costs of infectious disease during the early years (Crimmins and Finch, 2006a). According to our hypothesis, the reduction of infections, together with improved nutrition, would enhance early growth, leading to taller adults. Infections have high energy costs from fever and other host defense responses that re-allocate nutrients at the expense of growth (Fig. 1.2B). Infections account for most mortality before age 2 when the rate of growth is also greatest (Fig. 4.5). The increase of adult height during improving conditions is included in the Fogel-Costa hypothesis of "technophysio evolution" (Fogel and Costa, 1997; Fogel, 2004). The crucial infection-nutrition relationships are discussed later for modern health-poor populations (Section 4.6.5).

4.4.2. Size at Birth and Adult Height

Adult height is strongly influenced by size differences that arise during development. Sex differences emerge after 32 weeks of gestation. By term, boys are 150g

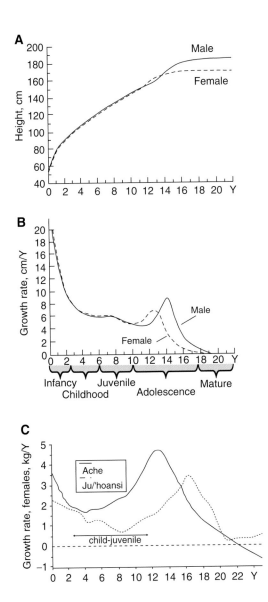

FIGURE 4.5 Growth rate curves. A. Total height normative curves for healthy children. The fastest growth ceases by age 3 y. (Redrawn from Bogin, 1999b.) B. Growth rate, normative, cm/y. The adolescent growth spurt is earlier in girls. (Redrawn from Bogin, 1999b.) C. Growth rates for Aché (solid) and Ju/'hoansi (dotted) females, kg/y. (Redrawn from Walker et al, 2006a.) These pre-industrial people have different growth rates by 2–3 years. The Aché are forager farmers (Paraguay) (Hill and Hurtado, 1996) with adolescent growth spurt peak velocity at 13; menarche at 14; first child at 17.7; adult height is 149 cm; Ju/hoansi are foragers (Botswana/Namibia) with adolescent growth spurt peak velocity at 16; menarche at 16.6; first child at 18.8; adult height is 150 cm.

heavier than girls on average. This sex difference continues postnatally with 500g differences by 12 m (Thomson et al, 1968). In the largest study of birth size (length and weight) so far, (393,570 Norwegian males 1967–1979) (Eide et al, 2005), the majority of births were >45 cm with normal gestation ages of 39–41 weeks; adult height closely followed birth length in each birth weight class (Fig. 4.6A, B). Among those short at birth (<45 cm, 2% of all births), the birth length did not predict adult height (Fig. 4.6A). Birth length accounted for up to 9% of adult height variation. Together, the birth weight and length accounted for 15% of adult height variation. Thus, most (85%) adult height variations were not accounted for by birth size.

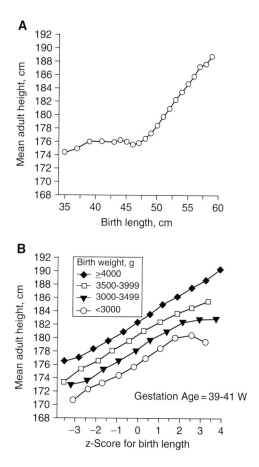

FIGURE 4.6 Adult height and birth length in Norwegian males. (Adapted from Eide et al, 2005). A. Adult height is proportional to birth length for >45 cm. B. Adult height stratified by birth weight classes; plotted against z-score for birth length (SD about mean).

Twins are particularly vulnerable to growth retardation from environmental hazards because of their small birth size. Finnish twin cohorts born before 1928 showed lower heritability of height, with progressive increases in heritability approximately in parallel with national economic improvements (Silventoinen et al, 2000). Other studies cited show lower heritability of height in twins from health-poor populations. Currently, Finnish twin adult height has a high heritability of about 90% (GenomeEUtwin cohorts) (Silventoinen et al, 2003a,b). These estimates may be also confounded by multigenerational effects of the environment, by which smaller mothers have smaller babies. The resolution of these gene-environment interactions is complicated by gene imprinting (Section 4.9).

4.4.3. Criteria for Growth Retardation

The focus on birth weight as a predictor of adult health and aging is motivated by two influences on mortality: (I) Small babies are more vulnerable to postnatal infections and higher mortality (Boulet et al, 2006; Karn and Penrose 1952); (II) smaller birth weight from <2500 g into the normative range is associated with adult systolic pressure and with other risk factors for cardiovascular disease included in the metabolic syndrome (Table 3.2). In a large meta-analysis, neonatal systolic pressure was positively associated with birth weight (80 studies, 440,000 Ss worldwide) (Huxley et al., 2000). The coronary risk of adults is increased by catch-up growth. Moreover, heavier babies (macrosomia) are also at risk for becoming obese as adults with metabolic disorders, particularly if their mothers were obese or had diabetes (Section 4.6). Much is still obscure about blood pressure regulation across the life span.

Most birth weights in the developed countries are >3000 g, with <10% below 2500 g—e.g., Norway (Fig. 4.7) (UNICEF, 2004). The criterion of low birthweight as <2500 g (5 lb, 8 oz) was proposed by Arvo Ylppö in 1919 and became widely used (World Health Organization, 2005a). The criterion weight for macrosomia is >4000 g. Not surprisingly, mortality risk curves vary between populations with different norms of birth weight (Rooth, 1980; Rooth and Ericson, 1980). In the developing world, particularly in rural areas and city slums, average birth weights are lower by up to 900 g (Table 4.2). India and Bangladesh are extremes with 30% of births <2500 g. The U.S. incidence of low birth weight in White non-Hispanics was 8.4%; and in Blacks, 4.8% (Hoyert et al, 2006). Birth length follows a similar distribution in Norway (Fig. 4.6B).

Low birth weight arises from two main causes: (I) impaired fetal growth (intrauterine growth retardation) and/or (II) prematurity (preterm delivery, before 37 weeks). The relative importance of growth retardation and prematurity differs by the level of national development and the average income, which determines the quality of the diet, hygiene, housing, health, etc. In health-poor developing countries, retarded fetal growth accounts for most of the low birth weights, and prematurity has a minor contribution. In modern, health-rich countries of Europe and the Americas, low birth weight is <10% and is mainly due to prematurity

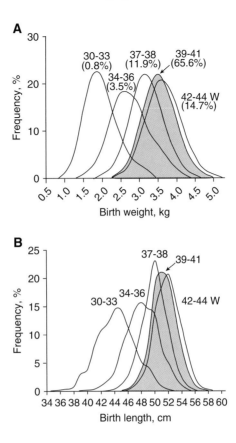

FIGURE 4.7 Birth frequency distributions by gestational age at birth. Norwegian boys 1967-1979 (393, 570 singleton births), followed to 1999. (Redrawn from Eide et al, 2005.) The shading identifies the majority weight and height classes. The parentheses indicate percent of all births in each gestational age class. A. Birth weight frequency distribution by gestational age at birth. B. Birth length.

(Villar and Belizan, 1982). Maternal age also strongly influences the incidence of low birthweight, with a U-shaped curve highest at early and later ages across ethnic groups (Ananth et al, 2004).

There is debate on the choice of threshold for low birthweight because of major differences between populations. Rooth (1980) suggested a new criterion normalized to the distribution as 2 standard deviations below the mean for countries with different mean birth weight. This is equivalent to a z-score of minus 2.

TABLE 4.2 Maternal Birth Weight and Size

Population	Birth Weight, Mean, g	% <2500 g	Maternal Size, Height (m); BMI, kg/m^2
poor urban Indian	2763[1]	>30[2]	1.6; 20.4[1]
middle-upper class Indian[3]	3060		1.61; 20.4
rural Gambia[4]	2980	17	1.59; 20.7
	seasonal minimum, 2750		
rural Guatemala[5]	2549	34	1.43; 25.9
U.S.[6]	3500	7.8%	1.73; 24.8

1. (Stein et al., 1996); Mysore, South India, born 1934–1954 measured at age 47 y.
2. (Yajnik et al, 2003; Yajnik, 2004a,b).
3. (Piers et al, 1995); Indian women, living in London; non-vegetarian.
4. (Ceesay et al., 1997); West Kiang region, 1984–1990.
5. (Mata, 1978); Santa Maria Cauque; 1964–1972, Tables 5.2, 6.3, 7.5.
6. NHANES III.

This relative criteria also adjusted for the neonatal mortality, which was less than expected in some countries for the absolute weight class. Implicit in this proposal is the controversial possibility that lower birth weight is an adaptation to local conditions (Section 4.8).

4.4.4. Maternal Metabolism and Fetal Growth

Direct evidence for adaptation of fetal growth to local conditions is the remarkable variation of maternal fat deposition and basal metabolic rates (BMR) during pregnancy (Prentice and Goldberg, 2000). Fat deposition during pregnancy ranged from large increases of maternal weight in health-rich Swedish and Dutch women (>10 kg) to the net losses in rural Gambian women in an extremely 'health-poor' population afflicted by malnutrition, malaria, and other infections (Fig. 4.8A). Birthweights ranged correspondingly, from Sweden (3300 g) to rural Gambia (2980 g) (Table 4.3).

The BMR normatively increases during pregnancy but can *decrease* in the 'health-poor' (Fig. 4.8B). Swedish women have large increases in BMR early in gestation with further increases later when fetal mass accelerates. Their total body weight gain approaches 14 kg, of which 3.5 kg is fat (Lof et al, 2005; Lof and Forsum, 2006; Prentice and Goldberg, 2000). These large net gains in body tissue require net increase of energy (+523 MJ, or about 120,000 kcal) (Prentice and Goldberg, 2000). In great contrast, the rural Gambian women incur lower BMR early in pregnancy to an extent that offsets the later increase in BMR, so that there is a net energy reduction or 'energy sparing' during pregnancy (−30MJ, −7000 kcal). The 50% smaller weight gain (6.4 kg average) corresponds to the 300 g lower birthweight and smaller maternal fat gain of <0.5 kg (Lawrence et al, 1987; Poppitt et al, 1993; Poppitt et al, 1994). Food supplements partly corrected the decreased

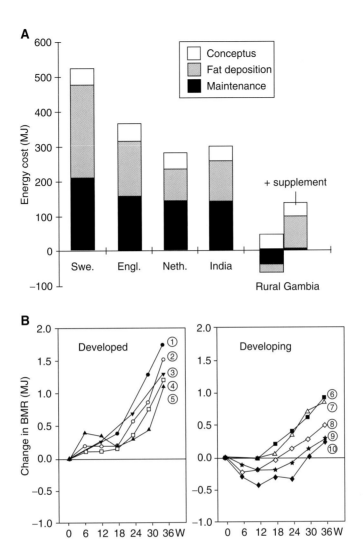

FIGURE 4.8 Energy costs and metabolism during pregnancy. (Redrawn from Lawrence et al, 1987; Poppitt et al, 1994; Prentice and Goldberg, 2000), measured in metabolic chambers (20–80 women in each country). A. Energy costs partitioned as conceptus, maternal fat deposition, and maintenance (basal metabolism) in selected samples from countries representing the affluent and health-rich (Sweden, Netherlands), transitional populations (middle-upper class Indian), and health-poor with malnutrition and high infectious loads (rural Gambia). Note the net loss of fat in Gambia, which was counteracted by nutritional supplements (Fig. 4.12). B. Metabolic rate during pregnancy. Left panel, health-rich samples increased progressively during pregnancy: 1, Sweden; 2, England; 3 and 4, Netherlands; 5, Scotland. Right panel, metabolic rate in health-poor populations increased much less and later in pregnancy. 6, Philippines; 7, Thailand; 8, Gambia sample A; 9, Gambia A, supplemented; 10, Gambia sample B, normal. These poor rural Gambian women show decreased basal metabolism during pregnancy.

TABLE 4.3 Birth Season Effects on Mortality in Gambia
TABLE 4.3 A Mortality

Age Group	Hungry Season (Wet)	Harvest Season (Dry)	Odds Ratio of Premature Death
Birth Weight[*]	2808 ± 41 g	2944 ± 42 g	
Neonatal mortality[+]	7% total births	9–10% total births	
15–35 y[#]	8.3% (38/460)	2.4% (10/415)	3.65
36–45 y[#]	13.2% (9/68)	1.4% (1/69)	10.4

[*](Prentice et al., 1987); [+](Moore et al, 2004a); [#](Moore et al, 1997).

TABLE 4.3 B Causes of Death Ages After Age 15 Years

Cause (Total Deaths)	Hungry Season (49)	Harvest Season (12)	All %
infections[*]	21	7	46% (28)
other, not infections[*]	21	4	43% (25)
unknown[*]	7	1	20% (8)
chronic degenerative disease[+]	0	0	0

[*]From data in (Moore et al, 1997). Infections include 3 cases of preeclampsia, which is associated with malaria placenta (C.E. Finch assignment); 1 case of hepatoma, which is regionally locally associated with hepatitis B virus; 1 case of rheumatic heart disease; 1 case of constrictive carditis associated with tuberculosis. Other not infections includes; maternal (excluding preeclampsia), 6 cases; cancer, 2; kidney failure, 3; epilepsy, 3; accidents, 5; miscellaneous, 3.
[+]Statement in (Moore et al, 2004)

BMR (9 vs. 10). Other populations show intermediates in an evident adaptive continuum. In poor rural Philippine women, the BMR increased throughout gestation, but without increased food intake; nonetheless, 1.3 kg of fat was deposited; reduced physical activity may be the major strategy in this energy sparing. Birth weights averaged 2885 g (Tuazon et al, 1987). Moreover, 'well-nourished and healthy' middle- to upper-class Indian women have progressive increases in BMR during pregnancy that are close to the 'health-rich' European and English women, with increased BMR and fat deposits (3 kg) *and* food intake (Piers et al, 1995). Birth weights of 3060 g are 300 g above poor urban Indians (Table 4.2), reflecting better nutrition and probably lower infectious load. Because the placenta consumes 30% of maternal energy in healthy pregnancy (Tycko, 2006), the placental growth and metabolism may also be altered by maternal malnutrition and disease. These findings again point to the crucial role of energy allocation (Fig. 1.2B) in reproductive success. The hierarchy of restricted energy allocation during development is not known in detail at the cellular level in brain or other organs.

Humans appear to differ widely in the distribution of fat at birth. One typology is described in South India (Yajnik, 2004). Urban poor Mysore infants are unusual in two regards: (I) They are among the smallest worldwide, with mean birth weight of 2700 g, just above the criteria for low birth weight. More than 30% have birth weight <2500g. (II) They are born 'thin but fat.' Despite small bellies (abdominal circumference), they had normal skin fold thickness (trunk fat) and normal head circumference. Relative to English standards, the Mysore infants had relatively more fat and relatively less muscle. These potentially important differences in fat distribution are not evident from the gross birth weight, nor described by the ponderal index or abdominal circumference[5] (Williams et al, 2000). In view of the importance of different anatomical fat depots to adult risk of diabetes and vascular disease (visceral vs. abdominal fat) (Chapter 2), a detailed anthropometric characterization of human fat diversity is urgently needed. Evolved specializations in fat may be found in traditional foraging societies with different patterns of postnatal growth and development (Section 4.9, Fig. 4.5C). The steatopygea of southern African Hottentots is well known to anthropologists, but scarcely studied with modern approaches. Time is running out to define the basic biology of these relict populations.

The total energy cost of pregnancy correlates strongly with adiposity before pregnancy (*r*, 0.80) and with weight gain during pregnancy (*r*, 0.94) (Prentice and Goldberg, 2000). Around the world, thin women tend to gain less body fat during pregnancy. The extreme example may be the near absence of fat deposits in rural Gambian women. In the conventional view, low birth weight and maternal thinness, particularly in health-poor developing countries, is attributed to undernutrition ('involuntary' diet restriction). However, the prevalent infectious diseases also drain energy, as shown by the increase of birth weight after mothers were given anti-malarial drugs (Section 4.5).

Human populations also differ widely in postnatal growth and maturation rates that are postulated to be evolutionary adaptive responses to mortality rates (Walker et al., 2006). Analysis of 22 groups, including foragers, defined trajectories of fast growth relative to the adult size, with earlier menarche and first reproduction (Fig. 4.5C). Fast development was associated with higher post pubertal mortality in subadults, possibly due to poor nutrition and/or infectious load. Yet others had growth rates equaling U.S. standards, but still reaching smaller adult size. Some groups had delayed growth spurts, relative to developed nations, while others did not show a clear adolescent growth spurt. These remarkable variations could be due to local environmental influences of nutrition and infections, as well as genetic influences on growth and menarche, as observed in twins (Section 5.2).

---

[5]Other birth size estimates of body fat are the *ponderal index* ($kg^{1/3}$/length; approximating the body mass index) and the *abdominal circumference*.

4.4.5. Birth Size and Adult Vascular and Metabolic Disease

The coronary arterial diameter may directly determine the risk of ischemic occlusions. Smaller diameter coronary arteries in adults present more stenotic atherosclerotic lesions. The bottom tertile of coronary diameters had 50–300% more stenotic lesions than the top, varying by the particular coronary artery (sonography of 884 Ss, N.Y.C.) (Nwasokwa et al, 1996). Similarly, in cardiac stent patients, the risk of restenosis varied inversely with vessel diameter in several studies (e.g., Kastrati et al, 2006). These observations concur with a "maxim of interventional cardiology . . . bigger is better" (Nwasokwa et al, 1996). That is to say, larger coronary arteries have fewer critical stenotic occlusions after transplantation or introduction of stents. Restenosis and primary atherosclerosis share a key mechanism of endothelial smooth muscle cell proliferation.

Slower flow in smaller diameter arteries may be proatherogenic as an outcome of Poiseuille's law that volume flow varies as the 4th power of the radius. Arterial blood flow velocity and turbulence have major effects on the proliferation of endothelial cells and the expression of inflammatory genes that influence the location of atheromas in different arterial beds (Section 1.5.3.2). This is directly observed in vein transplants in which slower flow causes more hyperplasia in clinical observations and canine models (Dobrin et al, 1989). According to this argument, the higher flow in a smaller diameter coronary at the same anatomic location will be more proatherogenic. Faster flow may also reduce the dwell-time of adherent LDL particles, monocytes, and platelets. Thus, minor developmental differences in arterial diameter could have exponentiated consequences later in life. However, this neat argument may be challenged by sex differences: Women have less clinical vascular disease than men at each adult age, yet their arterial size should be smaller. Data are needed.

Arterial development may be altered in association with low birth weight. At age 9 years, coronary artery diameters varied in proportion to birth weight (Fig. 4.9) (Jiang et al, 2006). For each standard deviation (SD) unit increase in birth weight, the coronary artery diameter increased 0.1 mm. Information is also emerging on neonatal arteries. Neonatal aortic walls were 9% thicker in birth weights averaging 2713 g relative to controls averaging 3762 g; normalized for weight, the smaller babies had 45% thicker walls (Fig. 4.10) (Skilton et al, 2005). Moreover, fetal lipid aortic deposits (Chapter 1, Fig. 1.15A) vary inversely with birth weight (Fig. 4.10B), (Napoli et al, 1999b). Cord blood HDL cholesterol (vascular protective) varied directly with birth weight, while LDL cholesterol (proatherogenic) varied inversely (birth weight range 2625–4420 g; 480 infants) (Ophir et al, 2004), consistent with associations of low birth weight and prenatal atherosclerotic lesion size. Maternal lipids were not reported. These observations generally support the associations of low birth weight to adult coronary disease. However, low birth weight can arise from diverse causes that each could have different links to adult vascular disease.

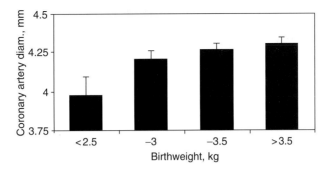

FIGURE 4.9 Influences of birth weight on arterial properties of children aged 9. Aortic diameter varied with birth weight (United Kingdom 216, both sexes). Adjusted for sex, gestational age, and height and weight of child and mother (Redrawn from Jiang et al, 2006).

Blood lipid and metabolic vascular risk factors are associated with birth weight and the ponderal index, but conclusions are less firm than for blood pressure. Placental cord and adult blood lipids may be more weakly linked to birth weight than adult systolic pressure. Each 1 kg lower birth weight is associated with 2 mg/dL higher total cholesterol. Not surprisingly, no consistent associations of birth weight were found with LDL or HDL cholesterol or triglycerides (meta-analysis of 79 studies) (Huxley et al., 2004). Moreover, identical twins, whose birth weight is typically <2500g at term, have normal lipid values as adults that do not differ from single births, despite the huge catch-up growth (Tuya et al, 2006).

C-reactive protein (CRP), a major vascular risk indicator (Fig. 1.16A), may have stronger associations with birth size than the lipid risk factors. In the MIDSPAN Family Study (Scotland, 30–59 years), the most obese adults showed the strongest inverse correlation with CRP across all birth weights (Fig. 4.11) (Sattar et al, 2004). Each 1 kg increase in birth weight predicts 11% decrease in adult CRP in men and women. The association of low birth weight with elevated risk for vascular and metabolic disease in later life could involve other inflammatory pathways besides CRP.

Adult metabolic disorders have more consistent links. In a systematic review, low birth weight was associated with adult glucose-insulin dysregulation in about 75% of 233 reports (Newsome et al, 2003): fasting glucose (15/25 reports), fasting insulin (20/26), clearance of a glucose load (20/25), and prevalence of diabetes type-2 (13/16). In general, those born small who later grew obese as adults had the highest risk for adult vascular or metabolic disorders (metabolic syndrome).

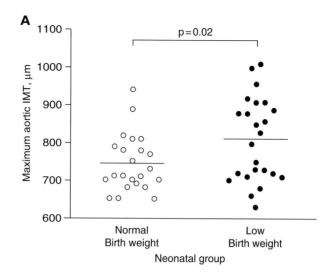

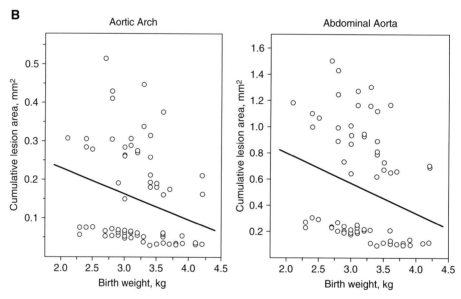

FIGURE 4.10 Neonatal aorta and birth weight. A. The neonatal aortic wall was 9% thicker in a group averaging 2713 g birth weight (low for Caucasians) relative to controls averaging 3762 g by ultrasonography. Normalized for weight, smaller babies had 45% thicker walls/kg (Skilton et al, 2005). These data were adjusted for current body size and maternal size prepregancy; the significant inverse relationship persisted with exclusion of the lowest group <2500 g (10 Ss). The smaller babies were designated as growth retarded in this report but were considered healthy. B. Arterial lipids (cumulative lesion area covered by lipid staining) varied inversely with birth weight. From samples in (Napoli et al, 1999a), kindly provided by Wulf Palinski.

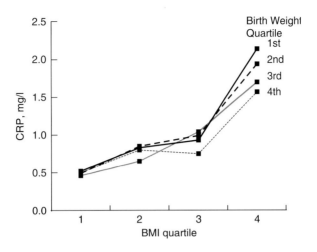

Birth Weight, Adult BMI and Adult Blood CRP

FIGURE 4.11 Birth weight is inversely associated with adult blood C-reactive protein (CRP). MIDSPAN Family Study (central Scotland, 1663 Ss, aged 30–59 y) (Sattar et al, 2004). Each 1 kg increase in birth weight was associated with 11% decrease in adult CRP in men and women. Birth weight was positively associated with adult BMI.

For example, a Swedish cohort born 1920–1924 showed weak inverse correlations between the ponderal index at birth and glucose tolerance at age 50 (r, −0.07); correlations were stronger in the tertile of BMI (r, −0.19) (Lithell et al, 1996). At age 60, the top fifth in ponderal index (fat babies) had 3-fold more diabetes than the others (12% vs. 4%). Adults of small birth weight show decreased insulin sensitivity and impaired insulin release (Levy-Marchal and Czernichow, 2006; Ong, 2006).

Low birth weight is not the only cause of adult metabolic dysfunctions. *Larger* birth weight is also associated with adult metabolic dysregulation (Kramer, 2004; Newsome et al, 2003; Yajnik, 2004). The varying strengths and directions of these effects across populations imply complex contingencies in the links of birth weight, high or low, to adult metabolism, with U-shaped and other multiphasic interactions.

Since catch-up growth in those born small is also a risk factor of adult metabolic disorders, it may be more important as an indicator of future disease than birth weight *per se* (Barker et al, 2005; Hales and Ozanne, 2003; Levy-Marchal and Czernichow, 2006; Ong, 2006). These effects emerge early. As discussed in Section 4.3 for the Pre-WWII Helsinki cohort, slightly smaller birth size, thinness at age 2, and catch-up growth by age 11 increased the risk of coronary events as adults (Fig. 4.1C) (Barker et al, 2005). In a south Indian population, growth rates at ages

4–8 were strongly associated with insulin resistance at age 8, with the greatest effect seen in children who were small at birth but grew faster (Yajnik, 2004a,b). Experimental animal models support these conclusions (Gluckman, 2005; Hales and Ozanne, 2001; Hales and Ozanne, 2003). For example in rats, 30% diet restriction during pregnancy lowered birthweight by 35% and altered postnatal behavior: If given high-fat diets, the offspring of diet-restricted dams rapidly became obese and inactive (Vickers et al, 2005). Famine exposure gives further insights (Section 4.7).

4.4.6. Twins: Small Size at Birth and Catch-up Growth, but Normal Longevity

Twins are an important exception to the generally adverse effects of low birth weight and catch-up growth. Twin birth weights are typically <2500 g, due to growth retardation of 800–900 g and prematurity by 2–3 wks (Leon, 2001; Phillips et al, 2001; Rosello-Soberon et al, 2005). Monozygous twins have even lower birth weights by 100–200 g and higher perinatal mortality. The twin growth retardation is apparent in the third trimester by about 32 wks (when sex differences in fetal growth are detected), but may begin earlier (studies diverge). Postnatal catch-up growth is strong by 24 m and normal height is reached by age 9 y. Adult twins have normal height and weight distributions. Danish twins did not vary in adult cardiovascular mortality or all-cause mortality from the general population (Christensen et al, 2001). Nor did twins differ in atherogenic profiles of lipids (Tuya et al, 2006) or higher blood pressure (de Geus et al, 2001). Some, but not all, studies found higher diabetes and glucose intolerance in adult twins (reviewed in de Boo and Harding, 2006).

These findings suggest that the prenatal growth retardation experienced by twins has a different biology than in singletons (Leon, 2001; Phillips, 2001). As discussed below, exposure to inflammogens like maternal smoking and infections like malaria cause fetal growth retardation. Another key difference is that the next generation offspring of twins has normal size at birth, whereas women who were small at birth themselves tend to have smaller babies (Ounsted, 1986; Phillips et al, 2001) (Section 4.7). The type of chorion (outer fetal membrane) may be important. But the larger effect remains: The remarkable catch-up growth of twins from 800 g deficits at birth has fewer, if any, of the consequences to adult health than experienced by singleton births with birth weights much closer to the norm (Fig. 4.1C). One may ask how much fetal growth retardation in singleton births is due to subclinical infections or other perturbations of the maternal inflammatory environment.

4.5. INFECTION AND UNDERNUTRITION ON BIRTH WEIGHT AND LATER DISEASE

Postnatal growth is highly sensitive to recurrent infections that were nearly unavoidable before the 20th century and are now much diminished in the health-rich developed countries. Infections can attenuate growth by draining energy through fever and anorexia during acute phase responses. Childhood infections are estimated to cost up to 30 g deficits in weight gain per day, if food is not sufficient (McDade, 2003).

4.5.1. The Tangle

The energy available for growth is determined by the balance of input from nutrition and the allocation for host defense and physical activity (Section 1.3, Fig. 1.2B), homeostatic adaptations that prevail throughout development. Maternal infections diminish the nutrients available for the 'fetal supply line' and may do so even if food is freely available. Maternal malnutrition, moreover, increases vulnerability to opportunistic infections. Both maternal malnutrition and maternal infections tend to retard fetal growth. At birth, a retarded or prematurely born fetus is more vulnerable to opportunistic infections and has more difficulty nursing. Infections of neonates and children retard growth, even if food is freely available, because of anorexia during acute phase responses. Even well-fed children are vulnerable to infections and growth retardation. Again, malnutrition decreases resistance to many infections. Thus, the analysis of malnutrition in limiting growth is inextricably entangled with the host defenses and synergies with infection and inflammation. Other causes of growth retardation include maternal exposure to smoke and stress.

Interactions of nutrition and infection are recognized as the key to interventions to maternal and children's health in health-poor populations of the developing world. However, few researchers have recognized their potential importance in the healthier populations being studied for causes of adult disease. I suggest that subclinical infections may have a much larger role. The divergence between twin and singleton births in growth retardation discussed above could be due to subclinical infections or other inflammatory conditions.

4.5.2. Maternal Infections and Nutrition

Maternal infections are well known to cause fetal growth retardation. One of the best understood examples is in rural Gambia. These subsistence farmers are thin and obesity is rare, unlike urban Gambia (van der Sande et al, 2001): average BMI is 20.7, while 20% have BMI <18.5 and are at the margins of survival. There are remarkable seasonal cycles of low birth weight (8% range of variation) and higher mortality (Fig. 4.12A), which are driven by malnutrition and infections (Ceesay et al., 1997; Moore et al., 2001, 2006). A 'hungry season' during rains lasting 4–5 months, June–October, is followed by a longer dry season, December–April, with the harvest in April and May. The dry months of December to April have the highest birth weights and fewest premature births. The seasonal minimum of 2750 g birth weight approximates the annual mean in South India (Table 4.2).

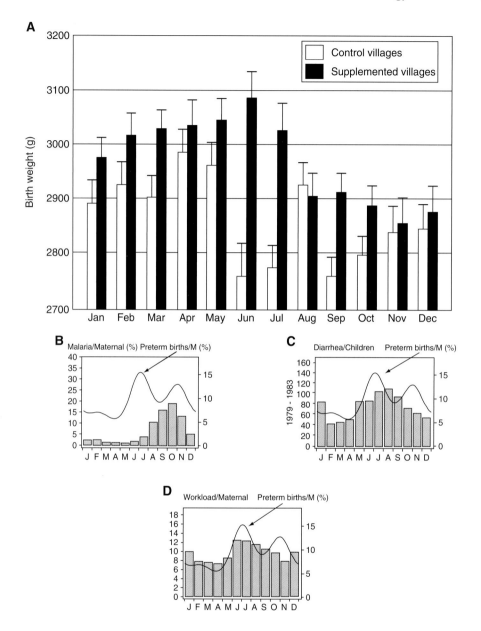

FIGURE 4.12 For legend see page 265.

In Gambia during the hungry (wet) season of chronic negative energy balance, pregnant and lactating women lose up to 50% of body fat (−1.2 MJ/d). Women, even if pregnant, are expected to do physically demanding field work during the harvest. The fetal growth retardation develops later in gestation (after 37 wk, 1–3 wk before birth (Prentice et al, 1987). Thus, the retardation may be regarded as an 'acute' outcome of an impaired maternal nutrient supply, from maternal nutrient deficits and/or placental transfer toward the end of gestation. In contrast to these large effects on fetal growth and survival, the birth season did not alter body size of young children or adults (from longitudinal data on height, weight, waist-hip ratio, skinfold thickness). Thus, even in this highly stressful environment, catch-up growth eliminates the seasonal growth deficit seen in the birthweight. Nonetheless, childhood growth is slower than the norm. At age 8, children's leptin levels are 2 ng/ml plasma, about 80% below an Italian comparison group, which is consistent with their thinness and poor nutritional state (Moore et al, 2002). Leptin is important as an immunomodulator (Section 1.3); e.g., leptin injections stimulated phagocytosis in starved mice infected with *Streptococcus* (*Klebsiella pneumoniae*) (Mancuso et al, 2006).

Infections are less rampant during the dry season, particularly diarrhea (Poskitt et al, 1999) and malarial parasitemia (Rayco-Solon et al., 2005). Two phases of premature births and low birth weight can be resolved. Phase I coincides with hard labor during the harvest (Fig. 4.12B, C, D). Phase II coincides with peaks of diarrhea and parasitemia. The relationship of these infections to growth retardation and prematurity is not resolved (the malaria data are from lactating women; diarrhea data, from children). However, some link of infections to fetal growth is likely because malaria directly infects the placenta (Crocker et al, 2004) and retards fetal growth in association with impaired placental blood flow (Fig. 4.13A, B). *Helicobacter pylori* (Section 2.9.1) is also associated with growth retardation in these rural Gambians (Thomas et al, 2004).

Nutrition and infections synergize in these seasonal effects. Diet supplements increased birth weights (Ceesay et al, 1997; Prentice et al, 1987) in one of the

FIGURE 4.12 Reproduction and diet supplements in Gambian subsistence farmers who incur a 'hungry season,' during seasonal rains. A. During the year, birth weight varies 8%. Nutritional supplements to pregnant women given during the rainy season had the greatest impact on birth weight. The supplements provided 4250 kJ/1750 kcal (protein 22 g; fat, 56 g; sugar, amount not designated) and minerals (calcium, 47 mg; iron, 1.8 mg) (Redrawn from Ceesay et al, 1997). B. Maternal malaria (bar graph) and preterm births (<37 wk solid curve). Parasitemia was highest in the late rainy season September–November, when preterm births show a second peak. Redrawn from Rayco-Solon et al. (2005). C. Preterm births (<37 wk) (solid curve, from above) and diarrhea (children, 1979–1983), redrawn from data of Poskitt et al. (1999), Fig.1. The prevalence of diarrhea of children in the community, which may be considered an indicator of gastro-intestinal infections, also coincides with peak prematurity. D. Maternal workload (bar graph) and preterm births (solid curve, from above) also show overlapping seasonal peaks. Redrawn from Rayco-Solon et al. (2005).

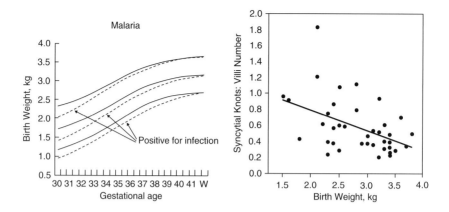

FIGURE 4.13 Growth retardation in pregnancy during infection with malaria in sub-Saharan countries. A. Birth weight in malarial pregnancy is lower across the weight range (Malawi), but did not influence gestation length. (Gestational age centiles, 10th, 50th, 90th; 4104 pregnancies) (Kalanda et al., 2005). B. Birth weight varies inversely with the density of placental lesions from malarial infestation of the placenta (Gambia) (syncytial knots; 31 placentae; $r = 0.5$, P<0.05) (Crocker et al., 2004).

most striking successes of nutritional interventions. In a randomized control trial over 4 y, supplements of protein, fat, iron, and calcium were given midgestation for 82 d. The supplement had most benefits to birth weight and survival during the wet season, but little effect during the dry season when food is more abundant. Women supplemented during wet season pregnancies had larger birth weights by 230 g average (Fig. 4.12A), while the incidence of low birth weight <2500 g decreased 3-fold (23.7% to 7.5%). Mortality also decreased remarkably: stillbirths (−50%) and neonatal deaths (−35%). Moreover, the metabolic rate during pregnancy was increased. As discussed above (Fig. 4.8B), the basal metabolic rate (BMR) decreases early in pregnancy in these Gambian women, a pattern opposite to the increased BMR in well-nourished women. The nutrient supplements partly restored the BMR (Fig. 4.8C, *right panel,* 9 and 10) (Lawrence et al, 1987b) and increased birth weight about 230 g (Fig. 4.12A) (Ceesay et al, 1997). The birth weight distribution curves are shifted by nutrient supplement uniformly to the right in the wet season, but dry season supplements only improved the lowest weight <2500 g (Fig. 4.12A) (Prentice et al., 1987). The greatest birth weights in these populations are still 300 g or more below the median in healthy populations, e.g., Norway (Fig. 4.7A). This difference suggests a threshold of nutrient balance for fetal growth retardation, also observed in the Dutch Hunger Winter (Section 4.7; Fig. 4.15C, discussed below). Thus, three seasonal factors may synergize in growth retardation: the stress of hard physical work, active infections, and undernutrition. The effectiveness of the supplement did not differ by the level of maternal nutrition or weight–height interactions (Prentice et al., 1987), suggesting the greater role of active infections and physical stress.

4.5.3. Smoking and Aerosols

Smoke and aerosols are unregistered factors in these and most other studies of growth retardation. As described in Section 2.4, aerosols are important major causes of inflammation in adults. Low birth weight from intra-uterine growth retardation is associated with maternal smoking (Bakketeig et al, 1997; Lambers and Clark, 1996; Mitchell et al, 2002; Naeye, 1981), particularly with lower socioeconomic status (Dubois and Girard, 2006). Third trimester maternal smoking had the greatest effect, with 2-fold more low birth weight babies. Smoking dose effects on lowering birth weight are well known (Garn et al, 1978; Lieberman et al, 1994). In a smaller sample, children of maternal smokers were heavier at age 3 y; here, the critical period was the first trimester (Oken et al, 2005). Among many the mechanisms being considered in fetal growth retardation, nicotine crosses the placental barrier and may be 15% higher than in fetal than maternal blood (Lambers and Clark, 1996).

Air pollution may also be a factor in fetal growth retardation (Yang, 2003). In the developing world, urban and rural households are often very smoky, from heating fuel, which can cause 'hut lung' and other chronic respiratory conditions (Gold et al, 2000) (Section 2.4). Fecal aerosols from omnipresent domestic animals can induce systemic inflammatory responses, as observed in the elevated blood inflammatory proteins (CRP, complement C3) in sewage and garbage workers (Section 2.4).

4.6. INFECTION AND NUTRITION IN POSTNATAL DEVELOPMENT AND LATER DISEASE

The common childhood affliction of diarrhea is used to show mechanisms in growth retardation (next section) that are at work in the shorter life spans in health-poor populations.

4.6.1. Diarrheas in Growth Retardation

Diarrheas are major causes of childhood growth retardation and mortality in health-poor populations of the developing world (Lutter et al, 1989; Martorell et al, 1975; Poskitt et al, 1999; Rowland et al, 1977; Scrimshaw, 2003; Thapar and Sanderson, 2004). Energy deficits of diarrhea are 400–900 kcal/d (Hoyle et al, 1980; Lutter et al, 1989). Diarrheas cause 'pathological caloric restriction' by impairing food digestion and nutrient absorption and draining systemic energy in acute phase responses (Fig. 1.2B).

Infections are the main cause of diarrheas, particularly rotaviruses, and pathogenic forms of *E. coli* and epidemic cholera (Thapar and Sanderson, 2004). The intestinal flora also shifts in chronic diarrheas, with bacterial invasion of the jejunum (Mata et al, 1972), which is normally sterile (Section 2.4). Diarrhea decreases the intestinal transit time, as well as decreasing intestinal absorption of nutrients by damage to the microvilli and nutrient transporters. Bacterial endotoxins can enter the circulation and can stimulate antibody production (Campbell et al, 2003a,b; Voravuthikunchai et al, 2005), discussed below.

Chronic diarrhea also triggers acute phase responses including elevated CRP and IL-6 (Liu et al, 2005; Yeung et al, 2004) and inducing fever, which independently of diarrhea, can increases basal metabolism 25–100% (Section 1.3.3, Fig. 1.2B). Further compounding the energy drain, the anorexia of fever can reduce food intake by 20% (Butte et al, 1989; Lutter et al, 1989; Martorell et al, 1980). Adding further insult, diarrheas increase the risk of infection, reducing catch-up growth (Guerrant et al, 1992). Gene variants that influence inflammation and lipid metabolism may be important: Children with diarrhea who also carried apoE4 alleles showed better cognitive development (Oria et al, 2005) (Section 5.7.5).

The association of diarrhea with growth retardation is well known in health-poor populations, as shown in four examples. (I) Severe growth retardation (<3 SD below mean) was associated with 2-fold more total days of diarrhea and more frequent and longer episodes (Fontaleza, Brazil) (Guerrant et al, 1992). (II) Loss of growth was proportional to the number of diarrhea days (Bogota, Colombia) (Lutter, 1989; Martorell et al, 1975). (III) Nutritional supplements given to children with diarrhea eliminated growth retardation (Lutter et al, 1989). The total energy deficits from average 78 d of diarrhea before age 3 y (70,200 kcal total) approximate the nutritional supplements that eliminated the growth deficits (109,500 kcal total). However, in children without diarrhea, diet supplements did not improve growth. This finding suggests why diet supplements have variable benefits to growth. Lastly (IV), measles can precipitate diarrhea. Rural Guatemalan children in the 1960s had a high early prevalence of measles by age 2 y, accompanied by acute diarrhea, weight loss, and 5% mortality (Scrimshaw et al, 1966). Diarrhea was more frequent in undernourished children. Nutritional supplements nearly eliminated mortality and growth retardation during measles. Scrimshaw also documents that, in well-nourished populations, measles is rarely fatal and is rarely accompanied by diarrhea. In 19th century England, when malnutrition was common, diarrhea was 'a usual accompaniment of measles'; this historical reference supports the association of early mortality and adult height in 19th century England (Crimmins and Finch, 2006a).

4.6.2. Seasonal Effects

We return to rural Gambia, where the birth season also has strong influences on adult mortality. As described above, those born in the hungry season had markedly higher seasonal death rates as neonates (first year). The hungry-season mortality bias persists to early adulthood (Table 4.3A) (Moore et al, 1997), with 10-fold higher risk of death after age 15, among which >40% are attributed to infections (Table 4.3B). Mortality from gastroenteritis and measles is more strongly associated with birth season than from malaria and acute respiratory infections (Moore et al, 1999;

Moore et al, 2004). So far, the non-infectious causes of death have not differed by season of birth (Table 4.3). However, chronic infections and inflammation can cause cardiomyopathy, e.g., sudden death from clinically silent Chagas' disease, caused by *Trypanosoma cruzi* (Baroldi et al, 1997). Thus, some mortality attributed to acute infections could also involve cardiomyopathy from chronic infections.

The large seasonal mortality bias can be traced to the early months of life when infections are rampant in the hungry season, as discussed above. Most (75%) Gambian children suffer from gastroenteritis (enteropathy), which impairs intestinal transport of nutrients. The mucosa is damaged with villous atrophy and elevations of $CD3^+$ T cells and cytokine-expressing monocytes (TNFα, IFNγ) by several-fold or more (Campbell et al, 2003a). Infant diarrhea is also common (7.3% of time, ages 3–15 m) (Campbell et al, 2003b). After normal postnatal growth up to 8 weeks, growth falls off sharply relative to norms. Moreover, unlike the normal decrease of intestinal permeability during the first year, these children have increased intestinal permeability with microbial leakage, as shown by serum elevations of bacterial endotoxin and IgG endotoxin antibodies. The growth impairments were correlated to varying degrees in each child by plasma endotoxin and IgG levels and gut permeability. Plasma C-reactive protein (CRP) and other acute phase proteins are also elevated in Gambian children, particularly before age 5 (Campbell and Kuo, 2003; Filteau et al, 1995). The increase of CRP during normal aging in health-rich populations might also be due to increased gut leakage of endotoxin during aging, suggested by evidence that aging rats have increased intestinal permeability (Section 2.3). The Gambian enteropathy is hypothesized by (Campbell et al, 2003a) to be acquired from unhygienically prepared weaning foods. Household hygiene is hard, if not impossible, to maintain during the rainy season for obvious reasons. The children failed to respond to nutritional interventions and had impaired digestion of lactose.

More generally, mucosal damage from poor hygiene is implicated as a major global cause of growth impairment and malnutrition. The link between early enteric infections and later vulnerability in infections could be included in Fig 1.2A. The high exposure to enteric antigens suggests a mechanism in the chronic antigenic stimulation of naive T cells, as has been associated with cytomegalovirus (CMV) infections that increase vulnerability to infections later in life in developed countries (Section 2.8). Ongoing studies may show whether diet supplements during pregnancy reduce the seasonal bias of deaths after age 15. So far, birth season in Gambia has not altered adult metabolic or/and vascular disease risk factors (Moore et al, 2001). The low incidence of cardiovascular risk factors in this rural population is consistent with the absence of obesity, the physically demanding lives, and the poor nutrition (van der Sande et al, 2001).

These seasonal effects in the later 20th century give insights into seasonal cycles of mortality that were once more extreme than in health-rich modern populations of Europe and North America. For those born in the early 20th century, spring season cohorts from Northern Europe lived 3–6 m longer than autumn births (Doblhammer and Vaupel, 2001). Australian mortality was also cyclic for the corresponding growth season, with a phase lag of 6 m. Besides seasonal variations in nutrition suggested by these authors, infections also vary seasonally. The higher prevalence of infections in the winter coincides with cyclic availability of bulk nutrients and vitamins to the general public.

Seasonal effects on immune function are proposed in an important expansion of the fetal origins hypothesis to include maternal effects on immune system development that influence adult vulnerability to infections (Collinson et al, 2003; Moore et al, 1999). As discussed above, the original study of Barker and Osmond also showed strong correlations of early and later mortality due to infections (Table 4.1). In Gambia, the neonatal thymus gland is about 10% smaller in the hungry-season. Correspondingly, a longitudinal study in the nearby country of Guinea Bissau showed associations of thymus size with infant mortality due to infectious disease (Aaby et al, 2002). A smaller thymus could cause developmental deficits in the initial endowment of naive T cells, and thus faster immunosenescence (Section 2.9). Undernutrition is considered the main seasonal factor in these African countries, because malarial parasitemia was not common in these women and because the timing of malarial transmission is not concurrent with the effects (Collinson et al, 2003). However, maternal parasitemia may be occult in peripheral blood because the placenta sequesters parasitized erythrocytes (Arbeille et al, 2002) (Section 4.4). Maternal cortisol elevations are probably prevalent during the hungry season, caused by negative energy balance from undernutrition (Section 3.3) and compounded by the nutrient drains from infection.

4.6.3. Serum Immune Response Markers of Chronic Infection in Health-Poor Children

Elevated CRP may be widespread in the developing world. The Tsimane of Amazonian (low-land) Bolivia are being studied because of their rare status as forager-agriculturalists with minimal access to modern medicine. The Tsimane may be as close representatives as still exist in the 21st century to pre-historic forager populations (Godoy et al, 2006; McDade et al, 2005; Gurven et al, in prep.). Their life expectancy is 42 y with infant mortality of 12% (Fig. 4.14A). These children have a high prevalence of elevated CRP—e.g., age 2–4 y, 23% had CRP >5 mg/L (McDade et al., 2005), a level which may be considered a clinical indicator of vascular disease in adults ('high risk CRP') (Chapter 1, Fig. 1.16). Tsimane may have elevations of CRP throughout their lives (Fig. 4.14 B). The proportion of 13% aged 2–15 y with high CRP >5m/L is far higher than health-rich populations in developed countries. In the U.S., about 7% of children aged 8–16 y had CRP elevations above a clinical threshold of 0.22 mg/L (NHANES III sample; different CRP cut-offs arise from different assays). Children with high CRP have growth retardation particularly if malnourished (preliminary analysis cited in McDade et al, 2005). Moreover, the prevalence of elevated CRP is several-fold higher than in the U.S. up to age 42 (Tsimane life expectancy) (Gurven et al, in prep.). In effect, Tsimane show 2-fold more years lived with high-risk CRP than in the

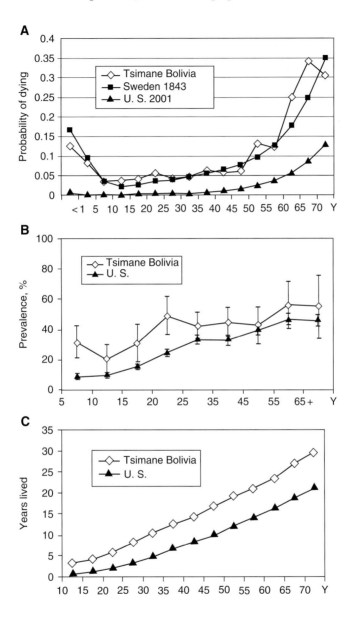

FIGURE 4.14 Tsimane mortality and CRP (Gurven et al, in prep.). A. Mortality rates of Tsimane, Sweden in 1843, and United States in 2001. B. Prevalence of high-risk plasma CRP (>5 mg/L) in Tsimane and United States (single blood sample) (U.S. data from NHANES III). C. Years lived with high-risk CRP at each age.

U.S. up to this age (Fig. 4.14C). Repeat samplings are ongoing to evaluate whether CRP elevations are sustained over one or more years.

Adult immune responses are compromised by early exposure to unhealthy environments. In rural Filipino adolescents (Cebu Longitudinal Health and Nutrition Survey, CLHNS) (McDade et al, 2001a,b; McDade et al, 2004), successful response to typhoid vaccine was 44% in a group with the healthiest history (normal birth weight, long breast-feeding, rapid growth, higher BMI). In contrast, in those with poorer health by these criteria, only one-third as many (14%) responded to the vaccine. In all of these trait combinations, lower birth weight (<10th percentile for gestational age) was associated with poor later response to immunization. Immunoglobulin E (IgE) levels in adolescents were inverse to the number of childhood infectious episodes, mostly gut and lung (McDade et al, 2004). These findings support the hygiene hypothesis of allergies, which associates the elevation of IgE in atopic immune diseases (asthma, hay fever, eczema) with reduced antigen exposure during childhood (Strachan, 1989). Strachan's original hypothesis emphasized household density, cross-infections, and hygiene and was expanded to include other infections and inflammogens, pre- and postnatally (Tantisira and Weiss, 2001). Bacterial endotoxin may be protective for atopic diseases, even during adult exposure (Douwes et al, 2004).

4.6.4. Infections During Development

In malarial pregnancies, low maternal weight before pregnancy was the largest factor associated with low birth weights (Kramer, 1987). Maternal malaria, as noted above, retards fetal growth (Fig. 4.13) (Kalanda et al., 2005) and may account for 5% of low birth weights in exposed populations (meta-analysis of 895 studies) (Kramer *op. cit.*). Maternal malaria also increased the risk of spontaneous abortions, stillbirths and preeclampsia, a systemic inflammatory condition associated with placental pathology (Menendez, 1995). The real prevalence of malarial impairments of fetal growth may be higher than estimated because maternal blood parasitemia can be low or undetectable, as noted previously.

Although maternal transmission of malaria to the fetus is rare, there are many direct effects through maternal support (Beeson and Duffy, 2005; Brabin et al, 2004; Crocker et al, 2004; Duffy and Fried, 2005; Menendez, 1995) shown in four aspects: (I) Maternal anemia from lysis of parasitized maternal erythrocytes causing degrees of hypoxia; (II) maternal hypoglycemia; (III) direct damage to the placenta by adherent parasitized maternal erythrocytes ('placenta malaria'). The parasitized maternal erythrocytes accumulate in pockets on the placenta and damage the villi that transfer maternal nutrients in association with inflammatory reactions and increased IL-8 and IFNγ, deposits of fibrous proteins, and necrosis ('syncytiotrophoblast degradation' and 'fibrinoid villar necrosis'). Birth weight varied inversely with the number of 'syncytial knots' on the placenta (Fig. 4.13B), suggesting graded impairments of nutrient transfer (Arbeille et al, 2002). (IV) The hypoglycemia of pregnancy is worsened by malaria, consistent with the high metabolic demand of fever and host defense responses to parasitemia (Menendez, 1995). Anti-malarial treatment (Maloprim) begun at midgestation increased birth weight by 153 g, confirming a prior study (Menendez et al, 1994). Nutritional supplements alone also remarkably improved birth weights during the malarial season in Gambia (Fig. 4.12A), consistent with the compensating for the nutrient drain of malaria.

TNFα gene variants are associated with susceptibility to malaria in Gambia and other populations, and are also associated with fetal growth retardation and insulin resistance (Casano-Sancho et al, 2006). For example, TNFα promoter alleles, −308G/A, alter susceptibility to malaria (Knight, 2004; Ubalee et al, 2005), hepatitis virus B (Niro, 2005), and septicemia (Nakada et al, 2005; Sipahi et al, 2006). These alleles also influence TNFα synthesis and possibly adiposity, insulin resistance, and hypertension (metabolic syndrome) (Table 3.2). In non-infected pregnancies, these alleles also influence fetal growth (Section 4.9). The genetics is complex, because the TNFα gene resides among other immunoregulatory genes of the highly polymorphic MHC complex (Section 1.3.2).

Although the above low birth weight group (2300 g mean) in rural Gambia was chosen to exclude 'infectious etiology" (Casano-Sancho et al, 2006), subclinical infections may be elusive. For example, in developed countries periodontal disease is associated with small birth weight, premature delivery, and other adverse outcomes of pregnancy: a meta-analysis showed higher risk of adverse outcomes in 18/25 studies, while 3 clinical trials showed that periodontal treatments lowered the risk of low birth weight by 57% (Xiong et al, 2006). In rodent models, the oral pathogen *Campylobacter rectus* (gram-negative) induced placental inflammation (Offenbacher et al, 2005). Similarly, systemic LPS injections (Gram-negative endotoxin) induced placental inflammatory responses including elevated amniotic fluid IL-6 and IL-10 (Beloosesky et al, 2006). This study also showed the close link of oxidative stress to inflammation: The anti-oxidant N-acetyl cysteine (NAC) attenuated the IL-6 elevations in the amniotic fluid and maternal serum, whether given before LPS or up to 2 h after.

4.6.5. The Cost of Infections to Postnatal Growth: Evidence from Migration and Antibiotics

Examples just discussed show that infections stunt the growth of children in health-poor populations in direct relation to the intensity and duration of infections. When children from these backgrounds grow up in a better environment, the improvement can be large within one generation. The children of rural Guatemalan immigrants to the U.S. in the 1990s are 8–10 cm taller at ages of 5–12 y, relative to a Guatemalan reference population in 1998 (Bogin, 1999a; Bogin, 2002). About 70% of the total increase is due to leg length, which may be particularly sensitive to infection and malnutrition. Similarly, Ache children (Fig. 4.5C) that were adopted and lived in the U.S. had faster motor development, walking 9 m earlier, and grew 10 cm taller (Hill and Hurtado, 1996, p. 220).

Likely causes of improved development in the U.S. include access to better medical care during pregnancy and early childhood (the W.I.C. Program includes vaccinations and antibiotics; better sanitation and clean water; and nutrition, especially free school breakfast and lunch). Concurrently in Guatemala, the rural villagers have not shown such large increases between generations, although conditions are improving (Mata, 1978; Rivera and Ruel, 1997). In a well-studied group of Guatemalan villages (INCAP Study), birth length was 2 cm less than the U.S. reference and growth up to 3 y was markedly retarded, with infants <12 months showing the greatest impairments (Martorell et al, 1975; Rivera et al, 1997). The gap of 10 cm at age 3 y was almost as large as the adult difference of 13 cm gap below the U.S. mean. Diarrhea consistently impaired growth up to 3 y with a dose response such that each 10% more diarrhea days impaired growth by 0.2–0.7 cm. Respiratory conditions independently reduced growth, but less than diarrhea (Martorell et al, 1975). Children aged 6–7 y experienced 115 d of illness/year. The birth weights and incidence of infectious disease should be analyzed in the U.S. immigrants.

Intrauterine infections have an unknown role in growth retardation. In rural Guatemala and probably many other health-poor settings, intrauterine infections are indicated by elevations of immunoglobulins IgG and IgA, and complement C3 (acute phase protein) in both umbilical cord blood and maternal blood (Lechtig and Mata, 1971a,b, 1972; Mata, 1972). In the absence of chronic maternal infections (tuberculosis, rubella), fetal IgA is very low (Allansmith et al, 1968; Berg, 1969). Elevations of fetal cord blood IgA, IgG, and C3 have been attributed to fetal immune responses to infections; by midpregnancy, the fetus can make C3 and IgM (Berg and Nilsson, 1969; Lechtig and Mata, 1972; Mata, 1972) (Section 4.5).

Even without overt infections, postnatal growth can be retarded by chronic inflammatory conditions. Juvenile diabetes, juvenile rheumatoid arthritis, and uremia share the feature of retarded growth and elevated plasma IL-6 and lower IGF-1 in the absence of GH deficiency. In mice engineered for high systemic IL-6 expression, IL-6 elevations in the absence of infections cause skeletal muscle atrophy soon after maturation (Tsujinaka et al, 1995). One hypothesis is that IL-6 elevations suppress GH signal transduction via the SOCS family proteins (suppressors of cytokine signaling) that modulate GH receptor activation (Lieskovska et al, 2003). Protein synthesis may be impaired by elevated glucocorticoids in maternal stress (Jackman and Kandarian, 2004). Malnutrition, like diet restriction (Fig 3.2A), elevates blood cortisol as an adaptive homeostatic response to increase glucose availability through gluconeogenesis (Fig. 3.10). Diarrhea also increases blood cortisol (Zin Thet et al., 1992), which may be either or both a stress or gluconeogenic response. In a rat model of sterile diarrhea, cardiac muscle protein synthesis was inhibited (Hunter et al, 2001), possibly linking infant diarrhea with later cardiovascular disease (Buck and Simpson, 1982).

Other evidence pointing to the cost of infections comes from antibiotics. The major increase of adult height after the mid 20th century in Japan and other developed countries coincided with mass production of antibiotics (Ternak, 2004). The

10 cm added to height of Japanese men by the 1980s is hard to explain by improved nutrition alone. Liberal use of antibiotics may also be a factor in the obesity epidemic. While there cannot be controlled experiments in humans, antibiotics are widely used for growth promotion in the fowl and swine, with up to 30% greater growth during maturation (Lochmiller and Deerenberg, 2000).

Another model is germ-free animals (rodents, fowl, swine), which usually grow faster (Lochmiller and Deerenberg, 2000). Although germ-free status can eliminate bacteria and parasites, it does not eliminate viruses (Section 2.2.2). Mouse colonies can also differ in postnatal growth rates because of different enteric organisms. Transfer of microbiota at weaning also conferred the donor colony characteristic growth rate (Dubos et al, 1966). The intestinal microbiome is extremely diverse and interacts throughout life with systemic functions (Eckburg et al, 2005; Ley et al, 2006). Commensal bacteria are essential for immune system development, yet cost the host by draining resources that attenuate growth below its maximum. The energetic cost to the organism in the commensal bacterial load can be regarded as a set of trade-offs, which are part of the evolutionarily 'design' that allows the immune system to be programmed by ecological information (McDade, 2003).

4.6.6. Unknowns

Much remains unexplained about low birth weight that is not simply accounted for by poor maternal nutrition and infections. Some women have a series of low birth weight babies, despite apparent health. In a huge sample from Norway, women whose first child was <2500 g had 5-fold higher risks of second low birth weight (Bakketeig et al, 1979, 1997). These associations were not explained by maternal smoking or medical complications of pregnancy. Fetal growth was attenuated throughout, possibly more at the end of gestation in those with repeatedly retarded fetal growth than in those with sporadic retardation. Maternal weight and diet were not analyzed.

These examples show the complexity of the nutrition-infection interaction on developmental links to later health and aging. The seasonal variations in nutrition and infections with long-term consequence to adult health and mortality may seem exotic and even irrelevant to researchers on aging processes in much healthier populations in the developed countries. I suggest that they are highly relevant because subclinical infections occur in even the healthiest populations (the prevalence of subclinical infections in pregnancy is not well characterized). The role of maternal infections seems particularly important to further define as a cause of fetal growth retardation. Another major question is the epigenetics and genetics of birth size. Could small size be an evolutionary response to energy limitations or other diet deficiencies that allows an adaptive phenotype? This controversial concept is discussed together with epigenetic imprinting of maternal and paternal genes that influence fetal growth in Sections 4.8 and 4.9.

4.7. FAMINE

Famine exposure in 19th century Finland and Sweden and during World War II is being studied intensively for effects of malnutrition during development on later aging. In addition, there is evidence for epidemics of infectious disease that have not been much considered in these analyses. Overall, the impact of famine and epidemic disease during development on lifespan and chronic diseases of aging seems relatively modest, as summarized in Table 4.4. Up to age 57, prenatal exposure to the Dutch famine has not altered adult mortality (Painter et al., 2005a). Nor has birth weight been found to have a major influence on adult health in the 'Dutch Hunger Winter' cohort.

4.7.1. World War II (WWII)

The 'Dutch Hunger Winter' of November 1944–May 1945 occurred during German reprisals, which imposed severe food deprivation upon the civilian population, including about 40,000 pregnant women with surviving children (Burger et al, 1948; Stein et al, 1975) (Table 4.5A, note 1). By the beginning of WWII, the Dutch were considered well nourished (Bogin, 2005; Stein et al, 1975).

TABLE 4.4 Summary of Main Famine Effects on Adult Disease and Mortality and Link to Birth Weight

Event (see text for references)	Birth Weight Link
Swedish famine, 1809–1849 1.2-fold higher death from stroke; no overall change in mortality	no birth weight data
Finnish famine, 1866–1868 no effect on mortality 17–80 y	no birth weight data
Dutch Hunger Winter, 1944–1945 1. no effect on mortality, age 17-57 2. obesity increased (+90%) from exposure in first and second trimesters 3. coronary disease by age 55 y: 3-fold higher in first trimester exposure. 4. blood vascular risk factors LDL:HDL-C in first trimester exposure 5. systolic pressure up to age 50 varied inversely with birth weight: 2.6 mm decrease in bp per kg birth weight. 6. adult 50–100% more respiratory disease, any trimester exposure 7. mild glucose intolerance at 50 and 58 y; inverse birth weight association. 8. postnatal famine exposure: breast cancer increased 2-fold	 no no yes no yes
Leningrad Siege, 1941–1942 1. exposure age 9–15 y: 1.5-fold more hypertension, 1.4-fold more ischemic heart disease, and 1.65-fold more stroke ages 67–74 y 2. no increased glucose intolerance or dyslipidemia at 52–53 y 3. no increase of obesity	no birth weight data

Early in the German occupation before the Hunger Winter, the official ration was 1700–1800 kcal/d, with allowances for pregnancy and nursing (Table 4.5A, note 2) (Fig. 4.15). This ration was about the same or slightly less than in the Minnesota Starvation Experiment, which was sustainable for barely 6 m under much better conditions of temperature (Section 3.2.3; Table 4.5B). The official rations varied regionally, reaching recognized starvation levels (<1500 cal/d) in some urban areas for about 6 months, and diminishing to as low as 400 kcal/d in Amsterdam. However, this

TABLE 4.5 A Caloric Intake during the WWII Dutch Hunger Winter

Period[1]	Rations	
May 1940–December 1943 German Occupation	1800 kcal/d	
December 1943–October 1944 German Reprisals	gradual decrease from 1800 to 1400 kcal/d	
	Famine Zone (west)[5]	Control Zone (north)
26 November 1944	June–August 1944, 1512 kcal/d	1512 kcal
	September–November 1944, 1414	1450
	December–February 1945, 740	1345
	March–May 1945, 670 Amsterdam (400–800)	1392
12 May 1945 (Liberation)	Restoration and Rebound	
	June–August 1945, 1757 kcal/d	1755
	September–November, 2083	2083
	December–February 1946, 2270	2273
	March–April 1946, 3200	3200

1. The Dutch population was considered well nourished at outbreak of war. During the German occupation after May 1940, official rations were about 1800 kcal/d (7650 kJ), which gradually decreased after December 1943. In 1944, Netherlands was still under German control, except for a liberated zone south of the Rhine. Then in November, the German occupation imposed an embargo on transported goods including food in reprisal for a general strike by railroad workers ('German Reprisals'). The Western urban area (Amsterdam, Rotterdam) suffered the worst food shortages. In contrast, rations were larger and more supplements were available in the northern and southern agricultural areas and their cities (Enschede, Gronigen), designated for study as the 'Northern and Southern famine control areas'.

2. Emergency supplements were sometimes officially available to those who had lost >25% of normal body weight (Burger et al., 1948). As the food shortage worsened, the criterion was raised up to 40% weight loss (Burger *op. cit.*, p.21). Special needs were recognized (footnote 5). Additional 'extra-legal' food was sought from charitable organizations, foraging trips to the agricultural areas, and on the black market (Burger et al, 1948; Roseboom et al, 2001b; Stein et al, 1975). These supplements may have nearly doubled the official rations, according to a detailed survey made just after liberation (Burger *op. cit.*, pp. 76–77). This 'extra-legal' food clearly delayed and blunted the full effects of starvation that would have otherwise been predicted throughout the country by mid-1944, when official rations had decreased from 1800 to 1400 kcal/d. For comparison, most in the Minnesota Starvation Experiment developed visible edema on 1800 kcal/d within 4–6 m (Keys et al, 1950, p. 956; Keys, 1994). However, edema of starvation was not reported until January 1945, 13 m after the official ration fell below 1800 kcal/d (Burger *op. cit.*, p. 20; Stein et al, 1975, p. 45). Not long after, hunger edema was widespread. Thus, the real food intake for most of 1944 must have exceeded the strict 1800 kcal/d in the Minnesota Starvation ration by several hundred calories. Another burden not experienced in Minnesota was the cold interior of homes and workplaces.

3. There were major SES differences during the war and even after liberation; e.g., in Amsterdam in June 1945, the poor class had 55% less milk than the upper class (Burger *op. cit.*, Tables 13 and 14 of Appendix in Vol. II). The poor also had up to 5-fold more diarrhea (Burger, *op. cit.*, Table 6).

4. Average, 3 mo (Roseboom et al, 2001a,b; Stein et al, 1975); Amsterdam, December 1944–May 1945 (Painter et al 2005a).

5. When possible, children up to 1 y were 'protected' by official rations of ≥1000 kcal/d, with composition "always above the Oxford Nutrient Survey" (Painter et al, 2005a; Burger *op. cit.*, p. 22). Pregnant and lactating women and men required to do heavy physical labor were also eligible for official supplements. However, the allotted rations were difficult for most to obtain, and supplements to women were not available during the worst of the famine (Painter et al, 2005a) (Stein et al, 1975, p. 50).

TABLE 4.5 B Infant Mortality and Famine

	Famine District	Control District
stillbirths (cohort)	20/1000	35/1000
<6 d	15	15
7–29 d	before famine (B): 5–10	B: 5
	during famine (F): 20	F: 10
30–89 d	B: 10	B: 15
	F: 30	F: 30
90–364 d	B: 10	B: 30
	F: 40	F: 60

The higher mortality in the control district may be associated with epidemics that swept southward in 1944–1945 (Stein et al, 1975).

TABLE 4.5 C Comparisons with Other Studies of Starvation and Diet Restriction

	Food Intake, kcal/d
typical Western diet	2000–3000
South Asian[*]	2110 average; 1810, lowest range
Minnesota, 1944[**]	1800
Biosphere, 1991–1993[***]	1750–2200
Caloric Restriction Society 2004[+]	participants, 1112–1958
	controls 1976–3537

[*] FAO norms for South Asia (Chandrasekhar and Ghosh, 2003).
[**] Minnesota Starvation Experiment: (Keys et al, 1950; Keys, 1994).
[***] Biosphere 2: (Walford et al, 2002); approximate mean values.
[+] Caloric Restriction Society (Fontana et al 2004; Meyer et al, 2006). See Section 3.2.3.

average food intake was unevenly available, and total daily caloric intake was estimated at nearly twice the official rations through undocumented 'extra-legal' food (Table 4.5A, note 2). Nonetheless, several hundred thousand became emaciated, and malnutrition-related death rates soared, particularly among the elderly. About 10,000 died because of hunger and associated causes (Stein et al, 1975, p. 167). Fuel for heating was scarce and the difficulties of staying warm increased the stress of the food shortages. Hygiene declined for lack of soap and warm water. Infectious disease rose sharply throughout the Netherlands. Skin abscesses and other infections were common. Although mortality of infants and children increased (Table 4.5B), it was attributed to the cold and infections (dysentery, diptheria); with few exceptions, infants were given sufficient food to avoid emaciation (Stein et al, 1975, p. 52, pp. 93–94). Despite the severity of diet restriction, vitamin deficiencies were rare (*op cit*, p. 77). Thus, the extent of starvation varied widely, particularly affecting the poor who had limited goods to trade for food and less access (Table 4.5A, note 3).

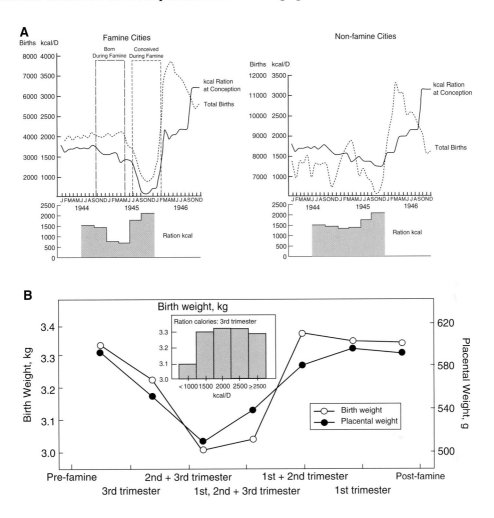

FIGURE 4.15 Reproduction and caloric intake during The Dutch Hunger Winter (WWII). (Adapted from Stein et al, 1975.) Caloric intake according to the official ration may generally underestimate actual consumption (Table 4.5A, note 2). A. Calories at conception and number of births in famine and non-famine cities (northern area). B. Birth weight and placental weight by trimester of exposure in famine cities. Inset, birth weight by official ration in third trimester suggest a threshold effect <1500 kcal/d.

(Continues)

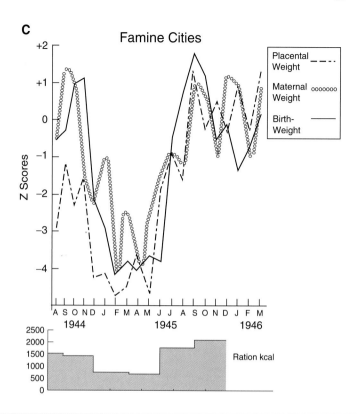

FIGURE 4.15 (continued) C. Birth weight, maternal weight, and placental weight in famine cities; the bar graph below approximates caloric intake in famine cities. Caloric intake accounted for 58% of the variance in birth numbers in the famine cities: Change of 100 kcal/d altered monthly births by 10%. The caloric threshold for impaired fertility is about 1500 kcal/d (official ration); below this threshold, the ration kcal/d and number of births had stronger correlation (r, 0.92). The decline of births conceived during the famine was delayed about 2 m after official rations fell below 1500 kcal/d, in both the famine cities, where the drop was greater, and in the control cities. (Redrawn from Stein and Susser, 1975b.)

Zena Stein, Mervyn Susser, and colleagues looked for evidence of impaired mental development from famine exposure by the trimester of pregnancy, which developed criteria for path analysis and cohort data formats that are still widely used. Everyone should read their classic monograph, *Famine and Human Development* (Stein et al, 1975). The Dutch famine cohort includes 2254 live births, November 1943 through February 1947, with data on birth and placental weight; maternal weight postpartum; stillbirths and mortality up to age 18; and head circumference and body length at birth (Stein et al, 1975; Stein et al, 2004a,b) (this Stein, Aryeh, is Zena's nephew). Contrary to expectations, there was no increase of mental retardation, or of cognitive impairments in young men exposed to famine before birth or shortly after. However, famine exposure clearly increased developmental defects and psychiatric disorders. These unique data reveal critical periods for energy deficits during human development that influence adult health and reproduction, some effects extending to the next generation.

Few physical effects of prenatal famine exposure during early life have been described in those who survived to adulthood. Height and BMI were normal (Lopuhaa et al, 2000), as was female fecundity (Lumey et al, 1995). However, 90% more obesity was found in young men exposed to famine during trimesters 1 and 2, relative to 'famine control regions' (Ravelli et al, 1976). Birth weight does predict systolic pressure up to age 50 (inverse correlation, 2.6 mm decrease/kg) (Roseboom et al, 1999) approximating the global meta-analysis value of 2 mm/kg noted above (Section 4.2) (Huxley et al, 2000). Vascular blood lipid and clotting risk factors increased with first trimester exposure (Painter et al, 2005b; Roseboom et al, 2000). The ratio of LDL:HDL cholesterol was slightly elevated, but not associated with birth weight (Fig. 4.16B). Adult blood pressure, while not related to caloric intake during pregnancy, was sensitive to the protein carbohydrate ratio in the third trimester (Roseboom et al, 2001d). Maternal diet composition had a stronger influence on systolic pressure than birth weight. In the third trimester, each 1% increase in protein:carbohydrate ratio *lowered* adult systolic pressure 0.5 mm Hg.

Then 30 y later by age 55, first trimester exposure was associated with 3-fold more coronary artery disease (Roseboom et al, 2000) (Fig. 4.16A). As expected, the subgroup of adults with more body fat, higher systolic pressure, and impaired glucose tolerance had more coronary disease. Even so, birth weight,

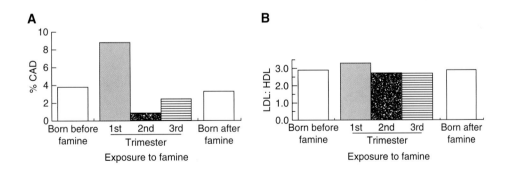

FIGURE 4.16 Famine exposure in utero and later metabolic and vascular characteristics. A. Coronary artery disease (CAD) (Roseboom et al, 2000). B. LDL:HDL cholesterol, P<0.05, Bonferoni corrected; adjustment for adult BMI removed the significance of this association; there was no birth weight association (Roseboom et al, 2000).

maternal weight, and SES have not shown links to coronary disease in this population. Nor has prenatal famine exposure influenced adult mortality up to age 57, of which 20% deaths are attributed to coronary disease and 40% to cancer (Roseboom et al, 2001; Painter et al, 2005a). However, the success of modern clinical interventions for vascular risk factors must be considered in the apparent lack of famine impact on mortality. The above evidence for increased coronary disease and obesity suffice for a 'cohort morbidity' effect of prenatal famine.

Urinary albumin elevations ('microalbuminuria,' an index of kidney dysfunction) at age 50 were 1.7-fold more prevalent for midgestation famine exposure, relative to the other trimesters or the non-exposed (12% vs. 7%) (Painter et al., 2005b). Microalbuminuriacs had more electrocardiographic abnormalities (25% vs. 14%), higher systolic blood pressure (135 vs. 125 mm Hg), poorer glucose clearance (40% vs. 16%), and higher glycated hemoglobin (HbA_{1c}, an index of elevated glucose and systemic oxidative stress; Section 1.4.2). At ages 50 and 58 y (repeated testing), none of those exposed in any trimester had abnormal glucose regulation (de Rooij et al, 2006). In the standard oral glucose tolerance test, 120-min glucose levels were below the clinical threshold for pre-diabetes. Nor was there any difference in diagnosed diabetes in relation to famine exposure during pregnancy. Respiratory symptoms (wheeze, cough) and obstructive airways disease were 50–100% more frequent in those from second trimester exposure (Lopuhaa et al, 2000). Here again, birth weight was not a factor.

Birth weight declined definitively in the famine area with the onset of famine, with smaller decreases in the control areas (Fig. 4.15C) (Stein et al, 1975). Famine exposure in the third trimester accounted for 64% of the variance in birth weight. At the most affected times, mean birth weights of 3011 g had fallen by 9% below the postfamine norm. Note that this decrease is still 10% above the 2700 g baseline of South Indian current birth weights discussed above. The diet threshold for smaller birth weight may be 1500–1750 kcal/d (Susser, 1991); again, this may underestimate the real consumption (Table 4.5A, note 2). Later pregnancy was the most susceptible to effects on the birth weight: third trimester (−9%); second trimester (−4%); first trimester, no effect (A. Stein et al, 2004). The protection of fetal weight during maternal malnutrition is remarkable.

Birth weight was also linked to maternal weight changes during pregnancy and decreased when maternal gain was ≤ 0.5 kg/wk (Stein et al, 1995). Statistical resolution of the causal pathways (caloric intake to maternal weight and/or to birth weight) is not easy. Non-famine controls did not show strong links of caloric intake and birth weight. Only below some caloric threshold was the link of caloric intake to maternal weight gain to birth weight significant (Susser, 1991). Smaller birth weight was not due to shortened gestation, nor was gestation length altered. Those in the famine 'control regions' exposed to milder diet restriction (Table 4.5A) maintained normal birth weights of about 3400 g. Maternal weight postpartum was most impacted by caloric deficits in the third trimester: Each 100 kcal/d intake predicts maternal weight change of 0.37 kg postpartum, explaining 77% of the variance. Famine exposure in first and second trimesters had little effect on maternal weight.

Head size (circumference), like birth weight, was smaller in third trimester famine exposure (Stein, 1975, p. 104; Stein et al, 2004). Small head size may be a marker for risk of later neurodegeneration. Alzheimer patients showed an excess of small heads above age-matched elderly controls in two studies (Borenstein et al, 2005; Mortimer et al, 2003). The Dutch hunger populations did not show adverse effects of small head size on mental status up to age 18 (Stein et al, 1975).

To summarize effects of birth weight on later health, low birth weight had small effects on glucose tolerance (de Rooij et al, 2006). Although no associations with cardiovascular disease have been detected (Roseboom et al, 2000), later effects may be anticipated because of effects on systolic pressure, which varied inversely with birth weight up to age 50; a 2.6 mm decrease/kg increased birth weight (Roseboom et al, 1999).

Postnatal exposure to famine has shown immediate and delayed effects on reproduction. Reproduction decreased sharply at all ages during the famine (Stein et al, 1975). Menstrual irregularities occurred in 50% of women (Burger et al, 1948, p. 77) and were more common in the poor. At the worst time, births decreased by 65%. Stillbirths and perinatal mortality increased with third trimester exposure. The decline of births conceived during the famine was delayed by 2 m after the reduction of official rations below 1500 kcal/d, both in the famine cities, where the drop was greater, and in the control cities (Fig. 4.15A). This asynchrony could represent the depletion of endogenous body reserves required for fertility, or the depletion of food hoards, or both. A strong SES gradient of impaired fertility (Stein et al, 1975, p. 79) corresponds to the worse health and nutrition in the urban poor. With improved food, fertility immediately recovered, with a transient surge of births in 1946 that doubled the prefamine incidence (Fig. 4.18).

Early exposure to famine impaired adult reproduction in unexpected ways. First, no critical age of exposure was evident for later effects on reproduction. Second, women exposed to severe famine before puberty were 14% less likely to have a first or second child and had more reproductive problems requiring surgically induced menopause (Elias et al, 2005). Third, menopause was slightly earlier, showing 'dose effects' in proportion to the level of famine exposure during childhood (Elias et al, 2003). Menopause was 1.83 y earlier in those exposed to famine at ages 2–6 y. Later exposures had progressively less effect on menopause. These effects are opposite in direction to effect of diet restriction (DR) in rodents, which slows ovarian oocyte loss (Chapter 3, Fig. 3.18). However, the mouse exposure to DR was much longer in proportion to the life span (50%). Lastly, and the most curious, is a transgenerational effect: In the next generation from women exposed to famine in the first trimester, the grandchildren's birth weights are markedly lower in the second and later births (Lumey, 1997), despite the lack of effects of first trimester exposure on birth weight. These and other transgenerational effects are discussed in Section 4.8.

Postnatal famine exposure increased cancer up to 250% in proportion to the severity of famine, with breast cancer accounting for most of the effect (Fig. 4.17A) (Elias et al, 2005; van Noord, 2004). The average age of famine exposure was post pubertal (15–20 y). The increase of breast cancer would not be predicted by the earlier mean age of menopause. Delayed menarche, which was observed throughout the war, particularly in those aged 14, might also be protective (van Noord and Kaaks, 1991). However, other risk factors, IGF-1 and IGF binding protein-3 (IGFBP-3), showed modest elevations in proportion to the severity of famine exposure at ages 2–20 (Elias et al, 2004) (Fig. 4.17B). Elevated IGF-1 and IGFBP-3 may enhance the risk of breast cancer (Chapter 1), particularly after age 50 (Rinaldi et al, 2006). Because diet restriction decreases IGF-1 and IGFBP-3 (Chapter 3), it was hypothesized that the elevations represent a neuroendocrine disturbance. In contrast to breast cancer, colon and prostate cancer showed weak reductions (Dirx et al, 2001; Dirx et al, 2003). van Noord (2004) is correct in viewing the famine exposure and cancer relationship as very different from diet restriction in the laboratory because of the rebound eating and weight gain when food became available.

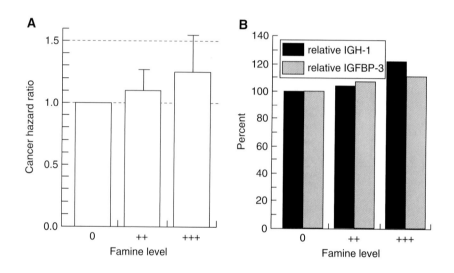

FIGURE 4.17 Postnatal famine, breast cancer, and IGF. From the 'DOM cohort' study of breast cancer (Diagnostic Onderzoek Mammacarcinoom, Utrecht and surrounding regions; 1974–present); a subgroup participates in the European Prospective Investigation into Cancer and Nutrition (Prospect/Epic Study). A. Total cancer risk of women aged 2–33 y during the famine and 41–73 y at interview. Mean adjusted hazard ratio (95% confidence intervals) (P = 0.30). Breast cancer was the predominant site (35.5% of all cancers); when breast cancer was removed from the analysis, no other cancer was significantly associated with famine; breast cancer alone did not show significant associations (Elias et al, 2005). B. Serum IGF-1 and IGFBP-3 in postmenopausal women exposed to famine at ages 2–20 who were free of breast cancer (Elias et al, 2004) at mean ages 62–63; the women did not differ in body mass index and did not use sex steroid replacement or insulin therapy (N = 87). Relative to unexposed levels: IGF-1, 133 ng/ml; IGFBP-3, 3171 ng/ml. IGFBP-1 and -2 showed weak decline (not significant, not shown).

These cohorts are being followed closely. Adults exposed to famine in the first trimester had 2-fold higher self-reported poor health (Roseboom et al, 2003). In longitudinal studies, self-rated health strongly predicts future longevity (Mossey and Shapiro, 1982) and adds further statistical power to blood risk indicators such as blood albumin and leukocyte levels (Jylha et al, 2006). Vulnerable subgroups may be defined, especially among those with self-rated 'poor health.'

Besides undernutrition, I suggest infections may also have an impact on future outcomes of aging in the Dutch cohorts. Acute gastrointestinal and respiratory infections are recognized as major causes of civilian deaths during and immediately after the war (Stein et al, 1975, p. 181). Mortality of infants and children from infections increased strikingly during 1944–1946 throughout the country (Stein et al, 2004a,b). Stillbirth rates and first-week deaths rose higher than 'control' than in the 'famine areas' (Stein et al, 1975, p. 152). A rubella epidemic spread country-wide in 1943 and the first half of 1944, and was implicated in a surge of congenital heart disease (*op. cit.*, p. 225). Although this epidemic preceded the full famine, the already diminished food rations may have increased vulnerability to infections. Severe typhus epidemics arose locally during the end of the war, with 3-fold increase in cases in 1944 versus 1941–1943 (Burger et al, 1948; Hemmes, 1945).[6] Bacillary dysentery also increased several-fold during the war. Many households kept increased numbers of household rabbits and goats for food, which increased bacillus-carrying flies (*op. cit.*, p.112). Diarrhea was common, 25% across ages and social classes (Burger et al, 1948, p. 77). Diptheria may have caused the most casualties, with 20-fold increase of morbidity 1943–1944 (*op. cit.*, p. 120). Puerperal fever increased 2-fold 1940–1944 (*op. cit.*, p. 127). Tuberculosis death increased up to 3-fold by the winter of 1945 (*op. cit.*, p. 403). After liberation, there was an increase of stillbirths spreading from North to South, "…compatible with the spread of a maternal infection that had greater impact in nutritionally deprived areas (Stein et al., 1975, p. 154; also p. 163). "…Taken together with reports of rampant infections, these [mortality] patterns suggest that debility produced by prenatal stressors predisposed infants to…postnatal infections current at the time of epidemic mortality" (*op. cit.*, pp. 185, 224). The surge of infections during increased food availability recalls the Murrays' observations in refeeding of starving Africans (Section 3.2.4).

Given the greater privations of the lower social classes, we might expect distinct morbidity subgroups during future aging. The possible impact of these infections on adult health has not been included in subsequent analyses, as far as I can find. One approach might be screening for antibodies to endotoxin, such as found in Gambians with chronic gastroenteritis (Campbell et al, 2003a,b) (Section 4.6.2). Acceterated immunosenescence may be predicted (Section 2.8).

Leningrad (St. Petersburg) experienced an even more terrible famine, 1941–1942 from the German blockade (Siege of Leningrad). Conditions were so dire that

---

[6]Paulus van Noord kindly found this archival source and translated key sections.

almost half of the population died, far more than in the Netherlands (Antonov, 1947; Pavlov, 1965; Stanner et al, 1997). In addition to dire malnutrition, the population was subjected to the stress of ceaseless bombardment and shelling (Antonov, 1947; Bell, 2004), not experienced by the Dutch. During the worst phase November 1941–February 1942, rations averaged 300 kcal/d. This diet was mostly carbohydrate and much less in amount and composition than in the Dutch Hunger Winter (Table 4.5A). Nutrition gradually improved after the siege.

During the first half of 1942, birth weights dropped by 500 g, and half of the live-born weighed <2500 g (Antonov, 1947). Birth weight information by personal recall indicates a 700 g deficit: intrauterine exposure, 2700g, not exposed 3200 g (Stanner and Yudkin, 2001). Nonetheless, 4% of births were >3500 g above the median normal weights, implying that some had privileged access to food during the siege.

Vascular risks are higher in men who were exposed to famine during ages 9–15 ('around puberty') (Sparen et al, 2004). Relative to a wartime reference group outside the siege zone, the famine-exposed had 1.56-fold more hypertension (>160 mm Hg), 1.39-fold more ischemic heart disease, and 1.65-fold more stroke in 1999 (ages 67–74; my calculation). However, exposure at earlier or later ages had less or no effect. Effect of famine exposure during trimester of pregnancy has not been reported. Exposure to famine during pregnancy versus infancy did not alter coronary artery disease indicators, glucose intolerance, or dyslipidemia at age 52–53 (Stanner and Yudkin, 2001). Nor did early famine exposure influence height and weight at age 52, relative to those outside Leningrad. Overall, cardiovascular mortality was slightly higher than in controls, not besieged, who experienced milder undernutrition.

Effects of the Leningrad siege and Dutch Hunger Winter are similar in the decrease of birth weight and increase of vascular disease at middle age. However, there are important differences: Leningrad survivors have not shown intrauterine effects on vascular disease, but this may represent the success of medical interventions. Obesity and overweight in adults were not increased from the Leningrad siege. An important gap is the lack of reliable data from Leningrad on birth weight and postnatal growth. In other populations, as discussed above, catch-up growth is linked to adult obesity and vascular disease. Table 4.4 summarizes similarities and differences.

4.7.2. 19th Century Famines

Famine was horribly recurrent and widespread in many countries that are now highly developed and well nourished. In 18th century Finland, for example, crop failures occurred about twice a decade, slightly improving by the mid-19th century (Pitkanen, 1993). The 'Great Finnish Famine of 1866–1868' was made even worse by a series of intermittently poor crops, beginning in 1857 (the 'decade of misery') (*op. cit.* p. 51), which caused about 150,000 excess deaths. The lower SES landless class suffered the most from starvation and disease (Ikonen, 1990;

Pitkanen, 1993).[7] About 100,000 left their homes in treks of endless begging (Hakkinen, 1992). Moreover, infections raged throughout Finland, particularly typhus and dysentery (Table 4.6): typhus rose 30-fold above prior levels and was still 5-fold higher the year after (Pitkanen, 1993). In 1865–1866 infant mortality transiently doubled to 400/1000 (Vuorinen, 2006). Nonetheless, these severe health challenges show remarkably little impact on adult mortality. Those born during the famine who survived to age 17 had mean lifespans of about 43 more years (Kannisto et al, 1997). Their mortality rates did not differ up to age 80 from those born 1866–1868, relative to those born 4 years before or after the famine. Kannisto and colleagues (1997) noted that the postfamine conditions in the 19th century were worse than in the 20th century. Nonetheless, there could have been cognitive and physical impairments, as in the 1918–1919 Influenza Pandemic. My comparison of fertility shows the great difference in these postfamine environments. The postfamine fertility (Fig. 4.18) showed much smaller rebound in the Finns (<1.5-fold increase), barely regaining 1861 fertility levels; whereas the Dutch fertility boomed immediately by 4-fold. This huge difference could be caused by poor diet and persistent infections in the rural Finns. The average Finnish diet in the 1860s was 2300 kcal/d, reaching 3000 kcal/d only after 1890 (Heikkinen, 1996).

It is cogent that most Finns were rural farm workers, with endless heavy daily physical work loads. The diet available to most in 19th century Finland, even in good crop years, would be considered uneven in micronutrients and energy and was almost certainly below Dutch norms after WWII (Marja Jylhä, pers. comm.). The rebound physical growth of famine-exposed Dutch infants after the major improvement of food is considered a major factor in the subsequent increase of metabolic disorders, as discussed above. Considering the smaller fertility rebound after the Finnish famine as an index of more modest improvements in a basically stringent diet, it is likely that there was also less rebound growth. The combination of poor diet and the infections might both be synergizing factors in the small fertility rebound.

Another example is from Överkalix parish in Sweden, which suffered intermittent crop failure from 1809–1849 (Bygren et al, 2000). Although exposure to famine during pregnancy did not influence overall mortality up to age 70, sudden death from stroke was 2-fold higher in those exposed to variable food supply during pregnancy (these deaths were 11% of the total). Thus far, stroke incidence has not been reported in the Dutch famine population. There is also evidence for transgenerational effects from alternating famine and feast years (Kaati, 2002): Surfeit of food during the paternal grandfather's growth period increased his *grand*children's mortality from cardiovascular and diabetes by 2-fold. Male germ line gene imprinting of IGF-2 is a possible mechanism (Section 4.10).

In sum, episodes of famine (with or without epidemic infections) experienced during development in several northern European populations have not

---

[7]Marja Jylhä kindly found these sources and summarized key information.

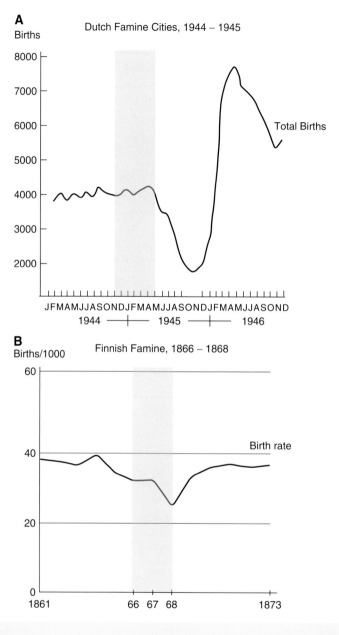

FIGURE 4.18 Birth numbers and famine. A. Dutch 'Hunger Winter' 1944–1945 (redrawn from Fig. 4.4). B. 'Great Finnish Famine', 1866–1868. Note the larger rebound of births in the Dutch. (Redrawn from Kannisto et al, 1997.)

shown major effects on subsequent mortality or life expectancy. Further analysis may show how episodic malnutrition and infection have different impact on arterial disease and immunosenescence than chronic life-long exposures, such as persist in health-poor populations of Africa and Asia (Section 4.6). Survivors of the 1919 Great Influenza Pandemic might also yield valuable information.[8] But these 20th century populations can not be compared with the earlier Finnish and Swedish populations discussed above and those in (Finch and Crimmins, 2004; Crimmins and Finch, 2006a,b) because of advances in public health and medicine in the 20th century, and because of the confounds of smoking (Finch and Crimmins, 2005). One general feature seems clear: Early growth impairments from whatever cause, when followed by catch-up growth, increase the risk of adult vascular disease and diabetes. We are just beginning to appreciate the multiple pathways by which development can influence outcomes of aging.

4.8. MATERNAL PHYSIOLOGY, FETAL GROWTH, AND LATER CHRONIC DISEASE

The adverse conditions that retard growth in health-poor populations with shorter life expectancy also give some clues to growth retardation in developed countries. The mechanisms linking the maternal environment to chronic diseases are poorly known and certainly extend far beyond immediate effects on birth weight. The main current focus is on how maternal nutrient physiology alters metabolic setpoints that favor greater postnatal obesity, leading to metabolic syndrome risk factors for vascular disease. Maternal diet restriction and diabetes-obesity have opposite effects on prenatal growth, but appear to converge postnatally to favor catch-up growth and overgrowth, and increasing the risk of the metabolic syndrome (Chapter 3, Table 3.2). Several other aspects of maternal physiology have received less attention: maternal cholesterol and maternal stress; and how any or all of these factors impose growth limitation on fetal structures, including kidney and the arterial bed architecture and elastin. In addition, I argue that maternal infections warrant greater attention because of direct pathogen impact

---

[8]The Great Influenza Pandemic of October 1918–January 1919 is being analyzed by Douglas Almond and colleagues for U.S. regions. This information became available too late to integrate into the text. In brief, the birth cohort exposed in utero had one year shorter life expectancy by the 1980s (Almond, pers. comm.). Vascular diseases and diabetes are higher, and self-rated health worse than in flanking cohorts (Almond and Mazumder, 2005). Lifetime education and income are lower (Almond, 2006). Because these findings generalize across U.S. regions, maternal malnutrition is less likely than maternal infections as the main influence on development. The impact of postnatal infections is unclear.

TABLE 4.6 Deaths from Infectious Disease During the Decade of the Great Finnish Famine (Famine Years in Bold)

	Total Deaths	Typhus	Dysentery	Pulmonary Tuberculosis	Smallpox	Measles (Rubella)
1862	48,639	1,437	878	4,660	302	2,439
1863	51,556	1,574	771	4,594	307	4,179
1864	39,914	2,038	728	4,460	321	852
1865	45,743	3,747	835	4,788	3,033	1,215
1866	**61,894**	**14,151**	**1,229**	**5,253**	**4,264**	**1,327**
1867	**69,774**	**21,026**	**1,038**	**5,895**	**3,103**	**808**
1868	**137,720**	**59,582**	**7,855**	**8,048**	**4,159**	**2,322**
1869	42,474	7,471	848	4,674	712	727
1870	31,071	2,819	615	6,758	205	172

(From Pitkanen, 1993, Table 5.1). 'Typhus' deaths may be underestimated because some medical officers of the time separately classified deaths from dysentery and other secondary causes of typhus. The old name 'typhus" represents three diseases, each caused by a different bacterium with common symptoms of fever and headache: louse-borne typhus ('epidemic typhus') due to *Rickettsia prowazakii* was probably spread by desperate and parasite-ridden refugees from the famine zones. However, the endemic typhus (*R. felis*) is transmitted by mice and fleas. Typhoid fever (typhus abdominalis, enteric fever) is caused by *Salmonella* bacteria and may be distinguished by abdominal pain and higher fevers.

on feto-placental function and because the pathogens themselves and maternal host defense responses compete with the fetus for energy and nutrients. Moreover, tobacco smoke and other environmental inflammogens alter fetal growth through unknown pathways that may interact with others above.

Maternal and fetal blood do not directly mix; gases and nutrients are exchanged across the feto-placental-maternal barrier. Maternal glucose enters the placental circulation, but maternal insulin is excluded. Fetal oxygen is much lower than the maternal, particularly early in gestation when the embryo is highly sensitive to oxidant damage. Many other factors may intervene between maternal and fetal blood nutrients that can alter growth and that can alter fetal development without altering the birth weight (Cetin et al, 2005; Regnault et al, 2005). Fetal growth is controlled by insulin-like growth factors (IGFs) that enhance the uptake of AA and glucose. Fetal IGF production does not depend on pituitary secretion of growth hormone (GH), unlike the postnatal regulation. Fetal blood amino acid (AA) levels exceed those in maternal arteries. Most maternal plasma AA levels decrease after the first trimester, when fetal growth is accelerating, whereas fetal plasma AA levels are normally higher than the maternal. The placenta is highly sensitive to the maternal condition of nutrients, stress, and infections, and is directly attacked by malaria, among other pathogens associated with retarded fetal growth (Section 4.5.2).

Fetal blood levels of amino acids (AAs) may be lower in growth-retarded fetuses. A large sample of growth-retarded fetuses 26–40 weeks (<10th percentile for gestational age; Milan, Italy) had umbilical vein blood AA levels about 30% below maternal arterial levels for most AA (Cetin et al, 1996). Yet, the maternal plasma AA levels in these cases were about 50% *higher* than in normal pregnancies, confirming (Economides et al, 1989) and others cited by (Cetin et al, 1996). Thus, fetal growth can be retarded despite the evident lack of maternal deficits in AA, which implicates placental dysfunction. Fetal growth retardation has been largely attributed to maternal malnutrition by the Barker group, but pathological conditions may also be suspected, particularly preeclampsia, toxemia, or infections. Preeclampsia is a toxic condition of pregnancy associated with placental inflammation (Jauniaux et al, 2006; Matthiesen et al, 2005), in which some maternal AAs are increased (Lopez-Quesada et al, 2003). Again, some of these AAs are elevated in models of endotoxemia, e.g., acute response of rats to LPS (Hallemeesch et al, 2000). In view of the diverse conditions that can afflict pregnancies and placental functions, particularly in unhealthy environments, it seems rash to attribute growth retardation simply to malnutrition.

Birth size has a strong tendency to be repeated in the next generation for both small and large size extremes (Klebanoff et al, 1997; Ounsted, 1986). For example, 20th century Swedish mothers were more likely to give birth to small babies if the mothers were born small for gestational age (2.68-fold higher) or if the mothers had low BMI (1.24-fold); influences of adult height were not reported (Selling et al, 2006). The maternal line shows a 'prepotency' of influences on fetal growth of greater impact than the paternal (Ounsted, 1986). The effects may extend for three generations: In 20th century UK, each 10 cm of the grandmother's height added 53 gm to her grandchildren's birth weight (Emanuel et al, 1992). These effects are coming to have major importance because of maternal obesity, which may impose a generalized set of burdens on the fetus with later consequences.

Birth weight increases with maternal weight, with few exceptions (Dietl, 2005; King, 2006; Oken and Gillman, 2003; Sebire et al, 2001). Birth weights over 4000g (macrosomia) increase the risk of elevated BMI of adolescents and, in some studies, increase the risk of type-2 diabetes (King, 2006; Oken and Gillman, 2003). Maternal obesity and diabetes before pregnancy are independent risk factors in macrosomia (Sebire et al, 2001). Fetal macrosomia also increases fetal death and other birth complications (Jolly et al, 2003). Moreover, children of normal birth weight who were exposed to gestational diabetes had an increased risk of obesity and glucose intolerance (Malcolm et al, 2006). On the other hand, growth retardation and low birth weight are lessened in maternal obesity (Sebire et al, 2001).

Obesity increases the risk of gestational diabetes with hyperglycemia to 6–30%, many-fold above the risk in all pregnancies of 1–3%. The normal increase of insulin resistance during the third trimester is greater in obese women (Table 4.7), which may promote a cascade of greater postprandial elevations of glucose and other nutrients that enhance fetal growth and adiposity (King, 2006; Ramsay et al, 2002). Maternal hyperglycemia later in pregnancy increases fetal growth, whereas first trimester (embryonic period) hyperglycemia is associated with slower growth. Gestational diabetes has differential effects on fetal growth, with

TABLE 4.7 Lipid and Inflammatory Factors in Obese Pregnancy, Third Trimester; Median Values (Interquartile Range); * Significant Difference

	Lean	Obese	Obese:lean (%)
Body mass index (BMI)	22.1 (20–24)	31 (29.1–34)	+140%[*]
Cholesterol, total (mmol/L)	6.35 (5.87–6.95)	6.25 (5.6–7.0)	0
Cholesterol, VLDL (mmol/L)	0.52 (0.31–0.64)	0.75 (0.6–1.0)	30%[*]
Triglycerides (mmol/L)	2.17 (1.9–2.6)	2.7 (2.3–3.2)	120%[*]
Insulin (mU/liter)	6.15 (4.47–9.5)	14.2 (11.3–27)	230%[*]
Leptin (ng/ml)	23.4 (12.4–30.9)	56.8 (46.2–65.2)	240%[*]
CRP (mg/ml)	2.13 (0.89–3.29)	4.45 (3.09–6.78)	210%[*]
IL-6 (pg/ml)	2.1 (1.7–2.8)	3.15 (2.36–3.59)	150%[*]

(From Ramsay et al, 2002). Healthy, normotensive. Ages: lean, 20–24 y, median 22 y; obese, 25–34 y, median 31 y. BMI, first trimester. Leptin correlated more strongly with fasting insulin (r = 0.74), than with CRP (r = 0.53).

increased fetal adipocyte formation, inferred from greater abdominal circumference, and impaired bone growth, as indicated by shorter legs (Lampl and Jeanty, 2004). Gestational diabetes and obesity may increase the risk of diabetes and obesity, which are major risk factors in vascular disease (Boney et al, 2005; Malcolm et al, 2006); e.g., maternal obesity during pregnancy increased the risk of childhood obesity up to 4-fold (Berkowitz et al, 2005).

Maternal obesity increases metabolic fuels used by the fetus, particularly glucose. In contrast, maternal diabetes increased certain fetal blood AAs (Cetin et al, 2005). The increased obesity may be an intensification of the normal increase of circulating nutrients needed for the increased fetal growth later in gestation. Hyperlipidemia also develops (Table 4.7), with elevated VLDL cholesterol, CRP and IL-6, and triglycerides. Gestational diabetes accelerates atherosclerosis (carotid artery thickening) in the mother herself (Tarim et al, 2006). In these cases, VLDL was elevated, while total cholesterol and LDL were not. Some impact on fetal arteries might be expected in view of the greater fetal atherogenesis in maternal hypercholesterolemia (Fig. 4.19, discussed below).

Materno-fetal hyperglycemia and hyperinsulinism are hypothesized to alter the postnatal setpoints for appetite and metabolism in the hypothalamus of the developing brain (Dorner, 1976; Horvath and Brunins, 2006; Plagemann et al, 2006; Ong, 2006). Altered hypothalamic leptin regulation is also implicated in obesity, which is associated with leptin insensitivity (resistance) (Chapter 3). In a rat model of maternal diabetes, fetal glucose was elevated 5-fold (Singh et al, 1997). The elevated maternal insulin did not alter fetal glucose, which is expected because maternal glucose, but not insulin, crosses the placental barrier. Hypothalamic neuropeptide Y (NPY) was lowered in the fetus exposed to maternal hyperglycemia, whereas isolated maternal hyperinsulinemia had no effect. NPY is strongly implicated in neuroendocrine setpoints (Section 3.3.1) and could be a mechanism in fetal programming by maternal glucose.

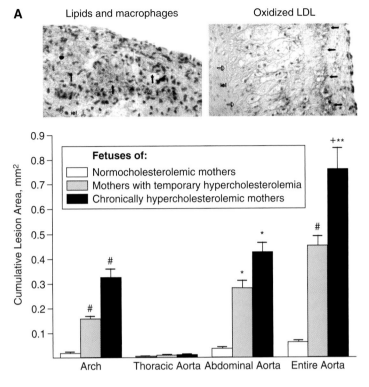

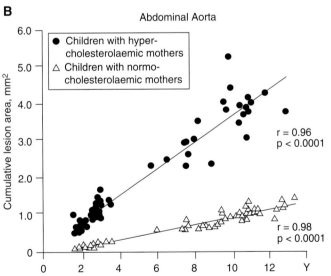

FIGURE 4.19 Fetal arteries from hypercholesterolemic mothers have accelerated atherogenesis (Napoli et al, 1997; Napoli et al, 1999a). A. Bigger fatty streaks and more intimal layer lipid accumulations with oxidized LDL and macrophage/foam cells. B. Children of hypercholesterolemic pregnancies had faster accumulations of arterial lipid, despite normal blood cholesterol.

Inflammation is also at work in obese pregnancies. As King (2006) emphasized, obese women bring higher basal levels of many inflammatory factors to their pregnancy. Table 4.7 compares healthy normotensive obese and normal weight women. In the third trimester, obese women had >2-fold elevation of plasma CRP and leptin, and 50% higher IL-6 (Ramsey et al, 2002). In another study, obese women with elevated IL-6 during pregnancy had fatter babies (Radaelli et al, 2006). Moreover, their neonatal lean body mass varied inversely with maternal insulin-like growth factor binding protein-I (IGFBP-I). Rat models support a direct link of maternal systemic IL-6 to fetal adipogenesis. IL-6 is transported across the placenta into the fetal circulation, whereas IL-1 and TNFα are not (Zaretsky et al, 2004). Thus, the effect of exogenous IL-6 and TNFα to increase fetal adipose depots by ≥30% (Dahlgren et al, 2001) could be mediated by different pathways, in which maternal elevations of IL-6 act directly on fetal adipogenesis, whereas elevations of TNFα would be indirect.

Maternal diabetes also markedly increases the risk of infections, as shown in many studies. Group B *streptococcus* colonization of the vagina was 3.5-fold higher for diabetic women (Ramos et al, 1997). Group B *streptococcus* is found in 10–30% of women and is a significant cause of neonatal morbidity. Vaginal fungal infections were 4-fold more prevalent in diabetic pregnancies (Nowakowska et al, 2004). These findings are consistent with the higher incidence of infections in diabetics, which may be a direct consequence of elevated glucose (Section 3.2.4).

Preeclampsia, another inflammatory condition associated with obesity, is characterized by hypertension and toxemia (Jauniaux et al, 2006; King, 2006). The placenta becomes oxidatively damaged and releases debris into the maternal circulation, causing systemic inflammatory responses, with elevations of cytokines IL-6 (4-fold) and IL8 (>10-fold) (Jonsson et al, 2006). Lipid changes include increased oxidized LDL and decreases of paroxinase (PON1) (Jauniaux, 2006; Uzun et al, 2005), which are also observed in lipid remodeling during infections (Section 1.5.4). Consistent with this proatherogenic lipid profile, preeclampsia increases subsequent maternal cardiovascular death by about 3-fold (Roberts and Gammill, 2005). Preeclampsia is associated with many inflammatory and infectious conditions, including elevated blood (Qiu et al, 2004); malaria, which infects the placenta (Section 4.4.4, above); cytomegalovirus infections (CMV); and periodontal disease (Jauniaux, 2006).

As a further example, maternal elevations of cholesterol may be directly linked to the earliest stages of atherogenesis in fetal arteries (Section 1.3, Fig. 1.15). In normal pregnancies, maternal plasma cholesterol is modestly elevated, up toward the current clinical criterion of 200 mg/dL (Table 4.8) (Herrera et al, 2006; Napoli et al, 1997; Saarelainen et al, 2006; Woollett, 2005). However, some pregnancies develop moderate to extreme hypercholesterolemia >300mg/dl (the prevalence is not well defined). A unique set of fetal and postnatal arteries from normal and hypercholesterolemic pregnancies in Naples, Italy, was assembled by Napoli, Palinski, and colleagues (Napoli et al, 1997; Napoli et al, 1999a,b; Napoli and Palinski, 2001). Mean birth weights in normal hypercholesterolemic and normal groups were identical, and there was no evidence of malnutrition.

TABLE 4.8 Maternal Plasma Cholesterol

	Normal (27% subjects)	Hypercholesterolemia Pregnancy Induced (33%)	Hypercholesterolemia Pre-existing (40%)
before pregnancy	155 ± 28, mg/dl	178 ± 30	292 ± 41
pregnancy	175 ± 20	325 ± 44	385 ± 50

From (Napoli et al, 1997) and (Wulf Palinski, pers. comm.). Women from Naples, Italy (N=82) of similar age (mean 28 y) and dietary and smoking habits. Maternal and fetal cholesterol were significantly correlated (r = 0.37, p<0.02), but correlations were stronger when analyzed by fetal age up to 6 months (r = 0.88, P <0.01; accounting for 77% of the variance vs. 14%). These statistics support the clinical understanding that maternal and fetal cholesterol *at birth* are not well correlated. In the two hypercholesterolemic groups, plasma lipoxides and cholesterol were strongly correlated, as expected. Also see Fig. 4.19. Maternal blood lipids (but not lipoproteins) are transported across the placental barrier (Herrera et al, 2006). Cholesterol and non-esterified fatty acids are directly transferred to the fetus, while transport of long-chain polyunsaturated fatty acids (LC-PUFA) is mediated by placental receptors. In humans, maternal cholesterol may contribute more to fetal cholesterol during early development.

Maternal hypercholesterolemia increased the accumulation of fetal *and* postnatal arterial lipids (Fig. 4.19A, B). Fetal arteries from hypercholesterolemic mothers had bigger fatty streaks and more intimal layer lipid accumulations with oxidized LDL and macrophage/foam cells (Fig. 4.19A). The nascent atheromas apparently grow larger in an environment of maternal hypercholesterolemia and oxidized lipids (see Table 4.8 note for interactions of fetal and maternal cholesterol). Moreover, the children of hypercholesterolemic pregnancies had faster accumulations of arterial lipid (Fig. 4.19B), despite their own normal blood cholesterol. As discussed in Section 4.3, atherosclerotic lesion size was inversely correlated with birth weight in children of normal cholesterol mothers only (Fig. 4.10) (Napoli et al, 1999a). Animal models of maternal hypercholesterolemia also increased fetal atherogenesis (Napoli et al, 2002; Palinski and Napoli, 2002; Yamashita et al, 2006) and increased expression of genes associated with atherogenesis, e.g., SOD3 and FGF binding protein (Napoli et al, 2002). Although it is difficult to accumulate such cases of maternal hypercholesterolemia and fetal postmortem material, high-resolution ultrasound imaging may further develop these findings.

The impact of maternal cholesterol on fetal arteries may be one of the strongest examples of 'fetal origins' hypothesis, but a different version than originally proposed. Maternal obesity may become of great general importance in the developed nations as a transgenerational factor predisposing to obesity and early chronic diseases. The obesity-linked condition of preeclampsia also favors premature maternal cardiovascular disease.

4.9. GROWTH IN ADAPTIVE RESPONSES TO THE ENVIRONMENT

As discussed above, fetal development is highly sensitive to the maternal systemic and uterine environments. Diverse phenotypic variations in arterial, endocrine, and neural systems have multifarious links to adult health. Evidently, many attenuated developmental phenotypes are compatible with subsequent reproductive success. Otherwise, we would not see the large populations of small people whose birth weights can be reasonably inferred to have also been small for innumerable generations. The remarkable variations of maternal metabolism during gestation (Section 4.4.4) also make this clear. On one extreme are Swedish women, with progressive increases of metabolism throughout pregnancy and 14 kg of body weight gain (Fig. 4.8B). Rural Gambian women are at the other extreme in this study, with decreased maternal basal metabolism during most of gestation and smaller body weight gain of 6 kg, also shown in Fig. 4.8. Their ability to maintain pregnancy is remarkable, given the burden of malnutrition, infectious disease, and physically demanding work. Humans may have evolved special homeostatic adaptive mechanisms not known in the great apes to maintain successful pregnancies at this level of duress. Despite the smaller birth size and higher incidence of stillbirths than in developed countries and despite the poor diet and high load of infections, this traditional society shows no sign of reproductive collapse. Similarly, the 2700 g average birth weights in Southern India suggest similar adaptations (metabolic data not reported).

The ergonomics of growth approximates caloric availability in these differing environments and shows the tight margin of this adaptation. The current average daily intake in Southern India is about 2100 kcal/d and the "lowest range of food" is 1810 kcal/d (FAO norms for South Asia). By various estimates, 30–60% of Indians are below the FAO norm (Chandrasekhar and Ghosh, 2003). The 1810–2100 kcal/d intakes are close to the margin of energy needed for sustained physical labor. The trade-value (equivalent purchase cost) of these calories as 3 kg wheat matches the smallest wage that Indian day laborers are willing to accept (Seckler et al, 1984; Clarke and Haswell, 1970). The 3 kg wheat at 3150 kcal/kg wheat yields 9450 kcal, which the day laborer would share with his household (average 5.3 dependants), equivalent to 1783 kcal/d per individual. Recall from the Minnesota starvation experiment (Section 3.2.3 and above) that this caloric input is at the level of 1800 kcal/d (Table 4.3B), which caused drastic weight loss and imminent death by starvation within 6 m. Although Indian laborers weigh about 25% less than the Minnesota volunteers at the start of the starvation experiment (52 vs. 69 kg), their caloric input may be just above starvation levels. Nonetheless, this small margin of caloric safety has still enabled sufficient life expectancy and reproduction for rural population growth in the 19th and 20th centuries. There may be other metabolic adaptations, besides those during pregnancy in malnourished women (Section 4.4.4, Fig. 4.8).

Further, Beaton (1989) calculated the energy involved in the greater growth in developed countries. Depositing 1 kg of tissues during 1 y requires 5000 kcal of energy at 5 kcal/g tissue for normal growth (13.5 kcal/d; FAO/WHO). Maintaining this 1 kg of tissue also costs about 5000 kcal/y. Then compare Swedish women, weighing 55 kg, with poor Indian women, weighing 40 kg. The 15 kg body weight difference would require 75,000 additional kcal/y, which is about 10% of the 766,500 kcal annual average intake (average daily intake 2100 kcal/d; FAO norm for South Asia). Thus, a major increase in energy availability would be needed to maintain the Swedish body weight, which could be achieved by reducing the load of infections, as well as increased food.

These variations in growth and metabolism (Gambia vs. Sweden) may be considered alternate pathways within the evolutionary reaction norm of phenotypic variations (Stearns and Koella, 1986; Walker et al, 2006). Others have considered small birth weight as an adaptation to the low nutritional energy available over the life history (Beaton, 1989; Ounsted, 1986; Walker, 2006). In considering small birth size and small adult size as adaptations to the energy available, I do not suggest that these lives should be considered optimal or benign from humanistic or ethical perspectives. These people suffer hunger, infections, and many other stigma and insults of low SES. While the concept of 'small but healthy' (Seckler, 1984) is challenged by the reality of malnutrition and many infectious diseases, long-term evolutionary processes may have enabled successful postnatal maturation despite fetal growth retardation. In our pre-history, adult size decreased by 15% after 50,000 years ago (Chapter 6, Fig. 6.7).

We do not know how many generations in improved environments are required to eliminate prior environmental effects. While data are fragmentary, they show fast responses to improvements. As discussed in Section 4.6.5, in only one generation, the children of Guatemalans who immigrated to the United States in the 1990s grew 8–10 cm taller. The birth weight trends for these children are not known, but would be expected to improve. In the second generation of Indian immigrants to the UK, birth weights were 280 g (8%) heavier than the first in 1989 (Dhawan, 1995). Comparisons of two generations of Illinois residents 1950–1990 showed modest increases of birth weight in the second generation (Chike-Obi et al, 1996).

Transgenerational effects of the environment are well recognized in animals. Zoos around the world record the increased size and fecundity of primates in successively healthier generations from feral origins. Rhesus monkeys have been observed for 5 generations after import from India to the Wisconsin Primate Laboratory. Birth weights of females increased by 8% after the third generation (Price and Coe, 1999; Price et al, 2000a). Surprisingly, male birth weights were unchanged in these same lineages, which might be consistent with gene imprinting, as discussed below. Maternal weights were also unchanged. The matrilineal associations of birth weight extend to half-sibs for both small and large birth weight. The age at first birth decreased progressively by 6 m per generation, associated with earlier attaining of adult weight. These changes might be further informed by individual records of health and infectious load.

Effects of food restriction, micronutrient deficiencies, and maternal obesity-diabetes with three or more transgenerational effects are well described in animal models (Aerts and Van Assche, 2006; Campbell and Perkins, 1988; Reusens and Remacle, 2006). In an exemplary study, rats from malnourished pregnancies were cross-fostered on normally fed nurses (Zamenhof et al, 1971a,b). As adults, their brain cell density (DNA content) was lower. The offspring of mating with normally fed controls still had lower brain cell density. Importantly, these effects were transmitted maternally and not found in males from the same litters. Such maternal transmission suggests gene imprinting, as discussed in the next section.

These models test the many hypotheses of fetal origins of adult disease on different organ systems, aptly described as the 'fetal matrix' (Gluckman, 2005). The fetal oocyte is another element in this matrix with potential transgenerational environmental effects. Oocytes are fully formed before birth in the fetal ovary, as recently confirmed (Eggan et al, 2006). Thus, the egg from which we stemmed was present in our mother's ovaries before her birth, exposed to our grandmaternal environment (Finch and Loehlin, 1998).

These reversible variations in fetal growth are matched by the varying schedule of growth and maturation in traditional foragers, e.g., in the timing of the adolescent growth spurt and age at first birth (Walker et al, 2006) (Fig. 4.5C, legend). The progressively earlier age at menarche and greater adult size in the past 5–10 generations in Europe and America are comparable to the differences seen in these foragers (Floud et al, 1990; Tanner, 1962; Tanner, 1981). In the larger national populations, the historical changes are clearly environmentally driven. New mutations influencing growth are unlikely to have major roles in this number of generations. However, there could be different allele frequency distributions of genes that alter growth during these historical changes or between the forager populations with different developmental schedules.

More generally, the plasticity of schedules for growth and reproduction for rapid responses to the environment is seated in the ability of these systems to respond soon after their differentiation. The male and female secondary sex characteristics that emerge at puberty, e.g., pubic hair, can be induced in neonates by sex steroids (Leung et al, 2005). Thus, life history scheduling depends on two main parameters (Finch and Rose, 1995): (I) the developmental acquisition of receptors and other cell machinery that enables response to hormonal and neural signals at the next life history stage; (II) the arrival of the appropriate stimuli. The gonads are able to produce sex steroids far before puberty. The hypothalamic-pituitary axis, in turn, can produce sufficient gonadotrophins to support precocious puberty; or depending on nutrition, stress, and health, puberty may delayed for years. The hypothalamic-pituitary-gonadal axis is also sensitive to metabolic hormones and cytokines, including leptin and insulin and hypothalamic TGF-α and TNFα (Gamba and Pralong, 2006). The system level of regulation allows rapid evolution of the reproductive schedule. If each component had its own genetically controlled clock, change would be very slow (Finch and Rose, 1995). This 'physiological architecture' enables the manifested plasticity in the timing and extent of adaptive responses to energy resources.

4.10. GENOMICS OF FETAL GROWTH REGULATION

The variations of growth, pre- and postnatal, are mediated by the genome in two fundamental mechanisms: genetic variations encoded in DNA base sequences and epigenetic variations, which are reversible, including gene imprinting, which alters the expression of the parental genes.

4.10.1. Inherited Genetic Variations

Inherited genes clearly contribute to the tendency of small mothers to have small babies (Knight et al, 2005) but have less influence than environmental factors. In 20th century Sweden, genetics contributed 33–46% of the incidence of small-for-gestational-age births (Svensson et al, 2006) [familial and twin studies, based on the Swedish Multigeneration Register of 8.5 million children born since 1932 with links to the biological parents and at least one set of grandparents]. This range of heritability approximates that of life expectancy in these and other populations from health-rich populations (Section 5.2). In other populations with high burden of disease and malnutrition, genetic influences on birth weight would be even more masked by the adverse environment.

Two gene candidates have come to light that have plausible links to inflammation and nutrition in fetal growth. The TNFα promoter alleles, discussed in Section 4.6.4 for influences on malaria resistance, also influence fetal growth. The −308 G/G homozygotes had 2.3-fold higher risk of being small-for-gestational age, with lower birth weight across the full birth weight range (Casano-Sancho et al, 2006). In very low birth weight infants, the −308 alleles were associated with different durations of required breathing support (mechanical ventilation) (Bokodi et al, 2005). The lower TNFα expression in −308 G/G carriers may influence fetal growth, because TNFα is mitogenic for myocytes and possible adipocytes (Casano-Sancho et al, 2006). Responsiveness to endotoxin by TNFα alleles could directly link maternal infections to birth weight. In mice, LPS increased TNFα in maternal blood and amniotic fluid, increased lipid oxidation (TBARS) in maternal and fetal liver 2-fold, and caused fetal growth retardation and death (Xu et al, 2006).

The apoE receptor-2 was implicated in small birth weight by an SNP screen of candidate genes for preeclampsia in Black women (SNP, single nucleotide polymorphisms in 129 candidate genes chosen for possible associations with fetal growth retardation and preeclampsia) (Wang et al, 2006). The apoE2 allele, which is protective for adult vascular disease, was underrepresented in small birth weight in a multi-ethnic study (Infante-Rivard et al, 2003). It is thus possible that apoE2 may protect against low birth weight, which is a risk factor in adult heart and metabolic disease. Preeclampsia has not been associated with any apoE allele.

These two gene candidates in regulating fetal growth return us to the possibility that environmental conditions could alter allele frequency by differential survival, within a few generations. The 10-fold decrease in early mortality during the 19th and 20th centuries could have allowed survival of those with allele sets that would have been eliminated in the not-too-distant generations that were conceived and born under harsher conditions.

4.10.2. Gene Imprinting: Inherited but Epigenetic Influences on Development

Fetal growth is highly dependent on IGF-1, IGF-2, and insulin, and their receptors. IGF-2 at its receptor IGF-2R in particular is influenced by epigenetic gene imprinting, in which one parental allele of a gene is silenced or not transcribed in somatic cells. Of the tens of thousands of mammalian genes, fewer than 100 are imprinted. Other genes that regulate growth are over-represented in this small group Akt-1/2 (Fig. 1.3A,B), metabolite transporter (Slc22a18), and cyclin-ckd inhibitor (Cdkn1c) (Reik et al, 2003; Smith et al, 2006; Tycko and Efstratiadis, 2002; Tycko, 2006). The longevity pathway links of IGF-1 and Akt-1/2 thus may extend to fetal growth regulation through imprinting. Nematodes and insects also employ imprinting by parent-of-origin, but genes that influence longevity (Fig. 1.3A) have not shown imprinting.

Imprinted genes are clustered in human chromosome 11p15.5 and 15q11–13 and the corresponding mouse chromosome. In addition, mice have imprinting of X-chromosome genes not known in humans. The silent imprinted gene, while not expressed in somatic cells, continues to be transmitted through the germ line. Imprinted genes are silenced by enzymatic methylation of cytosines, which can alter accessibility of the gene to transcription regulators by altering chromatin packing. Acetylation and phosphorylation also mediate imprinting and its converse, loss of imprinting (Kaneda and Feinberg, 2005; Mancini-Dinardo et al, 2006). The complexity of imprinting mechanisms continues to emerge.

Imprinting may be a fundamental epigenetic mechanism in the regulation of fetal growth by the parental genomes (Devriendt, 2000; Solter, 1988). Embryos derived from only one parent fail, despite having complete diploid genomes: Parthenogenetic embryos derived from maternal genes fail to develop the trophoblast and other extra-embryonic components, becoming teratomas; conversely, androgenetic embryos develop only the extra-embryonic tissues, becoming hydatidiform moles. In the Beckwith-Wiedemann syndrome, the fetus grows abnormally large and differentially; neonates are hypoglycemic and, if they survive, have a high incidence of Wilms tumor and other childhood cancers. The Beckwith-Wiedemann syndrome is caused by segmental trisomy and other defects of chromosome 11p15, where IGF-2 is located (DeChiara et al, 1991). IGF-2, the first imprinted gene identified, regulates the growth of both placenta and fetus (Smith et al, 2006; Tycko and Efstratiadis, 2002). Gene knockout experiments for IGF-2 and some other imprinted genes also show the importance of maternally expressed genes to placental growth and fetal development (Tycko and Efstratiadis, 2002). IGF-2 with a placental specific promoter activates placental trophoblast cells through AKT phosphorylation and is a regulator of amino acid transport.

The parental contributions to imprinting differ among the imprinted genes: IGF-2, which promotes growth, is mainly expressed from the *paternal* allele; its receptor, IGF-2R, which inhibits growth, is expressed from the *maternal* allele. Some maternally expressed genes encode placental transporters of amino acids and other solutes. While all known imprinted genes are active in the placenta, not all imprinted genes control growth. These parental asymmetries in the imprinting of key metabolic genes suggest counterbalancing evolutionary strategies and are interpreted as an outcome of fetal-maternal competition for resources (Haig, 1993; Haig, 1996). From the 'selfish gene' perspective, success of the paternal genome has depended on evolution of mechanisms that favor its genes in competition with maternal genes for nutritional and other resources during development. The maternal genome, according to this model, counterattacks by expressing genes that inhibit growth. The exclusive paternal expression of IGF-2 is countered by the exclusive maternal expression of IGF-2 receptor, which suppresses growth by trafficking IGF-2 for lysosomal degradation.

Imprinted genes have major influences on mammalian development by controlling placental growth, and thence the nutrient supply to the fetus, but also fetal growth itself (Angiolini et al, 2006). Placental nutrient flow is influenced by multiple imprinted genes, including *IGF-2* (Constancia et al, 2005) and *PHLDA2* (Salas et al, 2004), as well as other genes that have not shown imprinting, e.g., *TOR* (Fig. 3.10) (Jansson, 2006). Moreover, imprinted genes influence maternal postpartum behaviors, including nursing (Davies et al, 2005; Isles and Holland, 2005). Gene imprinting is implicated in low birth weight, preeclampsia, and other pathological conditions (Haig, 1993; Tycko, 2006). For example, *PHLDA2* (maternally silenced) had increased expression in the placentas of growth-retarded human fetuses (McMinn et al, 2006). Loss of imprinting of *PHDLA*, which increases its expression, also caused fetal growth retardation in mice (Salas et al, 2004). The importance of loss of imprinting extends to cancer, as observed for IGF2, which shows increased cellular expression in colorectal and other cancers (Kaneda and Feinberg, 2005). There is no direct evidence for maternal infections and placental or fetal gene imprinting. However, preeclampsia, which is associated with malaria and other infections (see above), can involve maternally expressed imprinted genes expressed in the placenta (Oudejans et al, 2004).

Neonatal behavioral experiences can also modify neuroendocrine gene imprinting functions with potentially important later effects as shown by Meaney and colleagues. Experimental handling of rat pups altered adult levels of plasma corticosterone and glucocorticoid receptor (GR) in the hippocampus, a critical locus of feedback control of the adrenal cortex (Meaney et al, 1988). During aging, the handled rats had lower corticosterone and less hippocampal neuron loss. As noted in Section 2.5.2, hippocampal neuron loss during aging was more prominent in earlier rodent colonies. Further studies show that maternal grooming also alters hippocampal GR gene methylation at a binding site for the NGFA-1 binding site (Weaver et al, 2007). These findings suggest that infections that alter neonatal-maternal behavioral interactions could have consequences to adult brain functions in the vulnerable hippocampal neurons.

Gene imprinting may be sensitive to nutrition. Mice fed a diet deficient in methyl donors (low in folic acid, methionine, and vitamin B12) showed loss of imprinting of the maternal IGF-2 allele, with decreased cytosine DNA methylation and increased gene expression. The effect persisted after restoration of a balanced diet for 100 days (Waterland et al, 2006). Thus, childhood dietary deficiencies can have persisting effects on gene imprinting, with potential importance to fetal growth. The scope of dietary imprinting is unknown but could be of major importance. Maternal protein-deficient diets that cause growth retardation also alter placental amino acid transport by the transport 'system A' (Malandro et al, 1996), which includes imprinted genes. Imprinting effects from early nutritional conditions may have caused the transgenerational effects of famine on grandchildren noted above on birth weight (Section 4.7.1) (Lumey, 1997) and on mortality from cardiovascular disease/diabetes (Section 4.5.2 (Kaati et al, 2002). As discussed in Section 4.9, in monkeys during adaptation to captivity, female but not male birth weights increased (Price, 1999; Price and Coe, 2000), suggestive of imprinting. Moreover, the trends of small mothers to have small babies for several generations could also involve imprinting (Section 4.6). Future studies may consider infections that directly affect the placenta and cause fetal growth retardation, such as malaria (Fig. 4.13) and HIV (McDonagh et al, 2004).

4.11. SUMMARY

Review of Barker's initial papers, 1986–1991, shows the important evidence that infections in birth cohorts were correlated with adult mortality to nearly the same extent as birth weight. Immunosenescence, accelerated by chronic antigenic stimulation, may contribute as much to adult mortality as the vascular risk factors. Adult height, which is determined by fetal and postnatal growth, was identified by Barker as protective for vascular events. It is robustly confirmed that taller people live longer, as seen in the historical increase of height and longevity. Crimmins and I hypothesize that both the increases of height and longevity resulted from the overall decrease of infection and inflammation (Crimmins and Finch, 2006a).

Birth weight is an important indicator of maternal health and nutrition, and predicts health of the adult in a U-shaped distribution. Low and high birthweight babies show higher vascular risk factors in the metabolic syndrome as adults. High birth weight (macrosomia) is more common in obese and diabetic mothers. The future of maternal effects will be dominated by maternal obesity and diabetes. Such pregnancies increase not only the risk of the same conditions in their offspring, but also the risk of infections.

I have questioned the focus on maternal malnutrition as the main cause of low birth weight. Twins typically have birth weight 800 g below single births in well nourished mothers, yet usually catch up by age 9 y. Because adult twins show many fewer levels of the vascular risk factors than low birth weight singletons, I suggest a different pathobiology is at work than in twins. Could maternal infections cause a substantial portion of low birth weights, even in health-rich countries? Subclinical maternal infections may be more prevalent than recognized. Survey of maternal blood for endotoxin antibodies might yield clues (Campbell et al, 2003a,b).

Infections and poor nutrition clearly synergize to cause low birth weight in health-poor tropical populations. Maternal metabolism is remarkably different in these poverty-struck populations. Unlike well-fed mothers, health-poor mothers fail to increase basal metabolism during pregnancy and gain 50% less weight. This may be a metabolic adaptation to the energy challenge. In rural Gambians, who experience a hungry season with high infections, food supplements during pregnancy increased birth weight by 230 g, but only partly restored the maternal metabolic upregulation. Moreover, birth weights are still 300 g or more below the median in healthy populations. Prevalent malaria is a factor in low birth weight by directly infecting the placenta, while diarrheas cause postnatal growth retardation. These children also suffer chronic gastroenteritis, with endotoxin leaking into the circulation. Those born in the hungry season of high infections had higher adult mortality from infections than those born 4–6 m earlier. The presence of endotoxin and IgG antibodies in adults (Campbell et al, 2003a,b) suggests useful markers for other populations in association with vascular disease. Even in health-rich populations, maternal infections may have unrecognized roles in fetal retardation.

Moreover, widening international trade can spread infections. As will be developed in Section 6.4, we live in a globally confluent microbial system. Moreover, modern health-rich populations are only 2–3 generations removed from highly infectious environments. With few exceptions, nutritional supplements of malnourished populations improve pre- and postnatal growth. However, broad generalizations are unlikely to be sustained because of the heterogeneity of populations in infectious disease load and nutritional history. Individual variations in intestinal flora may reflect host genome-environment interactions in the life history of nutrition and pathogen exposure.

Infection-nutrition interactions in health-poor tropical populations may be pertinent to ongoing studies of famine and malnutrition in the 19th century and World War II. Many studies show relationships of adult health to caloric deficits at different times in pre- and postnatal development. Moreover, infections were also raging in the Netherlands at that time, as well as in the Finnish Famine of the 19th century. Survivors of the WWII famines have shown modest trends for glucose dysregulation, but inconsistent effects on cardiovascular disease (present in the Dutch Hunger Winter, exposed first trimester; absent in Siege of Leningrad). However, breast cancer is notably increased (up to 250%) and the age of menopause decreased (up to 1.8 y) in those exposed postnatally to famine (each change shows its own critical time). Overall, the effects of maternal starvation on development seem relatively mild in populations that had been relatively healthy and well nourished. However, exposure to infections predicts accelerated immunosenescence (Section 2.8).

Clearly, many factors at work during development can modify outcomes of chronic aging conditions. Besides infections, inflammation, and nutritional factors from the environment, genetic factors are at work. For example, TNFα promoter alleles, which influence susceptibility to malaria, may also influence fetal growth, adult adiposity, and other metabolic syndrome risk factors. Other genetic variations in inflammatory responses may be viewed as balancing selection in the context of nutrition, infection, and delayed health consequences.

Another genetic effect on development is through imprinted alleles of the insulin/IGF pathways that may be modified by diet. But there is another major source of variation, through chance events during development, illustrated by the wide variation in ovarian oocyte numbers that, in turn, determine the onset of reproductive senescence (Finch and Kirkwood, 2000). The next chapter considers these chance variations as a factor in the low overall heritability of the life span.

The evidence assembled shows major roles of infection and inflammation on human development. Similar associations were described in Barker's original papers (1986–1991). I hope to have challenged the focus on maternal nutrition in the Fetal Origins theory to include the omnipresent burden of infections and inflammation, which contribute on the same level of magnitude to adult chronic diseases with inflammatory processes.

Genetics

5.1. INTRODUCTION

Genetic influences on aging and longevity are now added to the discussion of environmental influences on nutrition and host defense mechanisms from prior chapters. Arterial disease, diabetes, obesity, and Alzheimer disease may be modified by some of the same alleles of lipoprotein and cytokine genes. In some respects, inflammatory processes in these chronic diseases are amplifications of processes ongoing throughout life in the absence of specific diseases. Environmental causes of infectious and inflammatory processes and pharmacological interventions may also be sensitive to allelic variations. Diet restriction (DR) and obesity-diabetes represent opposing degrees of inflammation. DR shows anti-inflammatory effects whereas obesity and diabetes are proinflammatory. In each condition, the relation to inflammation alters the progression of arterial and Alzheimer disease in rodent models. Developmental influences on adult disease processes include nutrition and infection. Enhanced fetal growth from maternal obesity and diabetes is increasingly recognized in association with insulin-like growth factors that are also gene candidates for longevity. The fly and worm mutants give genetic clues to processes that broadly regulate development and aging. Before delving into details of these gene variants, I outline a perspective about the limitations of genetic determination in the phenotypes of aging and then consider sex determination, which is the largest genetic effect on human longevity.

5.2. SOURCES OF INDIVIDUAL VARIATIONS IN AGING AND LIFE SPAN

The genetic analysis of life span has recognized the extensive non-heritable individual variations within a species. In the inbred fly, mouse, and worm, the heritability (V_H) of life span ranges 20–50% (Finch and Tanzi, 1997; Finch and Kirkwood, 2000). Twin V_H for life span is about 25% (Skytthe, 2003; Christensen et al, 2006). According to the hypothesis that the reproductive schedule is a major factor in the evolution of life span (Section 1.2.8), it is cogent that age at menopause shows a higher range of V_H, 45–86% (Towne et al, 2005; Kirk et al, 2001; Murabito et al, 2005; de Bruin et al, 2004). Other life history traits fall closer to the V_H of lifespan: age at menarche, V_H of 45–50% (Towne et al, 2005; Kirk et al, 2001; Snieder et al, 1998). Birth weight, which is a determinant of adult health (Chapter 4.10) has V_H 33–46% (Svensson et al, 2006), slightly less than menarche. The balance of the variance in life span, 50–80%, is usually considered 'environmental (V_E), and attributed to chance variations from external and internal factors.

Even in the highly protected lab environment, worms and other experimental models display great individual variability in aging. In a theory developed with Tom Kirkwood, a portion of the non-heritable variance in life span arises from chance developmental variations (non-heritable constitutional variability, V_C) (Finch and Kirkwood, 2000, p. 11; Kirkwood et al, 2005). For example, highly inbred self-fertilizing worms hatched in the same culture dish differ individually (constitu-

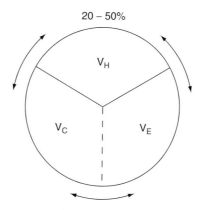

FIGURE 5.1 Variance in life span may be partitioned into three components: V_H, V_E, and V_C (Finch and Kirkwood, 2000, p. 11). My original figure. The heritable component of life span V_H is 20–50% in flies, worms, and human twins (Finch and Tanzi, 1997). The majority of the variance in individual life span is non-heritable and may be partitioned as mortality due to the external environment V_E (environment in classical quantitative genetics) and V_C (random individual constitutional factors that arise from chance variations at a cell and molecular level). An unknown proportion of the non-heritable variations is due to developmental noise. The phenotype also diversifies during aging through structural DNA changes in somatic cells (mutations, telomere shortening) and epigenetic changes (loss of imprinting, derepression) that progressively accumulate during aging.

tionally) in the rates of feeding, locomotion, and egg laying, and in their life spans, over a 2- to 3-fold range. Surprisingly, the coefficient of variation[1] for worm life span (34%) in the homogeneous culture dish is almost 2-fold larger than for identical twin life spans (19%) in the open world (Finch and Kirkwood, 2000, p. 15). We do not have good estimates of the random developmental contribution to life spans because of interactions between V_C and V_E (Fig. 5.1). The classic quantitative genetics model subsumes V_C under V_E (Falconer, 1996),[2] which may obscure important independent classes of interactions with V_H and V_E. Nonetheless, individual genotypes determine the range of reactions and responses.

---

[1]The coefficient of variation (COV) is a dimensionless number that normalizes the variance to the mean. For life span, X, the COV is calculated as the standard deviation, SD/X.
[2]"[L]arge amount of variability is . . . due neither to heredity nor to tangible environmental conditions" (Wright, 1920, p. 328). "Some of the intangible variation . . . may arise from 'developmental' variation . . . which can not be attributed to external circumstances, but is attributed . . . to accidents or errors of development" (Falconer, 1996, p. 135).

Chance external factors include accidents, infections, poor diet, predation, weather, etc. (Fig. 5.1). Chance internal factors include bystander damage from free radicals to cells and molecules, chance variations in cell numbers during development, and stochastic variations in gene expression. For example, chance variations in a worm heat shock gene transcription (hsp-16.2) present in young worms predict individual variations in life span, over a 2-fold range (Rea et al, 2005). The molecular origins of these differences could involve random variations in the assembly of multi-component transcription factors and their movements on DNA, which are described by the stochastics of diffusion (Brownian motion) (Finch and Kirkwood, 2000, pp. 58–65; Chang et al, 2006; Hu et al, 2006).

Variations of neuronal connections arise during development in *C. elegans*, despite the invariance of cell numbers as shown in two detailed studies. Motor-interneurons "might have gap junctions in one animal and chemical synapses in another . . . often synapses on the dorsal side of the nerve ring appear more sloppy." (Albertson and Thompson, 1976, p. 319). I suggest that the individual variations in pharyngeal pumping and food ingestion at hatching could arise from such neurodevelopmental variations in the pharynx. Some worms may be developmental phenocopies of the *eat* mutants described below, which have different pharyngeal pumping rates that correlate with life span. The ventral nerve cord also shows individual variations in dendritic processes and synaptic connections that could influence locomotion (White et al, 1976). Advances in optical techniques can access this level of variation in cell ultrastructure and gene expression over the life span of individual worms.

Mammals also have individual variations in cell numbers that influence outcomes of aging (Finch and Kirkwood, 2000, pp. 83–91). An instructive example is ovarian cell variations, which impact on reproductive senescence and related pathology. Ovaries of inbred mice vary 3-fold between individuals at birth in the number of primary follicles and oocytes (Gosden et al, 1983). Thus, inbreeding does not suppress individual variability of reproductive and other phenotypes (Phelan and Austad, 1994). The variations within a strain approximate the variations between strains in the average oocyte number and in the timing of reproductive senescence (Finch, 1990, p. 330; vom Saal et al, 1994). Human ovaries from unrelated stillbirths had the same COV as inbred mice (Finch and Kirkwood, 2000, p. 24). The ovarian oocyte pool was shown to determine the age of reproductive senescence in elegant experiments with graded partial ovariectomy (Nelson and Felicio, 1986). Variations in age at menopause also have a non-heritable component. The heritability of coronary disease and osteoporotic fractures could include a component from ovarian cell variations during development, which determines the number of estrogen-producing follicles surviving to mid-life. Recall from Section 2.10.4 that estrogen may be protective for atherosclerosis. Similarly, the number of follicles at birth may determine the risk of later-life genito-urinary tract infections, because the composition of microbial flora is highly sensitive to estrogen deficits (Devillard et al, 2004; Heinemann and Reid, 2005; King et al, 2003).

Developmental variations in the cerebral arterial bed warrant attention in relation to stroke damage. Identical twins can be discordant for cerebral aneurysms (Astradsson and Astrup, 2001; Puchner et al, 1994). Inspection of the angiograms of the non-involved parts of the carotid gives the impression of considerable variation in branching. A similar range of variations is seen in sketches of the orbito-frontal arteries of unrelated individuals (Whitaker and Selnes, 1975). Hypothetically, the same thrombosis in the varying sub-branches would cause different degrees of infarction and circulatory blockage in these individuals. A topological analysis of twin angiograms for branching properties (Pries et al, 1996) might give further insights into cognitive difference between twins, currently attributed variations in neuronal circuit architecture. The extensive differences in onset age of Alzheimer disease could also have a component in the arterial bed architecture: Identical twins in concordant pairs differ by an average of 4.5 years in dementia onset, with the range up to 16 years (Gatz et al, 1997).

The levels of adipose tissue at birth also vary between individuals. Differences in the expression of the imprinted genes MEST and BMP3 in fat depots of C57BL/6J mice predict the level of obesity in response to high fat diets (Koza et al, 2006). Besides the variations in gene expression that may arise autonomously, as in the heat shock gene of worms described above, mammals with multiple fetuses show an additional source of variation from fetal neighbor interactions. As analyzed by vom Saal, the sex of the neighboring fetus influences sex steroid levels during development that account for individual differences in reproductive and neuroendocrine system development (Finch and Kirkwood, 2000, pp. 158–171; vom Saal, 1989; vom Saal et al, 1994). The 3-fold differences between identical twins in weight gain on high fat diets (Bouchard et al, 1990) could represent other fetal interactions.

Adding to these developmental variations, individuals further differentiate during aging due to epigenetic drift or somatic cell variations in an individual from changes in the levels of gene expression (Martin, 2005). The imprinted *Igf2* autosomal gene, which is repressed in young female mice (Section 4.9), becomes activated during aging with tissue specificity (Bennett-Baker et al, 2003). The X-linked *Atp7a* showed similar progressive activation. These changes are not correlated between tissues in the same animal, implying that they arise sporadically (cell autonomously) in each tissue. DNA methylation, which is a major mechanism of imprinting, is also altered during aging. Blood leukocytes of identical twins show much greater differences in DNA methylation with aging in CpG islands in the promoter of C14orf162 and in chromosomal methylation patterns (Fraga et al, 2005). The differences with aging were greater in twins that had different lifestyles and environments. Mosaic features of somatic cell aging are also shown in the diploid cell models of senescence (Chapter 1). The scale of these epigenetic changes may be 100-fold greater than somatic DNA mutations, as discussed by Bennet-Baker et al (2003).

I'm sure to have tried the patience of some readers in deliberating on individual variance before addressing the proper 'genetics' of aging. But the genetics

of longevity must consider the different types and levels of variance in the interactions of gene-environment (G *x* E) and gene-gene (G *x* G) during aging. These
interactions are qualitatively different than in younger organisms because of two
major postnatal divergences in the genome: 'epigenetic drift,' as just discussed,
and DNA structural instability. Somatic cell genotypes diversify within each individual during aging because of DNA instability in mitochondria and chromosomes, and especially in the telomeric shortening that also alters gene expression
(Bahar et al, 2006) (Chapter 1). These findings suggest that genetic influences
have some intrinsic upper limit due to epigenetic and structural variations in individual genomes during aging that would arise even if the environment was
ideally invariant.

5.3. SEX DIFFERENCES IN LONGEVITY

In humans, the sex chromosomes are *the* major genetic determinant of longevity
differences within populations. This simple fact is often overlooked in discussions of genetic influences on aging. In most countries, women have greater life
expectancy (LE) (Gavrilov and Gavrilova, 1991), whether measured at birth (total
LE), or LE after age 1 (Teriokhin et al, 2004), or as years lived in full health
(DALE, or disability adjusted LE equivalent to the 'healthy life expectancy')
(Mathers, 2001). Currently, women live an average of 3.9 y longer than men (late
20th century global average from 227 countries and territories) (Mathers et al,
2001). The human female has lower mortality during all phases of life (Crimmins
and Finch, 2006b; Newman and Brach, 2001; Suthers et al, 2003).

In general, the female advantage scales in proportion to the mean (Fig. 5.2A),
which plots male and female life spans against the mean life span of both sexes
for each country (Teriokhin et al, 2004). Some extremes are shown in Table 5.1
and Fig. 5.2B, C. At the low extreme, Zimbabwean women live 2.81 y *less* than
men. At the high extreme, Lithuanian women live 12.05 y longer. African men
had only 37 y of health (DALE), whereas western European women averaged
70 y, a 2-fold difference (Mathers et al, 2001). For populations with life expectancies >80 y, women live ≥ 5 y longer.

The female advantage is present at birth and holds across most ages, as shown
for female:male mortality ratios in Sweden, mid-18th century to present
(Drevenstedt et al, in prep.) and in many other countries (Gravrilov and
Gavrilova, 1991; Horiuchi, 1999; Teriokhin et al, 1994). Despite fluctuations,
some explicable by wars, the baseline age-specific sex mortality ratios are soon
regained. The Gompertz acceleration of mortality (ascending line after age 40)
has a relatively constant slope across these historical Swedish periods, despite
the 10-fold range of mortality at each age (Fig. 2.7) (Drevenstedt et al, in prep.).
Although other countries and periods may show greater variations in the
Gompertz slope (Gavrilov and Gavrilova, 1991), in nearly all populations the
female mortality curves are displaced to lower values. That is, aging in
demographic terms appears to begin later in women.

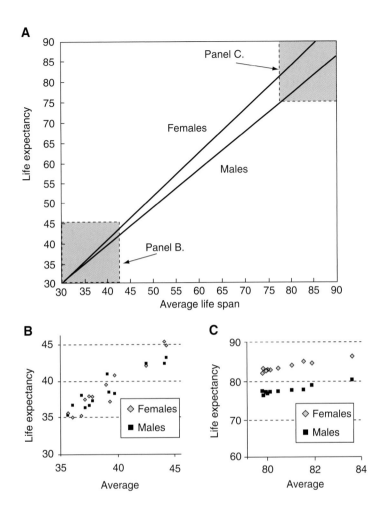

FIGURE 5.2 Human life spans from global average from 227 countries and autonomous territories (late 20th century public data). Redrawn from (Teriokhin et al, 2004). Calculated as life expectancy after age 1. A. The female advantage of life span increase with greater life expectancy. Male and female life expectancy graphed against the mean life span (unweighted mean of both sexes, male-female mean life span half-sum). B. Life expectancy <45 y: Female:male ratio 1.003 ± 0.014; calculated from data in (Teriokhin, et al, 2004). C. Life expectancy >79 y: Female:male ratio 1.086 ± 0.004.

TABLE 5.1 Sample of Extreme National Demographic Profiles

	Life Span (LS) Calculated as Life Expectancy After age 1 Year[a]			Environmental Mortality per Year (Gompertz-Makeham Coefficient, A)			Healthy Life Span (disability Adjusted Life Expectancy, DALE) Average of Both Sexes[b]
	Female	Male	Difference/ Ratio	Female	Male	Difference/ Ratio	
Andora	86.61	80.62	5.99/1.07	0	0	0.0004/5.00	72.3
Japan	84.28	77.76	6.52/1.08	0	0.001	0.0001/1.10	74.5
Lithuania	75.69	63.64	12.05/1.19	0	0.006	0.0025/0.59	64.1
Sweden	82.66	72.22	10.44/1.14	0	0.001	0.0005/1.45	73
U.S.A.	80.25	74.55	5.70/1.08	0	0.002	0.0002/1.08	70
Gambia	56.39	52.45	3.94/1.08	0.011	0.0116	−0.0005/0.96	48.3
Malawi	37.57	36.5	1.07/1.03	0.015	0.015	−0.0001/0.99	29.4
Mozambique	35.1	36.76	−1.66/0.95	0.025	0.023	0.002/1.09	34.4
Zambia	37.97	37.4	0.57/1.02	0.023	0.0224	0.0006/1.03	30.3
Zimbabwe	35.31	38.12	−2.81/0.95	0.025	0.0218	0.0032/1.15	32.9

a. Examples reformatted from (Teriokhin et al, 2004). The environmental mortality is calculated as the Makeham term M in the Gompertz-Makeham equation for mortality as a function of age x: $m(x) = M + I\exp(\alpha x)$, where the age-independent first term M represents environmental causes of death, I is the initial mortality rate, and α is the Gompertz constant of mortality rate acceleration (Section 1.2.1, Table 1.3). Sex differences in life span are explained by sex differences in A (Teriokhin et al, 2004), which approximates the initial mortality rate I (Table 1.3) and (Finch, 1990, pp. 663–666). The Gompertz slope coefficient α for birth cohorts is relatively stable across human environments (Finch and Crimmins, 2004; Jones, 1956) (Fig. 2.7A).
b. (Mathers et al, 2001).

The female advantage in life expectancy at birth in industrialized countries was about 2–3 around 1900, with further progressive increases. However, later in the 20th century, the female advantage shrank in some countries (Horiuchi, 1999). These trends are attributable to changes between the sexes in behavioral risks, mostly cigarette smoking, but also to alcohol consumption and occupational hazards (Horiuchi, 1999; Pampel, 2002; Waldron, 1985). Nonetheless, the female advantage culminates in the dominance of women among centenarians (Robine and Vaupel, 2001; Robine et al, 2006). The growth of the oldest age group beyond 90 is a demographic novelty that emerged after 1850 and continues growing remarkably in health-rich populations. Centenarians are increasing exponentially, doubling every 6 years, faster than any other age group. Sex differences of life span in late 20th century countries are strongly associated with sex differences in the Gompertz equation 'initial mortality rate' coefficient, I (Table 5.1, legend; Table 1.3) (Teriokhin et al, 2004). The female advantage persists across the 20-fold range of environmental mortality in different countries (Gompertz-Makeham coefficient M) (Table 5.1).

However, at life spans <45 y, the female longevity advantage is less robust and wobbles (Fig. 5.2B) (Table 5.1). The age 45 cut-off is crucial to understanding the evolution of the human life span, because life spans are typically 30–40 y (Fig. 1.1A) in pre-industrial countries (Oeppen and Vaupel, 2002) and in the remaining small groups of forager-hunter gatherers (Gurven and Kaplan, 2007). For example, Ache foragers living in the forest before contact had lower female mortality and longer life expectancy at age 20 (female 39.8 y, male 34.2 y) (Hill and Hurtado, 1996, p. 196), but few other groups have been described. Birth rates are also much higher in these health-poor populations (Easterlin and Crimmins, 1985; Teriokhin et al, 2004), where infections are major causes of death. Only when early mortality from infectious disease has been greatly diminished do we see large proportions of adults surviving to post-reproductive ages, with increasing female advantage in longevity. Evidently, the lower prevalence of infections in industrialized nations has diminished a major 'natural' cause of mortality. Thus, we may consider that the recently growing female advantage at later ages is a post-Darwinian phenomenon that cannot be attributed to natural selection of genotypes for superiority in reproduction. However, health-poor populations with high mortality remain under greater Darwinian selection because of highly prevalent gastro-enteritis, HIV, malaria, worms and other parasites, TB, and other chronic and acute infections that are major causes of mortality (Chapter 4).

Gender differences in mortality are seated in the genetics of sex determination. The male phenotype depends strictly on the Y-chromosome sex-determining locus (SRY), which encodes a transcription factor required for testes development (Barsoum and Yav, 2006). In the absence of a fetal testis, mammalian female organs develop as the default phenotype. Of the genes carried by the two X chromosomes present in females, one of the two alleles is usually randomly inactivated during development (X-inactivation is different from gene imprinting; Section 4.10). However, about 15% of X-linked genes escape inactivation and are expressed to some extent in adult cells (Carrel and Willard, 2005). Thus, female and male genomes differ in the following major attributes: Y-chromosome genes that are absent from the X chromosome; the heterozygote advantage of women for harmful recessive alleles that are not offset in males; and, the expression in women of both copies of some X-linked genes.

Sex differences in postnatal mortality are not obviously explained by sex hormone levels and involve the cultural complexes described as gender differences. The prenatal sex difference in mortality is less subject to cultural influences because the fetal sex is not clearly recognizable by the mother without modern technology. However, ultrasonic imaging indicates greater male wakefulness (Robles de Medina et al, 2003) and earlier female oral-motor development (Miller et al, 2006a). Humans experience irreducible gender effects on mortality risk through their social roles and status at all ages. Gender-dangers include childbirth in women and fighting in males. Independent of these risk situations, sex differences are recognized in morbidity that are the result of differences in organ structure during development. Osteoporotic fractures begin to increase during aging 5–10 y earlier in women than in men. Why heart disease mortality also lags behind in women is still obscure, despite sex differences in many vascular event risk factors, including blood lipid and blood pressure regulation. Males are more vulnerable to infections in many studies. During the first year, male infants were 20% more likely to die from infections than females (U.S. births, 1983–1987) (Read et al, 1997). Other studies, pro and con, are summarized by (Wells, 2000). Whatever the 'intrinsic' role of biological sex, the gender issues in health from culture and behavior are always present and hard to resolve, especially in health-poor populations. Despite these uncertainties, we may anticipate a convergence of the physiological and genetic basis for the sex differentials in mortality.

Many other species have major sex differences in life span (Finch, 1990; Kirkwood, 2001; Tower, 2006). A comprehensive analysis of more than 1000 groups of rodents showed 5% greater maximal longevity of the female in rats, but no sex difference in mice (Rollo, 2002). Sex differences in longevity may also be influenced by the resistance to infections: In general, female rodents survive most pathogenic infections better than males (Pasche et al, 2005). Infections in the early era of husbandry may have contributed to some sex differences in life span of mouse strains (Storer, 1966). Among five species of *Drosophila*, the females had small differences in mortality acceleration rates (Gompertz slopes), whereas male interspecific differences include both the slope and baseline mortality rate (Promislow and Haselkorn, 2002). Metabolic rates differ 3-fold between species and tend to be higher in the females, but do not correlate highly with life span. Sex effects on age-specific mortality differ between fly lines and are influenced by population density (Khazaeli et al, 1995).

Sex differences in rodent and fly mortality are associated with reproductive stresses (costs) (Chapman et al, 1998; Phelan and Rose, 2005) that are minor in modern human populations (Aiello and Key, 2002; Hrdy, 2000). As predicted by evolutionary theory. Virgin flies live longer than mated females, even though egg production was unaltered (Fowler and Partridge, 1989). Fighting during mate selection increases male mortality, while production of large numbers of eggs is energetically costly. In the worm, germ cell ablation increased life span, discussed below (Fig. 5.4), whereas in the fly, germ cell ablation may decrease life span (Barnes et al, 2006). Of course, the absence of germ cells can alter endocrine functions in other ways. Generalizations are premature.

Many sex-specific cases of trade-offs in immunity and reproduction can be interpreted in terms of antagonistic pleiotropy (Tower, 2006). Contact with seminal fluid shows a trade-off in flies; while being toxic to females, seminal fluid prevents mating with other males. One toxin in seminal fluid is the protease inhibitor Acp62F (Wolfner, 2002). Seminal fluid also contains antimicrobial peptides that may protect from venereal transmitted infections, as seen in other insects (see below) (Khurad et al, 2004). Sex differences in nutrition-infection interactions may be anticipated, because of sex differences in response to diet restriction in flies (see below, Fig. 5.6) and the sex differences in vulnerability to infections discussed above. The selective vulnerability of male flies in *Drosophila bifasciata* and *D. psuedoobscura* to the bacterium *Wolbachia* might be a good model (Veneti et al, 2004). Many fly strains carry this rickettsial bacterium as an intracellular symbiont, which is transmitted maternally. *Wolbachia* may participate in reproductive isolation mechanisms in natural populations, mediated by male-specific mortality.

Furthermore, transgenic manipulations of life span are influenced by the sex of the genetic host in fly strains and differ by background genotype. Targeted overexpression of human superoxide dismutase (SOD) in fly motorneurons generally increased life span, with sex-specific effects that differed between long-lived wild-caught fly strains (Landis and Tower, 2005; Spencer et al, 2003). Insulin-producing neurons contribute to the sex differences in motor activity (Belqacem and Martin, 2006). Some mutants that inhibit insulin-like pathways increase the female life span more than the male (Tu et al, 2002a).

5.4. METABOLISM AND HOST-DEFENSE IN WORM AND FLY

Metabolic genes influence longevity from single-celled yeast to worms, flies, and mice (Fig. 1.3A) (Kenyon, 2005; Finch and Ruvkun, 2001; Longo and Finch, 2003). Many of these genes belong to systems of hormone signaling, including insulin-like peptides, insulin-like growth factors (IGF), and sterols. Variants of insulin-like genes also influence inflammation. In some cases, these hormones enhance survival during states of reduced metabolism, which are coupled to increased stress resistance. Depending on the species, development may be arrested in hypometabolic states.

5.4.1. Metabolic Gene Signaling

All animals have multiple insulin-like peptides that mediate growth during development and postnatal metabolism and feeding behaviors (Nassel, 2002; Wu and Brown, 2006). The invertebrate insulins are almost exclusively neurosecretions, whereas vertebrate neuronal insulin expression is minor relative to pancreatic ß-cells. IGF-1 is widely expressed in brain, liver, and other tissues (Bondy and Cheng, 2004). The invertebrate insulins have many specialized functions, and some conserved activities in glucose regulation. The fly has glucose receptors in the corpora cardiaca, which receives insulin as a neurosecretion and responds to hypoglycemia, as does the pancreas (Kim and Rulifson, 2004). Genetic ablation of the insulin-secreting medial neurosecretory cells in fruit flies increased hemolymph glucose 3-fold, as expected (Broughton et al, 2005).

Current models of insulin/IGF-like signaling in nematodes include the sequence of biochemical steps from the insulin-like receptor DAF-2 to the transcription factor DAF-16 (Fig. 5.3). Sensory neurons secrete an insulin-like peptide that activates an insulin-like receptor (DAF-2), followed by a phosphorylation cascade through phosphatidylinositol (PI) from AGE-1 (a PI-3OH kinase, Fig. 1.3). After further steps,

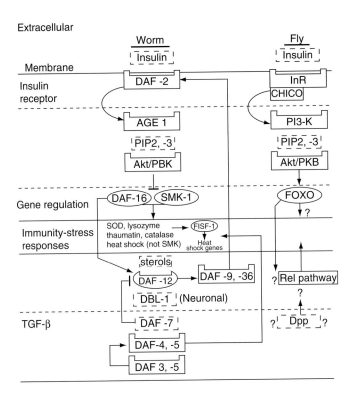

FIGURE 5.3 Metabolic signaling and immunity in worm (*Caenorhabditis*) and fly (*Drosophila*), based on mutant effects. Adapted from graphs and information in (Gerisch, 2004; Hertweck, 2004; Kurz and Tan, 2004; Libina et al, 2003; Mak and Ruvkun, 2004). Note that most of these predicted pathways are based on mutant effects and the orthologous proteins have not been isolated and analyzed biochemically. Both fly and worm have insulin-like peptides which activate insulin-receptors with ensuing kinase cascades and downstream effects on transcription. These pathways are known in more detail for worm than fly. The TGF-β pathway in worm (DAF-7 peptide) converges with insulin signaling and sterols at DAF-12. The fly orthologue of TGF-β is the Dpp peptide in fly, which interacts with the Rel pathway during early development. Because Rel/NfKB homologues are major transcriptional regulators of immune genes in the fly, it is plausible to consider Dpp-Rel interactions in adult immunity and aging. The GATA transcription factor (not shown here) regulated the expression of anti-microbial peptide genes independently of the Toll system (Senger et al, 2006).

the transcription factor DAF-16 translocates to the cell nucleus to modulate genes that are hypothesized to enhance longevity by increasing stress resistance (Morley and Morimoto, 2004). The phosphorylation of DAF-16 inhibits its translocation to the nucleus, e.g., in loss of function mutant AKT-1 kinases. Mutants impairing DAF-

16 activation are shorter-lived. DAF-16 nuclear translocation is highly sensitive to a narrow range of phosphorylation so that genetic defects can have widely different consequences ranging from extended longevity to developmental arrest (Imae et al, 2003). Other longevity mutants are found in the sirtuins, mTOR, and other gene systems that may serve as intra-cellular sensors of individual cell energy.

Despite this great progress, only one invertebrate insulin has been isolated and directly studied. An insulin cross-reacting peptide was semipurified from the brain of *Calliphora* (blowfly) and acted like vertebrate insulin in increasing glucose uptake in two assays: *in vitro* glucose uptake by rat fat cells and *in vivo* uptake from *Calliphora* hemolymph (Duve et al, 1979; Duve et al, 1982). Unexpectedly, in fly embryo cells, human insulin inhibited glucose uptake and glycogen synthesis but stimulated the pentose phosphate pathway (Ceddia et al, 2003). No worm insulin has been isolated and directly tested for functions. The mechanisms deduced for all the worm and fly longevity mutants by indirect evidence may be revised as the biochemistry becomes further developed.

Relationships among the ancient metabolic systems of insulins, sirtuins, and target of rapamycin (TOR) are outlined in Fig. 1.3A and Fig.3.9. Additionally, the AMP kinases (AMPK), the Per-Arnt-Sim protein domain kinases (PASK) and the hexosamine pathway could be involved because of their sensitivity to glucose and other nutrients. The yeast 'silent information regulator-2' ('sir-2') gene family (whence *sir-2–uins*) was recognized to repress the mating-type loci and extend the reproductive life span (Hekimi and Guarante, 2003). Sirtuins are NAD+-dependent deacetylases with many protein substrates (Blander and Guarante, 2004). The NAD-dependence couples sirtuin activity to cell nutritional status through the [NAD]/[NADH] ratio (Lin and Guarante, 2003). SIR2 increases chromatin condensation (heterochromatinization) by deacetylating local histones and interacting with proteins bound to 'silencer' DNA sequences (Blander and Guarante, 2004; Rusche et al, 2003). SIR2 is induced by resveratrol (a polyphenolic sirtuin activator and anti-oxidant) (Cohen et al, 2004; Longo and Kennedy, 2006). Resveratrol also shows anti-fungal activity, consistent with its presence in grapes (Jung et al, 2005; Sinclair, 2005), and is an immunosuppressant in transplantation experiments. Sirtuin activators are referred to as STACs.

SIR2 may have different roles in the longevity model of yeast aging (Section 1.2.6) (Longo and Kennedy, 2006). A current controversy concerns the role of SIR2 in the increase of yeast life span by diet restriction. SIR2 functions differ between the experimental yeast model (replicative senescence vs. aging; Section 1.2.5), which may be due to the different levels of media glucose used by the experimenters.

Human SIRT1 deacetylates histones and a remarkable range of key regulators, including ku70 and other mediators of apoptosis and DNA repair, the transcription factors FoxO[4] and p53, and even cytoskeletal α-tubulin (Blander and

---

[4]FoxO (forkhead) genes have alternate names: FoxO1, also FKHR; FoxO3, also FKHRL1; FoxO4, also AFX. FOXO is the mammalian forkhead orthologue of worm DAF-16.

Guarante, 2004; Borra et al, 2004). FoxOs regulate glucose metabolism and resistance to oxidative stress. FoxO is acetylated by CBP (cAMP response element-binding protein-binding protein) and deacetylated by SIRT1, which coactivates FoxO1 (Daitoku et al, 2004). The FoxOs respond to diet and insulin; e.g., fasting increased FoxO4 by 35% in muscle (Imae et al, 2003). FoxO3 and FoxO4 increased in muscle of aging rats (Furuyama et al, 2002).

TOR (target of rapamycin) acts as a nutrient sensor in mammalian and yeast cells (Gray et al, 2004; Long et al, 2004; Lorberg and Hall, 2004; Powers et al, 2006a; Proud, 2004). Rapamycin is a natural antifungal and immunosuppressing antibiotic. TOR nutrient sensing depends on its complex with RAPTOR (regulatory associated protein of TOR). Deficits of leucine or other amino acids activate TOR and in turn attenuate protein synthesis and metabolic quiescence. Rapamycin-treated cells appear starved. TOR kinase inhibits protein synthesis by phosphorylating the elongation factor (eEF2), which is activated by insulin. In flies, TOR signaling through elongation factor binding protein (4E-BP) also acts as a metabolic brake to control fat metabolism (Teleman et al, 2005). Unlike the fly, the worm *C. elegans* is insensitive to rapamycin. This insensitivity may be adaptive because rapamycin is produced by a soil bacterium *Streptomyces hygroscopicus* (Long et al, 2002).

5.4.2. Immunity and Metabolism

Innate immune defenses to infections are highly specialized and vary widely between phyla (Fig. 5.4) (Brennan and Anderson, 2004; Martinelli and Reichhart, 2005; Mylonakis and Aballay, 2005). Four key functions are involved in host defenses: (I) pathogen recognition; (II) activation of cell and systemic machinery to inactivate, isolate, or remove the pathogen; (III) activation of somatic repair processes; and (IV) mobilization of energy, as needed for acute or chronic responses. The ergonomics of host defense (Fig. 1.2B) has not received much attention in current molecular studies of invertebrate immunity. Many common pathogens are detected and bound by specialized pathogen receptor proteins that recognize 'pathogen associated molecular patterns' (PAMPS) (Section 1.3) (Medzhitov and Janeway, 2002). These complex interactions are represented in Fig. 5.4 as black triangles interacting with abstract pathogen receptors.

Nematode immunity is very different from that in insects. Lacking a pumped circulation, nematodes do not rapidly deploy the mobile phagocytes and anti-microbial proteins of insects and vertebrates. Nematode bacteriocidal agents are presumed but have not been described. Insect bacteriocidal mechanisms include induction of anti-microbial peptides, e.g., defensin, among more than 20 others with specificity for various bacteria and fungi (Table 5.2). Many of these peptide genes show increased expression during aging in flies (Landis et al, 2004; Pletcher

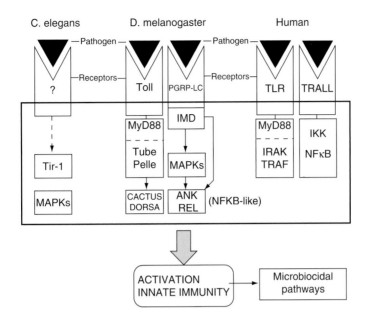

FIGURE 5.4 Elements of innate immunity, vastly oversimplified, representing *C. elegans, D. melanogaster* and human. Adapted from (Martinelli and Reichhart, 2005; Mylonakis and Aballay, 2005; Oda and Kitano, 2006). The pathogen ligands are represented as black triangles, which are bound by the membrane receptors on macrophages or other cells that are front-line defenses. The outlined box encompasses myriad signal transduction machinery that engages complex kinase inter-actions, e.g., MyD88 in the fly and mammals, but absent from worm. The output activates various microbicidal pathways that induce acute phase proteins, anti-microbial peptides, free radicals, phago-cytosis, and cell death. At least 10 regulatory layers can be conceptualized in mammals, with mod-ules that allow exquisite conditional regulation of immune output according to information on the physiological state: energy reserves, burden of tissue damage, and pathogen load. IKK, IκB kinase; Imd, immune deficiency pathway; IRAK, interleukin 1 receptor-associated kinase; MAPK, mitogen-acti-vated protein kinase; MyD88, myeloid differentiation primary response gene 88, which recruits and activates IRAK and other kinases; NF-κB, nuclear factor κB, transcription factor that regulates many immune system genes; Pelle, kinase with roles in embryogenesis and adult immunity; PGRP-LC, pep-tidoglycan recognition proteins; Tir-1, Toll/interleukin-1 resistance domain protein (*C. elegans*) and orthologue of human SARM; TLR, Toll-like receptors (11 in mammals), which bind diverse pathogenic ligands; *TRAF*, tumor necrosis factor receptor-associated factor; Tube, an adaptor protein downstream of Toll, recruits MyD88 and Pelle (kinase).

TABLE 5.2 Host-Defense Genes with Increased Expression[a] in Aging *Drosophila*

Agent	Activity[a]
attacin	anti-bacterial, Gram-negative[b,c]
cecropins	anti-bacterial, Gram-negative[c]
defensin	anti-bacterial, Gram positive[b,c]
diptericin	anti-bacterial, Gram-negative[d]
drosocin	anti-bacterial, Gram-negative[b]
drosomycin	anti-bacterial, Gram neg. and pos.; anti-fungal[b]
Hsp70	in the endocytic complex; associated with Toll-like receptors[b]
metchnikowin	anti-bacterial, Gram-positive and anti-fungal[b]
Pgrp-lc, peptidoglycan recognition proteins	pathogen receptors for Gram-negative bacteria; activate Relish/imd pathways and phagocytosis; 13 genes and splice variants[c,d]
relish	NF-κB-like transcription factors required for induction of anti-microbial genes[c]
Toll receptors	signal transduction downstream of pathogen receptors (Pgrp-1); mammalian orthologues bind microbial peptides, e.g., Toll-4 binding of LPS[c]

a. The relative size of age changes is generally not provided by the cited papers, due to the uncertainty in microarray analysis of background estimates. RNA blot images give the impression of many-fold increase during aging in whole body extracts. b. (Landis et al, 2004); c. (Pletcher et al, 2002); d. (Seroude et al, 2002).

et al, 2002) (Section 1.8, Fig. 1.24). These defenses are also integral to successful mating because pathogens are transmitted venereally in insects (Khurad et al, 2004). Seminal fluid also contains anti-microbial peptides that protect from venereal infections. The sex-peptide of male *Drosophila* seminal fluid rapidly induces defensins and other peptides that are at low levels in virgin female flies (Peng et al, 2005a). In male flies, sexual activity decreased the clearance of pathogenic *E. coli* in proportion to the frequency of female contacts, suggesting trade-offs for reproduction at the expense of life expectancy (McKean and Numey, 2001).

The pathogen receptor machinery differs between fly, worm, and human, but does share some elements of subcellular signaling machinery (Fig. 5.4). The insect immunity gene responses employ transcription factor binding sites resembling those of vertebrate immunity, including GATA srp-like, NF-κB/Rel-like, and Stat (Wertheim et al, 2005). The ancient Toll receptors are widely used core regulators of immune responses. Toll activation in flies induces numerous host defenses, including genes encoding anti-microbial peptides (Table 5.2) and gene mediating phagocytosis, hemolymph coagulation, and production of free radicals used for cell signaling and cytotoxicity. In fly embryos, the Toll pathway is critical to establishing the embryonic dorsoventral axis. I suggest that the employment of Toll in early development may also activate host defense genes to protect the energy-rich larvae.

Toll-like receptors (TLRs) differ widely between phyla. In mammals, TLR4 directly binds LPS endotoxin, whereas the fly primary pathogen receptors are the peptidoglycan recognition proteins (PGRPs) and Toll is downstream. In the worm, the only Toll-like receptor (TOL-1) is not on a known pathogen-stimulated signaling pathway. While TOL-1 deletion did not alter resistance to pathogenic bacteria, TOL-1 deletion did slightly shorten life span of worms fed on the mildly pathogenic *E. coli* OP50 strain (Kim and Ausubel, 2005). The worm also lacks NF-κB-like transcription factors and the MyD88 effector but does share with flies and mammals the PMK-1 (p38 mitogen-activated protein kinase) in its immune circuits.

Kim and Ausuble (2005) propose that the ancestral metazoan immune signaling system was a PMK-1/p38 element that interacts with TIR-1/SARM, another immune element of arthropods, nematodes, and the vertebrates. From a genomic perspective, the conserved PMK signaling elements in immune circuits are a regulatory 'kernel' of ancient signaling functions in host defenses for 600 million years or more (Davidson, 2006; Davidson and Erwin, 2006). It would not be surprising if other nematodes had different roles of Toll-like receptors and employed NF-κB and MyD88.

Heat shock-induced proteins (HSPs), which increase resistance to oxidation and other stress, are also active in host defense through chaperoning of phagocytosed pathogens. In mammals, HSP chaperone functions extend to anti-bacterial host defense mechanisms for HSP70, which is part of a complex of proteins that interact with the Toll-receptors that remove bacterial fragments by endocytosis (TLR2, gram-positive bacteria; TLR4, gram-negative bacteria) (Asea, 2003; Triantafilou and Triantafilou, 2003). HSP-TLR interactions have not been shown in flies or worms. Because temperature (behavioral fever) is used as a host defense to inhibit microbial infections in insects (Blanford and Thomas, 1999), as in vertebrates, HSP responses may be protective for fever-induced protein denaturation.

Energy reserves are fundamental to immunity. Host defenses are usually energy demanding and require rapid and possibly long-term mobilization (Section 1.3.3). Energy allocation during host defense may trade off short-term survival at the expense of growth (Fig. 1.2B and Section 4.6). At a cell level, macrophage production of superoxide is dependent on glucose transport and oxidation (Kiyotaki et al, 1984), and activation of macrophages induces glucose transporters and increases glucose and fructose transport (Malide et al, 1998). At the physiological level, diet restriction (DR) attenuates NF-κB dependent gene expression changes, which are widely used in host defense (Pletcher et al, 2002). In mammals, DR has anti-inflammatory effects, and moreover, can impair instructive immunity and decrease resistance to infections (Section 3.2.4). Leptin, which is secreted by adipocytes as a metabolic hormone and regulator of feeding behavior, is also major immunoregulator (Section 1.3.3), e.g., mice starved to impair immune responses to *Streptococcus* (Klebsiella) had rapid immune restoration by leptin injection (Mancuso et al, 2006).

Immune and fat cells may be ancient partners. Fat depots accumulate macrophages, which may be a source of the increased plasma CRP and IL-6 associated with obesity (Chapters 1 and 4). Specialized adipocytes in lymph nodes are resistant to starvation and may supply the follicular dendritic cells of instructive immunity with fatty acids (Pond, 2005). Moreover, the insect fat body is the major site of anti-microbial peptide production and secretion (Brennan and Anderson, 2004; Mylonakis and Aballay, 2005). Connections of immunity through MAPK signaling in lipolysis (Carmen and Victor, 2005) may be integrated in inflammatory responses to produce the energy need for biosynthesis and fever. TNFα-induced lipolysis, for example, involves MAPK activation (Souza et al, 2003). Insect fat body oenocytes may also be connected to immunity.

Trade-offs from energy allocation to immune functions are well known in human growth (Fig. 1.2B; Chapter 4). Many invertebrates also show these trade-offs by reduction in fecundity and lifespan, when anti-microbial defenses are activated (Zerofsky et al, 2005). Overexpression of the pathogen receptor protein PGRP (Fig. 5.4) in the fat body shortened life span of both sexes by about 20% (Libert et al, 2007). PRGP overexpression also increased anti-microbial peptide levels and resistance to pathogenic bacteria. In young flies, the induction of antimicrobial peptides by heat-killed bacteria also decreased egg production. This may be attributed to decreased yolk protein synthesis from resource re-allocation for synthesis of antimicrobial peptides, which may reach 5 μg/ml in the haemolymph. The *relish* fly mutant, which lacks the NF-κB required for induction of genes encoding antimicrobial peptides, maintained egg production during immune stimulation (Kim et al, 2001). Fly larva are vulnerable to wasp 'parasitoid' infections. Eggs laid by wasps inside larvae are encapsulated and killed by blood haemocytes. Selection for wasp resistance increased the density of circulating hemocytes in adult flies, which can attack the parasite eggs (Kraaijeveld et al, 2001). However, resistant lines had poorer survival during diet restriction (competition for food), suggesting a trade-off for host defense (Kraaijeveld and Godfray, 1997). Parasitoid-resistance was also indirectly selected by rearing in crowded conditions (Sanders et al, 2005). High larval density limits food (density-dependent diet restriction), but also increases exposure to excreta.

Social insects show further complexities in trade-offs with immunity that come from their coexistence with a complex microbial biome (Evans and Armstrong, 2006; Evans and Pettis, 2005). The hive is a constant target of invasive colonization by bacteria and fungi by its warmth and nutrients. The cost of immune response to colonies infected by the 'foulbrood' *Paenibacillus* was indicated by reduced larval production in proportion to the induction of the antibacterial gene abaecin (Evans, 2004). As another example, immune activation of worker bees by endotoxin (LPS) shortened life span 50% if bees were starved, but had little effect with well-fed bees (Moret and Schmid-Hempel, 2000). Long-lived queens are fed royal jelly, which is the major nutrient source needed for yolk production. The royal jelly includes the defensin-like royalisin among its 'swarm' of antimicrobial peptides (Fontana et al, 2004).

Vitellogenin in the hemolymph is also associated with immunity. In worker bees, hemolymph vitellogenin co-varies with the number of the phagocytic hemocytes and resistance to oxidant stress (Amdam and Omhott, 2002; Amdam et al, 2004). Oxidative protein damage varied inversely with levels of vitellogenin, whether constitutive or manipulated (Seehuus et al, 2006). Major changes in immunity arise during foraging activities when mortality is accelerated due to environmental hazards and possibly from increased bacterial load (Amdam et al, 2005). During foraging, vitellogenin and hemocytes decrease sharply. These major changes are reversed by forcing workers to revert to hive tasks. This striking finding suggests that in the high-energy demanding phase of foraging, immunity is suppressed as a life history trade-off. Again, we see the critical role of energy reserves in trade-offs of host defense and longevity. A worm experiment described below also suggests a cost for vitellogenin production.

The antioxidant activity of vitellogenin may be mediated by an SOD-like domain with homology to bovine Cu/Zn SOD (Tokishita et al, 2006). Vitellogenins and the vertebrate apolipoproteins belong to an ancient class of large lipid transfer proteins (LLTP) that branched prior to the divergence of protostomes (nematode-insect lineage) and deuterostomes (chordate lineage) (Babin et al, 1999). There may be shared mechanisms of lipoproteins in the interactions of immune and vascular functions with longevity.

5.5. THE WORM

5.5.1. Overview

In the lab worm *Caenorhabditis elegans*, cell aging changes are less characterized than those of development (Section 1.2.4). During its relatively long postreproductive phase, feeding and movement gradually slow, and mortality rates accelerate. Wads of partially digested bacteria accumulate in the pharynx and gut (Section 2.3.2, Fig. 2.5C) (Herndon et al, 2002). Bacterial clouds that form around body orifices of aging worms suggest a weakening of anti-microbial defenses (Vanfleteren, 1998). Many anti-microbial genes are also induced. When food is limited during development, worms may arrest in non-feeding larval stages (*dauer* larvae) that also extend life span. Diet restriction (DR) by strongly decreasing the titer of bacterial food increases adult worm life span by up to 60% (Houthoofd, 2006; Klass, 1977). DR worms are thin and less fecund. The longest life spans are achieved by growth on liquid axenic culture, which causes a thin DR-like appearance. Axenic cultured worms are more resistant to stress and temperature and have higher catalase and SOD activities that resemble responses to DR (Houthoofd et al, 2002).

Age-1, the first gerontogene identified on a chromosome, increased life span by about 50%, together with delayed slowing of movements and slower acceleration of mortality (Gompertz slope) (Johnson, 1990). *age-1* and other mutants that cause obligatory dauer larval arrest also have longer adult phases. Although the chromosomes that carried *age-1* and other mutants were identified, these strong genetic effects on longevity were skeptically received. Until recently, many doubted that single mutations could cause much increase in life span by actually slowing aging, because of assumptions that aging results from complex interactions among numerous genes (Johnson, 2005). The strength of these single gene effects on longevity may depend on the highly protected lab conditions.

Mutants in more than 50 genes are known to modify *C. elegans* life span (Hekimi and Guarente, 2003; Lee et al, 2003; Olsen et al, 2006). Many of the mutants alter the basic dyad of metabolism and innate immunity. Many of these genes are shared in eukaryotic aerobic organisms, whether single-celled or multi-cellular tissue grade (Barbieri et al, 2003; Gems and Partridge, 2001; Finch and Ruvkun, 2001; Kenyon, 2001; Lee et al, 2003; Longo and Finch, 2003; Tatar et al, 2003). Several neuroendocrine pathways with vertebrate orthologues influence worm life spans: 'insulin/insulin-like growth factor (IGF-like)'(metabolism), TOR pathway (nutrient sensing); and 'TGF-β-like' (inflammation). These pathways are associated with transduction of sensory signals that can induce dauer larval stages and converge on the orphan nuclear receptor DAF-12, which binds steroid-like ligands (Fig. 5.3) (Motola et al, 2006), discussed further below. This convergence of insulin and TOR in regulating both the dauer state and life span implies deep links between metabolism, host defense, and life span. The TGF-β-like pathway could join insulin and TOR in regulating aging processes through its role in innate immunity (Kurz, 2004; Nicholas and Hodgkin, 2004).

Several concerns are noted. The interpretation of the mutant effects is largely based on sequence similarity to mammalian genes, and the biochemistry and physiology of these pathways is not directly known. Moreover, the lab diet *E. coli* OP50, a mammalian enterobacteria, may be a confound (Section 2.3.2) (Garigan et al, 2002; Lithgow, 2003). *E. coli* strain OP50 as a food shortens life span, relative to a diet of heat-killed bacteria (Garsin et al, 2003; Mallo et al, 2002), or culture on liquid media (Houthoofd et al, 2002). Some long-lived mutants are resistant to the mild toxicity of *E. coli* OP50, as discussed below. Some consider that *E. coli* is not an optimal food and should be considered 'mildly toxic' (Section 2.3.2). However, these toxic effects do not emerge until later ages. In humans, chronic infections cause oxidative stress with mitochondrial dysfunctions, e.g., in blood leukocytes and myocardium during trypanosome infections (Chagas' disease) (Wen et al, 2006). It will be important to resolve whether the toxicity of *E. coli* OP50 is restricted to later ages because such an effect might interact with the other bacterial pathogens being studied (Scott Pletcher, pers. comm.). Given the intense artificiality of lab models, with 'wild-type' strains selected for rapid maturation and high fecundity than in the real wild-type of wild-caught mice (Section 2.3), it seems to me that delayed effects of lab diets on aging processes and life span are an important concern in experimental design and interpretation of mutant effects.

5.5.2. Slower Eating Increases Life Span

Induced mutants that increased life span in association with reduced food intake were the first stage that launched the genetics of worm aging and longevity (Klass, 1983). The initial five long-lived mutants had slower pharyngeal pumping as young adults and decreased food ingestion inversely to life span (r, 0.97). These same mutants were later studied by Friedman and Johnson (1988), who separated the *age-1* mutation from other mutations in the same strain that affected fertility (*fer-15*) and movement and pharyngeal pumping (*unc-52*). The *age* mutants also anticipated the *eat* mutants, which have reduced feeding rates in association with 30–50% longer lives (Lakowski and Hekimi, 1998). Mutants in more than 30 different genes have slower pharyngeal pumping due to various defects in pharyngeal development. Their 'starved' look with thin bodies and pale intestines resembles effects of diet restriction (Avery, 1993). Both diet restriction and the *eat-2* mutant elevate catalase and SOD and increase stress resistance (Houthoofd et al, 2002). Individual worms also differ in pharyngeal pumping, noted earlier. I suggest that the decreased food ingestion from slower pharyngeal pumping causes the equivalent of diet restriction and increases life span, as in the *eat* mutants. The spontaneous developmental variations in worms may be considered as individual phenocopies of pharyngeal mutants that increase life span.

5.5.3. Metabolism and Host Defense

A *daf-2* mutation that doubles the life span impairs an insulin-receptor-like protein, as discovered by Ruvkun (Kimura et al, 1997).[5] The year before, *age-1* was identified as orthologous to a phosphatidylinositol-3OH kinase (PI-3 kinase). In the mammalian insulin system (Fig. 1.3A,B), PI-3 kinase is downstream of a membrane-bound insulin receptor (Morris et al, 1996). These discoveries extended Kenyon's finding that *age-1* and *daf-2* share a pathway in modulating life span (Dorman et al, 1995). Both mutants increase resistance to oxidative stress and heat (thermotolerance), as do many of the other longevity ('gerontogene') mutants (Johnson et al, 2001a).

The nuclear receptor DAF-16 is downstream of membrane receptors in the insulin-signaling pathway (Fig. 5.3 and Fig. 1.3). When food is abundant, DAF-16 is not active as a gene regulator but can rapidly move to the nucleus during starvation, heat stress, and oxidative stress (Henderson and Johnson, 2001). DAF-16 regulates a remarkable array of genes that influence resistance to stress and to infections, which are constitutively induced in *age-1* and *daf-2* (Kenyon, 2005; Murphy et al, 2003) (Fig. 5.3). The insulin-like signaling system appears to

---

[5]The *age-1* and *daf-2* mutants are considered 'hypomorphic' or weak, in the old genetic terminology. In biochemical terms, these alleles reduce the activity of the encoded enzyme but do not eliminate it, as in knockout mutations.

serve as a major switch to increase stress resistance and immunity. *age-1* and *daf-2* are resistant to gram-negative pathogens more virulent than *E. coli* OP50[6] (Garsin et al, 2003). Moreover, the bacterial constipation of aging is delayed in *age-1* and *daf-2* (Garigan et al, 2002). When grown on *Bacillus subtilis*, a soil bacterium that may be a natural food, the *age-1*, *daf-2*, and background strain lived longer than on *E. coli* OP50. *daf-2* mutants have increased expression of genes encoding anti-bacterial lysozymes expressed in the intestine, saposin, and other host defenses (Kurz and Tan, 2004). An anti-fungal-like gene (thaumatin-related, F28D1.5) that increases 3-fold during aging has a delayed increase in the longer-lived *daf-2* (Golden and Melov, 2004). This delay in association with delayed constipation suggests the bolus of food may increase pathogen growth. Repression of several of these host defense genes with RNAi shortened the life span of *daf-2* mutants (Murphy et al, 2003). *daf-16* mutants did not alter the longevity effect of axenic media (without living organisms), implying that diet restriction may be insulin-independent (Houthoofd et al, 2003).

DAF-16 also represses vitellogenin expression, suggesting a trade-off of energy required for host defense at the expense of reproduction. This hypothesis is consistent with the reduction of early egg laying when DAF-2 was lowered in wildtype by RNAi; early egg production is considered a critical fitness trait (Jenkins et al, 2004). Worker honey bees also show trade-offs in vitellogenin expression, which is suppressed with other immune functions during the high mortality phase of foraging (Section 5.4.2).

Genes regulated by *daf-2* influence adult fat stores, metabolic rate, ROS production, and repair of oxidative damage (Finch and Ruvkun, 2001; Tatar et al, 2003). Worms expressing weak *daf-2* alleles accumulate fat deposits not seen in adults (Kimura et al, 1997). Dauer larvae, moreover, normally accumulate fat. In humans, morbid obesity results from an equivalent insulin receptor mutation (Kim et al, 1992; Kimura et al, 1997). The increase of life span in *daf-2* ('gain of function mutation') has parallels to diet restriction (Klass, 1983) (Chapter 3).

These insulin-signaling effects may be neuronally mediated. Cell-targeted expression of *daf-2* increased life span when expression was limited to specific neurons (Wolkow et al, 2000). Sensory neurons that mediate feeding (gustatory and olfactory) are implicated in nematode aging, with links to insulin-like pathways (Alcedo and Kenyon, 2004). Pre-synaptically active anti-convulsant drugs (ethosuximide) also extended life span, with delayed slowing of pharyngeal pumping and body movements (Evason et al, 2005; Kornfeld and Evason, 2006). Presynaptic actions are hypothesized to involve insulin-signaling in sensory neurons.

---

[6]Human bacterial pathogens also kill *C. elegans* in processes that are sensitive to many of the same bacterial virulence factors (Garsin et al, 2003) and that share the p38 MAPK pathway (Kim and Ausubel, 2005). Pathogenic species include Gram-negative *Psuedomonas aeruginosa* and *Salmonella enterica* and Gram-positive *Enterococcus faecalis* and *Staphylococcus aureus*.

Longevity influences of insulin-like genes are linked to gonadal activity. Germ cell ablation by genetic manipulations increased life span by 60%, without apparent cost to vigor (Fig. 5.5A, B) (Hsin and Kenyon, 1999). In the long-lived *daf-2* mutants, germ-line ablation further increased the life span up to 4-fold longer than intact wild-type, some remaining active 4 months (Fig. 5.5C). In the *daf-12* mutant, however, germ-cell ablation did not increase life span (not shown in this figure), implying a role for a nuclear receptor coupled to insulin-like signaling. Similar responses to gonadectomy were seen in *Pristionchus pacificus*, from another nematode family that may be 100 million years divergent. These results suggest basic interactions between germ cells and aging processes in nematodes that involve insulin-like pathways.

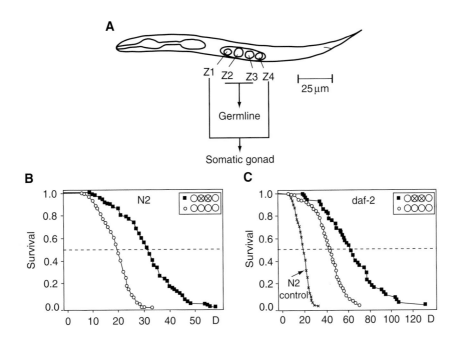

FIGURE 5.5 Germ cell ablation increases worm lifespan. (Adapted from Hsin and Kenyon, 1999.) A. Four cells comprise the gonad: the somatic gonad is formed from Z1 and Z4, germ line from Z2 and Z3. B. Survival of N2 ('wildtype') is increased by selective ablation of germ-line cells Z2 and Z3. If all germ line and somatic gonad cells are ablated, life span is not increased (not graphed). C. Survival of *daf-2* is increased by germ cell line ablation 4-fold. Unlike the wildtype, total gonadal ablation further increased life span (not graphed).

A TGF-β-like pathway may operate in parallel to DAF-2 for control of reproductive development by environmental cues (Gerisch and Antebi, 2004; Jia et al, 2002; Mak and Ruvkun, 2004) (Fig. 5.3). The vertebrate TGF-β peptides are major modulators of inflammation (Section 1.4). *daf-7* encodes a TGF-β-like ligand; *daf-4*, a type-II TGF-β receptor; *daf-9* influences DAF-2 expression in some tissues. *daf-12* encodes a transcription factor resembling the vitamin D- and androstane receptors of vertebrates (Antebi et al, 2000), which have major roles in the inflammatory responses, and binds steroid-like ligands, as noted above (Motola et al, 2006). DAF-9 and DAF-36 may produce lipophilic sterol-like ligands for DAF-12. P450 enzymes in flies and mammals have similarity to DAF-12, while DAF-36 resembles vertebrate ring-hydroxylating oxygenases (Gerisch et al, 2001; Rottiers et al, 2006). The TGF-β orthologue (DB-1) regulates anti-microbial defenses in intestinal cells, e.g., lectin-binding proteins and lysozymes, which are induced by the bacterial pathogen *Serratia marcescens* (Mallo et al, 2002). *dbl-1* mutants were highly vulnerable to *S. marcescens* and, correspondingly, lived much longer on heat-killed than live *E. coli* 50. *daf-9* appears to integrate the insulin-like and TGF-β-like pathways (Gerisch and Antebi, 2004; Mak and Ruvkun, 2004). *daf-9* and *daf-12* show reciprocal feedback interactions mediated by a DAF-12 response element (Gerisch and Antebi, 2004; Mak and Ruvkun, 2004).

Heat shock factors (HSF) have important roles in stress responses that modify aging and that interact with insulin-like pathways. DAF-16 and heat shock proteins mediate a remarkable phenomenon in which sublethal heat treatments of young worms increase thermotolerance *and* increase longevity, the 'hormesis' effect of stress (Cypser and Johnson, 2003). Dauer-defective mutants *daf-16* and other block this effect. The transcription factor, HSF-1, regulates more than 60 heat shock genes in many tissues and also acts downstream in the *daf-2* pathway. Life span was increased 40% by additional copies of *hsf-1*, while inactivation of *hsf-1* by RNAi reversed the longevity of insulin-like signaling mutants and shortened life span (Hsu et al, 2003). Bacterial constipation occured earlier after inactivating *hsf-1* (Garigan et al, 2002). Life extension in *daf-16* mutants also depended on an active *hsf-1* gene. HSF-1 may sit high in a gene network hierarchy, because there are more modest effects on life span of inactivating HSP-16 and other individual HSFs that are regulated by *hsf-1* (Morley and Morimoto, 2004). The spontaneous variations in HSP-16 levels which are associated with up to 4-fold differences in individual worm life spans (Section 1.2) (Rea et al, 2005) could be driven by spontaneous variations in *hsf-1* that may arise during development, possibly like the variations in pharyngeal pumping noted above.

The fly intestine shows convergence of insulin-signaling, immunity, and reproduction. Infection with the pathogenic bacterium *Serratia marcescens*, which caused degeneration of the intestinal epithelium, also decreased egg laying (Mallo et al, 2002). Increased longevity from *daf-9*, which integrates insulin-like and TGF-β-like pathways, required DAF-9 expression in the intestine, while expression in neurons had minor effect (opposite to *daf-2*). Similarly, *daf-16* expression in the intestine increased life span more than in neurons or muscle (Libina et al, 2003). Moreover, resistance to the bacterial pathogen *Pseudomonas aerogunosa* depends on intestinal cell expression of SMK-1, a transcription co-regulatory factor of DAF-16 (Wolff et al, 2006). Deletion of *smk-1* also suppressed the resistance of *daf-2* mutants to *P. aeruginosa*. In addition, intestinal cells detect and discriminate enteric pathogens though Toll proteins of host defense (Kim and Ausubel, 2005; Pujol et al, 2001). The act of ingestion in nematodes, as all other organisms, is closely tied to anti-microbial defenses. The link of infection to aging is also supported by the earlier onset of bacterial constipation and shorter life span of worms with lower *hsp-1* expression, discussed above.

The TOR metabolic pathway influences life span. Worms with CeTOR deficiency (*let363* mutant) increased life span 2-fold, as in *daf-2* mutants (Vellai et al, 2003). CeTOR deficiency impairs digestion, with some bacteria in the intestinal lumen remaining intact (Long et al, 2002). Gut cells atrophy and fill with lyso-some-derived vesicles. The ceTOR deficient phenotype is also produced by inhibiting translation initiation factors (eIF-4G, eIF-2), which mediate translation arrest by mammalian TOR. Insulin- and TOR nutrient signaling converge at DAF-15 (RAPTOR) (Fig. 5.3), suggesting a role of TOR signaling in diet restriction (Jia, 2004). Deficiencies of DAF-15 increased life span (Jia et al, 2004). The LET363 and DAF15 deficits caused extensive fat deposits, like *daf-2* mutants. TOR also interacts with the sirtuins (Fig. 5.3). The sirtuin activator resveratrol increased life span by about 20%, but did not alter feeding rates or fecundity (Wood et al, 2004). This effect was observed on diets of live or heat-killed bacteria, suggesting that impaired immunity was not involved. Recall that resveratrol has anti-fungal activities. The absence of resveratrol influence on feeding rates argues against a diet restriction-like mechanism.

These remarkable manipulations of life span are observed under highly protected lab conditions. However, long-lived mutant worms are less robust under more natural conditions than agar plates. When grown on natural soil, the survival of the mutant *daf-2* (e1368) was 65% less than wildtype, even if the soil was sterilized and *E. coli* added back (Van Voorhies et al, 2005). Nor would we expect long-lived dwarf mice to survive in the wild.

5.6. FLY

5.6.1. Overview

Drosophila melanogaster life spans are also increased by hypofunctional genes of insulin-like pathways (Fig. 1.3A and Fig. 5.3). Infections and host defense responses are evident during aging. Like worms, wild-type flies do not develop tumors during aging. However, aging flies develop myocardial instability, a dysfunction categorically absent from nematodes. Longevity is increased in weak mutants of *inr*, the single insulin receptor (Tatar et al, 2001), and of *chico* (Clancy et al, 2001), a protein which binds to the insulin-like receptor. Longevity is nearly doubled on some genetic backgrounds, with greater increase in females than males. The *inr* and *chico* mutants are both small, accumulate fat, and have reduced or delayed fecundity. These characteristics recur in dwarf mice through mutations in the insulin/IGF-1 signaling pathway (Fig. 1.3A). Development influences of insulin-like signaling on cell size and cell number are well known, e.g., through mutants of insulin receptor substrates CHICO, PI3K, and the tumor suppressor PTEN, a phosphatase that inhibits PI3K. Some *inr* mutants had slower accelerations of mortality during aging (Tu et al, 2002a) (Section 5.7).

5.6.2. Metabolism and Diet Restriction

Like the worm *C. elegans,* fly longevity is strongly influenced by neurosecretions. The median neurosecretory cells (mNSC), a cluster of seven neurons in the head, secrete drosophila insulins (*dilp 2, -3, -5)* into the circulation (Broughton et al, 2005). Genetic ablation of the mNSCs reduced fecundity and increased life span through reduced initial mortality (IMR) and delayed mortality accelerations, which had similar Gompertz slopes. Resistance to oxidative stress (paraquat) was also increased, but thermal sensitivity was not. Neuron ablated flies had 2-fold higher fasting blood glucose, consistent with a role of humoral insulin in glucose uptake. Targeted expression of dFOXO to the pericerebral fat body selectively lowered neuronal expression of *dilp-2* and increased life span and oxidative stress resistance (Hwangbo et al, 2004). Lipids were increased in the head and abdominal fat body. These findings are broadly consistent with life span extension through deficient insulin-like signaling in *ins* and *chico* mutants. Nutrient regulation of *dilp* transcription (Ikeya et al, 2002) could mediate effects of diet on life span, discussed below.

Insulin also interacts with other major hormones that regulate development and reproduction. Neurosecretory cells expressing *dilp-3* and *-5* project to the ring gland, which synthesizes ecdysone and juvenile hormone (JH), a lipid-like hormone. Ecdysone, a steroid-like hormone, regulates egg yolk production by the fat body (Truman and Riddiford, 2002; Tu et al, 2002b). *Inr* mutants have impaired ecdysone production and lower fecundity (Tu et al, 2002a). Mutants with impaired ecdysone synthesis or ecdysone receptors (*EcR*) lived longer, but without impaired fertility (Simon et al, 2003). The *inr* and *chico* mutants are also deficient in JH, which has powerful effects on development and aging that epitomize hormonal pleiotropy (Finch and Rose, 1995). Restoration of JH with methoprene attenuated the long life spans of *inr* and JH-deficient flies (Flatt et al, 2005; Tatar, 2001). JH also suppresses innate immunity and stress resistance, and may be a proximal mediator of trade-offs in insect life history.

TOR modulates insulin signaling via PI3K (Colombani et al, 2003). Inhibition of TOR activity in the fat body sufficed to increase life span (Kapahi et al, 2004). Similarly, life span was increased by manipulations of tuberous sclerosis complex genes (*Tsc1* or *Tsc2*), which directly modulate TOR, and the S6 kinase, which mediates downstream effects of TOR on translation initiation. The sirtuin gene system also influences life span (Wood et al, 2004). Resveratrol and other sirtuin activators (STACS) increased life span about 25% (see above). Egg production was slightly increased and body weight was not changed, which indicates maintained feeding. During diet restriction (DR), resveratrol did not further increase longevity, indicating a shared pathway. As in worms, the longevity effects of STACs depend on *Sir2* functions. Sir2 deficiency blocked the effects of DR on increasing life span (Rogina and Helfand, 2004).

An unexpected connection has emerged of Sir2 to p53, which is a powerful tumor suppressor in mammals. The fly homologue Dmp53 was known to regulate apoptosis during development. While p53 null flies had shorter life span, the targeted reduction of p53 in neurons increased life span by about 50% (Bauer and Helfand, 2006). DR, however, did not increase life span in neuron-targeted Dmp53 deleted flies, linking p53 to metabolism in flies as in mammals (see next section). As noted above, Sir2 deacetylase acts on p53. Cell ratios of [NAD]/[NADH] can regulate the activity of sirtuins, which couple deacetylation to NAD hydrolysis. Because mammalian p53 expression increases in some infections, e.g., *H. pylori* in association with gastric mucosa proliferation (Kodama et al, 2005), the microbial load of aging flies may be a factor in the effects of Dmp53 on life span.

Is there overlap or convergence of mechanisms in diet restriction (DR) and insulin hypofunctional mutants? In wildtype, DR reduced the 'short-term' mortality risk[7] when imposed at any adult age, but did not alter mortality acceleration (Mair et al, 2003). Life spans were compared for responses to a range of food 'doses' in a dilution series (Fig. 5.6A) (Clancy et al, 2002). The food dose response of *chico* relative to wildtype was right-shifted, with greater sensitivity to food deficits as starvation was approached, suggesting that *chico* mutants are already partly diet restricted. *chico* increased life span beyond the wildtype maximum, but at a higher concentration (0.9x food) than the wildtype (0.65x). Wildtype males responded differently than females (Fig. 5.6B) (Magwere et al, 2004) with much smaller increase of life span and no clear food optimum. DR delayed the Gompertz mortality acceleration in females. This study is exemplary in analyzing the full food dose response that shows overlapping responses of insulin-signaling mutants. The greater response of females to food dose is consistent with nutrient needs for egg production. The different male physiology could involve insulin-like systems that modulate trade-offs in reproduction and longevity (Finch and Rose, 1995; Mair et al, 2003; Mair et al, 2004; Rauser et al, 2004). However, the trade-off hypothesis remains to be rigorously tested by blocking specific male and female traits. Direct measurement of nutrient consumption is needed because it influences feeding behavior (Carvalho et al, 2005; Min and Tatar, 2006).

---

[7]Background mortality estimate, approximating the Gompertz-Makeham term, Table 5.1.

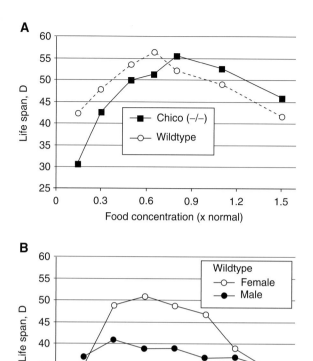

FIGURE 5.6 Nutrient caloric intake 'dose response' and life span in the lab fly. The units are relative to a standard yeast-sucrose media (1.0), adjusted with agar to the same consistency and moisture, and including antibiotics. (Redrawn from Magwere et al, 2004). A. Wildtype fly life span is decreased at low and high levels of food availability. The response of *chico* mutants (hypofunctional insulin system) was right-shifted, with shorter life spans at very low food, relative to the control, and longer life spans at higher food. B. Sex differences of life span in response to food availability. Females responded more than males. The Gompertz mortality acceleration rate constant was relatively unchanged in both sexes, whereas females had lower baseline mortality at reduced caloric intake (not shown).

5.6.3. Heart

A major surprise is the demonstration of myocardial aging in the fly (Wessells et al, 2004), which becomes increasingly vulnerable to arrest during forced electrical pacing (Fig. 5.7). Resting heart rates also slow progressively. Males have a faster pulse as young adults but converge to the female rate at advanced ages. Both heart rate and vulnerability to stress arrest are attenuated by manipulating insulin-like genes that also influence life span. The slow-aging mutants *inr* and *chico* had faster heart rates and less pacing-induced arrest. Moreover, myocardial aging was slowed by cardiac-specific expression of extra dPTEN and dFOXO, both insulin-signaling inhibitors. Despite the improved function by cardiac targeted *inr* and *chico*, life span was not altered. However, genetic ablation of neurons expressing *dilp-2, -3,* and *-5* slowed heart deterioration and also increased maximum life span with delayed Gompertz mortality accelerations. Conversely, cardiac expression of an extra copy of the wildtype *inr* gene slowed heart rate and increased pacing instability in young flies. These findings show the importance of insulin-like signaling at a local level to myocardial aging through local cell expression.

Myocardial cell degenerative changes are consistent with the myocardial instability described above. Aging house fly (*Musca domestica*) myocardium has fragmented myofibrils, degenerating mitochondria with fewer cristae, and autophagic vacuoles (Sohal and Allison, 1971a,b). Flight muscle shows similar cytolytic changes and the formation of giant mitochondria (Sohal et al, 1972). In aging human myocardium, mitochondrial DNA deletions increase with age in the absence of ischemic damage (Corral-Debrinski et al, 1992) (Section 1.2.2). Returning to *D. melanogaster*, age-related increases in oxidant damage are furthered by flight activity (whole fly assay): lipid oxidation (malondialdehyde, TBARS) and protein oxidation (carboxymethyllysine, CML, and other glyco-oxidation products) (Magwere et al, 2006). The accumulation of these glyco-oxidation products in aging flies implicates a role of haemolymph glucose and other reducing sugars (Section 1.4.2), and the insulin-like neurosecretions that regulate their levels. The myocardial mitochondrial degeneration and biochemical oxidative changes are consistent with oxidative stress during aging, and with the protective effects of inhibiting insulin signaling, which increases resistance to oxidative stress. In humans, insulin signaling systems are also a major focus in human cardiovascular and myocardial pathology (Fig 1.3B, Section 1.6.5).

Insect lipoproteins have not been studied in relation to heart function, but this possibility is indicated for apolipoprotein D (apoD), which is a fat transporter (lipocalin) associated with HDL particles in mammalian blood and is also expressed in neurons. The fly orthologue of apoD increased life span 20% when overexpressed (Walker et al, 2006b) and decreased life span similarly when deleted (Sanchez et al, 2006). There were corresponding differences in resistance to oxidative stress and starvation. Deletion also increased lipid oxidation. In mammals, lipocalin-2 mediates bacterial clearance and interacts with Toll receptors. ApoD is also induced in Alzheimer disease and by neuronal injury.

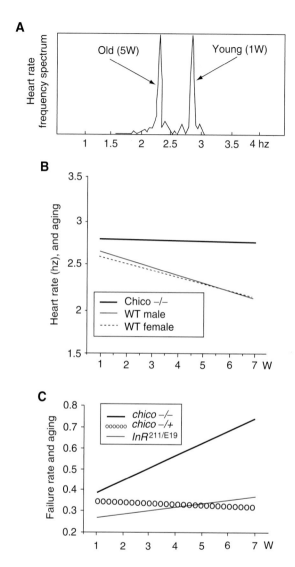

FIGURE 5.7 Heart functions in aging fly. (Redrawn from Wessells et al, 2004). A. Heart frequency spectrogram, showing shift to lower frequencies in flies aged 5 wk (senescent). B. Age slowing of the heart beat is progressive in males and females of the control strain (WT) C. Heart failure induced by fast external electrical pacing increases with aging in controls (WT), but long-lived mutants *chico* or insulin receptor (*inr*) did not show increased heart failure.

Ancient genomic mechanisms in heart development are worth pondering in relation to cardiac aging. In embryos of insects and vertebrates, the heart differentiates from bilateral precardiac mesodermal fields under the control of shared gene systems, including *HAND* (Han, 2006), *SMAD* (Euler-Taimor and Heger, 2006), *T-box* (Plageman and Yutzey, 2005), and *Wnt* (Eisenberg and Eisenberg, 2006). The shared ancestral lineage of flies (protostomes) and humans (deuterostomes) stems from a bilateran worm-alike ancestor 600 million or more years ago. From the current shared gene circuits in development, Davidson deduced its ancient regulatory 'kernel,' or core circuit in transcriptional regulation (Davidson, 2006, p. 219). The myocardial kernal uses TGF-β super-family ligands (Dpp/BMP) and a SMAD/TGF β class signal transduction factor to control orthologous regulatory genes (*Tin/Nkx2.5*) with autoregulatory feedback. These and other shared subcircuits have distinctive recursive loops that irreversibly lock down gene expression patterns during early development. Other interactions seen in vertebrates may be found in the fly heart, e.g., the cross-talk between TGF-β and IGF-1 in premyocardial cell proliferation (quail embryo) (Antin et al, 1996) and influences of IGF-1 on myocardial stem cells (human, rodent) (Chapter 1). The role of insulin signaling in both development and aging of the fly heart might have some shared circuit elements. There may also be a development-aging link through the links of TGF-β to host defense (Fig. 5.3). Embryos are vulnerable to bacterial infection and parasites (Section 5.4.2), and host defense gene systems may be important for successful development in the heart and other organs.

5.6.4. Infections, Host Defense, and Stress Resistance

Infections may influence aging in fly as well as worm.[8] Aging flies show large-scale induction of genes encoding anti-microbial peptides (Table 5.2) during aging (Section 1.8.2, Fig. 1.24) (Pletcher et al, 2002; Seroude et al, 2002) and extended by Tower (Landis et al, 2004) (Table 5.2). The increased anti-microbial gene expression progresses during the life span, up to 10-fold or more. Levels of drosomycin and metchnikowin varied inversely with remaining life span (Landis et al, 2004), which could reflect individual variations in endogenous pathogens. Immune impairments are shown by the slower clearance of *E. coli* infections in aging flies (Kim et al, 2001). The induction of anti-microbial peptides during aging supports the hypothesis (Chapter 2) that increased host defense activities during aging are caused, at least in part, by responses to invading pathogens.

Direct evidence partly confirms and partly negates these associations. The bacterial load of aging flies was recently shown to increase by several-fold (Ren et al, in prep.). As determined by culture and PCR assays of the body surface and interior,

---

[8]"[E]ssentially the same set of genes induced by infections was upregulated during aging . . . " (Landis et al, 2004). This " . . . suggests the intriguing possibility that infection is a primary cause of death in laboratory *Drosophila*" (Pletcher et al, 2002).

the fly microbiome includes two species each of *Acetobacter* and *Lactobacillus*, and *Staphylococcus hominus*. Elimination or reduction of the bacterial load by antibiotics or by axenic culture sharply decreased the induction of anti-microbial peptides during aging, consistent with their induction as a response to bacterial expansion. However, life span was not altered by eliminating the microbial load (Landis et al, 2004; Ren, *ibid*). Moreover in one experiment, elimination of gut bacteria appeared to shorten life span (details not given; T. Brummerl et al, cited in (DeVeale et al, 2004). Thus, in lab conditions, other aspects of aging are stronger determinants of mortality than the increasing microbial load. Nonetheless, in a special variant of *Wolbachia* infection, life span was increased by antibiotics. Many flies carry this rickettsial bacterium as a non-virulent intracellular symbiont, which is transmitted maternally and mediates reproductive isolation mechanisms, as discussed earlier, through male-specific mortality. The removal of *Wolbachia* generally decreases life span (Fry and Rand, 2002). However, one variant caused massive cell damage and life shortening, and in this special case, antibiotics restored normal life spans (Min and Benzer, 1997).

It may be possible with axenic models to resolve the role of oxidative stress to mortality in aging flies from the bacterial load. Recall from Chapter 1 that oxidative stress from growth in oxygen also induces anti-microbial peptide genes in young flies (Fig. 1.24) (Landis et al, 2004). The fly model should allow resolution of how oxidative stress stimulates inflammatory processes *independently* of pathogen caused oxidative damage (Query I, Section 1.1) and the role of inflammatory responses in oxidative bystander damage during aging (Query II).

Other stress-induced genes are also induced during aging, including heat shock proteins, one of which (HSP70) is associated with phagocytic complexes that remove microorganisms (see below). Metabolic genes are also induced that may increase energy availability. Aging flies have selective induction of genes for purine biosynthesis (all 12 genes in the pathway), whereas the genes of pyrimidine synthesis were not changed during aging (Landis et al, 2004). This distinction may be important, because purines are required for the primary energy substrates ATP and NAD(P)H. Both purines and pyrimidines are needed for DNA and RNA synthesis and for DNA repair. The selective induction of genes of purine synthesis suggests a resource allocation like the mammalian acute phase response to produce additional proteins and fever (see below).

Uric acid is another modulator of innate immunity and oxidant stress and is a powerful scavenger of oxygen and nitrogen ROS. In a sample of mammals, plasma uric acid correlated with life span (Cutler, 1984; Finch, 1990, p. 286). Deletion of xanthine dehydrogenase (XDH), which produces uric acid, shortened fly life span by about 20% (mean and maximum), with huge impairments in the clearance of *E. coli* infections (Kim et al, 2001). The importance of XDH to gut immune defenses is suggested by the higher ROS levels in the XDH mutant gut (+50%) relative to whole fly XDH (+15%).

Aging flies show strong increases in heat shock proteins (HSP), e.g., 10-fold induction of HSP22 and HSP70 mRNA and protein in the flight muscles and other tissues (King and Tower, 1999; Wheeler et al, 1995; Wheeler et al, 1999). As noted in Section 5.4.2, HSPs are mediators of host defense through chaperoning and clearance of phagocytosed pathogens. The major induction of HSPs during aging concurrently with anti-microbial genes (Table 5.2) suggests a coordinated host defense response to endogenous infections. Brief exposure to non-lethal heat increases life span by up to 5 d (Hercus et al, 2003; Khazaeli et al, 1997; Maynard Smith, 1958; Norry and Loeschke, 2003). HSPs have also been associated with longevity in outbred lines artificially selected for reproduction at later ages (Chapter 1, Fig. 1.12). HSP22 mRNA and protein were elevated up to 10-fold in the long-lived late-reproducing lines (Kurapati et al, 2000). The early- and late-reproducing lines also differed in allelic variants of two enzymes: phosphoglucomutase (Krebs cycle, Fig. 3.10) and SOD1. Resistance to starvation was also greater in late-reproducing flies (Leroi et al, 1994). The rapid shift in reproductive schedule and the Gompertz slope suggest that natural populations have gene variants under active selection for fluctuations in stress, from variations in nutrition, as discussed below.

Other host defenses may synergize with the HSPs and anti-microbial peptides. Bacterial infections induce secretion of the peptide TotA (encoded by *Turandot A*) by the abdominal fat body (Ekengren and Hultmark, 2001; Ekengren et al, 2001). While TotA has not shown antibacterial activity, its expression increases heat resistance. Anti-oxidant mechanisms also mediate host defense, to protect tissues from bystander damage from the ROS generated in response to pathogens (Section 1.3). Flies selected for long-life had elevated SOD and catalase at later ages and greater paraquat resistance (Dudas and Arking, 1995). The greater effect of SOD overexpression on shorter-lived lines is hard to interpret without data on histopathology and the microbial biome. Other complexities of SOD in fly aging are described by (Landis and Tower, 2005).

5.6.5. Natural Variations in Longevity Pathways

Drosophila species have natural variations involving genes described above for effects on longevity. Alleles of insulin-like genes are associated with geographic variation in body size. Flies in colder temperate zones are larger than in the tropics. When reared at the same temperature, temperate zone flies grow faster than the tropical (De Jong and Bochdanovits, 2003). Many populations have latitudinal clines in the frequencies of chromosomal inversions that contain gene of insulin-signaling and TOR pathways. Globally distributed ('cosmopolitan') inversions may carry haplotypes, or multiple alleles of different genes, that are co-adapted. Geographic clines are found in the co-variations among larval glycogen and adult weight. Temperate zone populations were proposed to be a 'thrifty' genotype with higher activities in insulin-signaling, leading to greater glycogen storage, which would be adaptive for survival during the winter and greater egg laying in cool spring climates, but with the trade-off of shorter adult longevity. Conversely, tropical populations have lower activity of the insulin pathway and reduced nutrient stores. The rapid responses of flies to selection for age at reproduction, discussed above, might involve these alleles in view of the delayed egg laying of long-lived insulin signaling deficient mutants, *inr* (Tatar, 2001) and *chico* (Clancy, 2001). Methuselah (*Mth*) gene sequences also follow geoclines (Duvernell et al, 2003; Schmidt et al, 2000). *Mth* encodes a GTP-binding protein of the secretin receptor family of signal-transducing membrane receptors. *Mth* mutants live 35% longer and are resistant to heat, oxidative damage, and starvation (Lin et al, 1998; Song et al, 2002; West et al, 2001). No natural allelic variations in SOD and catalase were found by complementation analysis (Geiger-Thornsberry and MacKay, 2004). This negative result does not conflict with the SOD allele differences in artificially selected long- versus short-lived flies discussed above.

This survey of the genetics of aging in flies and worms has focused on the main themes of infection and nutrition. I am pained to have neglected the work of many esteemed investigators.

5.7. MAMMALS

'Home again' to mammals, to discuss gene variants with functions that are known in much more detail than in insects and nematodes. Humans and other mammals share a core of cellular, physiological, and genetic characteristics in aging patterns (Section 1.2). Trends for obesity and insulin resistance are also common. A fundamental difference in mammalian aging from fly and worm is the role of abnormal cell growths, which have major roles in arterial disease and cancer. Although aging monkeys accumulate Alzheimer-like β-amyloid (Aβ) deposits, aging mice lack Aβ deposits, unless given human transgenes (Section 1.6.1). The discussion is organized by three functions: growth and metabolism, inflammation, and lipoproteins. The discussion of human genotypes emphasizes common polymorphisms to the neglect of rare or familial mutants that dramatically shorten life span in major diseases.

5.7.1. Growth and Metabolism

More than 15 mutations influence longevity in association with alterations in growth and metabolism (Fig. 5.8). This summary of manipulations of longevity from Table 5.3 plots the percentage change of weight and life span relative to controls (0,0). The graph also shows transgenic mutants described in Section 1.2.6, mice overexpressing catalase (MCAT) and another wth partial superoxide dismutase 2 deficiency (Sod2+/−) Table 5.3 lists rodent models by order of life span in four categories with detals in footnotes: (A) primary pituitary hormone defects; (B) GH/IGF-1 receptor defects; (C) other growth factor defects (p44/p53, p63, p66shc); (D) adipocyte-targeted defects (C/EBPβ, FIRKO). Table 5.3 and notes give more details and references. Generalizations must be tentative because many studies compare the effects of mutants with diverse genetic backgrounds that include

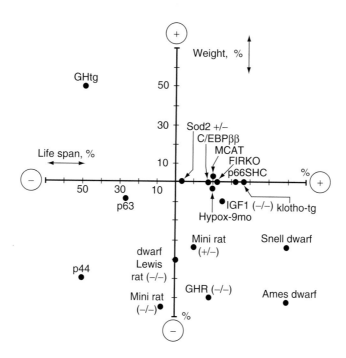

FIGURE 5.8 Life span and body weight in mouse mutants from Table 5.3, graphed as a scatter plot of rescaled data showing the % change in life span and % change in body weight for each study against controls (0,0). Sexes were averaged. Two other mutants are graphed that were discussed in Chapter 1: MCAT, overexpressing mitochondrial catalase (Schriner et al, 2005) and superoxide dismutase 2 partial deficiency (Sod2 +/−) (Van Remmen et al. 2003) (Section 1.2.6).

TABLE 5.3 Long-Lived Rodent Mutants Ranked in Order of Increased Life Span
TABLE 5.3 A Primary Pituitary Hormone Defects

Mutant; ref.	Change in Life Span	Body Weight (Young Adult)	Hormonal Defects	Fasting Plasma Hormones			Reproduction
				Glucose	Insulin	IGF-1	
Ames dwarf mouse Pit1[dw/dw;a]	F, +68% M, +49%	−67%,	no GH, TSH, PRL	lower	lower	> −99% lower	F, sterile M, low fertility
Snell dwarf mouse Prop1[df/df;b,c]	F, +42% M, +26%	−67%	no GH, TSH, PRL	lower	lower	> −99% lower	F, sterile M, low fertility
mini rat antisense GHtg[d]	+10%. tg/− −7.5%,tg/tg	−35%, tg/− −65%, tg/tg	−90% pituitary GH	normal (tg/−)	lower (tg/−)	−35%, tg/− −70%, tg/tg	
dwarf Lewis rat (dw/dw)[e]	M, 0% F, 0%	−40%, +/− −40%, −/−	−40% plasma GH	normal	normal	−40%, −/−	low fertility
excess GH (GH-tg)[f]	−45%	+50%	>10-fold GH elevation; corticosterone elevated				premature loss

(Continues)

TABLE 5.3 A (Continued)

a. Ames dwarf mouse: (Bartke et al, 2001; Brown-Borg et al, 1996; Tatar et al, 2003; Tsuchiya et al, 2004). The mean life span of *ad lib* fed Ames is 1062 d; current maximum is 1550 d (Ikeno et al, 2003) (Fig. 5.10). The Ames mutant (*Prop-1* gene, Ames dwarf) is upstream of the *Pit1* transcription factor and impairs differentiation of the anterior pituitary (Andersen et al, 1995). The mutant has been maintained on a genetically' heterogeneous background' for 20 y (Ikeno et al, 2003) The Ames dwarf has delayed neoplastic lesions and attenuated kidney pathology. The <1% normal IGF-1 was estimated from the radioimmunoassay sensitivity in consultation with Bartke and Chandrashekar (Chandrashekar and Bartke, 1993). The Ames dwarf shows increased insulin sensitivity but intolerance to glucose; insulin-stimulated phosphorylation of the insulin receptor is enhanced (Dominici et al, 2002).

b. Snell dwarf mouse: (Flurkey et al, 2002). Longevity of Snell dwarfs, relative to non-mutant litter-mates, depends on the genetic background (Brown-Borg et al, 1996; Liang et al, 2003). Life span is about 40% longer than the C3H/HeJ × DW/J)F1 background (Flurkey et al, 2001). Mean survival, dwarf, 1,178 ± 235 d versus background genotype, 832 ± 158 d. When Snell dwarfs are housed with normal males, life span was shorter than the normal; life spans were much longer when females were the cage mates, which is attributed to greater social stress in male company, or the greater access to body warmth in huddling with females (Vergara et al, 2004). Collagen cross-linking (tail-tendon breaking time) increased more slowly with age in the dwarfs. Knee-joint pathology during aging was also slowed (Silberberg, 1972). Spleen hypertrophy during aging is also attenuated (Flurkey and Harrison, 1990).

c. Snell dwarf history. The Snell dwarf was the first mutant dwarf identified (Snell, 1929). In an earlier phase of biogerontology, Fabris and colleagues described the Snell dwarf as a model for accelerated aging because of *short* life span, < 6 mo (Section 2.5.2) and early pathology (Fabris et al, 1972; Fabris et al, 1988). In a European colony, dwarfs developed cataracts, graying hair, kyphosis, and sagging skin by 4–5 m. Pneumonia or other infections, however, were not noted (Fabris et al, 1971a). These accelerated aging changes were blocked and life span was increased to >12 months by injecting lymphocytes from normal mice or by bovine GH (Fabris, 1972). The thymus gland deficiencies were attributed to deficits in GH (Fabris, 1971; Fabris et al, 1971b; Pierpaoli, 1969). Snell dwarfs were also short-lived in two U.S. breeding colonies. At Cornell U. Medical College (Winick, 1968), dwarfs died before maturing; survival was increased by limiting litters to 1–3 mice, which increased body weight, possibly by more access to milk and maternal care. All mice seemed to lose weight after weaning, implying pathogenic infections. I can add the personal observation that animal facilities were suboptimum at Cornell in 1970-1972, my first academic appointment. Graying is atypical of aging in mice (Finch, 1973b). At the National Cancer Institute (NCI) (Chen et al, 1972), dwarfs were also short-lived, although some survived to 12 mo. This colony had a high incidence of tumors, unlike modern colonies. However, obesity was observed, as in currently colonies. In great contrast to these three colonies, dwarfs in two other colonies from that period were longer lived. Dwarf mice at Washington U. lived up to 41 mo and were studied as models of retarded skeletal aging (Silberberg, 1972; Silberberg, 1973). In Glasgow U., dwarf mice lived at least 8 mo and without cataracts, or other aging markers; potential survival to later ages was not followed (Shire, 1973). We cannot know what conditions differed critically between these short- and long-lived dwarf colonies. The high incidence of lymphomas and leukemia in the NCI colony could have had viral origins (Chen, 1972). Reduced infections and other husbandry improvements are more likely than genetic changes (Section 2.5.2). As discussed in the text, dwarf mice are sensitive to stress-induced immune deficiencies and wasting conditions (Foster, 2000). At the Jackson Laboratory, improved conditions included temperature control and reductions of infections (Section 2.4.2) (Kevin Flurkey, pers. comm.).

d. Mini rat antisense GHtg: (Shimokawa et al, 2002; Yamaza et al, 2004). Transgenic expression of anti-sense GH in pituitary. Heterozygotes (tg/−) lived 10% longer than the (tg/tg) homozygotes. Although plasma GH was not different, despite the major decrease in pituitary GH, detailed sampling might show a dampened pulsatile secretion of GH. Pathology at death of tg/tg—mostly neoplasia, particularly leukemia, which was never observed in −/− rats; lower incidence of pituitary tumors and kidney disease. Natural killer (NK) cell activity was lower, but normal T-cell responses to mitogens; the smaller spleens and thymus were scaled to body size

e. Dwarf Lewis rat (*du/dw*):(Sonntag, 2005). Dwarf Lewis rats carry a recessive mutation (not mapped or characterized) that has no effect on other pituitary hormones (Charlton et al, 1988; Ramsey et al, 2002). Augmentation of GH after puberty slightly increased the male life span (14%), with no effect on females. Lewis dwarfs have no abnormalities in other pituitary hormones, corticosterone, insulin, or glucose. Learning was impaired at all adult ages, but without obvious brain abnormalities.

f. GH transgenic over-producer Giant GH-transgenic mice. Life span: mean, 425 versus 733 d controls; maximum, 550 versus 1150 d controls (Bartke, 2003). Corticosterone is elevated (basal and ether-induced) (Cecim et al, 1996). Pathology includes premature enlargement of seminal vesicles and increased mammary tumors (Bartke, 2003; Steger, 1993). Fertility declines prematurely, by 5–7 mo (Cecim, 1995). Brain aging is accelerated, with elevated GFAP (astrocytic hypertrophy marker, Fig.1.7E, Fig.1.9 Section 1.8.1) and slowed turnover of hypothalamic dopamine, confirming similar age changes in normal C57BL/6J mice after 600 d in my lab (Finch, 1973a; Nichols et al, 1993; Rozovsky et al, 2005).

abbreviations:

GH, growth hormone (pituitary); GHR/BP, growth hormone receptor/binding protein; the GHR/BP gene encodes the GH receptor (liver) and its truncated form, the GH-receptor binding protein (serum protein, secreted by the liver); Ghrh: growth hormone releasing hormone (hypothalamus); IGF-1, insulin-like growth factor-1 (liver); IGF-1R, the IGF-1 receptor; IRS, insulin receptor; PRL, prolactin ; TSH, thyroid stimulating hormone.

TABLE 5.3 B GH/IGF-1 Receptor Defects

Mutant	Change in Life Span	Body Weight (Young Adult)	Hormonal Defects	Fasting plasma Hormones			Reproduction
				Glucose	Insulin	IGF-1	
IGF-1 receptor knockout mouse; Igf/1r[+/−;g]	F, +33% M, +16%	<−8%		normal	normal	+20% higher	normal
GH-receptor knockout GHR[−/−;h]	F, +33% M, +19%	−60%; growth slows by 4 w	GH, 5–10x higher;	−80% lower	−20% lower	≥−80% lower	F, low fertility; maturity delayed 4 w
little (lit) mouse, Ghrh[lit/lit;i]	F, +25% M, +23%	−33%	>99% lower GH; corticosterone elevated			−75% lower	
Klotho over-expression[j]	F, +20% M, +30%	normal	impaired insulin and IGF-1 receptor activation	normal lower	F, +50% M, norm		50% fewer pups
midi mouse, m/m[k]		−35%	low IGF-1			>−99% lower	F, low fertility

g. IGF-1 receptor knockout mouse (Holzenberger et al, 2003). *Life span* background strain *129*: female mean 568 d, max 810 d; male mean, 585 d, max 1000 d. *Life span* +/−: female, mean 756 d; female max, ca. 960 d; male, mean 679 d; male max 1020 d (not significant). Fasting glucose, normal; fed glucose, females, +12%; males, −4%. Glucose tolerance, males hyperglycemic (peak about 2× females). Normal body temperature.

h. GH-receptor knockout (GHR−/−): (Coschigano et al, 2003; Kopchick and Laron, 1999).The GHR/BP−/− mutation in the GH binding protein impairs the GH-receptor by blocking dimerization required for GH signal transduction in hepatocytes that secrete IGF-1. Homozygotes Igf/1r−/− are not viable. Life span changes averaged from the two background strains: *C57BL/6J*, female mean 821 d, female max 1100 d; male mean 765 d, male max 1000 d; GHR −/− female mean 956 d, female max 1250 d; male −/− mean 951 d male max 1200 d. *Ola-BALB/cJ*, female mean 759 d, female max 1250 d; male mean 656 d, male max 980d. −/− female mean 921 d, female max 1250 d. Male GHR −/− C57/BL/6J gained 5g slowly. Another transgenic introduced a GH antagonist peptide (GHA) that did not alter life span; although weaning weight was the same as the GHR−/−, the GHA gained weight progressively, unlike the GHR−/−, and nearly caught up to controls by 1 y. Food intake in both mutants was normal for body weight or higher.

i. little (lit) mouse (Ghrh[lit/lit]): (Flurkey and Harrison, 1990; Flurkey et al, 2001). Growth impairments are very modest. The low blood GH is caused by a pituitary receptor defect, which impairs responses to GH-releasing hormone (GHRH) from the hypothalamus. *lit/lit* males, 1,093 ± 186 d versus background, 886 ± 148 d; females, 1070 ± 127 d versus background, 857 ± 169 d. In *lit/lit* homozygotes, tail growth ceased after 7–10 mo, while body mass and skeleton continued to grow; postnatal tail growth may be a better bioassay for GH than body weight (Flurkey and Harrison, 1990). Corticosterone is also elevated (Alt, 2006) Spleen hypertrophy during aging is attenuated relative to wild-type. Heterozygotes *lit/+* grew normally.

j. Klotho over-producer: Klotho encodes an uncharacterized membrane protein with an extracellular domain shed into blood and cerebrospinal fluid that regulates insulin signalin (Kurosu et al, 2005). Klotho deficits shortened life span drastically: dramatic involutional, age-like changes arose after weaning and few survived to maturation (2 months) (Kuro-o et al, 1997). Pathology included arterial calcification at a level atypical of current aging mice (Section 2.5.2) and loss of subcutaneous fat. Conversely, transgenic overexpressors lived 20–30% longer (two lines); KL48 female, 830 versus 697 d, background; male: 940 versus 715 d background (Kurosu et al, 2005). The Klotho peptide was elevated 2-fold in plasma. Glucose clamp studies showed resistance to IGF-1 and insulin in male mice, and IGF-1 resistance only in females. Klotho inhibits activation of the IGF-1 and insulin receptor and suppresses insulin-receptor mediated signaling including interactions of the PI3-kinase (p85 subunit with the insulin receptor). Pathology was not reported.

k. IGF-1 hypomorph mouse 'midi' (Lorenzini et al, 2004); reported as abstract.

TABLE 5.3 C p53 Family Function Mutants

Mutant	Change in Life Span	Body Weight (Young Adult)	Hormonal Defects	Fasting Plasma Hormones			Reproduction
				Glucose	Insulin	IGF-1	
p44 (p53 isoform)[l]	−50%	−50%	activated IGF-receptors			+20%	early M. infertility
p63[+/−;m]	−22%	−5%					
p66[shc−/−;n]	+30%	normal		normal	normal	normal	

l. p44 (p53 short peptide) may integrate insulin/IGF-1 and proliferation signaling (Maier et al, 2004). On C57BL/6-SJL background. Survival curves give the impression of increased IMR and shorter MRDT. By 5 m, skeletal degeneration was considerable: mice became hunched (kyphotic) and osteoblasts were greatly reduced; the seminiferous epithelium degenerated, with complete male infertility; *in vitro* proliferation was also attenuated. Serum IGF-1 was normal or higher and the IGF-1 receptor elevated in tissues that proliferate throughout life. IGF-1 signaling was abnormal in some proportion to the level of p44 expression. Embryo cells showed enhanced phosphorylation of the FKHR transcription factor and diverse changes in FKHR regulated changes: two genes with increased activity are Mdm2, a ubiquitin ligase of p53 (and only activated by p53) and IGFBP-3 (IGF binding protein); in contrast Gadd45 activity was lower. These models reveal an important connection between IGF-1 and p53, but also to Sir2, which regulates p53 as a deacetylase (Marmorstein, 2004; Vaziri et al 2001). A larger p53 deletion *p53[+/m]* (first 6 exons and 20 kb upstream sequences including the *Efnb3* gene) did not alter body size but had similar pathological phenotypes with short life span, osteoporosis, and 'generalized organ atrophy,' which is a mysterious term (Tyner et al, 2002). Age-related tumors were absent in both p53 deletions.
m. p63 deletion: p63 is in the gene family of transcription factors with multiple isoforms that regulate cell cycle arrest and apoptosis (Keyes and Mills, 2006; Levrero et al, 2000). Unlike p53, mutations in p63 are rare in human malignancy and p63+/− does not increase tumors in the mouse. Loss of p63 induces cell cycle arrest with cell senescence phenotypes (Section 1.2.3), e.g., SA-ß-galactosidase induction. The p63+/− deletion heterozygote on a F1(129/C57B6) background appeared normal as young adult, but lifespan was shorter: median 95 wk versus 104 wk background; maximum, ca. 110 versus 156 wk (Keyes et al, 2005). Survival curves give the impression of increased IMR and shorter MRDT. Tumors were absent as observed in the p44/p53 deletions (note l). Skin cells had striking induction of two human fibroblast cell senescence markers, SA-ß-galactosidase and p16(INK4a), which also increase in human skin during aging (Ressler S et al, 2006). However, neither was detected in aging control mice. Aging mice had 'some lordokyphosis' (spinal curvature), which is common at later ages in background strains. Chronic infections were unusually common during aging: 52% had skin lesions, or infections (abscesses with bacterial inclusions); 12% had hemorrhage; other sites of infection in subcutaneous tissues, mouth and pharynx, genitourinary tract.
n. *p66shc* knockout mouse: (Migliaccio et al, 1999). Knockout of p66 (p66[shc−/−]) increased life span by 30%: control lifespan (129/sv), 750 d; *shc* +/−, 830 d; *shc* −/−, 970 d. Resistance to oxidative stress was increased *in vivo*: paraquat toxicity; lipid oxidation on high fat diet (Napoli et al, 2003b); and *in vitro*: DNA damage from UV-radiation, or H_2O_2 (Orsini et al, 2004; Migliaccio et al, 1999; Trinei et al, 2002). Sex differences include greater female resistance to paraquat; males have slight glucose elevation.

TABLE 5.3 D Adipocyte Targeted Defects

Mutant; ref.	Change in Life Span	Body Weight (Young Adult)	Hormonal Defects	Fasting Plasma Hormones			Reproduction
				Glucose	Insulin	IGF-1	
C/EBP[β/β] mouse; deficient fat storage[o]	+22%	normal	low white fat				
FIRKO mouse, Fat-specific insulin receptor knockout[p]	+18%	<25% total wt; −50% body fat	loss of insulin-signaling in fat only; normal food intake	normal	lower	normal	

o. C/EBPβ/β mouse: C/EBP (CCAAT/enhancer-binding proteins) are required for adipocyte differentiation and activates PPARγ (Chiu et al, 2004). β/β mouse is a knockin replacement of C/EBP α by C/EBPβ, thus carrying two copies. Life span β/β 28.9 mo; β/+ 23.7 mo. Fat storage is reduced, but without hyperlipidemia. Food consumption and core temperature are higher than controls. White adipose tissue had increased thermogenic mitochondria. Pathology of aging not known.
p. FIRKO mouse, fat-specific insulin receptor knockout: (Bluher et al, 2002; Bluher et al, 2003).

varying combinations of inbred strains.[9] The associations of size and longevity vary widely. A provisional conclusion may be drawn that dwarfism is neither necessary nor sufficient for longevity, as was also concluded for the fly insulin-signaling mutants.

5.7.1.1. Rodent Mutants with Altered Insulin Signaling and Fat Metabolism

Presaging the findings of long-lived fly and worm mutants, the pioneering work of Andrej Bartke showed that deficits in insulin and IGF-1 increase mouse life span (Bartke et al, 2002; Brown-Borg et al, 1996). The Ames, little, and Snell dwarf mice lack pituitary growth hormone (GH) and live longer than most background strains (Fig. 5.9) under protected conditions (Table 5.3A, note c). The lack of plasma GH consequently greatly attenuates the hepatic secretion of IGF-1 (Chandrashekar and Bartke, 1993), which is required for normal growth. Currently, more than five gene mutants that reduce GH/IGF-1 levels or signaling also increase life span; other mutations have little or no effect on life span (Table 5.3A) (Fig. 5.8).

The Ames dwarf lives about 50% longer than most lab mice and was the first mutation (*prop-1*) shown to increase longevity in a mammal. The Snell dwarf (*pit-1*) is just behind in longevity. Both male and female life spans are increased. With favorable husbandry conditions, the GH deficits increase life span more than diet restriction. The Ames and Snell dwarfs have low insulin and glucose. However, other disturbances are less desirable from a human perspective: hypothyroidism, low body temperature, and impaired reproduction. Obesity is prevalent with aging. Brain aging changes may also be slowed. Tumors are decreased, discussed below.

Causes of death during aging in these mutants are not generally reported. The Ames and Snell dwarfs are the best described. In the Ames mutant, neoplasia was the major attributed cause of death (67% vs 95% in the background strain) with delayed occurrence (Fig. 5.9B), corresponding to the increased life span (Fig. 5.9A) (Ikeno et al, 2003). Lung adenocarcinoma was the most common lesion and was less severe in the dwarfs. Glomerulonephritis was also lessened. The 15% decrease in 'total pathologic burden' is modest relative to effect of diet restriction in attenuating pathology (Section 3.2.2). Snell and 'little' mice have less

---

[9]The standard inbred mice that are used as background strains or 'wild-types' may carry mutations that influence outcomes of aging; e.g., several common mouse strains (CE/J, DBA/2J, FVB) carry a mutant inactive complement peptide C5a (Pasinetti et al, 1996) that may alter responses to diet (Section 3.5, footnote 9). For this reason, I prefer the terms 'background' or 'control' over 'wild-type'. Wild-caught mice are the only properly designated wild-type in aging studies and differ remarkably from standard strains in smaller size, longer life span, and resistance to diet restriction (Chapter 3, Fig. 3.3).

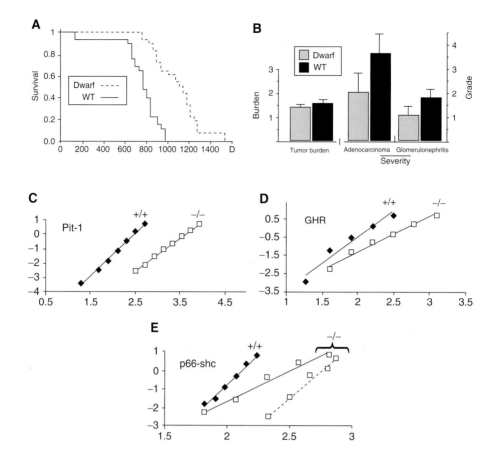

FIGURE 5.9 Mouse mutant life spans, pathologic lesions of aging, and mortality rates. A. Ames dwarf mouse survival, redrawn from (Ikeno et al, 2003). Survival curve, both sexes, from mice of Fig. 5.10 at completion of study. B. Lesion severity (25 controls, 21 dwarfs): tumor burden (average number of tumors); severity of adenocarcinoma; severity of glomerulonephritis. Mortality attributed to neoplastic lesions. In controls, 95% died from neoplasia, with 48% from adenocarcinoma of the lung. Dwarfs had about 28% fewer fatal neoplasms. Other fatal neoplasms include lymphoma, hepatocellular carcinoma, and hemangioma in liver and spleen. C. Mortality rates of selected mutants (Table 5.3), graphed as ln[$m(x)$] against age x. (Redrawn from de Magalhaes et al, 2005.) Table 5.4 gives the Gompertz mortality constants for initial mortality rate (IMR) and mortality rate accelerations calculated as the mortality rate doubling time (MRDT) (Section 1.2.1). Non-mutants +, mutants, –. Snell dwarf (*pit-1*), Pit-1 (–/–) data from (Flurkey et al, 2001). Life spans were 34% longer (average, M+F, Table 5.3), attributed to both lower IMR and longer MRDT relative to controls. D. GH-receptor knockout GHR(–/–), data from (Coschigano et al, 2003). Life spans were 20% longer. The IMR was lower than control, but MRDT was unchanged. E. p66^{shc} knockout, p66–shc (–/–) data from (Migliaccio et al, 1999). Life spans were 30% longer (av., M+F, Table 5.3), attributed to both lower IMR and longer MRDT. The dotted line is an alternate plot excluded the first three points, which illustrates the sensitivity of the analysis to the small numbers of animals available in most studies.

neoplasia and splenic hypertrophy (Flurkey and Harrison, 1990; Flurkey and Currer, 2004). Snell dwarfs had fewer lymphomas, plus milder kidney pathology and lens opacity (cataract score) (Vergara et al, 2004). The GH-receptor-knock-out also had less neoplasia (no details given) (Bartke, 2005). About 25% of old Ames dwarfs and 47% of the Snell dwarfs had no visible gross pathologic lesions at natural death, as seen in about 25% of aging F334 rats on diet restriction (Ikeno et al, 2003).

The Ames and Snell dwarfs have multiple pituitary defects and lack GH, TSH, and PRL. To evaluate the role of growth deficits and interactions with hypothyroidism, Snell dwarfs were injected with both GH and thyroxine (T_4) from 4–15 wk; a subgroup continued to receive T_4 (Vergara et al, 2004). Adult weight was partially restored, with greatest effect from continuing T_4. Survival curves did not differ between untreated dwarfs and those receiving GH/T_4 only early in life. However, continuing T_4 replacement decreased survival to levels close to the background controls.

Both Ames and Snell dwarfs have very low blood glucose, insulin, and IGF-1. Both become obese during aging, particularly males, which may reach 40 g, with corresponding increases in serum leptin (Flurkey et al, 2001). The 'little' mutation (*lit/lit*) in the GH-releasing hormone receptor (GHRH) restricts the pituitary hormone deficits to GH; however, the mice still become obese (Godfrey et al, 1993). Concurrent obesity and longevity as in these dwarfs may also co-exist in some human populations (Section 3, Fig. 3.4A) and in the fat accumulated by long-lived mutant flies. The *ad lib* food intake of Ames and Snell dwarfs is greater normal when calculated per g body weight (BW), but is normalized if calculated by $BW^{0.75}$ (metabolic BW) (Bartke, pers. comm.).

Ames and Snell dwarfs' learning ability declined little if at all during aging, unlike controls (Bartke, 2005). The Ames dwarf may have increased adult neurogenesis in the hippocampus, a brain region critical for memory (Sun et al, 2005b). Neuronogenesis in the adult brain is dependent on IGF-1 (Lichtenwalner et al, 2006) produced by local cells not dependent on serum GH; in the hippocampus, IGF-1 was normal (mRNA and protein) for the background strain. The brain also has autogenous GH expression, which is lower in the Ames dwarf (Sun et al, 2005a).

Diet restriction (DR) further increases the Ames life span in both sexes by about 30% (Fig. 5.10), which is relatively more than in the fly dwarf *chico* mutant (Fig. 5.6). Despite the obesity, the dwarf mouse metabolic mutants share some features of DR with lower blood glucose and insulin, increased resistance to oxidative stress, and trends to slower mortality acceleration (MRDT) (Bartke, 2002, 2005). Skin fibroblasts from the Ames, Snell, and GH-receptor mutants are resistant to H_2O_2, paraquat, and UV (Salmon et al, 2005). Increased expression of FoxO family transcription factors that regulate stress-resistance genes is hypothesized as downstream of attenuated insulin/IGF signaling in dwarfs, as in DR (Bartke, 2005).

The *lit/lit* and Snell dwarfs have slower immune maturation (Cross et al, 1992; Foster et al, 2000) and are more vulnerable to infections, stress-induced immune

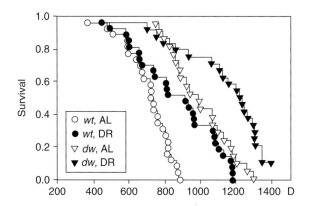

FIGURE 5.10 Longevity is increased by diet restriction (DR) of Ames dwarf mice.
Survival curve both sexes from mice of Fig. 5.9A showing that DR further increased
longevity by 30%. (Redrawn from Bartke et al, 2001.)

deficiencies, and wasting conditions (Foster et al, 2000). Immune system age
changes are slowed in Snell dwarfs (Flurkey et al, 2001), with smaller increases
of memory T cells (CD4, CD8) and smaller loss during aging of nHTL and pCTL
cells (mitogen-stimulated T cells that produce IL-2 or that differentiate into cytotoxic effectors, respectively). Ames dwarfs may have milder immune aging
changes in different markers: B and T cell numbers are normal, as is production
of antibodies to tetanus toxoid (Cross et al, 1992; Hall et al, 2002). However, *lit/lit*
mice have 3-fold higher mortality after infection with influenza virus (Alt et al,
2003). This may be a model for the higher mortality of hypopituitary humans
from respiratory infections, as shown in a large prospective study (Tomlinson
et al, 2001).

The IGF-1 receptor knockout benefits females; males were hyperglycemic in
glucose tolerance tests and lived slightly longer. Conversely, the GH-receptor
knockout mainly benefited male life span; glucose and insulin were much lower,
and female fertility was lower.

In an earlier phase of biogerontology, the Snell dwarf was described very differently as a model for accelerated aging because of its *short* life span, <12 m and
early onset pathology (Fabris et al, 1972; Fabris et al, 1988), including lymphomas that are currently rare (Chen et al, 1972) (Table 5.3A, note c summarizes
this important history). Reduced infections and other husbandry improvements
are more likely than genetic changes (Section 2.5.2).

Mortality rate analysis of some of these mutants indicates slower aging,
but statistics are weakened by the small numbers of mice in most studies

(Table 5.4) (de Magalhaes et al, 2005). In healthy rodent colonies, life span is mainly determined by the acceleration rate of mortality (Gompertz slope, or mortality rate doubling time [MRDT] (Section 1.2.1; Table 5.1 notes). However, decrease in the background mortality, or 'initial mortality rate' (IMR), will increase life span without slowing aging. Despite the statistical significance of mutant effects on life span, the Gompertz parameters did not differ (Table 5.4). The Ames dwarf (*prop-1*) had the clearest slowing of aging, with longer MRDT, confirming (Flurkey et al, 2001) (Fig. 5.9 C, D, E). This mortality profile implies a delayed onset of aging, without change in rate of aging, which represents a life history model predicted earlier (Finch, 1990, p. 26). The histopathology was also well characterized and was attenuated relative to background strain (Fig. 5.9B). The MRDT was also longer in the C/EBPβ/β fat storage deficient mutant, discussed below. Table 5.4 also shows the short-lived senescence accelerated mouse (SAM) (Takeda et al, 1981), with faster mortality accelerations (shorter MRDT) and the diet restricted F344 rat (longer MRDT) (Finch, 1990,

TABLE 5.4 Gompertz Parameters for Mouse Mutants and Diet-Restricted Rat

Gene/Intervention (Number of Animals)	Genotype	Change in Life Span	Initial Mortality Rate[+], IMR/y	Mortality Rate Doubling Time[+], MRDT, y
C/EBP (60)	CTL	22%[*]	0.52	0.27
	C/EBPβ/β		0.38	0.45[**]
Diet restricted F344 rat (230)	*ad lib* fed	30%[*]	0.031	0.17
	restricted		0.034	0.37[**]
GHR Growth hormone receptor-KO (26)	CTL	≥ +16%[*]	0.52	0.36
	KO		0.59	0.46
GHRHR little mouse (66)	CTL	≥ +23%[*]	0.19	0.29
	KO		0.15	0.28
Igf/1r[+/−]dwarf (37)	CTL	≥ +16%[*]	0.30	0.39
	KO		0.06	0.32
INSR FIRKO (127)	CTL	18%[*]	0.078	0.36
	KO		0.035	0.29
p66[shc−/−] (29)	CTL	30%[*]	1.7	0.11
	KO		0.29	0.25
PIT1, Ames dwarf (59)	CTL	≥ +49%[*]	0.020	0.23
	KO		0.0035	0.30[**]
PROP1, Snell dwarf, F.(29)	CTL	+42%[*]	1.29	0.75
	KO		0.74	0.35
SAM senescence - accelerated mouse (870)	CTL	−26%[*]	0.63	0.37
	SAM		0.77	0.21[**]

+, for definitions of IMR and MRDT, see Table 1.2.
[*], significant difference of life span, according to original reports (Table 5.3).
[**], significant difference of parameter in (de Magalhaes et al, 2005).
CLT, control strain, see Table 5.3.

p. 508). de Magalhaes et al. (2005) emphasize that different survival curves and mean life spans do not resolve whether the mutant actually slowed aging, and I fully agree. The slowing of aging must be determined by assessing mortality rate parameters and pathology. The sample must be sufficient for mortality statistics, usually at least 100 mice. Histopathology is always needed to define the nature of senescent mortality in each experiment. Few other reports in Table 5.3 even described gross pathologic lesions, and none noted the ubiquitous pituitary tumors of aging female rodents (Finch et al, 1984). An exemplary study is the mitochondrial catalase overexpressing mouse (Fig. 4.8, MCAT) (Section 1.2.6) (Schriner et al, 2005), in which life span was increased by right-shifting the Gompertz slope together with delayed and decreased organ pathology.

Hypophysectomy (surgical ablation of the anterior pituitary) gives another approach to pituitary hormones and aging, and can be accomplished with high survival in rodents as in humans. In Arthur Everitt's pioneering experiments, hypophysectomy at 2 m slowed many aging changes that are also slowed by diet restriction: major decrease in endocrine tumors and kidney lesions; less aortic wall thickening (Everitt et al, 1980). Life spans were increased by 16%, more than in the diet restricted rats of this study. Hypophysectomy at 15 m had less effect. These effects were verified in mice: Hypophysectomy at 1 m increased life span by 15% and at 9 months by 21%, with progressively less effect at later ages (Powers et al, 2006b).

Conversely, life span is shortened by 30% in transgenic mice that overexpress GH with plasma GH $\geq$ 1000-fold elevations. Excess GH may cause a progeria syndrome, with increased tumors, elevated corticosteroids, and impaired reproduction and immunity (Bartke, 2003; Hall et al, 2002; Steger et al, 1993). These adverse outcomes are at odds with the popularity of GH supplementation in some circles (see below).

Other mutants altering growth have modest effects on longevity (Table 5.3B) (Fig. 5.8). Mutants targeting GH/IGF-1 functions without other pituitary changes live slightly longer than background strains and are small-sized: GH-receptor knockouts (GHR$^{-/-}$) and IGF-1 receptor knockout heterozygotes (Igf/1r$^{+/-}$). The GH-receptor KO($^{-/-}$) has very low plasma IGF-1 (Kopchick and Laron, 1999); these mice are very insulin-sensitive (slightly lower to normal blood glucose, low insulin); however, GH is elevated (Andrej Bartke, pers. comm.; Coschigano et al, 2000; Coschigano, 2003). Gluconeogenic and stress-resistance genes are more active (Al-Regaiey et al, 2005). Diet restriction had no effect on median life span and increased the maximum of females only (Bonkowski et al, 2006b). This major contrast to Ames dwarf responses to DR (Fig. 5.9) implies the dependence of diet restriction responses on intact GH-receptor signaling. The GHR$^{-/-}$ mutant is a model for Laron syndrome in humans (next section).

The IGF-1 receptor mutant (Igf/1r$^{+/-}$) with 33% longer life span is studied as a heterozygote (homozygotes die at birth) (Holzenberger et al, 2003). Body weight is slightly lower (5–8%), with normal intake of food and water. Blood

IGF-1 is 32% higher, which may be a compensation for 50% lower density of IGF-receptors (brain, kidney, lung). While glucose-insulin regulation is nearly normal, IGF-1 signaling downstream of the receptor was decreased (50% lower phosphorylation of Akt and p66[shc] after IGF-1 stimulation). Body temperature is normal, unlike the Ames dwarf (Hunter et al, 1999). A new IGF-1 hypomorph, the midi mouse, has no detectable IGF-1, yet is only 35% smaller; its life span approximates the IGF-1R+/− (Christian Sell, pers. comm.; Lorenzini et al, 2004).

The *Klotho* gene[10] has added another link to insulin signaling. *Klotho* encodes a highly pleiotropic peptide that influences blood glucose and insulin signaling (Kurosu et al, 2005), enzymes that influence arterial disease (ACE and PAL-1) (Arking et al, 2005), and calcium metabolism (Lewin and Olgaard, 2006). KLOTHO-deficient mice have very short life spans, with dramatic involution by 2 months (Kuro-o et al, 1997). The gross pathology includes extreme arterial calcification atypical of current aging mice (Section 2.5.2) and loss of subcutaneous fat. Conversely, transgenic KLOTHO overexpressors lived 20–30% longer than the background strain (Kurosu et al, 2005). KLOTHO inhibits activation of the IGF-1 and insulin receptor and suppresses insulin-receptor mediated signaling, including interactions of the PI3-kinase (p85 subunit) with the insulin receptor. Body weight was normal with either KLOTHO deficits or elevations. The pathology of the KLOTHO-deficient mice was attenuated by inhibiting insulin signaling with a loss-of-function insulin receptor gene (IRS[+/−]), which recalls that Ames dwarf mice also show deficits of insulin and IGF-1 signaling (Bartke, 2006). In humans, the *klotho* polymorphism KL-VS with two coding changes may be associated with mortality risk (Arking et al, 2002; Arking et al, 2003; Arking et al, 2005). KL-VS heterozygotes were more prevalent than homozygotes at advanced ages in Ashkenazi Jews and Czechs, suggesting a survival advantage. There may be associations of KL-VS with blood pressure and HDL cholesterol and stroke.

Returning to rodent models, two dwarf rats show little or no difference in longevity. The Lewis dwarf has a recessive mutation (Charlton et al, 1988), which reduces body size by 40% in association with 40% deficits of plasma GH and IGF-1. However, life span is normal (Sonntag, 2005). Pathology showed counterbalancing changes: dwarfs had fewer fatal neoplastic diseases and milder kidney degeneration, whereas there was a high incidence of intra-cranial hemorrhage (an unusual lesion). Also puzzling is the 'mini' rat, which carries a transgene anti-sense GH (Shimokawa et al, 2002; Shimokawa et al, 2003). By comparison with wild-type (−/−), plasma IGF-1 and adult weight decreased by 35% per transgene copy (tg/, tg/tg). Despite size reductions comparable to the dwarf mice,

---

[10]Klotho (Clotho) is one of the three Greek Goddesses of Fate (the *Moirae*) who predestine the life span. In one version of this myth, *Klotho* spins the thread of life; *Lachesis* determines its length for each individual at birth; and, inevitably, the thread is cut by *Atropos*.

the homozygotes (tg/tg) had 15% shorter life spans. Transgenics had greatly decreased chronic nephropathy, but much more leukemia, a different balance of pathologies than in the Lewis dwarfs.

A new set of growth factor mutants affecting p44, p63, and p66-shk have altered aging phenotypes. These mutants, described below, alter activities related to the p53 oncogene, which, when not mutated, acts as a tumor suppressor. p53 is in a superfamily (p53/p63/p73) of transcription factors with multiple isoforms that regulate cell cycle arrest, metabolism, and apoptosis (Keyes and Mills, 2006; Levrero et al, 2000). In human tumors, p53 mutations are famous as the most common lesion, whereas p63 and p73 mutations are rare in human malignancy. p53 controls IGF-1 at the IGF-1 receptor as well as PTEN, which modulates IGF-signal transduction through Akt. Moreover, some p53/p63/p73 isoforms regulate transcription of IGFBP-3, which may be a vital link to somatic growth, inflammation, and metabolism. Reciprocally, SIRT1 regulates p53 transcription (Yang et al, 2006), which links p53 to nutritional status through NAD dependence of SIRT1 acetylase activity. As discussed above, flies also show a sirtuin-p53 link to life span and responses to diet restriction.

The p44 mutant mouse with a truncated p53 peptide, grows slowly, reaches only 50% normal size, and has 50% shorter life span (Maier et al, 2004) (Table 5.3D). Tumors were not reported. The IGF regulation is abnormal: Despite the slight elevations of IGF-1, there was notable activation of IGF-1R and Akt phosphorylation. The integration of p53 and IGF-1 points to deep-level controls of development and, possibly, aging.

The p63 deletion heterozygotes also had 22% shorter life spans, but were only slightly smaller (Keyes et al, 2005). Tumors were absent as observed in the p44/p53 deletions. Immune functions are impaired, with a much higher prevalence of spontaneous suppurative infections and hemorrhage than in the control mice or other colonies during normal aging.

The p66 'shick' knockout (p66[shc−/−]) is normal size and lives 30% longer (Migliaccio et al, 1999). The p66-SHC protein has an Src-homology2 (SH2) domain that is phosphorylated by the activation of cell growth factor receptors and mediates p53-dependent response to oxidative stress. The p66SHK protein, in turn, phosphorylates the transcription factor FKHR (DAF-16 orthologue), which regulates stress-resistance genes. IGF-1 is normal; no hormonal deviations were reported. Resistance to oxidative stress was increased and to oxidative kidney damage from diabetes, with possible greater benefit to females (see Table 5.3C, note n). Importantly, there was also increased resistance to atherosclerosis induced by fatty diet (Napoli et al, 2003a,b). Aortic wall aging was also diminished (cholinergic epithelial relaxation and NO release, which decline in aging) (Francia et al, 2004). Human variants of p66[shc] are rare (Sentinelli et al, 2006).

Two mouse mutants with altered fat cells have joined this longevous bestiary: the FIRKO (+12% life span) (Bluher et al, 2002; Bluher et al, 2003) and the C/EBPβ/β (+22% life span) (Chiu et al, 2004). FIRKO lacks the fat-specific insulin receptor, which decreases body fat by 50% and body weight by 20%. Despite higher food intake per gram body weight, blood glucose and glucose tolerance are normal. In FIRKO, unlike normal adults, body fat does not increase with age, nor does insulin resistance. Future comparisons could include knockouts of the insulin receptor in muscle (MIRKO) and liver (LIRKO); their insulin resistance may increase mortality (Rincon et al, 2004). Lastly, the C/EBPβ/β mutant carries a replacement of the C/EBPα gene, which alters adipocyte differentiation and blocks lipid accumulation (Chiu et al, 2004). Mitochondrial content and energy dissipation are increased. Mutants do not become obese on high fat diet. No details of aging or pathology were reported.

These exploratory studies are far from conclusive. Provisionally, I conclude that dwarfism is neither necessary nor sufficient for longevity, shown in Figure 5.8. Attenuated insulin-like signaling may be permissive of longevity in low stress environments. As discussed above, dwarf mice may be more vulnerable to wasting conditions and infections. Thus, attenuated insulin and IGF-1 signaling may be necessary, but not sufficient for increased life span in rodents, and possibly humans.

5.7.1.2. Human Hereditary Variations in Metabolic Genes

Would the mild to severe metabolic deficits in these rodent mutants also influence human longevity? At the least, inherited dwarfism and GH deficiency are compatible with normal life spans. In one of the first reports, isolated recessive GH deficiency was found in West Virginia kindred, with some dwarfs up to age 77 y, by self-report (Rimoin et al, 1966), which would have exceeded the life expectancy for that region and time.[11] Mutations causing GH-receptor insensitivity are found in the Laron syndrome, first described in Israel (Laron, 2005). Several different GH-receptor mutations have GH signaling defects and elevated GH (Laron, 1999). Growth is impaired and adults are obese, glucose intolerant, and may be mentally retarded depending on the mutation (Shevah et al, 2005). In rural Ecuador, about 70 individuals share a point mutation in the GH receptor (*E180* splice mutant in Exon 6) (Rosenbloom et al, 1999). These inbred and isolated communities include descendants of Jewish *conversos* from the Spanish Inquisition. The *E180* mutation also occurs in Israel (Shevah et al, 2005). Findings are intriguing but incomplete. Adult dwarfs have elevated GH and very low IGF-1. Total cholesterol and LDL cholesterol may be elevated (Rosenbloom et al, 1999). Death from heart disease of a man at 55 and woman at 67 was considered

---

[11]The demography of aging has advanced since the embarrassing reverses of the 'Supra-centenarians of the Caucasus,' who on a second visit gave quite different ages (Leaf, 1990). The gullibility of a reporter who showed a picture of supposed birth certificates of the alleged 'Centenarians of the Andes' was uncovered by the sharp eye of Doris Finch, who recognized them as death certificates (Finch, 1976C). Criteria for age validation have become well developed (Robine and Vaupel, 2001; Wang et al, 1998).

"uncommon." There may be 2-fold higher childhood mortality from infections (19% died before age 7 y vs. 9.7% deaths of unaffected sibs, due to diarrhea, meningitis, and pneumonia). Intelligence is considered normal (Kranzler et al, 1998), as in other *E180* carriers (Shevah et al, 2005). Dwarf mice also have normal brain development, which does not depend on blood GH or IGF-1.

Two other groups with heritable GH deficiency were not treated with GH. A Swiss kindred with the entire GH-1 gene deletion lived about 25 y less than unaffected first and second degree relatives (Besson et al, 2003). The main causes of death in the dwarfs were "infectious diseases and heart problems," not different from unaffected sibs. Other dwarfs from Krk in Croatia carry a *prop-1*–like mutation causing deficits of GH and TSH, like the Ames mouse (Laron, 2005). Several dwarfs reported their ages as 70 y or older, and tombstones indicate others lived up to 91 y.

In sum, these preliminary findings do not allow firm conclusions about potential longevity effects of human mutant GH and IGF-1. More data are needed on the health history and cause of death in relation to the number of mutant gene copies. Glucose-insulin tolerance tests are needed. The Ecuadorian studies should continue to be very productive, but GH therapy will eliminate the dwarf phenotype sooner than later. However, for most elderly who do not have clinically recognized GH deficits, there is no recognized basis for GH supplements as a general 'anti-aging' intervention (Liu et al, 2007).

The race is on to find human gene variants that increase longevity through altered metabolism (Bartke, 2005; Katic and Kahn, 2005). Centenarians may have better glucose tolerance and a lower incidence of diabetes than those of average life span, as observed in small samples from southern Italy (Paolisso et al, 1996; Paolisso et al, 1997; Paolisso et al, 2001). Centenarians may also have body mass index in a lower range (Barbieri et al, 2004). In a larger Italian sample, blood IGF-1 levels tended to decrease age (Fig. 5.11) (Bonafe et al, 2003); nonetheless, some centenarians have higher plasma IGF-1 than young adults. Longitudinal sampling is needed to resolve this hetergeneity. The IGF-1R (receptor) homozygote A+/A+ was 30% more prevalent in the oldest (median age 99 y) than younger (median 60 y) and was associated with lower IGF-1. Nonetheless, about 30% of the oldest had elevated IGF-1, which cautions against sweeping conclusions.

The Leiden 85+ Study examined six insulin pathway genes (1576 Ss, born 1883–1914) (van Heemst et al, 2005a). The strongest association was of short height with the GH-1 allele (intron SNP): female, height difference of −2 cm (p < 0.007); male, −1.9 cm (p < 0.078). The GH-1 allele also decreased mortality in females (RR, 0.80, range 0.67–0.96). Hormone levels were not reported. No allele associations were found for height or mortality with alleles of GHRHR (GH-releasing hormone receptor in the pituitary), IGF-1, insulin, and IRS1, or with two stress resistance genes, *SOD2* and *UPC2*.

Genetic risk factors for type 2 diabetes should also be considered. The *TCF7L2* gene, a putative transcription factor, has alleles that showed strong dose risk effects in a case control study in Iceland, with T/T homozygotes having 2.4-fold

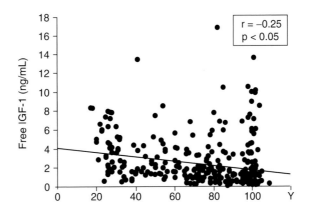

FIGURE 5.11 Blood IGF-1 levels over the adult life span. (Redrawn from Bonafe et al, 2003). All had normal liver, kidney, and thyroid functions; none was diabetic or had elevated fasting glucose (132 men, 364 women, 18–109 y; Italian Caucasians).

higher risk of diabetes (Grant et al, 2006). The T allele also predicted progression to diabetes during 3 years of observation with similar dose effects attributed to impaired pancreatic insulin secretion (Diabetes Prevention Program Study, DPP, 5847 Ss) (Florez et al, 2006). The diabetes-prone T/T allele may be the strongest genetic association with diabetes so far. The protective C allele should be examined for influences on longevity. The TCF7L2 gene is expressed in the developing pituitary and interacts with WNT signaling by binding to β-catenin downstream of PROP-1 (Douglas et al, 2001). Other candidates may be found in obesity. Kimura et al. (1997) noted that the *daf-2* worm mutant was the same as an insulin receptor mutation associated with morbid obesity. Most recently, an obesity marker single nucleotide polymorphism was mapped near the *insulin-induced gene-2* (*INSIG2*) (Herbert et al, 2006).

The genetics of diabetes gives a useful calibration for longevity gene searchers. Despite huge efforts, few general genetic influences have been found. As holds for all adult onset diseases, dominant familial genes are rare, and polygenic contributions of modest risk effects may be the norm (Florez et al, 2003). There may be few consistently strong genetic effects across human populations because of the huge number of allele combinations among the 30 longevity gene candidates scattered across the chromosomes (Christensen et al, 2006). Some may be mutually canceling, while others may synergize.

5.7.1.3. *Size and Longevity*

The association of small size and longevity is controversial. On one hand, Rollo's (2002) comprehensive meta-analysis of more than 1000 separate rodent groups, including diet restriction studies, showed statistically strong inverse correlations between maximum body size and maximal longevity (P < 0.00001). The regression coefficients account for 9–25% of the variance, depending on sex and species. As specific examples, in mice selected for different growth rates, the smallest also lived longer (Miller et al, 2000b; Miller, 2002b). It is interesting to compare the 10–15 g Ames dwarf with the 15–20 g wild-caught mice, which outlive the usual strains of inbred mice (Chapter 3, Fig. 3.3). (Here, we have a true genetic wildtype.) The Ames dwarf clearly wins, with 5 m longer average and maximum life spans than the wild mice.

However, not all of the longer-lived rodent mutants are small (Fig. 5.8). The IGF-1 receptor mutant is nearly normal in size, while the *C/EBPβ/β* and *MCAT* mutants are normal sized. Conversely, the mini and the Lewis dwarf rats have close to normal life spans, despite the reduction of body size in proportion to the Ames and Snell dwarfs. None of these mutants approach the Ames and Snell longevity.

Domestic dog breeds show strong inverse associations between plasma IGF-1 and body size versus longevity. Plasma IGF-1 ranges 10-fold across breeds, from the spaniel to the giant Newfoundland dog (Eigenmann et al, 1984; Eigenmann et al, 1988). Among these breeds, life spans vary inversely with adult size across a 3-fold range (Miller, 1999; Patronek et al, 1997). Similarly, some mouse strains at 15 m showed individual correlations of low IGF-1 with the remaining life span (Anisimov et al, 2004; Harper et al, 2003). The artificial selection of domestic dogs for size appears to parallel the rodent models, e.g., short-lived giant transgenic mice with high plasma GH (see above).

Nonetheless, robust and abundant evidence shows that human longevity has increased during the past 150 years at the same time as childhood growth increased (Section 4.4.1) (Crimmins and Finch, 2006a). Healthier children grow faster and are healthier and longer lived as adults. Small size is associated with smaller diameter coronary arteries that are at greater risk for occlusion, as is well known to vascular surgeons (Chapter 4.4.1). These observations are made in human populations exposed to challenges not experienced by lab models. These trends are also fully consistent with the allometric relationships of size and longevity in species comparisons of birds and mammals (Finch, 1990, Chapter 4) (Calder, 1984).

Nonetheless, in special cases larger size increases mortality risks. The statistics are convincing for inverse relationships of life expectancy to height in professional football and baseball players (Samaras and Elrick, 1999; Samaras et al, 2003a,b), and for premature mortality in sumo wrestlers (Section 3.4). A more general case is the association of breast cancer with higher body mass index and height (Barker et al, 1989a,b; Samaras et al, 2003a,b), e.g., the many-fold greater risk of breast cancer in Japanese women who grew up in Los Angeles versus Osaka (Henderson et al, 1984). As more humans live to greater post-reproductive, post-Darwinian ages, we should not be surprised to find many other exceptions.

5.7.1.4. *The Insulin-Sensitivity Paradox*

Nir Barzilai and colleagues describe the paradox that insulin insensitivity, e.g., metabolic syndrome increases human mortality, whereas mutant flies and worms with attenuated insulin-signaling live longer (Rincon et al, 2004). Adult humans with acquired insulin resistance (impaired insulin signaling) have increased chronic diseases (cancer, diabetes, hypertension, vascular disease) (Facchini et al, 2001). The adverse effects of insulin resistance in mammals versus the apparent benefit in fly and worm mutants may be explained by the different organization of insulin-signaling (Rincon et al, 2004). Recall from Section 5.4 that fly and worm insulin expression is largely restricted to neurons, whereas in mammals, insulin/IGF receptors are widely expressed in all tissues. Lacking information on the functions of most worm and fly insulin-like genes, it is not possible to make detailed comparisons with mammals. Even between flies and worms, different outcomes can be seen. Insulin receptor mutant worms with weak *daf-2* mutants accumulate fat (Kimura et al, 1997). This association is consistent with a human insulin receptor mutation that caused insulin resistance and hyperinsulinemia (Kim et al, 1992); the insulin receptor mutant increased life span in the worm mutant, but should decrease it in human insulin resistance. Body fat is also accumulated in flies with lower neuronal insulin mRNA (dilp-2), which should lower haemolymph insulin, but in this case life span is longer (Hwangbo et al, 2004). As noted to me by Bartke, lower IGF-1 may benefit mice more than humans because of the higher incidence of cancer in inbred mouse strains. The insulin-insensitivity paradox gives a useful platform for further discussion as additional species differences are recognized.

5.7.2. Inflammation

Inflammation gene variants are associated with mortality risks. Table 5.5 summarizes longevity gene candidates for inflammatory and lipoprotein genes, with chromosomal location. The histories of infectious exposure may have selected for certain combinations of alleles across different genes. For example, resistance to malaria may be mediated by hemoglobin variants *and* by the TNFα-promoter variant (−308) (Mombo et al, 2003). The genome projects may soon show the distribution of inflammatory gene haplotypes across human populations. IL-6 alleles at -174 may influence survival to advanced age. Further candidates may be sought in the genetic influences on plasma CRP, which is regulated by IL-6 and is a major risk indicator of vascular disease (Chapter 1, Fig. 1.16).

The IL-6 promoter has two alleles (−174G/C) that may be risk factors in longevity and vascular disease. Among Danes, the prevalence of G/G was 30% in the elderly, suggesting survival advantage (G/G allele: 25% below age 50, with

TABLE 5.5 Summary of Human Longevity Gene Candidates (see Text for References)

Gene/Chromosome; Function	Alleles	Age-Association
apolipoprotein C3 apoC3/Ch11q23; lipid binding protein mediating transfer of cholesteryl esters from HDL	−641C/A	C/C associated with centenarians
apolipoprotein E apoE/Ch19q13; cholesterol transport protein	+112C, apoE3 +112R, apoE4 −219G/T −419A/T	E4, shorter life span; higher risk of cardiovascular and Alzheimer disease T/T, myocardial infarct; G/G had higher plasma apoE and lower glucose A/A, higher apoE
cholesteryl ester transferase protein CETP/Ch16q21;	+405I/V −629C/A	+405V/V higher in centenarians combination of −629A/A and apoE4 may be 3-fold higher in Alzheimer; apoE4, did not synergize with +405I/V
interleukin-6 IL-6/Ch7p21; proinflammatory regulator	−174G/C	G/G, lower plasma IL-6, better survival to old age, vascular health, and resistance to bacterial meningitis
interleukin-10 IL-10/CH1q32; anti-inflammatory cytokine	−1082G/A	G allele elevated IL-10; elevated IL-10 may increases risk of diabetes
peroxisome proliferator-activated receptor gamma PPARγ/Ch3p25; transcription factor influences insulin sensitivity	Pro12Ala	heterozygote may increase male survival to later ages
paraoxinase-1 PON1/Ch7q21.3; protects LDL from oxidative damage	55L/M and 192R/Q	LR haplotype may increase survival to later ages

progressive increases to 32% at 100; 1710 Ss) (Christiansen et al, 2004). Finnish nonagenarians in a prospective study also had higher prevalence of the G/G allele of IL-6 (Hurme et al, 2005). Other studies indicate protective associations of 174G/G. Myocardial infarcts were 50% less frequent in older Italian G/G carriers (67 y mean) (Chiappelli et al, 2005). Older dialysis patients with G/G had lower diastolic blood pressure and left ventricular hypertrophy was 50% less frequent (Losito et al, 2003). G/G carriers were more likely to survive bacterial meningitis (Balding et al, 2003), which may be due to lower plasma IL-6 (Bonafe et al, 2001; Chiappelli et al, 2005). IL-6 elevations are risk indicators of vascular events (Chapter 1) and frailty (Ershler and Keller, 2000; Wilson et al, 2002; von Kanel et al, 2006).

IL-6 is also linked to plasma CRP by directly controlling CRP synthesis in the liver. Plasma CRP was lower in IL-6 −174G/G carriers (Ferrari, 2003). Moreover, plasma CRP levels showed strong heritability in association with IL-6 −174 G/G (Vickers et al, 2002). (The IL-1 and CRP genes are not chromosomally linked.) However, in younger ages, the IL-6 −174 G/C alleles have not been consistently associated with blood IL-6 levels (Qi et al, 2006). CRP levels are also influenced by alleles of IL-1 (Latkovskis et al, 2004) and of apoE (Austin et al, 2004; Rontu et al, 2006). CRP alleles at four different sites in the gene may influence plasma

CRP levels (Kovacs et al, 2005; Szalai et al, 2002) but have not been associated with vascular events (Zee and Ridker, 2002). The apolipoprotein E4 genotype is proinflammatory relative to apoE3 (Section 1.3.2), which may be one mechanism in the associations of apoE4 as a risk factor in Alzheimer disease, vascular disease, and frailty (discussed below).

TGF-β1 variants are also candidates in longevity. The missense allele +915C in the signal peptide of TGF-β1, which does not influence the plasma level, had lower prevalence in Italian centenarians (Carrieri et al, 2004). Survival advantages are consistent with the slower development of coronary vascular pathology after cardiac transplantation in a younger group of +915C carriers (Densem et al, 2000; Densem et al, 2004).

TNFα alleles (−308G/A) influence TNFα synthesis, as discussed in Chapter 3 for links to adiposity, insulin resistance, and hypertension. These TNFα alleles also influence fetal growth (Section 4.9) but have not been consistently associated with longevity or coronary disease.

IL-10 alleles may influence aging through levels of plasma IL-10, which interacts with atherosclerosis, diabetes, and infections. IL-10 secretion by leukocytes in response to LPS is highly heritable (MZ twin, 0.75 heritability) (Eskdale et al, 1998; Westendorp et al, 1997a,b). Of three IL-10 promoter alleles, −1082G/A had the most effect on plasma IL-10 (Lio et al, 2004). Elevated plasma IL-10 represses IL-6 and TNFα synthesis, which are risk indicators in atherosclerosis. Elevated IL-10 predicted diabetes (Leiden 85–Plus Study) (van Exel et al, 2002). Meningococcal disease mortality was predicted by leukocyte cytokine production in first degree relatives: High IL-10 leukocyte production was associated with 20-fold more mortality; low TNFα production, 10-fold more mortality (Westendorp, 1997a,b). However, IL-10 alleles have not been consistently associated with heart disease or life span (Lio et al, 2004). We may anticipate a complex genetics, because the close proximity of IL-10 and CRP on Chromosome 1 (Section 1.3.2) generates multiple haplotypes of these common alleles.

These scattered findings suggest potential benefits to longevity in some of the same gene inflammatory gene variants that influence vascular disease risk. The IL-6 and TGF-β1 alleles merit expanded screening.

5.7.3. Lipoproteins and Cholesterol Metabolism

Familial hypercholesterolemia was recognized 70 years ago as the cause of premature heart disease by Muller in Norway (Muller, 1938; Ose and Tolleshaug, 1989). The identification of LDL-receptor defects in a rare familial hypercholesterolemia by Brown and Goldstein (1974) has stimulated remarkable advances in vascular disease intervention and prevention, as well as the molecular mechanisms in normal vascular biology. However, lipoprotein system dominant mutants have minor contributions to vascular disease in most populations and account for <5% of variance in LDL cholesterol (Breslow, 2000). Nonetheless, elevated LDL cholesterol and low HDL cholesterol are strongly linked to vascular events and are becoming understood as complex environmental interactions of multiple genes (Knoblauch et al, 2004; Stengard et al, 2006). Further developments implicate several lipoprotein gene variants in human longevity and in human evolution (Chapter 6).

Apolipoprotein E (apoE) is the most common heritable variation in lipids with major associations of the apoE4 allele to heart disease, Alzheimer disease, and longevity (Mahley, 1988; Mahley and Rall, 2000). ApoE is a cholesterol transport protein that binds to the LDL receptor and is crucial to blood cholesterol levels, and for the transport of cholesterol for steroid synthesis and neuronal outgrowth. Coding changes that influence cholesterol binding in apoE2, -E3, and -E4 may account for 10% of the variance in total cholesterol and LDL-cholesterol (Breslow, 2000; Sing and Davignon, 1985). The apoE4 allele is associated with higher total blood cholesterol and LDL-cholesterol, e.g, LDL cholesterol is 10–20 mg/dl higher in E4/E3 than E3/E3, while E3/E2 are lower by the same amount. ApoE2 is associated with the uncommon familial type III hypercholesterolemia (E2/E2), but mysteriously, only 2% of E2/E2 develop this condition. When populations varying in apoE4 prevalence are considered, the level of E4 may account for 50% of the inter-population differences in *average* total cholesterol. Effects of E4 on triglycerides and HDL -cholesterol are more variable. Besides the structural differences in the apoE isoforms, apoE promoter variants influence blood apoE and other lipids, with differences by age and gender (Frikke-Schmidt et al, 2004; Stengard et al, 2006). Myocardial infarct risk may be higher in −219T carriers (Lambert et al, 2000).

ApoE4 is associated with shorter life span and was the first human 'aging' gene identified by its near absence in centenarians (Schachter et al, 1994). The effects of E4 approximate the sex differences in life span; e.g., Danish life expectancy was 7 y shorter in E3/E4 than E3/E2 genotypes (Fig. 5.12A) (Ewbank, 2004). Of the 25% heritability of life span in Denmark, about 3.5% is attributable to apoE alleles, which is equivalent to a substantial 15% of total life span heritability. ApoE alleles also influence later age mortality. For example, at age 85, the remaining life span of those diagnosed with cardiovascular disease varied 2 years by apoE alleles (Fig. 5.12B). ApoE4 decreases in prevalence at advanced ages because of survival effects (Fig. 5.13) (Gerdes et al, 2000; Rontu et al, 2006). Relative to the E3/E3 and E4/E2 genotypes, mortality in E4 carriers is 10–14% higher, while E2 carriers have 4–12% lower mortality (Gerdes et al, 2000). For these reasons, apoE4 is considered a frailty gene (Corder et al, 2000; Gerdes et al, 2000).

ApoE4 increases the risk of coronary heart disease by 42% (comprehensive meta-analysis of 48 studies representing 58,457 Ss) (Song et al, 2004). ApoE4 also increases the risk of Alzheimer disease (Fig. 5.14A) (Borenstein et al, 2005; Corder et al, 1993; Meyer and Breitner 1998; Poirier et al, 1993; Poirier, 2005; Roses, 2006) (Section 1.6). The E4 allele shows dose effects accelerating onset age (Khachaturian et al, 2004). ApoE4 carriers in end-stage Alzheimer disease have more severe cholinergic deficits, which are implicated in the early stages of memory impairments (Fig. 5.14B, C). Nonetheless, some centenarian E4/E4 homozygotes are not demented (Khachaturian et al, 2004; Sobel et al, 1995).

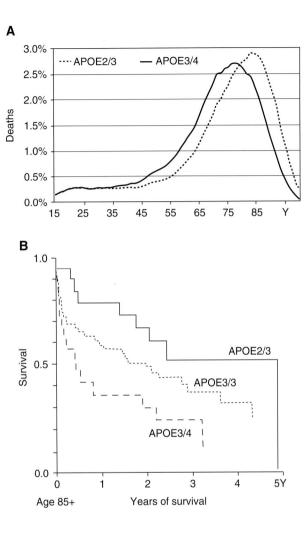

FIGURE 5.12 The apoE4 allele is associated with shorter life span and is considered a 'frailty' gene. A. Age at death of Danish E2/E3 and E3/E4 genotypes (both sexes, born in Denmark 1895–1899) for those who survived to age 15. Most common life span (peak of curve): E2/E3, 83 y; E3/E4, 77 y. (Redrawn from Ewbank, 2004.) B. Years of survival after age 85 with apoE alleles and diagnosed cardiovascular disease. Kungsholm Project cohort, a community-based study in a Stockholm neighborhood; 97 Ss with diagnosed heart disease. (Redrawn from Corder et al, 2000.)

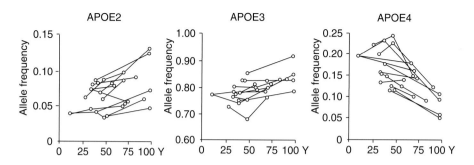

FIGURE 5.13 ApoE allele frequencies shift with advancing age. (Redrawn from Gerdes et al, 2000), based on 13 reports. The E4 allele decreases in frequency by about 50% after age 75, reflecting its promotion of frailty, arterial disease, and neurodegeneration. The initially rarer E2 allele increases in prevalence, converging to that of E4 by age 100.

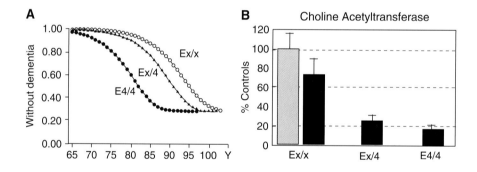

FIGURE 5.14 ApoE alleles in Alzheimer disease. A. The ApoE4 allele dose affects the onset age of Alzheimer disease but may not influence the ultimate risk. From the Cache County Utah observational study of 3308 community living elderly (90% of the population ≥ 65 y), which includes autopsy confirmation (Breitner et al, 1999; Tschanz et al, 2005). The '100-year life-time incidence' of dementia is 72%. Survivors to 100 may have lower subsequent risk of clinical dementia. While the Cache County elderly are relatively long-lived, these results are similar to apoE4 dose relationships and onset age in other populations cited in this article. (Redrawn from Khachaturian A. et al, 2004). (This Khachaturian is Ara, son of Zaven who was a founder of the Alzheimer disease field at the NIH). B. ApoE allele dose increases the cholinergic neuron damage at end stage Alzheimer disease, as estimated by choline acetyl transferase levels in the temporal cortex. (Redrawn from Poirier et al, 1995.)

Because some E4/E4 carriers reach advanced ages without dementia, apoE is not considered a genetic determinant, but rather a risk factor that influences the threshold for still mysterious early processes in neurodegeneration. The apoE4 allele show these adverse Alzheimer effects most consistently in temperate zone-derived populations and shows weaker association in Latinos and African Americans (Section 1.6.3).

ApoE3 is the most prevalent allele in human populations, while apoE4 varies over a greater range (Fig. 5.15). Reported extremes of apoE4 range from 49% (Huli, New Guinea) to 0% (Ache, Paraguay) (Demarchi et al, 2005). ApoE2 is the least prevalent allele, and least understood. Because of its low prevalence (<5%), apoE2 is not emphasized here. ApoE4 is more prevalent in Northern Europe than in the Mediterranean, and some aboriginal populations tend to have high E4 (Corbo and Scacchi, 1999; Gerdes et al, 1992; Panza et al, 2003; Demarchi et al, 2005). The European longitudinal apoE4 gradients also correlate with heart attack risk (Stengard et al, 1998). Besides Nordic caucasians, other groups with apoE4 prevalence >15% include Greenland Inuit, Central African pygmies, and Australian and New Guinea aborigines (Demarchi et al, 2005; Sing et al, 2006). Thus, there is no global generalization of apoE allele frequency with longitude or climate. The regional gradients suggest migration and possibly natural selection from interactions with nutrition and pathogen resistance (Section 5.7.4; Chapter 6).

Other lipoprotein system genes have variants that may influence longevity. Barzilai and colleagues are searching for centenarian candidate genes of vascular and metabolic disease in Ashkenazi Jews. Their first gene hit was cholesteryl ester transferase protein (CETP): in centenarians, the +405V/V alleles were 2-fold more prevalent than controls, implying survival effect (Atzmon et al, 2006; Barzilai et al, 2004). This association was confirmed in samples of Northern Italians, average age 89 (Vergani et al, 2006), but not in Italian centenarians (Cellini et al, 2005). The concurring two studies observed lower plasma CETP and elevated HDL, which is considered anti-atherogenic in human and animal studies. CETP is a lipid binding protein that mediates the transfer of cholesteryl esters from HDL. The multiple CETP alleles may account for 10% of variation in HDL (Knoblauch et al, 2004). A CETP promoter allele (−629C/A) interacts with apoE4 in Alzheimer disease (Table 5.5): The combination of apoE4 and 629A/A may be 3-fold higher in Alzheimer's; however, apoE4 did not synergize with +405I/V allele (Rodriguez et al, 2006).

The ApoC3 gene promoter allele −641 C/C homozygote was higher prevalence in centenarians (25%), than their F1 offspring (20%) or controls (10%) (Atzmon et al, 2006). The C/C genotype was associated with both longevity and lower plasma apoC, consistent with much evidence for elevated apoC as a risk of coronary disease. Plasma apoC3 is an exchangeable component of triglyceride-rich lipoproteins. By inhibiting lipoprotein lipase, blood apoC3 levels modulate the clearance of triglycerides after a meal, with low apoC3 associated with triglyceridemia. The centenarian apoC3 −C/C carriers also had favorable

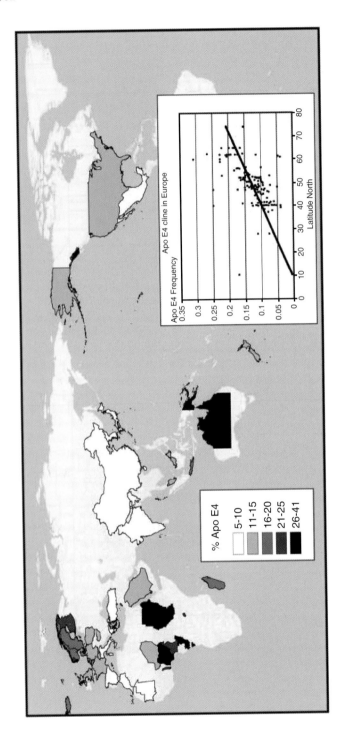

FIGURE 5.15 The geographic distribution of apoE4, shows remarkable global heterogeneity in the selected countries. Many regions show marked gradients of apoE2,3, and -4 (Panza et al, 2003; Corbo and Scacchi, 1999; Gerdes et al, 1992; Singh et al, 2006). Adapted from Singh et al, *op cit.*, Fig. 5. No data are shown for Russia and former Soviet republics, Canada, South America, most of Africa, or Indonesia. Countries show national averages, except for Australia which represents the aborigines within a central rectilinear zone (E4>26%) and other groups (mostly European) on the continent's edges (E4<15%). Note the high E4 in Papua-New Guinea. Adapted from Singh et al. *op cit.* The inset data kindly provided by Sarabijit S. Mastana, senior co-author of Singh et al, *op cit.* shows a 4-fold longitudinal gradient of apoE4 from northern Europe to the Mediterranean that corresponds to a gradient of heart attack risk (Steng et al, 1998). However, there is no global generalization of apoE alleles and longitude. This graph was developed by Jennifer Swift (USC Department of Geography).

insulin sensitivity. There is a direct link of apoC3 to insulin regulation through an insulin response element seated in the gene cluster of apoA1, apoC3, and apoA4. Promoter alleles that influence transcription rate (Dallinga-Thie et al, 2001) are among haplotypes of apoC3 implicated in type 1 diabetes (Hokanson et al, 2006).

The transcription factor PPARγ regulates genes in adipocyte differentiation, insulin sensitivity, and inflammation. Two alleles at codon 12 (pro/ala) have associations with insulin sensitivity and obesity in younger groups (de Rooij et al, 2006a; Moon et al, 2005; Muller et al, 2003; Ostergard et al, 2005) and with birth weight (Eriksson et al, 2003). The ala allele reduces transcriptional activity of PPARγ and may protect against type 2 diabetes. In very old Italian men (average 97 y), the pro/ala heterozygote was 2-fold more prevalent than in younger men; women did not show this association (Barbieri et al, 2004). The paraoxinases (PON1, -2, -3) are longevity gene candidates because of associations with heart disease (Marchegiani et al, 2006). PON1 protects LDL from oxidative damage, a by-stander effect (Section 1.4.1) and has alleles at two loci: 55L/M and 192R/Q. The LR haplotype may be slightly overrepresented in later ages, suggesting survivor effects (Rea et al, 2004).

ApoC3 also has parallels to invertebrate longevity genes through insulin-signaling and lipoproteins (Atzmon et al, 2006). ApoC3 transcriptional responses to insulin (see above) involve the transcription factor FoxO1 (Dallinga-Thie et al, 2001), an orthologue of worm *daf-16*. Moreover, levels of the lipoprotein vitellogenin influence immunity and oxidative damage in the honeybee (Section 5.4) and can influence the worm life span (Section 5.5). CETP, as a lipid binder, is in a family of proteins that bind bacterial endotoxins (LPS) and might itself be directly involved in host defense. In mammals, lipoproteins protect against oxidative stress, through associated anti-oxidants, β-carotene, discussed below. Blood lipoproteins are also remodeled during acute phase responses (acute phase HDL, Section 1.5.5). The complex lipoprotein system genetics includes haplotypes that may also influence diabetes and life span. This brief synopsis neglects other lipoprotein system gene candidates for roles in longevity, metabolic disorders, and vascular disease.

5.7.4. ApoE4 Interactions with Diet, Cognition, and Vascular Aging

Diet was not explicitly included in any of the above studies of genetic effects on longevity. Few lipoprotein gene variants have consistent effects on blood cholesterol responses to dietary changes (meta-analysis of >2500 studies) (Masson et al, 2003). ApoE4 carriers had the largest decreases of LDL cholesterol in response to reductions of dietary fat and cholesterol (nine studies); HDL cholesterol responded most in apoE4 carriers (3 of 4 studies) (Lopez-Miranda et al, 1994). The apoE promoter allele −219G/T in combination with apoE3/E3 did not influence the plasma LDL or HDL cholesterol responses to a diet shift from saturated to unsaturated fats (Moreno et al, 2005). However, glucose regulation in −219T/T genotype was relatively less sensitive to fat intake. The −219G/G carriers had lower glucose on all diets, confirming (Viitanen et al, 2001). Two other gene longevity candidates, apoC3 and CETP, also show allelic differences in LDL cholesterol responses to diet (Masson et al, 2003), but the active alleles are at different sites in these genes than those associated with longevity (apoC3, exon4 SsI; CETP, intron Taq1). Diet restriction of type 2 diabetics who were apoE4 carriers showed the most improvement in blood LDL-cholesterol (Fig. 5.16) (Saito et al, 2004). This observation recalls that mouse strains and mutants differ in responses to diet restriction; e.g., DBA/J (Fernandes et al, 1976) and GHRKO (Bonkowski et al, 2006b) show little, if any, increased life span.

ApoE4 carriers have faster carotid artery thickening after age 65 (Fig. 5.17A) (Haan et al, 1999), which is a cardiovascular risk indicator (Section 1.5, Fig 1.14). Carotid thickening may contribute to cerebral deterioration directly and indirectly. Cognitive decline after age 65 is accelerated in apoE4 carriers (Cardiovascular Healthy Study) (Fig. 5.17B) (Haan et al, 1999). ApoE4 carriers with diabetes, carotid atherosclerosis, or peripheral vascular disease showed the most cognitive loss. Similarly, E4 carriers in the healthy and high-performing elderly of the MacArthur Study of Successful Aging showed higher risk of

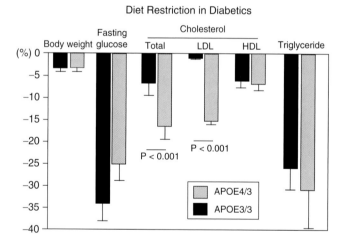

FIGURE 5.16 ApoE alleles influence response of obese diabetics to diet restriction (DR). Japanese male and female diabetics, about 60 y; BMI, 25 (moderately obese) were maintained on 25% DR for 14 d, from 33 kcal/kg body weight to 25 kcal, without altering cholesterol intake. Fasting glucose and triglycerides were lowered in all, whereas ApoE4 carriers had greater decrease of total and LDL cholesterol. (Redrawn from Saito et al, 2004.)

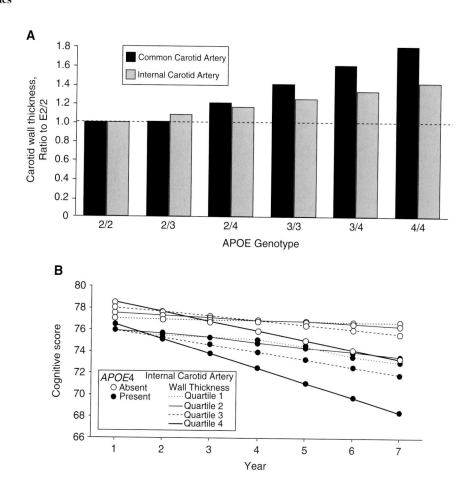

FIGURE 5.17 ApoE4 allele accelerates carotid atherosclerosis and cognitive decline, relative to apoE2/2. Cardiovascular Health Study, U.S. 5888 random Ss, 65+ y. (Redrawn from Haan et al, 1999.) A. Carotid artery thickening. Ultrasonic measurement of the mean thickness of common and internal carotid. B. Cognitive decline is increased during aging with apoE4. Each subject was tested at least twice by Modified Mini-Mental State Examination (3MSE) and Digit Symbol Substitution Test. ApoE4 carriers with diabetes, carotid atherosclerosis, or peripheral vascular disease declined the most. The majority (70%) did not show cognitive decline over up to 7 y.

cognitive decline and greater declines over 7 years (Hu et al, 2006b). The majority of elderly did not have measurable cognitive decline during 7 years in both studies. ApoE4 carriers in middle age already have reduced glucose metabolism in cerebral cortex regions (Reiman et al, 2005; Small et al, 2000) and use mnemonics extensively in compensation (Ercoli et al, 2006). Synapse density in the hippocampus granule neurons of cognitively normal elderly is also lower in apoE4 than E3 carriers (Ji, 2003). It is possible that these later deficits were present earlier.

Older apoE4 carriers with cognitive decline most likely included early Alzheimer disease and the syndrome of 'mild cognitive impairment' (MCI) (Section 1.6.3). ApoE4 is more prevalent in MCI than elderly controls and associated with greater hippocampal atrophy in proportion to the E4 allele dose; women may be more vulnerable to a single apoE4 allele than men (Farlow et al, 2004; Flatt and Kawecki, 2004; Fleisher et al, 2005). In the Cache County Study, elderly with MCI and other mild disorders were 2–5-fold more likely to develop Alzheimer disease if they were E4 carriers (Tschanz et al, 2006). These later life changes are departures from the slower and more general brain aging changes beginning during middle-age, which include synaptic atrophy and reduced blood flow (Chapter 1, Fig. 1.7). The transitions of the general brain aging changes to Alzheimer disease are not well resolved.

While apoE4 is the most common genetic risk factor for Alzheimer disease, it also synergizes with other rarer dominant genotypes to accelerate the age of onset, including the familial Alzheimer mutations in the amyloid precursor protein (APP), the presenilin mutations (PS-1 and PS-2), and in trisomy 21 (Downs syndrome). Moreover, a meta-analysis of the new AlzGene database indicates more than 10 potential other risk factor candidates, at least some of which interact with apoE alleles, e.g., apoC1, which is closely linked to apoE on chromosome 19 (Bertram et al, 2007). Combinations of risk factors on different chromosomes (Section 1.3.2) could reclassify some of the apparently sporadic cases of Alzheimer disease.

Cerebral metabolism may be slightly impaired as early as by age 30 in apoE4 carriers who have not shown clinical abnormalities (Reiman et al, 2004). Smaller head circumference increased the risk of dementia in E4 carriers 2-fold above non-E4 carriers (Borenstein et al, 2005). Because head size is driven by brain growth, we must consider the portentous question of apoE alleles on brain development. In a transgenic mouse with targeted substitution of apoE, the synaptic density was lower in E4 carriers than E3 (Wang et al, 2005a). Thus, it is possible that the lower synapse density in older E4 carriers (see above) and the trend to lower cerebral metabolism by age 30 represent developmental impairments.

ApoE alleles influence the effects of elevated plasma CRP and cholesterol, which are major vascular risk indicators. In the Finnish Vitality 90+ project (Rontu et al, 2006), plasma CRP and cholesterol varied with the apoE4 dose in opposite directions. We may anticipate additional complexities in the relationships of these risk factors to life span. In general, elevated plasma CRP and LDL-cholesterol are risk factors for vascular disease (Fig. 1.16), as is apoE4. In Finnish nonagenarians, however, some were observed to have elevated LDL-cholesterol, but low CRP. The apoE alleles partly explained the CRP-LDL status.

Plasma CRP varied inversely with the apoE4 allele dose, while LDL cholesterol increased with E4 dose. The inverse relation of the apoE4 allele dose to CRP in this age group differs from the proinflammatory associations of apoE4 in experimental and clinical contexts involving young ages (Section 1.3.2), suggesting a survivor effect that differs from the norm at advanced ages. CRP also co-varied with IL-6 over a 3-fold range, as expected from the direct control of CRP synthesis by IL-6 (Lehtimaki et al, 2005). Both reports excluded those with acute infections.

ApoE4 smokers may have higher risks of cardiovascular events than E3 smokers (Fig. 5.18) (Talmud et al, 2005). This finding if verified suggests that smoking, a powerful inflammatory stimulation, synergizes with apoE4 to accelerate atherosclerosis more than the apoE alleles (Fig. 5.17A). The incidence of atherosclerotic carotid plaques showed further synergies: apoE4, non-smokers, 1.7-fold higher risk than non-E4; E4-smokers, 3.7-fold higher risk (Djousse et al, 2002). In a different group (Caucasian diabetics), oxidized LDL cholesterol was 28% higher in E4 smokers than other genotypes or non-smokers (*op. cit.*). Furthermore, apoE4-smokers had lower serum β-carotene, an anti-oxidant (MacArthur Study of Successful Aging) (Hu et al, 2006b). One may speculate about the apoE alleles of Jeanne Calment, a regular smoker who achieved the record life span of 122 (Allard et al, 1998). The greater vulnerability of E4 carriers to oxidant damage from smoke should be examined for other proinflammatory aerosols (Chapter 2).

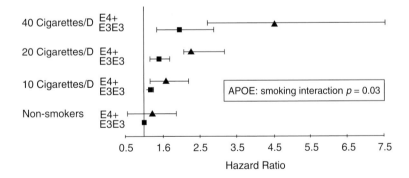

FIGURE 5.18 Smoking increased cardiovascular disease risk in apoE4 carriers from the Framingham Study (1668 Ss, 316 cardiovascular disease events). (Redrawn from Talmud et al, 2005.)

Alcohol consumption may also have different vascular risks by apoE allele. Modest regular alcohol consumption is recognized to lower risk of vascular events according to a J-shaped dose response. The coronary disease risk is about 30% lower with 1–2 drinks/d (Gronbaek, 2006), which is equivalent to 10–30 gm pure ethanol/d. Heavy drinking (>100 g/d) may increase the risk beyond heavy smoking. The mechanisms in alcohol benefit may derive from the consistently observed elevations of HDL cholesterol. However, there may be interactions of apoE4 and alcohol, because HDL elevations were smaller in apoE4 carriers of the NHLBI Family Heart Study (Djousse et al, 2004). In the Framingham Study population, apoE4 males had higher LDL cholesterol in proportion to alcohol consumption (controlled for energy intake, age, BMI, and smoking) (Corella et al, 2001; Ordovas, 2002). These effects of alcohol on LDL cholesterol could contribute to the greater 'frailty' of apoE4 carriers. Evidence is inconclusive about possible benefits from different types of alcoholic beverage and the content of resveratrol, an antioxidant and antibiotic (Section 5.4) (Baur and Sinclair, 2006; Gronbaek, 2006).

Could the benefits of exercise to vascular health and mortality (Section 3.4) be influenced by apoE alleles? Sedentary E4 carriers may have more atherogenic lipid profiles. However, findings on vascular correlates of exercise and the alleles vary between studies (Bernstein et al, 2002; Hagberg et al, 2000).

5.7.5. ApoE Alleles, Infection, and Reproduction

If apoE4 has so many adverse effects, what maintains this allele in all human populations? Collaborations with Robert Sapolsky and with Craig Stanford considered the role of apoE alleles in the evolution of the human reproductive schedule (Finch and Sapolsky, 1999; Finch and Stanford, 2004). The cognitive and vascular changes that are more severe in apoE4 carriers during middle age would impair the uniquely human multi-generational care giving. From other perspectives, Brian Charlesworth (1996) hypothesized that apoE4 is selected by some early life benefit, while George Martin (1999) proposed in a discussion of the Finch-Sapolsky article that apoE4 is a resistance factor for lipophilic pathogens. The 'Charlesworth-Martin' hypothesis thus considers that apoE4 may persist in human populations because of balancing selection with antagonistic pleiotropy. Balancing selection is a major factor in life-history gene evolution (Finch and Rose, 1995) (Section 1.2.8).

A strong case is emerging for the protective effect of apoE4 in infections by hepatitis C virus (HCV). ApoE4 carriers had milder liver disease in two independent studies (Fabris et al, 2005; Wozniak et al, 2002). The progression to hepatic fibrosis was worsened in proportion to E4 dose. Moreover, female E4 carriers progressed faster to fibrosis than males. Hepatitis virions associate with plasma LDL and HDL, and cell uptake is mediated by LDL receptor. We do not know if apoE isoforms alter virion transport or uptake.

Other examples indicate apoE allele interactions with the brain during childhood and later in life. In a Brazilian favela with poor hygiene, preadolescent apoE4 carriers had better cognitive scores (Oria et al, 2005). The apoE4 carriers had 15% fewer episodes of diarrhea and less *Giardia*. The cognitive benefits may be due to higher plasma cholesterol of E4 carriers, which might support brain neuronal outgrowth and myelination (Oria et al, 2005), particularly in lower birth weights (Garces et al, 2002). Although head circumference did not differ by apoE genotype in this study, childhood growth can be stunted by heavy diarrhea (Section 4.6). Later in life, Alzheimer disease shows a higher prevalence of apoE4 carriers with HSV-1 infections (Itzhaki, 2004). However, HSV-1 is neither necessary nor sufficient for Alzheimer disease. The HSV-1 load in Alzheimer disease may be a bystander consequence of HSV-1, which is a ubiquitous and opportunistic infection. ApoE4 carriers with Alzheimer disease also had higher brain load of *Chlamydia pneumoniae* (Gerard et al, 2005), which may represent opportunistic infections during brain degeneration, as indicated for associations of *Chlamydia* with arterial disease (Section 2.2.2).

The hypothesis that ApoE4 is maintained by balancing selection requires some evidence of associations with fecundity. The apoE gene is deeply linked to reproduction because the apoE protein is the major transporter of the cholesterol used by gonadal cells for sex steroid synthesis. However, apoE alleles have not shown consistent associations with sex steroid levels or age at menarche (about 10 papers, not cited). Adult fertility may differ slightly by allele according to mostly small samples from different populations: Danish men (Gerdes et al, 1996), women from Southern Italy (Corbo, 2004), African-Ecuadorian women (Corbo et al, 2004b). These European E3/3 carriers had slightly greater fertility than E3/4. In possible contrast, African-Ecuadorian women with E3/4 tended to have more children (significance only in a subgroup with 9–17 children). While this might suggest a later age at menopause in apoE3/4 carriers, others found little association of menopause and the apoE alleles: Iranian E4 carriers had earlier menopause by about 1 year (Koochmeshgi et al, 2004), whereas no E3/E4 difference in age at menopause was found in Down's syndrome (Schupf et al, 2003) or in large sample of German women (Tempfer et al, 2005). Postmenopausal plasma sex steroids do not differ consistently by apoE alleles, e.g., in a large U.S. study (Barrett-Connor and van Muhlen, 2003).

In sum, apoE4 allele benefits to hepatitis C virus infections support the Charlesworth-Martin hypothesis that apoE4 is maintained by balancing selection. The neurocognitive protection of apoE4 during childhood diarrhea could account for the higher prevalence of E4 in some equatorial populations (Fig. 5.15). The major effect of apoE alleles is on vascular and cognitive health during middle age and later. It is within this uniquely human 'aging' domain that the human apoE allele system evolved (Finch and Sapolsky, 1999; Finch and Stanford, 2004), discussed next in Chapter 6. Other allele systems with disease-longevity effects (Table 5.5) could also be interpreted by balancing selection.

5.8. SUMMARY

Genetic influences on aging in general populations are clear in the lower mortality risk of women throughout life. We do not know which genes on the sex chromosomes determine disease and mortality risks. The best characterized human 'aging' gene is apoE on chromosome 19 with two alleles, apoE3 and E4. The less common apoE4 allele consistently increases the risk of arterial disease and Alzheimer disease. Many other adverse effects characterize apoE4 as a frailty gene with an impact during mid-life and later. The persistence of the apoE4 allele may be due to balancing selection for pathogen resistance, as shown for hepatitis virus C and possibly other infections. Two lipoprotein system gene variants are associated with survival to advanced ages, apoC3 and CETP. All three genes influence blood cholesterol responses to diet. IL-6 alleles influence vascular disease and possibly survival to advanced age. The main gene candidates for longevity thus are lipoprotein and inflammatory system genes, which are strongly associated with vascular disease. Although the heritability may be minor in the individual variations, careful analysis of gene x environment interactions will be fruitful in identifying potential interventions, as precedented by responses to diet in the lipoprotein gene variants.

Animal model studies, however, have focused on a different set of genes, those connected with growth and metabolism. Mutants causing decreased insulin-IGF-1 signaling in the worm, fly, and mouse are long-lived and often accumulate fat. In humans, impaired insulin signaling (insulin insensitivity) is characteristic of diabetes, which increases mortality in association with vascular disease. Small size is not consistently associated with longevity and may increase vascular mortality. Historical improvements in adult life span are strongly associated with faster growth during childhood and larger adult height (Chapter 2). Future studies may develop further links of the insulin-IGF-1 model mutants to vascular disease.

Genetic influences on life span are now clearly seen in a physiological context that involves nutrition, hormones, and especially, interactions with pathogens in my view. A remarkable convergence and overlap of gene systems is emerging. Interactions of p53 and sirtuins with insulin signaling in responses to pathogens may be anticipated. Neuroendocrine seats of regulation of these complex interactions are also recognized by the clinical and experimental communities, in the importance of hypothalamic regulation of eating behavior and spontaneous activity, and in the neuronal expression of mutant genes that influence longevity of flies and worms. These recent findings support the concept that neuroendocrine systems can be pacemakers of aging (Dilman, 1971; Finch, 1973a; Finch and Rose, 1995; Finch and Ruvkun, 2001).

The longevity of the insulin system mutants may depend on a highly protected environment; e.g., hypopituitary humans and mice may have higher mortality from infections. Insulin resistance, as modeled in worms and fly mutants, also decreases resistance to stress and infectious disease in humans. Long-lived worm mutants with impaired insulin-like signaling were out-competed by non-mutants in two studies. We must consider the possibility that the long-lived mutants are a 'hot-house' phenomenon with genotypes that may not enhance longevity in dirtier and more complex 'real' environments. The next, and last, chapter considers the dirty and invasive environments within which humans evolved and which may be worsening through global warming and urbanization.

CHAPTER 6

The Human Life Span: Present, Past, and Future

6.1. INTRODUCTION

Human longevity may have evolved in two major stages. From an ancestral ape, 5 million years ago (MYA) or more, life spans doubled during the evolution of *H. sapiens* (Fig. 6.1, Table 6.1). We can not know the actual trajectory of change, which could have included fluctuations with decreases, as well as increases in life span during these several hundred thousand generations of Darwinian selection. Then, in less than 10 generations during the Industrial Revolution, life span doubled again, through processes that are seated in technology and culture, rather than genetic changes, particularly advances in hygiene, medicine, and public health, and improved nutrition and water (Section 2.5), which also increased adult height (Section 4.4).

Some aging processes have been slowed relative to the great apes, despite increased exposure to infectious pathogens, inflammogens, toxins, and cholesterol-rich foods. The slowing of aging and the increase of longevity despite greater inflammatory exposures is paradoxical: Arterial disease, Alzheimer disease, and some cancers involve inflammatory processes (Chapter 1) that may be accelerated by infection and inflammation (Chapter 2) and fatty diet (Chapter 3). Conversely, diet restriction, opposite of the human preference, attenuates many of these conditions. Frequent food shortages are likely to have been the norm. Maternal metabolism and fetal growth are depressed by malnutrition yet still allow sufficient adult reproduction (Chapter 4). Variants of genes of insulin-signaling and lipid metabolism (Chapter 5) may have facilitated these evolutionary changes.

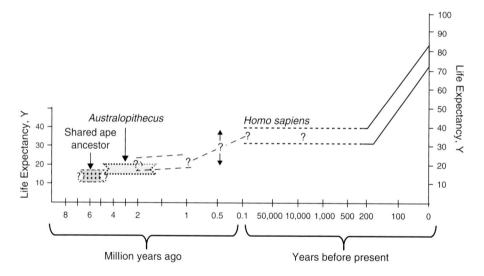

FIGURE 6.1 Evolution of the human life expectancy (LE), a speculative sketch of changes from shared ape-human ancestor 5–7 million years ago (MYA) to the 20th century. Also see Fig. 1.1 legend. The shared ancestor is predicted to have had LE like chimpanzees, 10–20 y LE at birth and a minority surviving beyond 40 (Table 6.1). *Australopitheus* and early *Homo* may have lived slightly longer than the great apes in proportion to their larger body and brain size (allometric relationships) (Table 6.1, Section 6.2.4). Skeletal evidence is insufficient to determine the age structure and LE of prehistoric populations (Section 6.2.4). The gradual increase of LE in the genus *Homo* reached 30–40 some unknown time after 0.2 MYA when anatomically modern *H. sapiens* emerged, and possibly before the initial spread into Eurasia. The suggested 30–40 LE y range for prehistoric *H. sapiens* is extrapolated from that of human foragers and other pre-industrial populations (Fig. 1.1A) (Table 6.1). The model age of adult death in those surviving to age 15 is about 70 in hunter-gatherers; 72, Sweden 1751; 85, U.S., 2002 (Gurven and Kaplan, 2007). In most of these populations, >25% of adult deaths are older than the mode. Further longevity increases after 1750 in industrializing countries follows the 'best case' curve of Oeppen and Vaupel, 2000 (Fig. 1.1A, right panel).

TABLE 6.1 Stages in the Evolution of the Human Life Span, Brain, and Body Size

Stage, YBP	Species	Life Span Median	Life Span Maximum	Brain, cc (95% CI)	Body, kg (95% CI)
I, 7–5 million	chimp-human ancestor[a]	13 y	50+ y	400	30–40
II, 4–3	*Australopithecus afarensus*	?	?	458 (335–580)	39 (32–45)
III, 1.2–0.2	*Homo erectus*[b] Early Pleistocene	?	?	1003 (956–1051)	61 (55–66)
IV, 0.6–0.1	*H. heidelbergensis*[b]	?	?	1204 (1130–1278)	71 (62–80)
V, 0.15–0.1	*H. sapiens*[b]/activity (Late Pleistocene)	30–40[e]?	80 y?	1418 (1384–1452)	64 (63–66)
75,000–36,000	/hunter-foragers[c]	?	?	1498	76
21,000- 10,000	/hunter-foragers[c,d] (Late Upper Pleistocene)	?	?	1466	63
<10,000	/sedentism-agriculture	?	?		
present	worldwide[d]	64 y	122 y	1349	58 (55–61)

a. The shared ancestor is predicted to have had a life expectancy (LE) at birth, approximating that of wild chimps (Section 6.2.2), range 10–16 y, with average 12.9 (av. female, 14.6, and male, 11.2) (Hill et al, 2001). Sizes from Skinner and Wood, 2006.
b. *H. heidelbergensis* is in a daughter lineage of *H. erectus* that spread after 600,000 YBP in Europe and possibly Asia, and is a possible shared ancestor of *H. sapiens* and *H. neanderthalensis*.
c. Hypothesized to resemble current hunter-foragers (Fig. 1.1A). About 60% of foragers survive to age 15, when their remaining life expectancy (q_{15}) is about 35+, or 2-fold longer than the chimpanzee q_{15} of 15 (wild) and 23 (captive): Foragers and pre-industrial small societies, mean 36.7 [30.6-41.7, 95% confidence intervals] calculated from Hiwi, 28; Hadza, 33; Kung, 35; Ache, 38; Yanamomo, 41; Tsimane, 42; data from Gurven et al, 2007. These LE's approximate those of preindustrial England, 1541–1741 (Oeppen and Vaupel, 2000): mean 36.7, [30.6-41.7, 95% CI] (Oeppen and Vaupel, 2000).
d. Global life span (LE at birth) from Fig. 1.1 legend; maximum life span, Jeanne Calment (Allard et al, 1998); brain and body size from (Ruff et al, 1997).
e. I chose not to present encephalization coefficient (EQ), a ratio of brain to body size, because of the lack of consensus on the allometric coefficient chosen and the variations between taxonomic orders (Balazs Horvath, 2007). Most analyses use EQ = brain mass/$(11.22 \times$ body mass$)e^{0.76}$, calculated from a broad sample of mammals (Martin, 1981). However, a more detailed analysis of primates showed the best fit to $e^{0.92}$ (Pagel and Harvey, 1988). It would be helpful to further resolve the EQ for the great ape clade and to account for the statistical uncertainties in size measurements (Auerbach and Ruff, 2004; Skinner and Wood, 2006). Two general trends seem clear during the last 2 million years: pre-*Homo* species had smaller bodies and brains, and the brain volume evolved faster than body height.

This chapter explores a new hypothesis that the pathogenic pathways in the chronic diseases of adult life were also critical to the evolution of longer human life spans *ab origine*. During evolution, our diet changed radically with major increase in cholesterol intake, as hunting and scavenging skills and technology advanced to allow a meat-rich diet. Moreover, humans were increasingly exposed to infections and inflammation from raw meat and later through high-density settlements with domestic excreta and smoky air. Besides containing enteric parasites and pathogenic bacteria, feces attract insects that are frequent vectors of infections. We do not know if the great recent reduction of infant mortality from decreased infections has modified the human gene pool by allowing survival of pathogen- or stress-sensitive genotypes.

The Queries of Section 1.1 will guide discussion of mechanisms fundamental to the evolution of human aging. Bystander damage from locally acting free radicals is emphasized to focus on proximal causes of molecular and cellular aging. These examples may be central to human evolution.

(I) Oxidative stress stimulates chronic inflammatory processes; e.g., glycotoxins in food that increase plasma oxidative markers also increase plasma CRP (human) and accelerate foam cell accumulation in aortic lesions (rodent) (Section 2.4.2.).

(II) Inflammation causes further bystander damage; e.g., particulate aerosols caused less lung damage in mice overexpressing extra-cellular SOD (Section 1.4.1).

(III) Diet and environmental pathogens influence chronic diseases with inflammatory components through bystander damage; e.g., *Chlamydia pneumoniae* accelerated arterial disease in hyperlipidemic rodents (Section 2.2.2).

Human evolution was dependent on attenuating bystander inflammatory damage to maintain health during the prolonged postnatal development and delayed onset of reproduction.

6.2. FROM GREAT APE TO HUMAN

6.2.1. Human Life History Evolution

During hominin[1] evolution, life spans have more than doubled. Based on the life spans of the current great apes (Finch and Stanford, 2004; Gurven et al, 2007), the shared ancestor may have had a life expectancy at birth of under 20 years (Fig. 6.1, Table 6.1). The even shorter life spans of prosimians and monkeys implies that trends for increasing longevity with multiple births per pregnancy (polytocy) co-evolved in hominids with a life history schedule of singleton births, extended maternal care, and prolonged maturation (Fig. 6.2).

Humans are distinctive among primates for the greatest longevity and most prolonged maturation. We also evolved a unique social system of multi-generational caregiving and resource transfer to the Young (Hawkes, et al. 1998; Hawkes, 2006; Hill and Hurtado, 1996; Hrdy, 1981, 2005; Lee et al, 2003; Kaplan and Robson, 2002). The evolution of human longevity is hypothesized to be an outcome of selection for low mortality during prolonged maturation that also selected for lower mortality in older individuals who comprise the critical multi-generational human social matrix. In

---

[1]The 'order' primate has two suborders: prosimians and anthropoids. The anthropoids (resembling man) include apes and monkeys. The hominoids includes the four extant genera of humans (*Homo*) and the great apes: chimpanzee and bonobo (*Pan*), *Gorilla*, and orangutan (*Pongo*). Hominins are a subdivision, encompassing all human ancestors from the last common ancestor with Pan, with humans as the only living representative. The expanding list of extinct hominins includes *Homo ergaster* and *H. erectus*, and the genera *Ardipithecus* and *Australopithecus* listed in text.

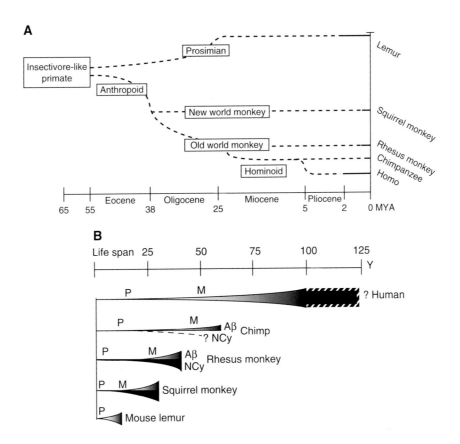

FIGURE 6.2 Human and primate evolution, life span, and Alzheimer-like changes.
A. Phylogeny. Solid lines indicate the depth of the fossil record; dotted lines indicate implied ancestors. Hominin lineages include early *Homo* (2 MYA), *Australopithecus* (4.5 MYA, extinct lineage), and possibly *Orrorin* (6 MYA, extinct lineage). Pongid lineages include *Pongin* (gorilla, 1 MYA) and *Sivapithecus* (12.5 MYA, extinct lineage). Pan lineages include chimpanzee (0.55 MYA), *Gorilla* (no fossils), and *Morotopithecus* (20 MYA, extinct lineage). From information in (Carroll, 1988; Grehan, 2006; Tappen and Wrangham, 2000). Earlier lineages are approximated: divergence of platyrrhines (New World monkeys) and catarrhines (Old World monkeys and hominoids), 40 MYA; ape (hominoid) and Old World monkey divergence, 28 MYA (median value in range of studies, ranging 20-47 MYA) (Kumar et al, 2005; Steiper and Young, 2006). B. Life history: P, puberty; M, menopause; Alzheimer-like neurodegeneration is represented by extra-cellular brain Aβ amyloid deposits and NCy (neurocytoskeletal changes with aging, which include neurofibrillary tangles), reviewed in (Finch and Sapolsky, 1999; Finch and Stanford, 2004).

addition to the special role of grandmothers hypothesized by Hawkes and colleagues, input to the young is often provided by less directly related older and younger members of traditional communities (alloparenting) (Hrdy, 1981, 2005).

The shared ancestor of humans and the great apes is obscure. It seems best not to designate the shared ancestor by genus or species name because few hominid species persist in evolutionary time for more than 3–5 million years. DNA sequence evidence consistently shows that humans are more similar to the chimpanzee than gorilla or orangutan (Chen and Li, 2001; Wildman et al, 2003). If DNA insertions-deletions (indels) are accounted for, then the overall similarity is about 95%, which equates to >40 million nucleotide differences (Britten, 2002). Gene expression profiles in the brain (anterior cingulate cortex) also concur with the 'sister grouping' of humans and chimps (Uddin et al, 2004). The time of divergence from a shared ancestor in Africa is estimated as 5–7 MYA (Kumar et al, 2005).

There are precious few fossils of hominins in the crucial time range 5–10 MYA (Fig. 6.2A): one possible chimpanzee fossil (0.55 MYA) and gorilla (1 MYA), but no orangutan. From 4.4–7 MYA (Upper Miocene), *Ardipithecus* and *Orrorin* in East Africa and *Sahelanthropus* in the present Sahara (Chad) are candidate ancestors of *Australopithecus* (4.1 MYA) and of *Homo* (1.8 MYA) (Brunet et al, 2002; Guy et al, 2005; White et al, 2006).

The poor resolution of these lineages and their inter-relationships have lead some scholars to challenge the definition of 'hominid' (Cela-Conde and Ayala, 2003). Many anatomical and behavioral traits of humans show greater similarity to orangutans than chimps (Grehan, 2006; Schwartz, 2004). Moreover, the chimp dentition resembles the orangutan more than other hominids (Pickford, 2005). Nonetheless, most agree that these early anthropoids were likely to have used bipedal postures. Bipedal movement on the ground and during arboreal foraging varies widely between chimp communities and may be a learned behavior (Stanford, 2006). Upper limb injury may also increase bipedalism, suggesting a different link of human evolution to risky behavior.

The unknown shared ancestor may have had a life expectancy of about 15 y, based on the life expectancy at birth of chimpanzee and other great apes (Table 6.1, note c). Maximum life spans are under 60 y in the wild and in captivity, with one likely exception.[2] Far more is known about chimpanzee aging than other great apes. Survival plots show major differences between chimpanzees and selected human populations with high mortality relative to health-rich populations (Gurven et al, 2007). Fig. 6.3A compares 'pre-industrialized' foragers (hunter-gatherers), acculturated foragers, and a reference high-mortality historical population, mid-18th century Sweden. Mortality rates (Fig. 6.3B) and the ratios of mortality in these groups (Fig. 6.3C) demonstrate the critical feature that at *all* ages, wild chimps have higher mortality than foragers. Humans and chimpanzees diverge further after sexual maturity. Wild chimps aged 15 live about 15

---

[2]A new record may be held by Cheeta, birth recorded in 1932 and living in the CHEETA Primate Sanctuary (Palm Springs) (Roach, 2003), but judge for yourself.

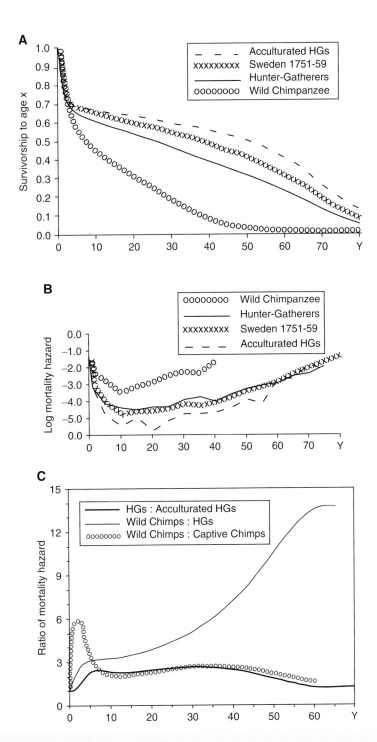

FIGURE 6.3 For legend see page 380.

more y. In great contrast, human foragers aged 15 live 40 or more y, with a modal age at death of about 70 (Fig. 6.1 legend) (Gurven and Kaplan, 2007). Thus, the chimp mean adult life span is about 60% shorter than foragers (Hill et al, 2001). I suggest that Paleolithic humans lived about as long as the current remaining foragers, 30–40 y. In the past 200 y, life span doubled again in health-rich populations (developed nations) (Fig. 6.1) (Table 6.1) (Chapter 2.4).

While humans have evolved remarkable longevity for a primate, this trend was already established in the apes, which live twofold longer than monkeys or prosimians (Fig. 6.2B). The four great ape species have single births spaced at long intervals, 4.5 to 10 y, with females becoming reproductive by age 10–15 (Fig. 6.4) (Wich et al, 2004; Goodall, 1986; Robson et al, 2006). Singleton births and prolonged maternal care characterize the four great apes, suggesting a long-standing trait of the hominid lineage of 10 million or more years. The postnatal development of humans thus further extends the canonical ape pattern of prolonged child care and postnatal development.

Great apes and humans also differ importantly in age at weaning and age at first birth (Sellen, 2006; Sellen, 2001; Wich et al, 2004; Kramer, 2004; Kennedy, 2005; Goodall, 1986). In natural fertility conditions, humans are weaned by 2–2.5 y, whereas chimps and other great apes delay weaning to age 5–10. The delayed weaning also delays the next pregnancy. The shorter intervals between successive births enables humans to reproduce more frequently, a crucial advantage that enabled progressive increases in early human population growth.

Human maturation is also prolonged. First births are delayed by 5 or more beyond the norm in great apes, and in some pre-industrial societies, occur as late as 20 (Robson et al, 2006; Wich et al, 2004; Gurven et al, 2006, 2007). Acquisition of skills for hunting extends the training period for full independence and adult competence beyond the maturation of other hunting mammals that are better equipped with specialized claws and teeth. Even after sexual maturation, further skills are acquired for hunting into the late 20s and possibly 30s (Gurven et al, 2006, 2007; Kaplan et al, 2000). It may not be trivial that modern professional training takes about as long as the acquisition of hunting prowess in foragers. Brain myelin maturation continues in humans into the third and fourth decades (Bartzokis et al,

FIGURE 6.3 (continued) Chimpanzee and human mortality across the life span. Three human populations have high mortality relative to modern industrial populations: Hunter-gatherers (foragers), acculturated hunter-gatherers (HGs), and pre-industrial Sweden 1751–1759. (Redrawn from Gurven et al, 2007). A. Survival curves. B. Log mortality curves showing the higher life-long mortality rates in chimpanzees. By age 5, all human populations have less mortality than chimps. Mortality accelerates later and less rapidly in humans. C. Mortality ratios of foragers (traditional and acculturated) and chimps (wild and captive). At all ages, wild chimps have higher mortality than hunter-gatherers, with accelerating differences after sexual maturity. Captivity decreases chimp mortality, particularly before age 10, but not to the lower levels in foragers.

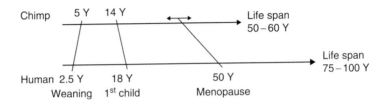

FIGURE 6.4 Chimpanzee and human life history compared, showing the major difference in age at weaning and age at first birth. In natural fertility conditions, humans are weaned by 2–2.5 y, whereas chimps and other great apes delay weaning up to age 5–10 (Kennedy, 2005; Sellen, 2006). Puberty and first births are delayed by 5 or more in humans. However, chimpanzee menopause may be earlier (Videan et al, 2006).

2003; Sowell et al, 2001), and may be critical to the later acquisition of high-speed complex processing of executive functions and emotional controls that enable hunting and other cooperative human activities (Finch and Stanford, 2004).

Reproductive senescence may be earlier in chimpanzees than humans, but evidence is mixed. On one hand, several chimpanzees (the famous Flo and her daughter Fifi of the Gombe study area) had successful pregnancies after age 40 (Finch and Stanford, 2004; Goodall, 1983). However, cycles may lengthen after age 30 (Videan et al, 2006), while continuing in some individuals up to nearly age 50, just before death (Graham, 1979; Gould et al, 1981). Tentatively, chimp perimenopause may begin earlier than in humans, but may last longer in some individuals into the human age range. The few aged chimp ovaries examined show definitive loss of ovarian oocytes as in human menopause (Gould et al, 1981). In any case, the higher mortality in chimps enforces a much shorter average reproductive duration than in humans.

Only the mother gives child care in the chimp and orangutan, while the male gorilla is protective and regularly plays with his kid (Table 6.2) (Allman et al, 1998). However, a few primates have extensive paternal roles in child care: The Siamang (lesser ape) and Titi monkey fathers carry their infants and develop close bonds with their offspring. The sex survival ratios are also correlated with the level of paternal behaviors. Chimp males have the lowest relative survival, while human males are the most favored among the great apes. One view of the ethnographic-anthropological evidence is that men mainly supply economic support, but give limited direct child care. Allman and colleagues hypothesize that the greater paternal role selected for increased relative life expectancy in these species.

These behavioral shifts in paternal roles suggest alterations in the Y chromosome that determine male phenotypes. Among the 60 active genes on the human Y chromosome, chimps incurred inactivating mutations in several genes that

TABLE 6.2 Sex Ratios of Survival in Anthropoids

Species	Survival Ratio, F/M	Male Care
Chimpanzee	1.42	rare
Orangutan	1.27	rare
Gorilla	1.13	protective, plays with kids
Human (Sweden 1780)	1.05	economic support, some care
Siamang (lesser ape)	0.92	carries infant in second year
Titi monkey	0.83	carries infant from birth

From (Allman et al, 1998). Ratios rounded off. Chimpanzee and bonobo fathers are also observed to play with infants (Enomoto, 1990). However, these males do not remain with the females or their children, unlike the gorilla, which stays with his harem, and may even protect infants from other members of the group, including juveniles (Whitten, 1987).

remain functional in humans (Hughes et al, 2005). The Y chromosomes also differ in the number of *alu* sequences and other repetitive 'mobile' elements and other non-coding sequences that influence gene expression (Kuroki et al, 2006). The great ape Y chromosomes show unusually extensive structural differences, indicating major reorganization in recent evolution: translocation of 100 kb DNA from chromosome 1 to the Y of a shared ancestor and, in humans, two subsequent inversions and a deletion (Wimmer et al, 2005). Although mutations in coding sequences are a main focus of genetic studies, chromosome reorganization can induce position effects in gene expression. The relationships of these mutational and structural changes to male phenotypes is unknown.

In addition to greater paternal involvement with longer male survival than is the norm, humans evolved multi-generational care giving lacking in great apes and other primates (Hawkes et al, 1998; Hill and Hurtado, 1996; Packer et al, 1998; Robson et al, 2006). Theoretical models show the importance of intergenerational resource transfer on mortality (Lee et al, 2003) and brain evolution (Kaplan and Robson, 2002). Our social networks allow earlier weaning and much shorter birth intervals, typically 2–3 years in natural fertility, relative to great ape norms. Traditional human societies provide child care and feeding, which allows rapidly succeeding pregnancies before the child is self-sufficient (Hrdy, 2005; Kaplan et al, 2000; Kaplan and Robson, 2002; Larke and Crews, 2006).

Also unlike the great apes, human birth is usually assisted. The increasing size of the human head requiring fetal rotation makes parturition more dangerous for mother and child, the human "obstetrical dilemma" from feto-pelvic disproportion (Rosenberg and Trevathan, 1996, 2002). In contrast, labor in the great apes "... *occurs speedily and rarely with difficulty....* [due to] *exceptionally wide birth canals...*" (Schultz, 1969, p. 154). By the pelvic geometry, Australopithecenes and early *Homo* up through 0.7 MYA had easy, non-rotational births (Rosenberg, 1996; Trevathan, 2000; Rosenberg and Trevathan, 2002; Ruff,

1996; Abitbol, 1996a,b). The increasing feto-pelvic disproportion would have increased mortality at a critical time in brain evolution (Section 6.2.4).

The 3-fold lower human mortality before maturation relative to chimps (Fig. 6.3C) has huge importance to evolution of the human life history by allowing even later maturation with sufficient survival (Fig. 6.4). The later onset of first births in humans, about 19–20 in traditional hunter-foragers (Robson et al, 2006; Walker et al, 2006a), would not allow sufficient reproduction if mortality was as high as in the great apes. Fossil evidence does not inform when this major demographic shift occurred.

Less contact with feces and lower density physical contact are further differences of major importance to the level of infection and inflammation. [These concepts are being developed in collaboration with Robert Sapolsky.] Great apes typically make individual night nests, into which they defecate and urinate in the morning before departure (Goodall, 1986, p. 208, p. 545; Carel van Shaik, pers. comm.). Night nest reuse is uncommon in chimps and orangutans, and both species fastidiously avoid contact with feces and urine. Their daily movements, personal hygiene, and the largely arboreal habitat would reduce exposure to infections from organisms supported by excreta that are nutrient-rich and biotrophic. Only mothers and their single child sleep next to each other, which also reduces exposure to communal infections. Moreover, groups are usually small, rarely as large as 30 individuals (ape communities change frequently by fission and fusion). Nonetheless, diarrhea and parasitic diseases are ubiquitous in feral ape populations (Goodall, 1986, pp. 93–96). Human societies have consistently even higher exposure to their excreta and other biotrophic wastes from their sedentism at higher density and numerous infants and small children. Even migratory hunter-gatherers typically maintain base camps for extended times that typically accumulate feces.

6.2.2. Chimpanzee Aging

Corresponding to the earlier mortality acceleration in chimps, physical signs of aging begin about 20 years earlier [see detailed reviews (Finch and Sapolsky, 1999; Finch and Stanford, 2004)]. Wild chimps often look decrepit by their adult life expectancy because of sagging skin, dental damage, and traumatic injuries from fighting and falls (Goodall, 1986, p. 104). At later ages, movements are slowed and tree-climbing is more difficult. Emaciation is common before death. Bone thinning (Lovell, 2000) and benign prostatic hyperplasia (BPH) (Steiner et al, 1999) are noted by age 40. Female reproductive cycles lengthen in the 30s with trends to increasing FSH and LH that are characteristic of peri-menopause (Videan et al, 2006). However, by ovarian histology, menopause with oocyte depletion may occur after 50 in some individuals, as in humans (Gould et al, 1981; Graham, 1979; Graham et al, 1979). In feral populations, most chimpanzees die before reaching menopause.

Another major species difference is that neurodegenerative changes are very mild by age 50. The few brains of chimps and orangutans examined had limited Aβ in plaques and arteries (congophilic angiopathy), but no neurofibrillary degeneration or large neuron loss (Erwin et al, 2002; Gearing et al, 1997). In contrast, macaque monkeys have earlier and heavier Aβ amyloid deposits by age 30, as does the gray mouse lemur by age 10 (reviewed in Finch and Sapolsky, 1999). These species differences must involve differences in amyloid metabolism (expression, processing, catabolism, and clearance) because all primates have the same Aβ peptide sequence (Section 1.2.2). Moreover, gene expression profiling showed little similarity in aging changes between chimp and human cerebral cortex (Fraser et al, 2005). The great apes may have fewer Alzheimer-type changes because their apoE is functionally more like apoE3 than apoE4 and possible dietary effects linked to the human intake of fat and metals from meat-eating (see below).

Lacking Alzheimer-like changes, chimps are vulnerable to arterial pathology [detailed summary of the scattered data in (Finch and Stanford, 2004), Table 6.3 and notes]: At autopsy of wild chimps shot for this purpose in the old Belgian Congo, 2/4 adults of unknown ages had aortic plaques (Vastesaeger and Delcourt, 1961). At the Yerkes Primate Center breeding colony, all adults had fatty lesions in the aorta and cerebral arteries, which were further increased by fatty diets (Andrus et al, 1968). At one time, chimpanzees were considered the "perfect model" for human arterial disease (Bourne and Sandler, 1973). Blood cholesterol was elevated to clinical levels in captive chimps and possibly in gorilla and orangutan (Table 6.3). Some studies, but not all (Finch and Stanford, 2004, pp. 14–15), observed extreme sensitivity to diet-induced hypercholesterolemia and to arterial disease. The older literature suggests that, even on 'normal diets,' sudden death from heart attacks and strokes may be common (Finch and Stanford, 2004, Table 1, footnote 3; Table 3B, and Appendix). Tooth wear is extensive and periodontal infections are common. According to many incidental observations, adult males are vulnerable to sudden cardiac arrest without evidence of coronary ischemia. Recall here the associations of periodontal infections and cardiovascular diseases (Section 2.3.1). In captivity, obesity is common, particularly in females on 'non-atherogenic' diets (Steinetz et al, 1996). We need detailed analyses of captive chimp vascular, myocardial, and

TABLE 6.3 Cholesterol Levels in Captive Great Apes (% of sample)

Blood Cholesterol	Chimpanzee[a]	Gorilla[b]	Orangutan[c]	Monkey[d]
High ≥ 240 mg/dl	34%	100%	100%	
Borderline 200–239	47%			
Normal <200	19%			100%

a. 17 groups of animals, 240 animals
b. 2 groups, 11 animals
c. 2 animals
d. 142 animals
Chimpanzee data summarized from (Finch and Stanford, 2004, Table 3A). The most detailed recent study of chimps is (Steinetz et al, 1996). Other species from (Srinivasan et al, 1976a,b).

dental pathology, and of blood lipids in relation to various diets, which often include animal fat and dairy products (Conklin-Brittain et al, 2002).

Monkeys also show vulnerability to lipid-rich diets in inducing accelerated vascular disease (Clarkson, 1998) and Alzheimer-like changes. Although no great ape has been studied for nutritional effects on neurodegeneration, in vervet monkeys fed for 5 y on a diet rich in saturated fats the deposition of Aβ was accelerated (Schmechel et al, 2002). Similarly, diets rich in cholesterol and fat induce Aβ deposition and other Alzheimer-like changes in rabbits and in transgenic mice with a human Alzheimer gene (Levin-Allerhand et al, 2002; Refolo et al, 2001; Shie et al, 2002). In cell culture models, added cholesterol increases Aβ production from APP by altering the subcellular distribution of BACE1 (Ehehalt et al, 2004; Kojro et al, 2001; Mills et al, 1999; Puglielli et al, 2001). Thus, the shift to cholesterol-rich diets in human ancestors could have accelerated the mild level of Alzheimer changes seen in the great apes. Provisionally, we may conclude from this varied literature that captive chimps are at least as vulnerable as humans to hypercholesterolemia and vascular disease on rich diets without regular demanding exercise.

6.2.3.   The Evolution of Meat-Eating

Diet is another major difference: Unlike humans, the great apes are primarily herbivores (Table 6.4), a long-standing characteristic of this clade for 35 million years (Milton, 1993; Stanford, 1999). While comprehensive dietary data are lacking, the typical caloric intake of chimps from animal tissues is about 5% of the total, which is far below human norms. Additionally, males in some chimp communities hunt and eat monkeys and other small mammals (Goodall, 1986; Boesch and Boesch, 1989; Stanford, 1998), with some averaging 70 g meat per day. Meat-sharing has a primarily social role in attracting females and in social favors by subordinate males. However, the regular consumption of meat is not essential to chimp survival, because some chimp communities have not been observed to hunt or to eat meat. And, in those communities, meat is rarely consumed by pregnant or nursing chimps (Finch and Stanford, 2004, pp. 8–12). Thus, hunting behaviors may be cultural and socially learned, as is the different tool use between chimp communities (Whiten et al, 1999; Sanz et al, 2004). Nonetheless, important nutrients are obtained from insects. Chimps in particular search for fatty termite larvae, using thin sticks for 'termite dipping', and females may ingest 65 g wet weight per day (McGrew, 2001). Bird eggs are also occasionally eaten. This consumption of fat is still much below human norms, e.g. fat is 15–25% of dry weight in the modern 'western' diet and 38–49% of foragers (Kaplan et al, 2000; Cordain et al, 2001; Cordain et al, 2002a,b; Conklin-Brittain et al, 2002; Eaton et al, 2002).

"Meat made us human" is Bunn's trenchant phrase (Bunn, 2007, p. 191). The meat-rich diet preferred by humans is strongly implicated in the evolution of the brain and complex social behaviors (Dart, 1953; Kaplan et al, 2000; Milton, 1993; Milton, 1999; Stanford, 1999). Meat provides a rich package of nutrients that greatly reduce the time spent in foraging. Chimps are occupied 75% of the

TABLE 6.4 Meat Sources of African Great Apes and Human Ancestors

	Pan[a] Chimp	Gorilla[a]	Pongo[a] Orangutan	Australopithecus[b]	H. ergaster[c]	H. neanderthalensis[d]	H. sapiens, Paleolithic[e]
cannibalization mammal	YES	NO	NO	?	?	YES	YES
skeletal muscle	YES	NO	NO	YES	YES	YES	YES
brain	YES	NO	NO	?	?	YES	YES
bone marrow	YES	NO	NO	?	YES	YES	YES
viscera	YES	NO	NO	?	?	?	YES
reptile- bird	RARE	NO	RARE	?	?	YES	YES
eggs	RARE	NO	RARE	?	?	?	YES
fish	NO	NO	NO	?	?	?	LIKELY
insect	YES	YES	RARE	LIKELY	LIKELY	LIKELY	LIKELY

Table directly from (Finch and Stanford, 2004). New entry for orangutan provided by Craig Stanford.
a. Organs consumed by chimpanzees (Stanford, 1999; Stanford, 2001). Both chimp sexes occasionally kill and eat the infants of other females in their group. Cannibalism is very rare in bonobos, gorillas, or orangutans (Goodall, 1986). Orangutans incidentally ingest insects with fruit and may randomly pluck them from leaves.'
b. *Australopithecus* 2.5 MYA extracted marrow from long bones, as indicated by induced fractures (e.g., (de Heinzelin et al, 1999). Some Australopithicenes (`robust taxa') had large chewing muscles and large, thickly enameled cheek teeth indicative of herbivory (e.g., (Andrews and Martin, 1991). Stone tools were very limited and crude.
c. Early *Homo* had smaller molars than *Australopithecus* (Andrews and Martin, 1991), suggesting less reliance on tough fibrous plants, consistent with evidence for tool use in obtaining meat by scavenging or hunting.
d. Neanderthals obtained most protein from animal sources (isotopic analysis, [*15]N), approximating that eaten by non-human carnivores (Richards et al, 2000).
e. Some modern hunter-gatherers, e.g., the Aché, save prey animal brains for their young children (Hillard Kaplan, pers. comm.).

waking day in searching for plant foods, which are mainly low-yield (Finch and Stanford, 2004, p. 8). The evolution of hunting and meat-eating thus made available high energy rich meals that take less time to digest, and that also reduce the necessity of all members of the group to spend every day of their lives in endless foraging. The huge increase in consumption of carrion exposed early humans to huge increases in cholesterol, but also to increased biohazards from infections and toxins. With Robert Sapolsky and Craig Stanford, I have developed the hypothesis that these huge shifts in diet and life history strategy were enabled by the evolution of 'meat-adaptive' genes, including the apoE alleles, which enabled increased longevity together with increased consumption of meat (Finch and Sapolsky, 1999; Finch and Stanford, 2004).

Besides its value to adults as an energy dense food, meat also provides a rich source of essential polyunsaturated fatty acids (PUFAs), which are required for normal brain development (Cordain, 2001; Cordain et al, 2002a,b; Eaton, 2002; Finch and Stanford, 2004, pp. 11–12). Arachidonic acid (AA) and docohexanoic acid (DHA) are made from different PUFA precursors (Section 2.9.5). Because PUFAs are scarce in plant material, their availability to children could decrease the risk of marginal neurological impairments from sporadic deficits. PUFA levels may influence brain development even on 'normal diets,' and in one study AA:DHA levels in mother milk strongly correlated with neonatal brain growth (Xiang et al, 2000). Vitamin B12 is also not provided by plant foods. It is cogent that some children given vegan-macrobiotic diets have a higher incidence of mild cognitive impairment and slower growth that is not corrected by supplements (Louwman, 2000; Van Dusseldorp et al, 1999). A lower risk of retarded development would have favored the acquisition of the skills for hunting and foraging.

By 2.6 MYA, mammalian prey bones were associated with *Australopithecus* at Oldovai Gorge in East Africa. Many bone cuts and breaks are consistent with the use of stone tools to remove flesh and crack long bones for marrow (Blumenschine and Pobiner, 2007; Bunn, 2007; Shipman, 1986; Asfaw et al, 1999; Shea, 2007). The lack of evidence for clubs or large weapons suggests that large carcasses were scavenged (Bunn, 2007). Cooperative transport of carcasses is suggested by the numbers of large bones at one site (FLK Zinj), which exceeded the regional density of these species. Brain and body size were slightly larger than in chimps (Table 6.1; see footnote for comment on encephalization coefficients).

The diet is inferred from the natural isotopic [^{13}C] composition of tooth enamel. *Australopithecus africanus* 3 MYA appears omnivorous, with greater isotopic similarity to hyenas than to grazers and browsers (Sponheimer, 1999; Sponheimer et al, 1999, 2007). These authors emphasize that the isotopic composition cannot resolve if the source of the isotope was directly ingested plant material or indirectly transferred through the flesh of an animal that ate the plant material. A wide variety of wild-plant foods was available in East and Southern Africa, including some with high nutritional values (Bunn, 2007; Peters, 2007; Sept, 2007). Australopithecenes had relatively larger teeth than all species of *Homo*, implying the greater importance of fibrous plants to their diet (Wrangham, 2007).

Early *Homo* by 1.8 MYA clearly used tools and, by isotopic evidence, was also an omnivore. By 1.8–1.6 MYA, *H. erectus* occupied a broad belt extending from East Africa to Java (Rightmire et al, 2006). In the recently developed Dmanisi site in the Caucasus (1.77 MYA), brain estimates are under 1000 cc, even as small at 600 cc; these size variations suggest sex differences (Rightmire, 2004). One toothless adult skull shows resorption of tooth sockets and extensive jaw bone remodeling, suggesting that this individual had impaired chewing for some years (Lordkipanidze et al, 2005). Survival in the cold climate of the Caucasus with such major impairments implies access to foods that don't require mastication, possibly mashes made from nuts or tubers, or soft tissues such as marrow and brain. There is no evidence for controlled use of fire for cooking, which would soften tubers for easier ingestion, until 0.5 MYA at the earliest (Wrangham and Conklin-Brittain, 2003; Wrangham, 2007).

Hunting technology advanced remarkably after 0.5 MYA, concurrently with further brain size evolution in *H. erectus* (Fig. 6.5). The earliest evidence of spears is 0.3–0.4 MYA in Schöningen (Gaudzinski and Roebroeks, 2000; Thieme, 1997). *H. erectus* in this region of Europe had brains of about 1000 cc. The Schöningen site

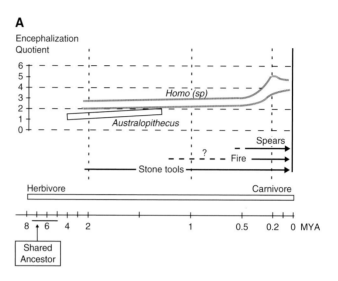

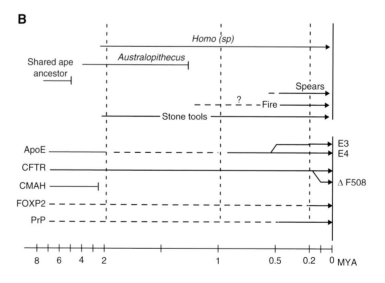

FIGURE 6.5 For legend see page 389.

finds include a remarkable series of long spears and other crafted wooden tools; flint scrapers; thousands of bones, many with cut marks; and fireplaces. Horse skeletons dominate over smaller bones of other mammals, birds, and fish. This evident ability to hunt a large herd animal and bring the carrion to one place implies that hunting was highly organized and suggests large-scale meat-eating; however, bone evidence does not inform on the frequency of meat-eating (O'Connell et al, 2002).

A daughter lineage of *H. erectus* may have lead to *H. heidelbergensis*, which had a larger brain (ca. 1200 cc) and is a possible shared ancestor of *H. sapiens* with *H. neanderthal* (Rightmire, 2004). Comparable skeletons of *H. heidelbergensis* have been found in Africa, but not *H. neanderthal*. Neandertals in Europe and Western Asia independently evolved large brains as large or larger than most modern humans (1200–1700 cc) and survived to 34,000 years before present (YBP) in the region of southern France (Hublin et al, 1996). The earliest anatomically modern *H. sapiens* skeleton dates to 195,000 YBP (Omo Kibish, Ethiopia) (McDougall et al, 2005). East Africa continues to be the most likely region of origin of modern *H. sapiens* (Ray et al, 2005; Grine et al, 2007).

By 100,000 YBP (Late Pleistocene), skilled extraction of bone marrow and brains is well documented (Gaudzinski and Roebroeks, 2000). Isotope signatures of neanderthal bones resemble those in non-human carnivores, suggesting that animal tissues were also their main protein sources (Richards et al, 2000). Cannibalism is evidenced by cut marks that could have been made during removal of marrow and the tongue. At one neandertal cave (Moula-Guercy, 100,000 YBP), all human crania and limb bones had cut marks and fractures (Defleur et al, 1999). Cannibalization is known only in chimps among the great apes, but may have

FIGURE 6.5 A. Evolution of tools and controlled use of fire in *Australopithecus* and *Homo*. B. Human meat-adaptive gene candidates. *ApoE* (apolipoprotein E) regulates cholesterol levels and transport. The 'bad' apoE4 isoform is associated with premature arterial degeneration, and Alzheimer disease is ancestral in the genus *Homo*, but differs from the chimpanzee (details in Fig. 6.6). The 'good' apoE3 isoform spread later in human evolution about 0.226 MYA, but before the initial migration from Africa (Fullerton et al, 2000). *CFTR* (cystic fibrosis transmembrane conductance regulator) has recessive mutants that cause cystic fibrosis, with incidence of about 1/2500. The ΔF508 mutant causes cystic fibrosis ($\geq$ 50% cases) and originated 0.05 MYA. The most common non-mutant CFTR allele resembles that in chimps and may be the ancestral allele (Bertranpetit and Calafel, 1996; Mateu et al, 2001). CFTR heterozygotes may be resistant to diarrheas (Table 6.6). *CMAH* (CMP-N-acetyl-neuraminic acid hydroxylase) modifies membrane sialic acids that influence viral attachment and may increase resistance to rotaviruses that cause diarrhea (Table 6.6). The inactivating mutation 2.7 MYA preceded the genus *Homo* (Chou et al, 2002). *FOXP2*, a transcription factor that influences brain development and acquisition of language, acquired two substitutions about 0.2 MYA, approximating the emergence of anatomically modern *H. sapiens* (Enard et al, 2002a,b). *Prp* (prion polymorphisms) increase resistance to prion infections in heterozygotes. The human alleles may have originated 0.5 MYA (Mead, 2003). (Adapted from Finch and Stanford, 2004, Fig. 1.)

been a long-standing human practice (Table 6.4). By 60,000 YBP in South Africa, plant fibers were apparently used to bind shaped stones to spear shafts (Lombard, 2005), which suggests further advances in hunting technology.

Humans also evolved distinctive fat depots. In pregnancies of captive chimps and other great apes, the newborn have remarkably less subcutaneous fat than characteristic of humans (Kuzawa, 1998; Robson et al, 2006; Schultz, 1969). Schultz also noted picturesquely "... newly born ... monkeys and apes resemble in their faces emaciated and toothless old men ... due to the lack [of] the padding of subcutaneous fat which appears in man before birth and normally persists throughout infantile life." (*op. cit.*, p. 114). In allometric comparisons with other mammals, human neonates are several-fold fatter for their size (Kuzawa, 1998). Frustratingly, none of the species compared with humans were primates. Moreover, Schultz's 'in the gross' observations of great apes could be misleading because visceral fat depots were not characterized. The needed data on primates can now be easily obtained with MRI.

The fat content of human infants increases further to a maximum of about 25% body weight by 6–9m, accounting for about half of the weight gain and more than half of total caloric intake (Kuzawa, 1998). The age of peak adiposity approximates the beginning of weaning, when transitional foods are introduced and when the risk of exogenous infections increases. The importance of neonatal fat is also shown in the babies of malnourished South Indian women, which had conspicuous subcutaneous fat, despite their low birthweight (Section 4.4.4). The uniquely human acquisition of breast fat before pregnancy may have evolved as a hedge for uncertain resources (Kuzawa, 1998; Robson et al, 2006).

In the great apes, breast development is delayed until pregnancy. Breast fat in particular is adaptive because it sustains nursing when resources are unpredictable. Skeletal evidence does not tell when breast fat began to be acquired before pregnancy in evolving human lineages. The great range of breast development before pregnancy is not obviously associated with subsequent milk production or success in nursing. Also recall the remarkable metabolic adaptations to energy limitations during pregnancy (Fig. 4.8). Humans have many individual variations in somatic fat deposits (abdominal, breast, steatapygic, and subcutaneous), suggesting genetic variations beyond the sex differences.

The fertility goddess figures of the Upper Paleolithic, such the Venus of Willendorf from 21,000 YBP on this book's cover[4], suggest an ancient ideal of fat, perhaps even an ideology, that represented survival advantages from stored nutritional reserves. Her broad hips also suggest easy child-bearing. Many other plump and broad hipped statues are found in Neolithic and Chalcolithic settlements throughout Europe and Western Asia (Hodder, 2004; Gimbutas, 1982). An intrigu-

---

[4]The roll of abdominal fat extends around the sides, while her buttocks are 'flat' (not steatopygic) (Witcombe, 2005). Note also her thin arms and short legs. Leg length in modern humans is sensitive to infection and malnutrition (Bogin, 1999, 2002) (Section 4.6.5). In health-rich modern populations, short legs may also be due to early puberly (Buckler, 1990; Wilt et al, 2004) (noted to me by Rene Jahiel).

ing statuette from a Çatalhöyük grain bin portrays a seated fat lady with plump limbs and pendulous breasts and belly (Hodder, 2006, Plate 24). Being 'overweight' by current standards may have caused far fewer ill effects within the shorter life spans of those days. Or, perhaps any consequences of obesity (Fig. 3.4) were outweighed by the greater reproductive success of women with ample fat reserves who could sustain nursing and for normal postnatal growth during seasonal fluctuations in food availability (Kuzawa, 1998; Sellen, 2006). The idea that plumpness and health coexist continues today in the pot-bellied Buddha statues found in many Asian households and shrines which represent prosperity and fertility.

6.2.4. Meat Adaptive Genes

The evolution of meat-eating poses an important puzzle. Given that diet restriction in lab rodents and monkeys slows aging processes associated with obesity and hyperlipidemia (Chapter 3), we may ask what genetic changes enabled human ancestors to shift to high fat content diet *and* to double the life expectancy. On many grounds, the major increase of meat-eating would be predicted to shorten, not lengthen, life span. If the atherogenic lipid profile of captive chimps is any index (Section 6.2.2), increased meat ingestion would have increased vascular-related deaths.

Meat-eating increased direct hazards not widely experienced by the herbivorous great apes: increased tissue toxins and infectious pathogens[5] (Table 6.5). Potential toxins from meat that are scarce in plants include cholesterol; iron and copper, from hemoglobin and myoglobin (both present in all vertebrate tissues); and phytanic acid in ungulate tissues. Infectious pathogens are unavoidable in

TABLE 6.5 Categories of Meat-Adaptive Gene Candidates

Human Genes	Benefit
Lipoproteins, apoE3	lower cholesterol; increase neuron growth
Detox genes: metals in red meat (Cu, Fe)	iron and copper damage neurons
plant toxins (phytanic acid)	protect brain development
Immune defense genes:	resistance to infections
prions in raw brains and marrow	
pathogenic viruses and bacteria	
parasites (malaria, trypanosomes,	
nematodes etc)	
Anti-oxidant genes	slowing of atherosclerosis
	less lung damage from smoke inhalation

---

[5]Meat-eating is also a biohazard to chimps. Ebola virus infections were acquired by wild chimps in proportion to the eating of Colobus monkeys (Formenty et al, 1999), a favored chimp prey (Stanford, 1998).

eating carrion. Wild mammals and birds carry prions, viruses, bacteria, blood-borne protozoans, and nematodes. Genomic analysis shows that the domestic tapeworm *Taenia* infested *Homo* as a host 0.8–1.7 MYA (Hoberg, 2002). The controlled use of fire, possibly before 0.5 MYA (Goren-Inbar et al, 2004; Wrangham, 2007), may have been important in pathogen control by cooking or smoking of meat. However, some pathogens are not killed by ordinary cooking; e.g., infectious prions can survive autoclaving at >120°C (Taylor, 1999).

Fire and cooking increase exposure to smoke, which must have been intense in the early cave dwellings, as well as in semi-permanent structures. In pre-industrial societies, open fires were used for warmth and insect control, as well as for cooking. Smoke inhalation causes lung damage with consequences to the level of aerobic activity that can be sustained and cardiovascular functions (Chapter 2). Moreover, the process of cooking and charring produces glyco-oxidation products (AGEs) that are proinflammatory (Section 2.4.2) (Vlassara et al, 2002). Fire is inflammatory, no pun meant. Each of these exposures may have selected for new gene variants not needed in the herbivorous apes.

The butchering and handling of carrion also bring hazards separate from ingestion. The Foré of New Guinea once suffered from the neurodegenerative disease kuru, a spongioform encephalopathy, acquired by women who handled raw brains of the recently deceased (Mead et al, 2003). The infectious agent in kuru is the prion, which causes the spongiform encephalopathies Creutzfeldt-Jakob disease in humans and of scrapie in herd animals (Liberski and Gajdusek, 1997; Prusiner and Hsiao, 1994).

The abundant bones in Paleolithic sites also imply extended human occupancy, which would increase exposure to infectious agents in carrion and human feces, and the insects attracted. In contrast, as discussed above, the great apes rarely occupy the same site for more than a day. The increased exposure to animal fat, new food toxins, and diverse pathogens in feces thus defines a new phase in the evolution of both lipoprotein metabolism and of host defense mechanisms.

Humans differ from the great apes in several lipoproteins that are candidates for meat-adaptive genes (Table 6.5) (Fig. 6.5B). The best case may be the cholesterol carrier apolipoprotein E (apoE), which is a regulator of blood cholesterol in reverse cholesterol transport (Section 5.7). ApoE also transports cholesterol for steroid synthesis and neuronal outgrowth. The main human variants, apoE3 and apoE4, differ in one amino acid (R112C) that alters lipid binding affinity and subcellular processing (Ji et al, 2006; Mahley and Rall, 2000) (Table 6.6). The apoE4 isoform was first identified in association with elevated cholesterol (Section 5.7.3).

Human apoE alleles evolved in two critical stages (Fullerton et al, 2000) (Fig. 6.6). In modern populations, apoE3 is the most prevalent allele (>50% in all populations; Fig. 5.15) and, relative to apoE4, increases life expectancy by up to 6 y (Fig. 5.12). ApoE3 also reduces age-related frailty from heart attacks, cognitive decline, and Alzheimer disease. During middle-age, apoE3 carriers have higher frontal cortex glucose metabolism and report less use or need of memnonics in daily activities. ApoE3 carriers have better recovery from head injury and may

TABLE 6.6 Gene Candidates for Resistance to Disease Associated with Meat-Eating

Animal Organ Component	Main Source	Disease Risk	Gene Candidate (note)
cholesterol unsaturated fatty acids	brain, fat, marrow, muscle	cognitive decline during aging; traumatic brain injury; Alzheimer disease; vascular disease	apoE4[a] apoE4[b] apoE4[c] apoE4[d]; Lp(a)[f]
infectious agents: viruses		dysenteries, hepatitis	apoE[e] CMAH[g] HLA[h]
prions	bone marrow, brain, viscera	spongiform encephalopathies	apoE3[e], HLA[h] Prp[i]
bacteria	viscera	cholera and dysenteries	CFTR[j] apoE3[e] HLA[h]
amoeba protozoa		dysenteries malaria	Hb[k], apoE[e]
nematodes			HLA[h]
metals: copper, iron, zinc	red meat, blood	vascular disease Alzheimer disease?	?[l]
phytanic acid	fish, ungulates, dairy	Refsum's disease, prostate cancer	PHYH[m]

Table directly from (Finch and Stanford, 2004).

a. ApoE4 also increases the risk of early Alzheimer disease (Section 5.7.3 text and references).

b. Traumatic brain injury and hemorrhagic stroke have worse outcomes in E4 carriers, with more memory impairments (Crawford et al, 2002; Liberman et al, 2002).

c. ApoE4 decreases cerebral glucose utilization during middle age and accelerates cognitive decline.

d. ApoE4 increases risk of heart attack by 40% and accelerates atherosclerosis (Section 5.7.3, text and references). Because apoE4 versus E3 carriers show more decrease of blood cholesterol in response to reductions of dietary fat and cholesterol, at least in the case of obese diabetics (Fig. 5.16) (Saito, 2004), they may be more sensitive to hypercholesterolemia on fatty diets.

e. ApoE3 increases liver damage to hepatitis C and may protect brain development from impairments in children with diarrhea (Section 5.7.5, text and references). Prion diseases have not shown consistent associations with apoE alleles.

f. Blood Lp(a) elevations are a mild risk factor in heart disease, up to 2-fold (Seed, 2001; Sharrett, 2001). Human Lp(a) levels vary >1000-fold between individuals under genetic control (Boerwinkle et al, 1992).

g. CMAH [CMP-N-acetylneuraminic acid (CMP-Neu5Ac) hydroxylase] is an enzyme that modifies CMP-neu5Ac (N-acetylneuraminic acid) to the hydroxylated CMP-NeuGc (N-glycolylneuraminic acid). CMAH and NeuGc are found in anthropoids but not humans (Chou, 2002; Crocker, 2001; Varki, 2001). The *CMAH* gene in humans was inactivated by deletion of exon 6 about 3.2 MYA (Hayakawa, 2006). Siglec-4a in myelin-associated glycoprotein shows species differences pertinent to white matter diseases such as multiple sclerosis and amyotrophic lateral sclerosis.

h. HLA-B27 allele is associated with reactive arthritis induced by diverse infections (Urvater, 2000). Reactive arthritis after enteric infections with bacteria is associated with *Mhc* haplotypes in gorillas and macaques (Finch and Stanford, 2004, Appendix). HLA-DQ7 is 75% less frequent in those with vCJD than normals (Jackson et al, 2001). *Onchocerca volvulus*, the nematode parasite that causes river blindness, is endemic in West Africa. HLA-DQ variants influence outcomes of infection (Meyer et al, 1994; Meyer et al, 1996); one haplotype associated with more severe disease in West Africa shows less malaria (Hill et al, 1991), implying balancing selection (Meyer et al, 1996).

i. The prion gene *PrP^c* influences transmission of infectious prions *PrP^sc* between species and the age of disease onset (Prusiner and Hsiao, 1994; Prusiner et al, 1999; Telling et al, 1996). Primates are relatively vulnerable to prion infections (Schatzl et al, 1995). The human *PrP^c* gene evolved two polymorphisms about 0.2 MYA ago that increase resistance to infection in heterozygotes (Mead, 2003).

j. CFTR (cystic fibrosis transmembrane conductance regulator) heterozygotes may be resistant to diarrhea from cholera and other dehydrating diseases transmitted by intestinal bacteria, as shown in a mouse model (Gabriel, 1994; Kirk, 2000).

k. Resistance to malaria from *Plasmodium falciparum* is mediated by variants of hemoglobin that cause sickle cell anemia; milder forms in heterozygotes are maintained by balancing selection. Variants in *G6PDH* and *HLA* genes (note h) confer relative resistance to malaria may have spread in association with agriculture (Hill et al, 1997; Rich et al, 1998).

(Footnote Continues)

TABLE 6.6 (Continued)

l. Muscle contains iron, copper, zinc, and other divalent metal ions, which are implicated in Alzheimer and vascular disease and infections (Bush and Tanzi, 2002; Finch and Stanford, 2004, Appendix). Trace metals enhance Aß aggregation (Huang, 2004). In the presence of soluble copper (Cu^{2+}), apoE4 enhances Aß aggregation relative to apoE3 (Bush and Tanzi, 2002). An iron-responsive element resides in the UTR of the amyloid precursor protein RNA transcript, which may have a role in APP metabolism (Rogers, 2002). The Aß peptide binds iron directly; the rodent amino acid differences from human and primate decrease iron binding and the chemical production of H_2O_2 (Boyd-Kimball et al, 2004). Because most plant sources have low metal concentrations, transitions to meat-eating would have sharply increased iron intake. Diet also influences metal bioavailability; e.g., iron absorption is inhibited by plant-derived phytase and tannins that bind free iron, whereas absorption is enhanced by vitamin C (Haddad et al, 1999). No chimp-human differences are known in iron transport proteins.

m. Humans have higher expression of an enzyme PHYH (phyantol CoA hydroxylase) that degrades phytanic acid, a branched chain fatty acid derived from fish and ungulate meat and milk products, which are rarely eaten by the great apes. Phytanic acid is absent from carnivores, eggs, and plants, although derived from chlorophyll (van den Brink, 2006). PHYH expression was higher in human than chimp (fibroblast gene expression profiling) (Karaman et al, 2003). Phytanic acid elevations in blood are associated Refsun's disease, a peripheral neuropathy, and possibly with prostate cancer (van den Brink et al, 2006; Xu et al, 2005).

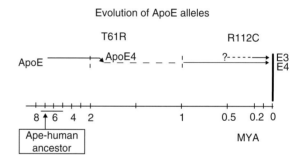

FIGURE 6.6 ApoE gene evolution. The apoE of great apes differs in a critical amino acids from the modern human apoE isoforms at position 61 (threonine to arginine, T61R). The great ape apoE is predicted to function in lipid binding like the modern human apoE3, as modeled in a transgenic mouse apoE4 (Dong et al, 1994; Raffai et al, 2001). At an unknown time, the mutation T61R occurred, yielding the human ancestral apoE4. The apoE3 isoform of the genus *Homo* arose subsequently (arginine to cysteine at 112, R112C) and spread ca. 0.226 MYA (Fullerton et al, 2000), which just precedes the first fossil of *H. sapiens* 0.195 MYA (McDougall, 2005). The lower range of date estimates (0.176–0.579 MYA) is confidently within the prevalence of *H. erectus (0.3–1.6 MYA)*, allowing the possibility that *H. neanderthal* shared apoE3 with *H. sapiens*. The subpopulation of *H. sapiens* from which apoE3 spread could be African or Eurasian. The apoE2 isoform (R158c) spread more recently. Directly from (Finch and Stanford, 2004, Fig. 2).

have higher bone density, which would protect against traumas in hunting and fighting, and age-related osteoporosis (Section 5.7.3). These anti-frailty effects of apoE3 would also have favored health in middle age and later. Middle-aged and older humans have unique roles in multi-generational care giving and mentoring (Gurven et al, 2006), including the grandmothering unique to humans (Hawkes et al, 1998; Packer et al, 1998; Robson et al, 2006).

ApoE isoforms also differ in effect on amyloid aggregation (Aβ peptide). In the presence of soluble copper (Cu^{2+}), apoE4 enhances Aβ aggregation relative to apoE3 (Bush and Tanzi, 2002). This interaction could promote amyloid degenerative processes from meat-eating, which introduces surges of copper, iron, and other metals at each meal. Even trace levels of copper in the drinking water increased Aβ deposits in animal models (Sparks et al, 2006b). Moreover, the Aβ peptide directly binds iron, which increases cytotoxic H_2O_2 production (bystander effect, Section 1.4.1), while the amyloid precursor protein (APP) transcript also has an iron-binding regulatory site (Rogers et al, 2002). The high metal content of senile plaques (copper, iron, and zinc are 2- to 5-fold above healthy brain neuropil) (Lovell et al, 1998) is implicated in the association of oxidative damage and amyloid burden (Bush and Tanzi, 2002). Other aspects of metal ingestion are described in Table 6.6, note l.

By DNA sequence analysis, apoE3 arose from a single point mutation in apoE4 and spread 0.226 MYA (Fullerton et al, 2000), just before the first fossil of *H. sapiens*. The 'bad' E4 allele was thus the ancestral human gene (Fig. 6.6) (Hanlon and Rubinsztein, 1995; Mahley, 1988). The dating estimates of apoE3 (0.176–0.579 MYA) partly overlap with *H. erectus* (0.3–1.6 MYA), which allows the possibility that *H. neanderthalensis* shared apoE3 with *H. sapiens* (Section 6.2.1). The subpopulation of *H. sapiens* from which apoE3 spread could have been African or Eurasian (this is not in conflict with an East African origin of modern *H. sapiens*). The great apes have a further functional base difference from the *H. sapiens* gene (T61R) (Fig. 6.6). This substitution is predicted to alter peptide folding, resulting in lipid binding functions like the modern human apoE3; these differences are modeled in a transgenic mouse apoE4 (Dong et al, 1994; Raffai et al, 2001). The great apes have other scattered base differences from human apoE (Table 6.7), which, by their location and effect on coding, are not predicted to influence peptide folding or lipid binding.

The single mutation leading to the ancestral apoE4 may have spread as a pathogen resistance factor. (Finch and Stanford 2004). ApoE4 carriers have less liver fibrosis during hepatitis C viral infections and maybe better cognitive development in children with enteric infections (Section 5.7.4). ApoE alleles also influence HDL remodeling during the acute phase response (Section 1.5.4). Acute phase lipid remodeling increases plasma triglycerides and other lipid energy resources needed in host defense, but also decreases the anti-oxidant activities of HDL. In a biochemical experiment, apoE4 caused greater release of serum amyloid A (SAA) from HDL (Miida et al, 2006), which, in turn, would increase uptake of cholesterol by macrophages, a key step in atherogenesis (Section 1.5). Thus, apoE4 by altering acute phase HDL remodeling would tend to promote vascular

TABLE 6.7 Apolipoprotein E: Polymorphisms in Humans and Species Differences

ApoE residue[1] (+signal peptide)	612 (79)	**112**[3] (130)	135[2] (153)	**158**[3] (176)
human: apoE2	R	C	V	C
apoE3	R	C	V	R
apoE4	R	R	V	R
Chimp	T	R	A	R
Gorilla	T	R	A	R
Orangutan	T	R	A	R

1. Amino acid residues numbered positions of the polymorphisms in the mature plasma protein, as used in this text and in (Finch and Sapolsky, 1999). The other numbering system includes the '+ signal peptide' of the full protein sequence (the 18 residue signal peptide is cleaved before secretion by the liver into the blood): data from National Center for Biotechnology (NCBI) http://www.ncbi.nlm.nih.gov/entrez). Table directly taken from (Finch and Stanford, 2004, Table 5).
2. Residue 61 strongly affects apoE structure through 'domain interactions' and is an important cause of species variations (Dong et al, 1994; Raffai et al, 2001). Chimpazee apoE with T61 is predicted to function in lipid binding like human apoE3, despite the R112 and R158 as in human apoE4.
3. Bolded residues identify the functionally important differences in the human alleles.

disease over longer durations in an infectious environment. ApoE also has a direct role in immunity in the presentation of lipophilic antigens (vander Elzen et al, 2005) (Section 5.7.5). These and other observations support the Charlesworth-Martin hypothesis (Charlesworth, 1996; Martin, 1999) that *apoE4* is maintained in human populations by balancing selection. We may also see how the evolution of longevity has involved selection for genes that influence oxidative damage from inflammation and infection (Queries II, III, and IV; Chapter 1).

Two other lipoprotein system genes differ between humans and chimps. The *Lp(a)* lipoprotein gene promoter differs between humans and chimps with strong effects on plasma levels of Lp(a), an LDL-like protein with links to thrombosis and vascular events though Lp(a) binding sites to fibrin in the clotting system (Belczewski et al, 2005; Doucet et al, 1994; Doucet et al, 1998). Chimpanzees typically have high plasma Lp(a), 2–4-fold above the human norm. In one colony, a majority of animals had plasma Lp(a) levels above a clinical threshold for cardiovascular risk (Doucet et al, 1994). The *Lp(a)* promoter has three nucleotide differences between chimp and human (Huby et al, 2001). Of unknown functional significance, the LDR-receptor gene of humans has an unusual Alu repetitive element in the 3′ untranslated mRNA not found in great apes, possibly from a rare gene conversion event (Kass et al, 1995; Kass et al, 2004).

Increased resistance to infections must have been a major importance to the reduction of mortality and increased life expectancy. Many gene candidates may be considered that influence resistance to infections transmitted by raw organs (Finch and Stanford, 2004). The prion diseases causing spongiform encephalopathies are particularly interesting examples and include 'mad cow' disease, first recognized in humans as *kuru* in New Guinea traditionalists (Foré) who handled and ate the brains of recently deceased relatives (Liberski and Gajdusek, 1997; Prusiner and Hsiao, 1994). Prion transmission is decreased by heterozygosity at the *Prp* locus

129M/V, which encodes the prion protein (Prusiner, 1999; Mead et al, 2003). Older Foré survivors of *kuru* are predominantly *PRNP* 129 heterozygotes, while homozygotes are more common in the younger generation (Mead et al, 2003). Homozygosity (M/M) also increases the risk of Creutzfeldt-Jakob disease (Lucotte and Mercier, 2005; Mitrova et al, 2005). Prion alleles differ widely in human populations and are in linkage disequilibrium, suggesting that balancing selection was associated with cannibalism, which was only recently suppressed. Chimp and human prion genes differ in six sites. The modern prion alleles may be dated to 0.5 MYA (Mead et al, 2003), which approximates the use of spears in organized hunting (Section 6.2.2). Contact with raw brains is not limited to cannibalism. Animal brains are considered a delicacy by many traditional peoples (Table 6.4, footnote e). Also recall that brain and marrow were extracted by early humans. Moreover, raw brains have been widely used for curing hides.

The sialic acids on cell membranes have major importance to pathogen resistance as sites for binding of viruses and bacteria (Angata and Varki, 2002; Varki, 2001). *CMAH* encodes an enzyme that modifies the sialic acid Neu5Gc (Table 6.6, note g). CMAH and NeuGc are found in other anthropoids but not in modern humans or Neanderthals (Chou et al, 2002). The *CMAH* gene in humans was inactivated by deletion of exon 6 about 3.2 MYA (Hayakawa et al, 2006), which predates the genus *Homo* and may have occurred in an Australopithicene (Fig. 6.5). Sialic acid binding immunoglobulins (SIGLECs) have also evolved differences from chimpanzees of potential importance in host resistance. SIGLEC-11 is expressed in human brain microglia but not in chimp or orangutan microglia (Hayakawa et al, 2005). Siglec-1 sequence differences may account for differences in tissue distribution of macrophages, e.g., chimps have higher titers of blood macrophages and fewer myeloid precursors in marrow than humans (Varki, 2001).

The evolved absence of Neu5Gc could increase resistance to rotoviruses, which cause diarrhea, and influenza viruses, both of which bind to Neu5Gc (Angata and Varki, 2002; Delorme et al, 2001). Children are especially susceptible to mortality from diarrhea (Fig. 4.2, Section 4.6). The absence of Neu5Gc could have also favored the later human cohabitation with domestic animals which are major reservoirs of pathogens.

Lactose tolerance was also evolved in association with the domestication of cattle and the increased use of milk as an adult food. Lactose, the main carbohydrate in milk, is hydrolyzed by intestinal lactase, which is universally expressed on intestinal enterocytes during early life (Swallow, 2003). However, lactose expression is transcriptionally suppressed in most populations before age 10. The resulting adult lactose intolerance typically causes diarrhea. Lactose tolerance, however, has arisen through at least four mutations in lactase gene promoter that arose independently in association with pastoralism during the past 9000 y (Tishkoff et al, 2006; Coelho et al, 2005). The spread of adult lactose tolerance is attributed to two factors: the benefit of milk as a new high energy food source for adults and the reduction of diarrhea as a side effect.

Besides the recognized danger of dehydration from diarrhea in hot climates, diarrhea also increases the local exposure to enteric pathogens.

The HLA system variants are also candidates for evolution of host resistance. This extraordinary complex cluster of a thousand genes (Section 1.3.2) modulates many aspects of antigen presentation to immune cells and includes cytokine and complement system genes. HLA haplotypes (combinations of alleles at different loci) are highly conserved, and some are shared with chimpanzees (O'Huigin et al, 2000; Venditti et al, 1996). Some class *HLA* I genes are more diverse in humans than chimps (Adams et al, 2001). HLA-DQ variants modulate responses to infections (Table 6.6, note h). The persistence of these ancient haplotypes is attributed to balancing selection, but the pathogens or environmental factors are not known.

Smoke inhalation from domestic fire causes lung damage, as noted above. Genes that increase resistance to smoke inhalation could include catalase, SOD, and other anti-oxidant genes, with increased expression (Cutler, 2005; Lopez-Torres et al, 1993). Recall that transgenic overexpression of SOD that decreases bystander damage to lung by fly-ash (Section 1.4.1) (Ghio et al, 2002b) and of transgenic catalase that increases mouse life span and delays atherosclerosis (Section 1.2.6) (Schriner et al, 2005; Yang, 2004a). Other candidates for resistance to inflammogens may be found in xenobiotic detoxifying enzymes, e.g., glutathione-S-transferase M1, which makes the key anti-oxidant glutathione (Fig. 1.11). The proinflammatory AGEs that are produced by cooking and charring may also be decreased enzymatically by amidoriases ('AGE-breakers') (Monnier and Sell, 2006) (Sections 1.2.6 and 2.4.2). On the other hand, AGEs may have been served as olfactory cues to tell when tubers were sufficiently cooked to destroy toxins (de Bry, 1994).

A further phase of 'meat-adaptation' occurred during the emergence of semi-permanent or seasonal assemblages which introduced new pressures on immune defenses and detoxification, and benefits of new hygienic behaviors. By 42,000 YBP, modern humans had reached the East European Plain (Don River site in Russia) (Anikovich et al, 2007). Caves, huts, and tents would have increased the exposure to infection and inflammation through carrion, excreta, garbage, and smoke from indoor fires. Hygiene must have been problematic with increasing population density, especially children in 'sphincter' training. Recall from above that the great apes have much lower exposure to biotrophic excreta; their night groups in close contact are usually small, 20 adults or less, wherein only mother and child sleep together. Because of vulnerability of the youngest to infections, it would be interesting to compare the proportions of infants and children per group in great apes and pre-industrial human communities and the prevalence of infections.

This putative phase of increased exposure to infections and inflammogens may coincide with the gradual reduction of human body size after 50,000 YBP (Fig. 6.7) (Ruff et al, 1997). Most agree that early anatomically modern *H. sapiens* were about 15% larger than current global averages (Kappelman, 1997). I hypothesize that this down-shift of size is due at least in part to the increasing load of

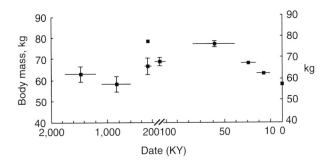

FIGURE 6.7 Body size changes in the genus *Homo* estimated from fossil limbs. Adapted from Fig. 2 and Table 1 of (Ruff et al, 1997). During the Upper Pleistocene, adult size decreased by about 3 kg per 10 KY (my calculation from data in Ruff et al, 1997). Although size estimates are subject to many uncertainties, e.g., in limb proportions (Ruff, 2006), the overall trend for decrease in size during the last 50 KY is generally accepted (Formicola, 2003; Kappelman, 1997). The single square (226 KY) represents the Jinniushan female just before the first *H.sapiens* fossil (195 KY, 78.6 kg, and 1.68 m tall; brain mass 1284 g; the largest paleolithic *Homo* female fossil) (Rosenberg et al, 2006).

infection and inflammation during transitions to sedentism with increasing population density. In modern populations, infections in early life attenuate growth, even when food is plentiful (Chapter 4). Exposure to infection and inflammation gradually increased with the beginning of the first high density permanent settlements ('towns') as the last Ice-Age ended. In the Jordan Valley, Natufian stone dwellings in semi-permanent or permanent settlements are dated from 13,000 YBP, before the domestication of crops and animals, and before pottery (Belfer-Cohen, 1991).

The Natufian culture shows progressive separation of garbage from inside the living and cooking space to designated middens (Hardy-Smith and Edwards, 2004). By the end of the Pre-pottery Neolithic B phase, 8000 YBP, interior living spaces were very clean, evidenced by sweeping and plastering (archeological sites of Beidha and Wadi El-Hammeh 27). Other important findings come from excavations at Çatalhöyük, a major town on the Anatolian plateau inhabited from 9500 to 8000 YBP, after the beginnings of crop domestication. Extensive findings by the Hodder team are summarized as interim reports (Hodder, 2005, 2006). Of great interest to our discussion are the hundreds of contiguous apartments that had definitive clean and dirty areas. Adjacent middens held diverse species of bones (Yeomans, 2005). Moreover, there is evidence for human feces in these middens from bile acid residues with human biochemical signatures of deoxycholate and lithocholate (Bull et al, 2005). The novel behavior of separating garbage and feces from the living spaces can be designated as 'urban proto-hygienic' and implies some understanding that infectious disease is linked to hygiene.

Despite the separation of clean and dirty spaces in the early Levantine towns, there were limits in clean living. Rodent infestations are evident, and insect swarms may be supposed. Inside smoke was dense in the apartments of Çatalhöyük, which vented smoke from the fireplaces through the access port on the roof of each unit. The skeletons of older adults buried within these apartments have sooty particulate deposits on the inside surfaces of upper ribs, presumably left by the drying lung tissue (Hodder 2006; Andrews et al, 2005; Molleson et al, 2005). The extent of the deposits suggests pulmonary impairments (anthracosis) (Birch, 2005), like 'hut-lung' disease (Section 2.4.1). A high burden of infection and inflammation is indicated by the excess of infants in the burials and by bone and dental evidence for slow growth and small adult size (men 1.63 m, women 1.54 m) (Molleson et al, 2005). DNA from skeletons in Çatalhöyük is being recovered and might be evaluatable for inflammatory gene allelic diversity (Sections 1.3.2 and 5.7.2).

Diffusion of hygienic concepts was slow and irregular. Other pre-industrial traditional people, Northwest Indians, for example, in the 18th Century did not exclude garbage from their living spaces (Hardy-Smith and Edwards, 2004, p. 284). In Roman cities, the toilet was typically located in the kitchen. Contact with human and animal excreta was unavoidable in rural and urban European households until recently, e.g., many traditional farm houses held animals on the ground floor with the family floor just above the manure (Barnes et al, 2006; Wright, 1960; George, 1984).

The domestication of mammals and birds would have created new reservoirs for disease and modes of transmission in all directions (Pearce-Duvet, 2006). Taeniid tapeworms, which have infested humans since 0.8 MYA or before (Hoberg, 2002), were evidently transmitted to cattle, dogs, and pigs during domestication 5,000–10,000 YBP. The three domestic *Taenia* species are derived from a common ancestor in Africa or Eurasia according to genomic data 0.78–1.81 MYB and may be the oldest parasite specific to the genus *Homo*. Malaria (*Plasmodium falciparum*) may also have preceded domestication (Pearce-Duvet, 2006), challenging the attractive hypothesis that domestication of fowl introduced malaria through host switching (Hill et al, 1997; Rich et al, 1998). Chimpanzees carry *P. reichenowi*, which is much closer to *P. falciparum* than the avian plasmodia (Waters et al, 1991; Waters et al, 1993). Expansions of agriculture are associated with the speciation of *Anopheles* mosquitoes in Africa (Pearce-Duvet, 2006). The strong associations of malaria with agricultural areas is hypothesized to have favored the spread of the sickle cell hemoglobin gene and the numerous other mutant hemoglobins by balancing selection (Hill et al, 1997; Livingstone, 1985; Pearce-Duvet, 2006; Rich et al, 1998). The many cystic fibrosis *CFTR* mutants may also be maintained by balancing selection (Table 6.6, note j). Cystic fibrosis causes abnormal mucus accumulation in intestine, lung, and skin that impair breathing, digestion, and sweating. *CFTR* mutants are common recessives in Caucasian populations (3–10%) and arise as independent mutations at many sites (Mateu et al, 2001; Mateu et al, 2002). The normal allele encodes a chloride (Cl^-) channel, activated by bacterial enterotoxins.

Hypothesized heterozygote advantages include reduced sweating, which might attract fewer mosquitoes, and decreased dehydration from diarrheal disease or from sweating in hot climates; however, supporting evidence is modest (Quinton, 1994). The spread of agriculture has had huge effects on human pathogen exposure through host reservoirs in flocks and herds that also increase transfer from feral populations (Pearce-Duvet, 2006). Thus, permanent settlements and the 'agricultural revolution' would have brought a further major increase in the burdens of chronic infection and inflammation.

Brain evolution also sharply accelerated in the genus *Homo* after 1.0 MYA concurrently with the record of increasingly sophisticated hunting tools and butchering. Brain evolution was crucial to the evolution of meat-eating; we may consider as 'meat-adaptive' the genes that enabled further brain developments (Finch and Stanford, 2004). A survey of genes expressed in the most rapidly evolving brain regions (human accelerated regions, HARs) identified a novel gene sequence in *HARF1* that evolved >1 MYA; this non-coding RNA is expressed in Cajal-Retzius neurons during cortical development (Pollard et al, 2006). White matter (myelinated pathways) increases also evolved during human cortex enlargement. The density of myelinated neuronal connections increased disproportionately relative to the great apes (Schoenemann et al, 2005), which enables high-speed exchanges between higher cortical centers that are critical to complex social decisions, as well as to spear throwing. The apoE3 allele favors slower myelin deterioration (Bartzokis et al, 2006), among other examples of apoE3 in delaying cognitive aging noted just above and discussed in Section 5.7.3. The increasing importance of older individuals to the uniquely human multi-generational care giving and mentoring not found in the great apes would be favored by healthier brains later in life with greater 'cognitive reserve' (Allen et al, 2005).

The spread of the apoE3 allele during the final stages of brain size increases (ca. 0.226 MYA) might have contributed to brain development as well as to cognitive functions later in life (Finch and Stanford, 2004). Besides its role in peripheral cholesterol metabolism, apoE transports cholesterol to growing neurons. Transgenic mice with targeted replacement of the mouse apoE gene with the human shows that apoE3 and E4 alter synaptic development. Neurons in apoE3 mice are more complex (dendritic arborization) and have more excitatory synaptic transmission than apoE4 mice (Wang et al, 2005a). Similar effects of apoE4 in human brain development are not yet documented but could be consistent with differences at later ages: non-demented E4 carriers had lower frontal cortex glucose metabolism (Reiman et al, 2005; Small et al, 2000) and more cortical synapses (Ji et al, 2003) (Section 5.7.4). Great care is needed in interpreting these data, which could be promiscuously used to support eugenic ideologies.

FOXP2 is another brain evolution candidate gene. This transcription factor of the FOXO gene family, which includes DAF-16, is expressed in neurons of brain regions that mediate language in humans and song in birds (Scharff and Haesler, 2005). FOXP2 acquired two mutations about 0.2 MYA (Enard, 2002), diverging from the highly conserved sequence in mammals. Because of rare familial mutations that cause speech abnormalities, the mutations of 0.2 MYA that approximate the earliest modern *H. sapiens* suggest a role of FOXP2 in human language capacity.

Two other genes expressed in the brain have variants that evolved and spread very recently. Variants of *MCPH1* (Microcephalin) and *ASPM* (abnormal spindle-like microcephaly associated) most likely arose <50,000 YBP, long after the initial emigration from Africa (Evans et al, 2005b; Mekel-Bobrov et al, 2005). The *ASPM-D* variant may be 6,000 years old, approximating the spread of cities and agriculture. Rare mutations in either gene impair brain size development, but it is not known if the common alleles, which differ across populations, influence cognition or behavior. There is debate about the role of selection in the spread of these variants, but the timing of spread is accepted as Neolithic (Currat et al, 2006).

6.2.5. The Increase in Life Expectancy

When did life expectancy of human ancestors begin to increase above the great ape baseline of 15–20 y? This inquiry does not assume that changes in life expectancy were linear or always progressive. In animals, life span can increase or decrease within 10-15 generations in response to predation or artificial selection (Section 1.2.8). One may start with the dental evidence for demographic shifts during the Middle to Upper Paleolithic (Pleistocene) (Caspari, 2004; Caspari and Lee, 2006). Younger and older adults may be distinguished by tooth wear and presence of adult molars (M3) that erupt at the end of the juvenile period. The Upper Paleolithic sample of modern *H. sapiens* 30,000 YBP in Europe had a ratio of old:young adults of 2.1, which was significantly higher than the <0.4 of old: young ratio for Middle Paleolithic 'early modern' *H. sapiens* in West Asia, Neandertal, other earlier *Homo*, and *Australopithecus*. Caspari and Lee (2006) suggest that the increased life expectancy implied by the 30,000 YBP European samples represents cultural developments after arrival from Africa and West Asia. Of course, paleodemographic estimates are problematic because of the incompleteness of age-group samples and uncertainties in age assignments based on wear (Hawkes and O'Connell, 2005; Skinner and Wood, 2006; Konigsberg, 2006; Hoppa and Vaupel, 2002). While this dental or skeletal evidence is not sufficient for estimating adult life expectancies, The Caspari-Lee analysis indicates that major increases in survival to adult ages occurred relatively recently in the Upper Paleolithic.

Two further arguments may be considered, both of which depend on the evolving size and suggest prior increases in life expectancy. First, larger animals tend to have slower development and to live longer as described by allometric relationships (Sacher, 1977; Calder, 1984; Finch, 1990, pp. 267–271; Charnov, 1993; Hawkes and Paine, 2006). Australopithecenes and other early hominids before 2 MYA were in the upper size range of chimpanzees, 20–40 kg (Skinner and Wood, 2006) (Table 6.1), implying modestly longer life spans (Fig. 6.2B). The genus *Homo* rose above this range with *H. habilis* (46 kg) and *H. erectus* (61 kg), followed by *H. heidelbergensis* 71 kg) and *H. sapiens* (64 kg). The range of uncertainty in adult sizes (Table 6.1, footnote e) precludes calculation of life span increases from allometric formulae.

As another approach, consider the possibility that life expectancy increased concurrently with the increase of brain size and the social cooperation. While social cooperation has been emphasized in relation to hunting (also seen in chimpanzees), three uniquely human behaviors are cogent to the evolution of mortality rates, and of life expectancies (summarized from Section 6.2):

1. All societies have multi-generational caregiving of mothers and their young children.

2. Human birth is almost always assisted, unlike that of the great apes. Humans have many difficulties in labor because of the larger human head size (Abitbol, 1996a,b; Ruff, 1995; Trevathan and Rosenberg, 2000; Rosenberg and Travathan, 2002).

3. Weaning is much earlier than in the great apes (Fig. 6.4). Across pre-industrial societies, the 2.5 y average age at weaning is several years earlier than in chimpanzees (4–6 y) or orangutans (7–8 y) (Sellen, 2006; Kennedy, 2005).

Early weaning allows a successive pregnancy before the child is fully able to forage independently. Access to energy dense meat is hypothesized to have facilitated early weaning (Kennedy, 2005). Survival before age 5 depends on provisioning and care by other adults (alloparenting), which enables their mother to become pregnant and give birth, often within a year of weaning. Alloparenting is general, if not universal, in human societies, with various care-giving by relatives of the parental generation, older siblings, or others in the community (Hrdy 1981, 2005). The 50% shorter inter-birth interval in humans gives a huge reproductive advantage that offsets the five-year longer maturation, relative to shared ancestors of the great apes with shorter life expectancy. Assisted birthing would also be developed in this scenario.

The trajectory of increasing life expectancy could have been interrupted or slowed by the enlarging head (Table. 6.1; Fig. 1.1, vertical arrow at 0.5 MYA). The evolving, apparently progressive increase in fetal head size and feto-pelvic dispro-portion would have increased both maternal and fetal mortality. Moreover, if male fetal growth and head size was greater than female, as in modern humans, the male infant mortality would have been greater (Alexander et al, 1999). The pre-dicted increase of maternal mortality and of infants, particularly males, during the final stages of brain size evolution could in turn have stimulated increased invest-ment in caregiving. Assuming that rotational birth began to evolve after 0.5 MYA with the major increase in brain size (Ruff, 1995), then the social complex of multi-generational maternal and child care and alloparenting would have been concur-rent. The evidence for cooperative hunting is also consistent with this timing.

The suggested importance of assistance to mothers and weanlings would join many other skills that are accumulated by mature and older adults, including the hypothesized importance of grandparents. The 70 y modal age at death of hunter-foragers would allow > $\frac{2}{3}$ of those reaching sexual maturity to become grand-parents (Fig. 6.1 legend) (Gurven and Kaplan, 2007). Hawkes and colleagues hypothesized that menopause was evolutionarily selected for the increased trans-fer of resources to the grandchildren (Hawkes et al, 1998; Hawkes, 2003). Survival to greater ages, through greater duration of adult health, would favor increased effective support from older individuals for the reproductive success of the young. However, mathematical life history models for the Aché (Paraguyan hunter-gatheres) did not find that benefits from the cessation of reproduction at menopause to the reproductive success of the daughtors and survival of grandchildren were sufficient to offset the cessation of reproduction at menopause (Hill and Hurtado, 1996; Rogers, 1993).

We need a comprehensive assessment of the many sources of inter-generational support that can enhance reproduction and reduce mortality. Kaplan and Robson (2002) used an economic capital investment model to show the co-evolution of brain size and longevity through trade-offs with delayed productivity. The increased mortality through feto-pelvic disproportion in early stages could be considered within this theory. Moreover, in Lee's mathematical model, intergenerational transfers can be the main force selecting age-specific mortality rates (Lee et al, 2003). Clearly, there are many alternative combinations of reproductive enhancement in the polymorphic multi-generational caregiving by blood relatives and alloparents that characterizes human societies (Hrdy, 1981, 1995; Marlowe, 2000; Peccei, 2001). We must consider next how these unique behavioral capacities were mediated by genetic influences on brain development. The evolution of language is likely to have been catalytic in expanding intergenerational transfers. Moreover, the new gene variants and their combinations (haplotypes) could have functioned at many levels of pleiotropy, as exemplified by apoE (Sections 5.7.4 and 6.2.3).

6.3. FOUR MAJOR SHIFTS IN HUMAN LIFE HISTORY FROM GENETIC AND CULTURAL EVOLUTION

The very recent increases in human life expectancy (LE) can now be placed in a sequence of four phases in the evolution of the unique modern human population age structure (Fig. 6.1). (I) ancestral demographic shift, ape to human LE; (II) recent reduction of early mortality after 1750; (III) recent increases of adult LE; (IV) modern reduction of fertility and delay of first pregnancy. The age structure in post-industrial populations is unique in the higher proportion of older age classes and the lower fecundity. These recent life history shifts have greatly changed the domain of natural selection:

(I) Judged by the current great apes, the shared human-ape ancestor had a 10- to 20-year life expectancy at birth (LE_0), 50% mortality by age 5, and adult mortality accelerations by age 20 (Fig. 6.3B) (Walker et al, 2006a). As a first approximation for early humans, we can look to the surviving forager-hunter-agriculturalists who have LE_0 of 30–40 y, 30% mortality by age 5, and mortality acceleration after age 40. Because the forager values also approximate those of pre-industrial Europe (Fig. 1.1A), we can also consider them to estimate LE during the 10,000 y of the neolithic agricultural and urban expansions during the Industrial Revolution. By all indications, early mortality remained high throughout this period when human populations expanded >20-fold from the beginning of neolithic (<10 million world-wide) to the mid-18th century (200 million) (Fogel and Costa, 1997; McKeown, 1976).

(II) Declines of early mortality before age 5 in the past 200 y have increased survival to maturity several-fold beyond those in feral populations of any other primate or vertebrate. Typical survival of great apes to maturity is <50%. The reduction of early age mortality in the industrializing countries is attributable to improved hygiene as much if not more than nutrition, because infant and child mortality is largely attributed to infections (Crimmins and Finch, 2006a; Finch and Crimmins, 2004, 2005). In Sweden, where death records are comprehensive since 1750 (Section 2.5), mortality was declining even before small pox was eliminated. Remarkably, inoculation programs were begun in Sweden by 1756 (Skold, 2000). Food production was increased by inbreeding and increasingly intensive agriculture, while food availability year round was increased by the growing national transportation networks of canal and rail (McKeown, 1976), collectively described as the 'techno physio revolution' (Fogel and Costa, 1997). Improved food relates to later childhood survival by reducing seasonal mortality in association with scarcity of fresh fruit and vegetables during the winter (Doblhammer and Vaupel, 2001). Seasonal mortality persists in some populations (Section 4.6.2) (Moore et al, 1997).

I wonder if the reduction of early age mortality by > 90% also relaxed natural selection for resistance to infection and its interactions with malnutrition. As a precedent, IL-10 production by leukocytes, which is strongly inherited, predicted mortality from meningococcal disease in the first degree relatives (IL-10 genotypes were not characterized) (Section 5.7.2) (Westendorp et al, 1997). Examination of IL-10 and other immune defense genotypes in early deaths in contemporary health-poor populations might give an estimate of selection in past populations. It might be possible to obtain DNA samples from stillbirths and childhood deaths for comparison with surviving children in the large families being studied in African and Asian clinics (Section 4.6). The relaxation of natural selection for immune gene variants of host resistance could increase vulnerability to infections later in life, if global public health and hygiene worsens (Section 6.4).

(III) Those who survived early mortality also had improved life expectancy in adult years in proportion to the reduction of early mortality in their birth cohort (cohort morbidity hypothesis) (Section 2.5.1) (Crimmins and Finch, 2006a). In 19th century Sweden, life expectancy at age 70 began to increase about 70 years after early mortality began to decline (Fig. 2.7C) (Finch and Crimmins, 2005). Inflammatory mechanisms connect early and later age mortality, e.g., through the arterial inflammatory lesions that are well defined before birth (Fig. 1.15A). The combination of decreased infectious load and access to energy rich foods contributed to greater early growth in unresolved ways that also lowered the age of menarche. The increase of LE_0 to 80 in health-rich populations thus has doubled the initial human life span achieved by natural selection. Survival to advanced ages of great grandparents spanning >4 generations is no longer extremely rare. Centenarians are the fastest growing age group (Robine and Caselli, 2005).

(IV) The reduction of early mortality and the increased availability of nutrition contributed to another major change throughout 20th century populations: the voluntary reduction in the number of children and delay of the first child, the 'Fertility Revolution' (Easterlin and Crimmins, 1985). The potential supply of births must exceed the family or community needs before contraception is sought. As food became cheaper in terms of labor, the duration of postpartum amenorrhea decreased, further increasing potential fecundity. These remarkable cultural shifts were enabled by women's access to education and contraception and in concert with improving health.

These cultural changes were enabled by prior genetic changes during human evolution that reduced early mortality in humans below that of the great apes and slowed aging by delaying mortality rate accelerations. At the same time, the age of menarche has shifted to earlier ages close to the great apes. This plasticity is seated in the neuroendocrine controls that regulate growth and development according to the energy balance, which depends on food availability, and the load of infection and inflammation. The reproductive schedule is highly plastic because most reproductive cell targets are genomically competent to respond to hormonal signals long before the usual age of maturation (Finch and Rose, 1995). The modern delay of reproduction to later ages does not depart from the long-established physiological architecture. The trend for later first births in certain populations to which many of the present readers belong, however, brings additional risks of mortality, e.g., from breast cancer (Ma, 2006). These special risks, moreover, are joined by a larger set of emerging mortality risks associated with increasing population, urbanization, and environmental deterioration.

6.4. THE INSTABILITY OF LIFE SPANS

6.4.1. Infections

The steady rise of life expectancy into the 20th century (Fig. 1.1A) does not apply to all populations. Russia is an important example of rapidly decreasing life expectancy (McKee and Notte, 2004) (Fig. 6.8) that has portentous implications for all current populations. Under the Soviet administration, in 1965, life expectancy in Russia was 65 for men and 73 for women, not far below the UK (69 y, men; 74 y, women) (Andreev et al, 2003). Ensuing complex health fluctuations may be explained by resource allocation (see Fig. 6.8 legend). During the collapse of the Soviet administration (1985–1991), Russian life expectancy fell sharply. By 2000, the UK–Russia differences in life expectancy were about 15 y for men and 12.5 years for women. Treatable causes of deaths account for about 3 y of the lost life expectancy, closely followed by ischemic heart disease. Regional mortality varies widely along urban-rural gradients. Meanwhile the UK life span continued to increase steadily by 1 y added per 6 calendar y. Note that sex differences in mortality persist even when health declined abruptly during

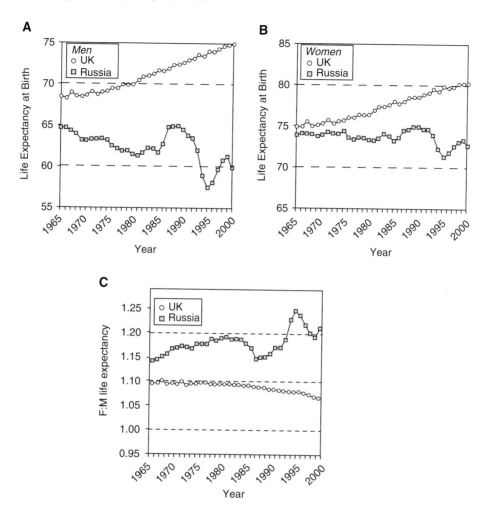

FIGURE 6.8 The declining life expectancy in Russia, 1965–2000, with the UK (Britain) for comparison. (From Andreev et al, 2003.) After WWI, health care advances were made especially in remote and rural areas. But then in the 1960s, resources were increasingly diverted to the military-industrial sector at the expense of health care. Isolation from medical and pharmaceutical advances increased. Transient improvements in life expectancy in the 1980s coincide with Gorbachov's anti-alcohol campaigns, with decreased hemorrhagic stroke. The Soviet political and economic collapse in 1991 triggered marked declines in health that are attributed to increased alcoholism and poverty. Heavy smoking and diets rich in fat and low in anti-oxidants are other long-standing factors in the high level of vascular disease. TB and other infections have increased and may be major factors in the higher mortality. A. Males, Russia versus UK. B. Females. C. Female:male (F, M) ratio.

the impending Soviet collapse. These differences are consistent with the global profile of greater male vulnerability (Section 5.2).

Increasing infections in post-Soviet Russia may be important in the increasing mortality. For example, tuberculosis (TB) is considered pandemic (Floyd, 2006; Toungoussova et al, 2006) and accounts for 75% of deaths from infectious causes (Andreev et al, 2003). TB deaths increased 2.5-fold from 1991 to 2001. Drug-resistant TB is increasing and exceeds 50% in some populations (Toungoussova et al, 2006). General risk factors for TB are crowded living conditions, consumption of raw milk, financial stress, and unemployment (Coker et al, 2006). TB is also a common co-morbidity (50%) in the widespread alcoholism and also found to varying degrees in HIV and hepatitis C (Krupitsky et al, 2006). These figures give the impression of declining public health and hygiene. Although infant mortality shows recent improvements, it is still higher than in industrial countries (Webster, 2003). The unreliable Russian pediatric mortality data (Webster, 2003) precludes examination of relationships to growth trajectories, which may differ between subpopulations like the observed historical changes (Section 2.5).

The Russian mortality catastrophe may guide thinking about public health in the United States and other industrialized countries where child health programs for non-citizens and indigent poor are receiving increasingly less political support. In all countries, the lower SES groups have a higher rate of endemic infections. Two examples from the migrant agricultural workers who handle the U.S. food are worth pondering: Seropositivity for hepatitis A virus (HAV) among a sample of Florida migrant workers' children was 81% by age 14, which is >5-fold above the U.S. average for these ages (Dentinger et al, 2001). This prevalence indicates the poor level of hygiene, which favors transmission by fecal-oral routes (Brundage and Fitzpatrick, 2006; Leach, 2004). Although most hepatitis A cases are asymptomatic, this level of seropositivity is a sentinel of poor hygiene that favors other infections. High-density housing is a factor in hepA transmission, which may contribute to the higher prevalence of tuberculosis in migrant workers. In California migrant workers, 11% had active TB, >100-fold above the general U.S. population (McCurdy et al, 1997).

Soon, the majority of people will live in urban environments that have not been planned or designed for the continuing influx (FAO, 2006; Moore et al, 2003). In 1970, about 35% of the world lived in urban areas, and by 2020 56% are expected. The developing countries in particular have urban populations with prevalent infectious disease, high exposure to environmental inflammogens, and poor nutrition. The health risks include polluted air and drinking water; insufficient water for bathing and hygiene; crowded housing and shared beds; inadequate disposal of garbage and sewerage; poverty and unemployment. Growth stunting is increased in these toxic environments. Domestic animals are also important pathogen pools in urban environments and in the contamination of produce in industrial farming. As the global climate worsens and rural industrialization progresses, small farmers are increasingly displaced and migrate to the coalescing megacities. The growing refugee camps also harbor increasing numbers of high-density, multi-generational health-poor populations. But the health-rich countries also have severely disadvantaged urbanites.

Major efforts are needed to monitor urban health and to prevent potentially catastrophic epidemic infections that can spread like the wind across the world. High-density population corridors extend the first ancient pathways of *H. sapiens* in East Africa and from the Mediterranean to South and East Asia. Although few data are available on health in most urban poor, it is instructive that the HIV pandemic has spread from urban populations into rural populations in Africa (Andoh et al, 2006) and Russia (Toungoussova et al, 2006).

Clean water, already in short supply for the health-poor, will be increasingly scarce and expensive (FAO, 2006). In 2000, only 15% of people had access to abundant water. The ongoing privatization of water will only worsen this situation. Diarrhea and other water-related diseases are scourges of childhood that often increase mortality in adult life (Section 4.6). Fecally transmitted *Shigella*, rotaviruses, and amoebiasis are major causes of dysentery and mortality. Typhoid fever, cholera, and nematode infections are also associated with poor water and sanitation. Half of the world (3.5 billion) is infected with roundworm (*Ascaris*), whipworm (*Trichuris*), or hookworm (*Ancylostoma* or *Necator*). The implicit relationships between the availability of clean water and life expectancy are seated in growth stunting from energy drain by parasites and microbial infections, and from weakened immunity from immune hyperstimulation, leading to premature immunosenescence (Section 2.8, Section 4.6).

Drug resistant TB, *Staphylococcus aureus, Streptococcus pneumoniae,* and other infections are clearly increasing. Thus, modern humans may re-enter a Darwinian regime with selection for resistance to infections. It seems unlikely that the modern health-rich populations will be exposed to the high level of early mortality (10–30% of neonates) that prevailed 200 years ago, with death of 10–30% of infants (Crimmins and Finch, 2006a,b). We will never know the role of genetic variations that may have increased mortality risks. However, there are many examples of gene variants that favor survival of infections. The sickle cell hemoglobin gene and others are well known to protect heterozygote carriers from malaria, while the IL-10 variants may enhance survival of meningitis (Section 5.7.2). The spread of drug resistant malaria and other pathogens may select for new genotypes of host resistance.

6.4.2. Air Quality

Declining air quality may be anticipated to impact on global longevity trends. The lung is vulnerable to chronic inflammation from airborne pollutants. Up to 5% of global mortality is attributed to indoor smoke (World Health Organization, 2002). It is not news that exposure is increasing to airborne pollutants from fossil fuels that are transported globally. But as the growth of cities continues, more humans will be exposed to additional adversity from polluted air. Urban areas are notorious for locally generated air pollutants from dense automotive traffic with minimal emission control and dust from unpaved roads. The burning of wood and charcoal ('biomass combustion') in inefficient household fires for cooking and warmth causes chronic pneumonia in children and chronic obstructive long disease (COPD) (anthracosis and 'hut-lung' disease, Section 6.2) (Diaz et al, 2006). These exposures began with the domestication of fire in the Paleolithic and intensified in the Neolothic. Tobacco use is also high in poor urban areas, while poor sanitation generates airborne endotoxins and odors. Some populations are exposed to industrial toxins and aerosols from deforested land. Industrial farming of poultry and cattle generates fecal aerosols. These myriad inhalants can cause chronic local and systemic inflammatory responses that compromise lung functions and increase COPD and vascular diseases (Chapter 2).

Two regional studies may represent global trends. In Edinburgh 1981–1995, mortality covaried with fluctuations in the density of black smoke (Prescott et al, 1998). Each increment of 10 $\mu g/m^3$ of smoke particles during the past 72 h increased adult mortality by about 1.5%, with cardiovascular and respiratory conditions as the main causes. Hospital admissions for cardiovascular conditions in the elderly were increased 4.8%. Similarly, seasonal variations in airborne particulates also correlated with hospital admissions in Indian cities (Kaushik et al, 2006). While few global statistics are available, there is little doubt that poor air quality is a growing contribution to mortality, particularly in urban populations.

Genetic risk factors for air pollution include glutathione-S-transferase M1 (GST), which makes the key anti-oxidant glutathione (Section 6.2). The null allele (GSTM1*0), which decreases anti-oxidant activity, is common in Europeans (70%). M1*0 homozygotes (equivalent to GSTM1 knockout) have impaired lung functions as children and a higher risk of asthma (Peden, 2005). Carriers from mothers who smoked during pregnancy had 2-fold higher risk of persistent wheeze (Gilliland et al, 2002). The increased oxidative damage in the lung from airborne inflammogens is directly linked to asthma, a chronic inflammatory condition (Queries II and III). Smoking may be anticipated to show synergies with other air pollutants. The transgenerational effect of maternal smoking on respiratory conditions may have later life consequences.

6.4.3. Obesity and Diabetes

At the same time as exposure to infections and inflammogens is growing in health poor populations, the prevalence of obesity is increasing rapidly (Flegal et al, 2002; Ogden et al, 2006) (Section 3.2.3). Between 1980 and 1999 in the United States, obesity doubled to 27.5% in men and 33.4% in women. Although adult obesity may be leveling off in some populations, it has continued to increase in children and adolescents by net increments in of 4–10%, depending on age, gender, and ethnicity. In the United States, overweight status in ages 2–19 increased from 13.9% in 1999–2000 to 17.1% in 2003–2004. In China, urban pre-school obesity increased from 1.5% in 1989 to 12.6% in 1997. The pandemic of worldwide obesity may be extending to health-poor and impoverished populations. In rural Gambia, obesity is still rare (Section 4.6) but is increasing in younger urban women (Siervo et al, 2006). We may anticipate that underweight babies who are exposed to Western diets will be at risk for vascular and metabolic diseases, as in the industrial countries (Fig. 4.1C).

There are strong indications of future decreases in adult health and life expectancy if the obesity pandemic continues. Based on NHANES 3 data, elimination of obesity at birth would increase life expectancy by up to 1 year (Olshansky et al, 2005) (Fig. 6.9). Health professionals broadly recognize costs to the healthy life span at many levels of function (Visscher and Seidell, 2001). Obesity increases morbidities and disabilities from cardiovascular disease, hypertension, impaired kidney function, peripheral neuropathy, and retinopathy. Mobility problems increase with joint wear. In the Framingham Heart Study, obesity shortened life expectancy and increased the number of years lived with cardiovascular disease by 2.4 y in women and 1.4 y in men (Pardo Silva et al, 2006). Obesity in adolescents is associated with decreased insulin secretion and impaired glucose tolerance and increased risk of type 2 diabetes (Marcovecchio et al, 2005; Weiss et al, 2006), which are among the vascular risk factors of the metabolic syndrome (Section 1.7, Table 1.8). Obese children have other adverse vascular indicators, e.g., 2-fold elevations of CRP, 35% higher

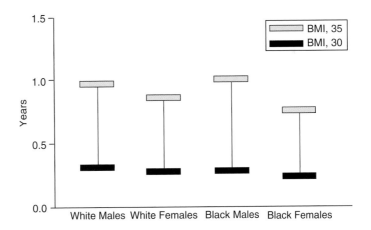

FIGURE 6.9 Obesity shortens the life expectancy by up to a year (U.S. 2000). (From Olshansky et al, 2005.) The potential gain in life expectancy at birth, if obesity were eliminated, was calculated by gender and ethnicity for BMI 30 (lower bar) to 35 (upper bar) relative to mortality risk in BMI of 24.

LDL/HDL and fibrinogen, 20% thicker carotid artery wall (IMT) (Meyer et al, 2006). Moreover, obese and diabetic mothers tend to epigenetically transmit these traits to their children, who have more preadolescent obesity and diabetes on sedentary and energy-rich diets (Chapter 5). Obesity-related health issues are stimulating national programs on healthy lifestyles that may soon be on the scale of the public health campaigns of the 19t^h century.

6.4.4. Prospects

The increase of U.S. life expectancy since 1980 was about 0.5 y, which is much less than the 1 y average added per 5 y of recent historical time (Fig. 1.1A). It is unclear if the increase of life expectancy is leveling off in the United States and other health-rich countries. Nonetheless, there is no way to guess the future. The Social Security Administration has consistently underestimated the increase in life expectancy (Olshansky et al, 2005). According to a widely cited calculation from the National Center for Health Statistics, the hypothetical elimination of cardiovascular and cerebrovascular diseases would increase life expectancy at birth by 6.73 y (Anderson, 1999). "[E]ven eliminating all aging-related causes of death [listed] on death certificates of the elderly will not increase human life expectancy by more than 15 years" (Olshansky et al, 2002, p. 293). Given the early onset and near universality of progressive atherosclerosis (Fig. 1.6), novel technologies and drugs may be required to eliminate vascular disease as a major cause of mortality.

However, two caveats may be considered: (I) These calculations are based on stated *single* causes of death. As aging progresses, multiple lesions are the norm in humans, as in rodents (Fig. 1.5). (II) Several subcritical lesions may synergize; e.g., congestive heart failure may be due to synergies of pulmonary hypertension (not fatal alone) and ventricular fibrosis (not fatal alone). About 25% of aging diet-restricted rodents have no defined gross pathology when autopsied (Section 3.2.2). Sudden death without gross organ degenerative conditions could arise from transient hypoglycemia, as in the 'dead-in-bed syndrome' of type 1 diabetics (Heller, 2002). A more comprehensive theory of mortality is needed that extends beyond the canonical histopathology to include data on physiological fluctuations. In fact, such data are being collected through personal mobile device monitoring of blood glucose and pressure.

Negative health trends throughout the world oppose further gains in life expectancy. In the more affluent populations, obesity is increasing, while ever more urban poor are immersed in dirty environments with infectious pathogens and inflammatory pollutants. Poor urban air quality does not only result from local industrialization, it is endemic because of inefficient fires used for cooking and exhaust from poorly maintained motor vehicles, among myriad other sources.

While remarkable advances may be made to eliminate polio and small pox, there has been smaller impact on HIV, parasites, and other infections, which remain a prevalent human experience. Rheumatic heart disease from streptococcus infections, now rare in health-rich populations (Section 2.2.1), continues to be a major cause of heart failure in Asia and Africa (Chockalingam et al, 2003; Mendez and Cowie, 2001; Rullan and Sigal, 2001). Moreover, medical interventions alone do not suffice in a poor environment: As discussed in Section 4.2, access to an excellent local clinic did not improve childhood growth in Guatemalan villages. Thus, the evident global environmental deterioration and the continued population influx to urban zones are exposing even more to adverse environments.

Further increases of life expectancy beyond 80 may be restricted to an elite who can afford to live in an optimum environment and lifestyle *and* who can afford biomedical advances including expensive drugs and regenerative surgery. In terms of demographic mortality profiles, most populations will continue to be subject to the Gompertz mortality acceleration, which prevails from age 40–80 (Fig. 1.1C, Fig. 2.7). The morbidities associated with obesity would be expected to generate Gompertzian mortality with advancing age, consistent with Fig. 6.8. A mortality rate plateau after age 90 emerged in the mid-19th century (Section 1.2.1), which introduced a post-Gompertzian subpopulation possibly unique in human history (Vaupel et al, 1998). Centenarians, while the fastest growing demographic group, cannot become more than an extreme minority of <0.5%, as long the Gompertz acceleration prevails globally.

Extreme longevity cannot become more prevalent without unprecedented improvement in the global load of infectious disease, unanticipated improvement in air and water quality, and unimaginable universal access to costly drugs and regenerative medicine. Despite the current advantages of the health-rich elite, the global systems of commerce, water, and wind prevent isolation of any group from the growing pools of infections and inflammogens. Consider this when you next dine in an elegant restaurant: You are but one handshake from staff who cannot afford to miss work because of illness.

6.5. SUMMARY OF CHAPTERS 1–6: MECHANISMS IN AGING AND LIFE HISTORY EVOLUTION

This exploration of aging has emphasized nutrition and inflammation in human aging processes. Inflammatory processes are well documented in arterial disease, Alzheimer disease, and obesity. Many of the disease-associated inflammatory processes are also found during normal aging without specific pathology. Fetal and neonatal arteries have microscopic aggregates of oxidized lipids in macrophages and focal inflammatory processes typical of later arterial lesions (Fig. 1.15). Inflammatory processes begun before birth may be further kindled by maternal conditions and unavoidable postnatal exposures to infections and inflammogens.

I have argued that general mechanisms of aging may be resolved as three interacting suites of mechanisms: (I) oxidant damage and inflammation; (II) damage to irreplaceable molecules and cells; and (III) physiological set points for food intake, locomotor activity, and blood metabolic hormones. The inflammatory origins of adult diseases may be more generalized than those presumed in 'fetal origins theory,' which emphasizes the role of maternal nutrition on adult cell numbers (kidney, muscle, and pancreas) and physiological set points (blood pressure, glucose, and stress responses) (Chapter 4). It seems that no single mechanism explains enough about aging. We must appreciate how multifarious environmental influences modulate the nuanced physiological systems of aging.

Humans and the lab models have generalized (canonical) aging patterns that are remarkably persistent across environments (Table 1.1). It is evident that many outcomes of aging result from the irreplaceability of molecules and cells that are generated during development, under the control of gene regulatory programs. Thus developmental established patterns of gene expression can be said to lock-in many aspects of aging. For molecules and cells that are replaced, aging damage may also accrue, depending on turnover rate (lifespan). The loss of elasticity during arterial aging is a consequence of accrued damage to its irreplaceable elastin through inflammation and oxidative damage. Elastin fibrils becomes progressively frayed and broken, while collagen and elastin become glycol-oxidized and cross-linked. Both changes contribute to the loss of arterial compliance and increased systolic pressure with aging (Fig. 1.6), which is a major mortality risk factor. Even before birth, fetal arteries are accumulating activated macrophages and oxidized lipids.

Thus, the fetal origins of adult vascular disease are seated in three intrinsic aging processes observed in optimal environments: aging of irreplaceable elastin; oxidation and cross linking of collagen and elastin from irreducible exposure to essential levels of glucose; and the accumulation of lipids and activated macrophages in fetal aortas. In addition, there are many influences from the maternal environment. The Barker theory of fetal origins has focused on maternal nutrition, which can influence the risk of obesity and diabetes (Sections 4.2 and 4.3). Physiological set points for appetite and responses to stress determine the risks of obesity and diabetes, and duration of stress responses. Metabolic disorders can accelerate the underlying endogenous arterial aging processes. In addition, I have emphasized the importance of infection and inflammation, which can also accelerate arterial aging processes (Section 2.2). The slowly progressive increase in human height and longevity over multiple generations since the 19th century may include transgenerational effects as well as the pace of environmental improvements.

Brain, kidney, muscle, ovary, and the adaptive immune system have limited cell regeneration in adults. Stems cells that can repair or regenerate arteries, brain, and muscle are attenuated by inflammation (Section 2.8). In clonal expansions during immunosenescence, telomere DNA loss is associated with increased vulnerability to infections (Section 2.8). Infections and immune activation can cause accelerated depletion of naïve T cells and increase the secretion of inflammatory factors by highly differentiated T cells (Section 1.5.3.1). We do not know if the presence of highly differentiated T cells in atheromas is a cause or effect of their instability. Fig. 1.2A illustrates the high connectivity within the matrix of aging.

We may anticipate a detailed quantitative framework of causal pathways for health and disease during individual life histories seated in differential gene expression. The pathways in Fig. 1.2A and Fig. 1.3 can be expanded to include environmental influences during development. The three Queries about inflammation, oxidative damage, and inflammation (Section 1.1) have pointed to a matrix of complex aging processes begun during development that interface with the external environment throughout life. These processes are modulated at almost every instant by biochemical events that are open to interactions and interventions through the external environment and internal milieu. The genetics of aging clearly influences individual responses to the environment, drugs, and nutrition.

However, we should not expect that aging outcomes are determined by tightly controlled gene regulatory circuits that lead to fixed cellular endpoints. Early development and cell differentiation are understood in terms of transcription factor sets that determine differentiated cell phenotypes (Davidson, 2006; Howard and Davidson, 2004). Embryo gene regulation in general leads to differentiation with restricted cell phenotypes. The core of developmental programming is logic circuits that irreversibly determine the successive patterns of gene expression leading to organogenesis and differentiation. Subsequent stages may vary widely between individuals depending on the environment, with social insect castes as a famous example. Variations of human birth weight may be considered as alternate phenotypes determined by maternal energy resources (Chapter 4).

In humans and other species with prolonged development and maturation, a different regulatory logic is activated that allows multiple outcomes with conditional switch points. We have seen this in the slowing growth by infection and malnutrition, and in the suppression of immune responses by energy restriction. The immune responses by pathogen receptors (Fig. 5.4) engage multiple regulatory levels, with checkpoints for input of physiological information after ligand binding. For example, the suppression of immune responses by starvation can be overridden by injection of leptin (Lord et al, 1998) (Chapter 3). Energy resources clearly regulate the later stages of development and maturation. Energy limitations induce the dauer larvae of worms and delay puberty in humans. The conditionality of these circuits is shown by the ability of leptin injection to override malnutrition and initiate puberty.

We must re-evaluate our use of clean experimental models that have recently given remarkable insights into the genetic regulation of aging. During adaptation to the lab, fly, worm, and mouse were selected for rapid growth and fecundity, following the paradigm that enabled the domestication of animals and plants. Elimination of most infectious diseases in lab animals was another major achievement that decreased experimental variability from sporadic infections and also increased life span. Recent wild-derived mice are smaller and mature later than standard strains; surprisingly, they also live even longer (Fig. 3.3). While lab rodents are not germ-free, their infectious burden is much more limited than in the wild. There are many parallels of animal husbandry to the public health and hygiene movement that improved human longevity during the past 200 years. But the open environment of humans has not eliminated exposure to pathogens.

As described above, human evolution has generated increasing exposure to infections and inflammogens. The great apes live in low-density migratory groups that move to a new night nest each day and so are rarely exposed to accumulating excreta. During several million years, human ancestors shifted gradually from plant-based diets to high meat intake, which increased exposure to atherogenic levels of cholesterol and to pathogens. In the past 10,000–20,000 years, humans increasingly settled in high density in close contact with domesticated animals, which further increased exposure to infectious pathogens, smoke, and other inflammogens. Despite some sewerage control in ancient cities, humans were adapted to high levels of infection and inflammogens. The progressive decrease in average weight over the past 50,000 years (Fig. 6.8) implies energetic costs to growth of this new life history. Variations between pre-industrial peoples in the rate of growth and maturation (Fig. 5.4C) (Walker et al, 2006a) could reflect different gene–environment responses to nutrition and inflammation. There may be many multiple alternate trajectories of human life histories in the ever-evolving human life spans. In populations under Darwinian selection, sufficient reproduction can be achieved by innumerable combinations of mortality rates and reproductive rates (Section 1.2.8).

I suggest that we need to develop animal models to incorporate the role of infections and inflammation in aging. A start has been made in the serendipitous finding that the some worm mutants with extended life span are also more resistant to pathogenic bacteria (Section 5.5.3). However, long-lived dwarf mice are more vulnerable to infections (Section 5.7.1.1). Little is known about the details of aging in humans exposed to high levels of infections and inflammogens. The long life spans enjoyed by the health-rich may soon be challenged by environmental deterioration and inevitable influx from the health-poor.

These huge questions are with the compass of ongoing biomedical research. I suggest that infections and inflammation be considered as part of the evolution of gene regulatory machinery for development. While the egg and early embryo may be relatively free from invading pathogens, larval stages are vulnerable and have well-developed host defenses. As noted in Section 5.4.2, the toll pathway that initiates embryonic fields in flies also regulates innate immunity. Pursuit of the mechanisms in aging thus has the same goals of understanding the 'regulatory genome' of development. Gene regulation corrects up to some range the random events encountered from the external environment and the internal milieu. Unlike the entelechy of development, there is no strongly selected unfolding program of outcomes in aging. Humans in particular have a remarkable range of behavioral, physiological, and pathological phenotypes throughout life.

Developmental aging research may reveal the implied conditional checkpoints in gene expression that determine aging patterns of the individual. Understanding these event-dependent aging processes may illuminate the central mystery in the biology of aging: how species of the same body plan, physiological architecture, and qualitative cell biochemistry can vary 10- to 100-fold in life span within a phylum.

BIBLIOGRAPHY

Aaby, P., Marx, C., Trautner, S., Rudaa, D., Hasselbalch, H., Jensen, H., and Lisse, I. (2002). Thymus size at birth is associated with infant mortality: A community study from Guinea-Bissau. *Acta Paediatr.* **91,** 698–703.

Abedin, M., Tintut, Y., and Demer, L. L. (2004). Vascular calcification: Mechanisms and clinical ramifications. *Arterioscler Thromb Vasc Biol.* **24,** 1161–1170.

Abitbol, M. M. (1996a). The shapes of the female pelvis. Contributing factors. *J Reprod Med* **41,** 242–250.

Abitbol, M. M. (1996b). *Birth and Human Evolution: Anatomical and Obstetrical Mechanics in Primates.* Westport, CT: Bergin and Garvey.

Adam, E., Melnick, J. L., Probtsfield, J. L., Petrie, B. L., Burek, J., Bailey, K. R., McCollum, C. H., and DeBakey, M. E. (1987). High levels of cytomegalovirus antibody in patients requiring vascular surgery for atherosclerosis. *Lancet.* **2,** 291–293.

Adams, E. J., Cooper, S., and Parham, P. (2001). A novel, nonclassical MHC class I molecule specific to the common chimpanzee. *J Immunol.* **167,** 3858–3869.

Adams, K. F., Schatzkin, A., Harris, T. B., Kipnis, V., Mouw, T., Ballard-Barbash, R., Hollenbeck, A., and Leitzmann, M. F.(2006). Overweight, obesity, and mortality in a large prospective cohort of persons 50 to 71 years old. *New Engl J Med.* **355,** 763–778.

Adams, N. R. (1976). Pathological changes in the tissue of infertile ewes with clover disease. *J Comp Pathol.* **86,** 29–35.

Adams, N. R. (1990). Permanent infertility in ewes exposed to plant oestrogens. *Aust Vet J.* **67,** 197–201.

Adan, Y., Shibata, K., Sato, M., Ikeda, I., and Imaizumi, K. (1999). Effects of docosa-hexaenoic and eicosapentaenoic acid on lipid metabolism, eicosanoid production, platelet aggregation and atherosclerosis in hypercholesterolemic rats. *Biosci Biotech Biochem.* **63,** 111–119.

Adelman, R. C. (1978). Endocrine regulation of enzyme activity in aging animals of different genotypes. In D. Bergsma and D. E. Harrison, Eds., *Genetic Effects on Aging,* pp. 355–364. New York: Alan R. Liss, Inc.

Aerts, L., and Van Assche, F. A. (2006). Animal evidence for the transgenerational development of diabetes mellitus. *Int J Biochem Cell Biol.* **38,** 894–903.

Aguado-Llera, D., Arilla-Ferreiro, E., Campos-Barros, A., Puebla-Jimenez, L., and Barrios, V. (2005). Protective effects of insulin-like growth factor-I on the somatostatinergic system in the temporal cortex of beta-amyloid-treated rats. *J Neurochem.* **92,** 607–615.

Aguilaniu, H., Gustafsson, L., Rigoulet, M., and Nystrom, T. (2003). Asymmetric inheritance of oxidatively damaged proteins during cytokinesis. *Science.* **299,** 1751–1753

Ahmed, M. N., Suliman, H. B., Folz, R. J., Nozik-Grayck, E., Golson, M. L., Mason, S. N., and Auten, R. L. (2003). Extracellular superoxide dismutase protects lung development in hyperoxia-exposed newborn mice. *Am J Resp Crit Care Med.* **167,** 400–405.

Aiello, L. C., and Key, C. (2002). Energetic consequences of being a *Homo erectus* female. *Am J Hum Bio.* **14,** 551–565.

Aisen, P. S., Schafer, K. A., Grundman, M., Pfeiffer, E., Sano, M., Davis, K. L., Farlow, M. R., Jin, S., Thomas, R. G., and Thal, L. J. (2003). Effects of rofecoxib or naproxen vs placebo on Alzheimer disease progression: A randomized controlled trial. *JAMA.* **289,** 2819–2826.

Ajjan, N., and Triau, R. (1975). Vaccination antimorbilleuse et allergie tuberculinique. *Pediatrie.* **30,** 29–44.

Akbar, A. N., Beverley, P. C., and Salmon, M. (2004). Will telomere erosion lead to a loss of T-cell memory? *Nature Rev. Immunol.* **4,** 737–743.

Akbar, A. N., and Fletcher, J. M. (2005). Memory T cell homeostasis and senescence during aging. *Curr Opin Immunol.* **17,** 480–485.

Akima, M., Nonaka, H., Kagesawa, M., and Tanaka, K. (1986). A study on the microvasculature of the cerebral cortex. Fundamental architecture and its senile change in the frontal cortex. *Lab Invest.* **55,** 482–489.

Akiyama, H., Barger, S., Barnum, S., Bradt, B., Bauer, J., Cole, G. M., Cooper, N. R., Eikelenboom, P., Emmerling, M., Fiebich, B. L., Finch, C. E., Frautschy, S., Griffin, W. S., Hampel, H., Hull, M., Landreth, G., Lue, L., Mrak, R., Mackenzie, I. R., McGeer, P. L., O'Banion, M. K., Pachter, J., Pasinetti, G., Plata-Salaman, C., Rogers, J., Rydel, R., Shen, Y., Streit, W., Strohmeyer, R., Tooyoma, I., Van Muiswinkel, F. L., Veerhuis, R., Walker, D., Webster, S., Wegrzyniak, B., Wenk, G., and Wyss-Coray, T. (2000). Inflammation and Alzheimer's disease. *Neurobiol Aging.* **21,** 383–421.

Al-Regaiey, K. A., Masternak, M. M., Bonkowski, M., Sun, L., and Bartke, A.(2005). Long-lived growth hormone receptor knockout mice: Interaction of reduced insulin-like growth factor i/insulin signaling and caloric restriction. *Endocrinology.* **146,** 851–860.

Albanes, D., Salbe, A. D., Levander, O. A., Taylor, P. R., Nixon, D. W., and Winick, M. (1990). The effect of early caloric restriction on colonic cellular growth in rats. *Nutrit Canc.* **13,** 73–80.

Albert, M. A., Danielson, E., Rifai, N., and Ridker, P. M. (2001). Effect of statin therapy on C-reactive protein levels: The pravastatin inflammation/CRP evaluation (PRINCE): A randomized trial and cohort study. *JAMA.* **286,** 64–70.

Albert, M. S. (2002). Memory decline: The boundary between aging and age-related disease. *Ann Neurol.* **51,** 282–284.

Albertson, D. G., and Thomson, J. N. (1976). The pharynx of *Caenorhabditis elegans*. *Philos Trans R Soc Lond B Biol Sci.* **275,** 299–325.

Alcedo, J., and Kenyon, C. (2004). Regulation of *C. elegans* longevity by specific gustatory and olfactory neurons. *Neuron.* **41,** 45–55.

Alexander, G. E., Chen, K., Pietrini, P., Rapoport, S. I., and Reiman, E. M. (2002). Longitudinal PET evaluation of cerebral metabolic decline in dementia: A potential outcome measure in Alzheimer's disease treatment studies. *Am J Psychiatry.* **159,** 738–745.

Alexander, G. R., Kogan, M. D., Himes, J. H. (1999). 1994-1996 U.S. singleton birth weight percentiles for gestational age by race, Hispanic origin, and gender. *Matern Child Health J.* **3,** 225–231.

Allansmith, M., McClellan, B. H., Butterworth, M., and Maloney, J. R. (1968). The development of immunoglobulin levels in man. *J Pediatr.* **72,** 276–290.

Allard, M., Lebre, V., and Robine, J. M. (1998). *Jeanne Calment. From Van Gogh's time to ours. 122 Extraordinary years.* New York: Freeman Press.

Allebeck, P., and Bergh, C.(1992). Height, body mass index and mortality: Do social factors explain the association? *Publ Health*. **106,** 375–382.

Allen, J. S., Bruss, J., and Damasio, H. (2005). The aging brain: The cognitive reserve hypothesis and hominid evolution. *Am J Hum Biol*. **17,** 673–689.

Allen, M. J., Laederach, A., Reilly, P. J., Mason, R. J., and Voelker, D. R. (2004). Arg343 in human surfactant protein D governs discrimination between glucose and N-acetyl-glucosamine ligands. *Glycobiology*. **14,** 693–700.

Alley, D. E., Seeman, T. E., Ki Kim, J., Karlamangla, A., Hu, P., and Crimmins, E. M. (2006). Socioeconomic status and C-reactive protein levels in the US population: NHANES IV. *Brain Behav Immun*. **20,** 498–504

Alling, A., and Nelson, M. (1993). *Life under glass*. Oracle AZ: Biosphere Press.

Allison, D. B., Miller, R. A., Austad, S. N., Bouchard, C., Leibel, R., Klebanov, S., Johnson, T., and Harrison, D. E. (2001). Genetic variability in responses to caloric restriction in animals and in regulation of metabolism and obesity in humans. *J Gerontol. Series A, Biol Sci Med Sci*. **56,** 55–65.

Allman, J., Rosin, A., Kumar, R., and Hasenstaub, A. (1998). Parenting and survival in anthropoid primates: Caretakers live longer. *Proc Natl Acad Sci USA*. **95,** 6866–6869.

Almanzar, G., Schwaiger, S., Jenewein, B., Keller, M., Herndler-Brandstetter, D., Wèurzner, R., Schèonitzer, D., and Grubeck-Loebenstein, B. (2005). Long-term cytomegalovirus infection leads to significant changes in the composition of the CD8+ T-cell repertoire, which may be the basis for an imbalance in the cytokine production profile in elderly persons. *J Virol*. **79,** 3675–3683.

Almond, D. (2006). Is the 1918 influenza pandemic over? Long-term effects of in utero influenza exposure in the post 1940 U.S. population. *J Polit Econ*. **14,** 672–712.

Almond, D. and Mazumeder, B. (2005). The 1918 influenza pandemic and subsequent health outcome: an analysis of SIPP data. *Am Econ Assoc*. **95,** 258–262.

Alt, J. A., Bohnet, S., Taishi, P., Duricka, D., Obal, F. J., Traynor, T., Majde, J. A., and Krueger, J. M. (2006). Influenza virus-induced glucocorticoid and hypothalamic and lung cytokine mRNA responses in dwarf lit/lit mice. *Brain Behav Immun*. **21,** 60–67.

Alt, J. A., Obal, F. J., Traynor, T. R., Gardi, J., Majde, J. A., and Krueger, J. M. (2003). Alterations in EEG activity and sleep after influenza viral infection in GHRH receptor-deficient mice. *J Appl Physiol*. **95,** 460–468.

Alzheimer, A. (1911). Uber eigenartige Krankheitsfalle des spateren Alters (On certain peculiar diseases of old age). *Zeitschrift fur gesamte Neurologie und Psychiatrie*. **4,** 356–385. Translation in *Clin Anat*. **8,** 429–431

Amano, T., Meyer, J. S., Okabe, T., Shaw, T., and Mortel, K. F. (1982). Stable xenon CT cerebral blood flow measurements computed by a single compartment—Double integration model in normal aging and dementia. *J Computer Assisted Tomography*. **6,** 923–932.

Amant, F., Moerman, P., Neven, P., Timmerman, D., Van Limbergen, E., and Vergote, I. (2005). Endometrial cancer. *Lancet*. **366,** 491–505.

Amantea, D., Russo, R., Bagetta, G., and Corasaniti, M. T. (2005). From clinical evidence to molecular mechanisms underlying neuroprotection afforded by estrogens. *Pharmacological Research*. **52,** 119–132.

Amarenco, P. (2005). Effect of statins in stroke prevention. *Curr Opin Lipidol*. **16,** 614–618.

Amarenco, P., Bogousslavsky, J., Callahan, A., 3rd, Goldstein, L. B., Hennerici, M., Rudolph, A. E., Sillesen, H., Simunovic, L., Szarek, M., Welch, K. M., Zivin, J. A., and Denis Diderot University, P. (2006). High-dose atorvastatin after stroke or transient ischemic attack. *New Engl J Med*. **355,** 549–559.

Amdam, G. V., Aase, A. L., Seehuus, S. C., Kim Fondrk, M., Norberg, K., and Hartfelder, K. (2005). Social reversal of immunosenescence in honey bee workers. *Exp Gerontol.* **40**, 939–947.

Amdam, G. V., and Omholt, S. W. (2002). The regulatory anatomy of honeybee lifespan. *J Theor Biol.* **216**, 209–228.

Amdam, G. V., Simäoes, Z. L., Hagen, A., Norberg, K., Schroder, K., Mikkelsen, Kirkwood, T. B., and Omholt, S. W. (2004). Hormonal control of the yolk precursor vitellogenin regulates immune function and longevity in honeybees. *Exp Gerontol.* **39**, 767–773.

Ananth, C. V., Balasubramanian, B., Demissie, K., and Kinzler, W. L. (2004). Small-for-gestational-age births in the United States: An age-period-cohort analysis. *Epidemiology.* **15**, 28–35.

Andersen, B., Pearse, R. V., 2nd, Jenne, K., Sornson, M., Lin, S. C., Bartke, A., Rosenfeld, M.G. (1995). The Ames dwarf gene is required for Pit-1 gene activation. *Devel Bio.* **172**, 495–503.

Anderson, R. N. (1999). U.S. decennial life tables for1989–1991, Vol. 4, no. 4. United States life tables eliminating certain causes of death. In *DHHS (PHS) 99-1150-4* Vol. 4, pp. 1–179. Hyattsville, MD: National Center for Health Statistics.

Anderton, B. H. (1997). Changes in the ageing brain in health and disease. *Philos Trans Royal Soc London. Series B, Biol Sci.* **352**, 1781–1792.

Ando, Y., Nyhlin, N., Suhr, O., Holmgren, G., Uchida, K., el Sahly, M., Yamashita, T., Terasaki, H., Nakamura, M., Uchino, M., and Ando, M. (1997). Oxidative stress is found in amyloid deposits in systemic amyloidosis. *Biochem Biophys Res Comm.* **232**, 497–502.

Andoh, S. Y., Umezaki, M., Nakamura, K., Kizuki, M., and Takano, T. (2006). Correlation between national income, HIV/AIDS and political status and mortalities in African countries. *Public Health.* **120**, 624–633.

Andree, C., and Sedivy, R. (2005). Discovery of a letter from Rokitansky to Virchow about subependymal corpora amylacea. *Virchows Archiv.* **446**, 177–180.

Andreev, E. M., Nolte, E., Shkolnikov, V. M., Varavikova, E., and McKee, M.(2003). The evolving pattern of avoidable mortality in Russia. *Int J Epidemiol.* **32**, 437–446.

Andrew, W., Brown., H. M., and Johnson., J. B. (1943a). Senile changes in the liver of mouse and man, with special reference to the similarity of the nuclear alterations. *Am J Anat.* **72**, 199–217.

Andrew, W. H., Brown, H. M., and Johnson, J. B. (1943b). Senile changes in the liver of mouse and man, with special reference to the similarity of the nuclear alterations. *Am J Anat.* **72**, 199–217.

Andrews, E., Jenkins, C., Seachrist, D., Dunphy, G., and Ely, D. (2003). Social stress increases blood pressure and cardiovascular pathology in a normotensive rat model. *Clin Exp Hypertens.* **25**, 85–101.

Andrews, P. and Martin, L. (1991). Hominoid dietary evolution. *Philos Trans Roy Soc London, Series B. Biol Sci.* **334**, 199–209.

Andrews, P., Molleson, T., Boz, B. (2005). The human buriels at Çatalhöyük. *Inhabiting Çatalhöyük: Reports from the 1995-1999 Seasons by Members of the Çatalhöyük Teams.* pp 261–278: McDonald Institute Monographs.

Andrus, S. B., Portman, O. W., and Riopelle, A. J. (1968). Comparative studies of spontaneous and experimental atherosclerosis in primates. II. Lesions in chimpanzees including myocardial infarction and cerebral aneurysms. *Progress in Biochemical Pharmacology.* **4**, 393–419.

Andziak, B., Buffenstein, R. (2006). Disparate patterns of age-related changes in lipid peroxidation in long-lived naked mole-rats and shorter-lived mice. *Aging Cell* **5**, 525–532.

Andziak, B., O'Connor, T. P., Qi, W., Dewaal, E. M., Pierce, A., Chaudhuri, A. R., Van Remmen, H., Buffenstein, R. (2006). High oxidative damage levels in the longest-living rodent, the naked mole-rat. *Aging Cell* **5**, 463–471.

Angata, T., and Varki, A. (2002). Chemical diversity in the sialic acids and related alpha-keto acids: An evolutionary perspective. *Chem Rev.* **102**, 439–469.

Angele, M. K., Schwacha, M. G., Ayala, A., and Chaudry, I. H. (2000). Effect of gender and sex hormones on immune responses following shock. *Shock.* **14**, 81–90.

Angiolini, E., Fowden, A., Coan, P., Sandovici, I., Smith, P., Dean, W., Burton, G., Tycko, B., Reik, W., Sibley, C., and Constãancia, M. (2006). Regulation of placental efficiency for nutrient transport by imprinted genes. *Placenta.* **27**, S98–102.

Anikovich, M. V., Sinitsyn, A. A., Holliday, V. T., Popov, V. V., Lisitsyn, S. N., Forman, S. L., Levkovskaya, G. M., et al. (2007) Early Upper Paleolithic in Eastern Europe and implications for the dispersal of modern humans. *Science.* **315**, 223–226.

Anisimov, V. N., Arbeev, K. G., Popovich, I. G., Zabezhinksi, M. A., Rosenfeld, S. V., Piskunova, T. S., Arbeeva, L. S., Semenchenko, A. V., and Yashin, A. I. (2004). Body weight is not always a good predictor of longevity in mice. *Exp Gerontol.* **39**, 305–319.

Anitschkow, N., and Chalatow, S. (1913). Uber experimentelle cholesterinsteatose und ihre bedeutung fur die entstehung einiger pathologischer prozesse. *Zentralbl. Allg. Pathol.* **24**, 1–9.

Anonymous. (1997a). Consensus recommendations for the postmortem diagnosis of Alzheimer's disease. The National Institute on Aging, and Reagan Institute Working Group on Diagnostic Criteria for the Neuropathological Assessment of Alzheimer's Disease. *Neurobiol Aging* **18**, S1–2.

Anonymous. (1997b). The sixth report of the Joint National Committee on Prevention, Detection, Evaluation, And Treatment of High Blood Pressure. *Arch Intern Med.* **157**, 2413–2446.

Anonymous. (2001). Executive summary of the Third Report of the National Cholesterol Education Program (NCEP) Expert Panel on Detection, Diagnosis, and Treatment of High Blood Cholesterol in Adults (Adult Treatment Panel III). *JAMA.* **285**, 539–553.

Anonymous. (2002). Collaborative meta-analysis of randomised trials of antiplatelet therapy for prevention of death, myocardial infarction, and stroke in high risk patients. Antithrombotic Trialists' Collaboration. *Brit Med J* **324**, 71–86.

Ansell, B. J., Navab, M., Hama, S., Kamranpour, N., Fonarow, G., Hough, G., Rahmani, S., Mottahedeh, R., Dave, R., Reddy, S. T., and Fogelman, A. M. (2003). Inflammatory/anti-inflammatory properties of high-density lipoprotein distinguish patients from control subjects better than high-density lipoprotein cholesterol levels and are favorably affected by simvastatin treatment. *Circulation.* **108**, 2751–2756.

Antebi, A., Yeh, W. H., Tait, D., Hedgecock, E. M., and Riddle, D. L. (2000). daf-12 encodes a nuclear receptor that regulates the dauer diapause and developmental age in *C. elegans.* *GenesDevelt.* **14**, 1512–1527.

Antin, P. B., Yatskievych, T., Dominguez, J. L., and Chieffi, P. (1996). Regulation of avian precardiac mesoderm development by insulin and insulin-like growth factors. *J Cell Physiol.* **168**, 42–50.

Antithrombotic Trialists' Collaboration. (2002). Collaborative meta-analysis of randomised trials of antiplatelet therapy for prevention of death, myocardial infarction, and stroke in high risk patients. *Br Med J.* **324**, 71–86.

Anton-Erxleben, F., Miquel, J., and Philpott, D. E. (1983). Fine-structural changes in the midgut of old *Drosophila melanogaster. Mech Ageing Dev.* **22**, 265–276.

Antonov, A. N. (1947). Children born during the siege of Leningrad in 1942. *Am J Pediatrics.* **30**, 250–259.

Anwar, A., Zahid, A. A., Scheidegger, K. J., Brink, M., and Delafontaine, P. (2002). Tumor necrosis factor-alpha regulates insulin-like growth factor-1 and insulin-like growth factor binding protein-3 expression in vascular smooth muscle. *Circulation.* **105**, 1220–1225.

Appay, V., Rowland-Jones, S. (2002). Premature ageing of the immune system: the cause of AIDS? *Trends Immunol.* **23**, 580–585.

Appt, S. E.(2004). Usefulness of the monkey model to investigate the role soy in postmenopausal women's health. *ILAR J* **45**, 200–211.

Apte, U. M., Limaye, P. B., Desaiah, D., Bucci, T. J., Warbritton, A., and Mehendale, H. M.(2003). Mechanisms of increased liver tissue repair and survival in diet-restricted rats treated with equitoxic doses of thioacetamide. *Toxico Sci.* **72**, 272–282.

Arafa, H. M. (2005). Curcumin attenuates diet-induced hypercholesterolemia in rats. *Med Sci Monitor.* **11**, BR228–234.

Arbeille, P., Caries, G., Tobal, N., Herault, S., Georgescus, M., Bousquet, F., and Perrotin, F. (2002). Fetal flow redistribution to the brain in response to malaria infection: Does protection of the fetus against malaria develop over time? *J Ultrasound Med.* **21**, 739–746.

Arita, M., Clish, C. B., and Serhan, C. N. (2005). The contributions of aspirin and microbial oxygenase to the biosynthesis of anti-inflammatory resolvins: Novel oxygenase products from omega-3 polyunsaturated fatty acids. *Biochem Biophys Res Commun.* **338**, 149–157.

Arking, D. E., Atzmon, G., Arking, A., Barzilai, N., and Dietz, H. C. (2005). Association between a functional variant of the KLOTHO gene and high-density lipoprotein cholesterol, blood pressure, stroke, and longevity. *Circ Res.* **96**, 412–418.

Arking, D. E., Becker, D. M., Yanek, L. R., Fallin, D., Judge, D. P., Moy, T. F., Becker, L. C., and Dietz, H. C.(2003). KLOTHO allele status and the risk of early-onset occult coronary artery disease. *Am J Hum Genet.* **72**, 1154–1161.

Arking, D. E., Krebsova, A., Macek, M., Sr., Macek, M., Jr., Arking, A., Mian, I. S., Fried, L., Hamosh, A., Dey, S., McIntosh, I., and Dietz, H. C.(2002). Association of human aging with a functional variant of Klotho. *Proc Natl Acad Sci USA.* **99**, 856–861.

Armbrecht, H. J., Strong, R., Boltz, M., Rocco, D., Wood, W. G., and Richardson, A. (1988). Modulation of age-related changes in serum 1,25–dihydroxyvitamin D and parathyroid hormone by dietary restriction of Fischer 344 rats. *J Nutr.* **118**, 1360–1365.

Armstrong-Esther, C. A., Lacey, J. H., Crisp, A. H., and Bryant, T. N. (1978). An investigation of the immune response of patients suffering from anorexia nervosa. *Postgrad Med Jl.* **54**, 395–399.

Arnaud, C., Burger, F., Steffens, S., Veillard, N. R., Nguyen, T. H., Trono, D., and Mach, F., (2005). Statins reduce interleukin-6–induced C-reactive protein in human hepatocytes: New evidence for direct antiinflammatory effects of statins. *Arterioscler Thromb Vasc Biol.* **25**, 1231–1236.

Arnold, J. W. (1961). Further observations on amoeboid haemocytes in *Blaberus giganteus. Can.J.Zool.* **39**, 229–236.

Arnold, J. W. (1964). Blood circulation in insect wings. *Memoires Entomol. Soc.Canada* No. **38**.

Aronow, W. S. (2003). C-reactive protein. Should it be considered a coronary risk factor? *Geriatrics.* **58**, 19–22.

Asea, A. (2003). Chaperokine-induced signal transduction pathways. *Exercise Immunol Rev.* **9**, 25–33.

Asfaw, B., White, T., Lovejoy, O., Latimer, B., Simpson, S., and Suwa, G. (1999). *Australopithecus garhi*: A new species of early hominid from Ethiopia. *Science.* **284**, 629–635.

Ashley, F., Kannel, W. B., Sorlie, P. D., and Masson, R. (1975). Pulmonary function: Relation to aging, cigarette habit, and mortality. *Ann Intern Med.* **82**, 739–745.

Ashman, R. B., Papadimitriou, J. M., Fulurija, A., Drysdale, K. E., Farah, C. S., Naidoo, O., and Gotjamanos, T. (2003). Role of complement C5 and T lymphocytes in pathogenesis of disseminated and mucosal candidiasis in susceptible DBA/2 mice. *Microb Pathogen.* **34**, 103–113.

Asikainen, S., and Alaluusua, S. (1993). Bacteriology of dental infections. *Eur Heart J.* **14**, 43–50.

Assa-Kunik, E., Fishman, D., Kellman-Pressman, S., Tsory, S., Elhyany, S., Baharir, O., and Segal, S. (2003). Alterations in the expression of MHC class I glycoproteins by B16BL6 melanoma cells modulate insulin receptor-regulated signal transduction and augment [correction of augments] resistance to apoptosis. *J Immunol.* **171**, 2945–2952.

Astor, B. C., Coresh, J., Heiss, G., Pettitt, D., and Sarnak, M. J. (2006). Kidney function and anemia as risk factors for coronary heart disease and mortality: The Atherosclerosis Risk in Communities (ARIC) Study. *Am Heart J.* **151**, 492–500.

Astradsson, A., and Astrup, J.(2001). An intracranial aneurysm in one identical twin, but no aneurysm in the other. *Br J Neurosurg.* **15**, 168–171.

Atamna, H., and Boyle, K.(2006). Amyloid-beta peptide binds with heme to form a peroxidase: Relationship to the cytopathologies of Alzheimer's disease. *Proc Natl Acad Sci USA.* **103**, 3381–3386.

Atkinson, R. L., Dhurandhar, N. V., Allison, D. B., Bowen, R. L., Israel, B. A., Albu, J. B., and Augustus, A. S. (2006). Human adenovirus-36 is associated with increased body weight and paradoxical reduction of serum lipids. *Int J Obes.* **29**, 281–286.

Atzmon, G., Rincon, M., Schechter, C. B., Shuldiner, A. R., Lipton, R. B., Bergman, A., and Barzilai, N.(2006). Lipoprotein genotype and conserved pathway for exceptional longevity in humans. *PLoS Biol.* **4**, e113.

Auge, N., Garcia, V., Maupas-Schwalm, F., Levade, T., Salvayre, R., and Negre-Salvayre, A. (2002). Oxidized LDL-induced smooth muscle cell proliferation involves the EGF receptor/PI-3 kinase/Akt and the sphingolipid signaling pathways. *Arterioscler Thromb Vasc Biol.* **22**, 1990–1995.

Aurelian, L. (2005). HSV-induced apoptosis in herpes encephalitis. *Curr Top Microbiol Immunol.* **289**, 79–111.

Austad, S.N. (1993). Retarded aging rate in an insular population of opossums. *J Zool* **229**, 695–708.

Austad, S. N. (2006). Patterns in mammalian aging: Demography and evolution. In J. M. Robinne, Crimmins, E., Horiuchi, S., Yi, Z., Eds., *Human longevity, individual life duration, and the growth of the oldest-old population. International Studies in Population, Vol. 4, Berlin:* Springer pp. 43–55.

Austad, S. N., and Kristan, D. M. (2003). Are mice calorically restricted in nature? *Aging Cell.* **2**, 201–207.

Austin, M. A., Zhang, C., Humphries, S. E., Chandler, W. L., Talmud, P. J., Edwards, K. L., Leonetti, D. L., McNeely, M. J., and Fujimoto, W. Y. (2004). Heritability of C-reactive protein and association with apolipoprotein E genotypes in Japanese Americans. *Ann Human Genet.* **68**, 179–188.

Avery, L. (1993). The genetics of feeding in *Caenorhabditis elegans*. *Genetics*. **133,** 897–917.

Awtry, E., H, and Loscalzo, J. (2000). Aspirin. *Circulation*. **101,** 1206–1218.

Azumi, K., De Santis, R., De Tomaso, A., Rigoutsos, I., Yoshizaki, F., Pinto, M. R., Marino, R., Shida, K., Ikeda, M., Arai, M., Inoue, Y., Shimizu, T., Satoh, N., Rokhsar, D. S., Du Pasquier, L., Kasahara, M., Satake, M., and Nonaka, M. (2003). Genomic analysis of immunity in a *Urochordate* and the emergence of the vertebrate immune system: "Waiting for Godot". *Immunogenetics*. **55,** 570–581.

Babin, P. J., Bogerd, J., Kooiman, F. P., Van Marrewijk, W. J., and Van der Horst, D. J. (1999). Apolipophorin II/I, apolipoprotein B, vitellogenin, and microsomal triglyceride transfer protein genes are derived from a common ancestor. *J Mol Evol*. **49,** 150–160.

Bachman, G. C. (2003). Food supplements modulate changes in leucocyte numbers in breeding male ground squirrels. *J Exp Biol* **206,** 2373–2380.

Bada, J. L., Schroeder, R. A., Protsch, R., and Berger, R. (1974). Concordance of collagen-based radiocarbon and aspartic-acid racemization ages. *Proc Natl Acad Sci USA*. **71,** 914–917.

Baer, J. T., Du Laney, T. V., Wyrick, P. B., McCain, A. S., Fischer, T. A., Merricks, E. P., Baldwin, A. S., and Nichols, T. C. (2003). Nuclear factor-kappaB activation in endothelium by *Chlamydia pneumoniae* without active infection. *J Infect Dis*. **188,** 1094–1097.

Bahar, R., Hartmann, C. H., Rodriguez, K. A., Denny, A. D., Busuttil, R. A., Dolle, M. E., Calder, R. B., Chisholm, G. B., Pollock, B. H., Klein, C. A., Vijg, J. (2006). Increased cell-to-cell variation in gene expression in ageing mouse heart. *Nature*. **441,** 1011–1014.

Bakketeig, L. S., Hoffman, H. J., and Harley, E. E. (1979). The tendency to repeat gestational age and birth weight in successive births. *Am J Obstet Gynecol*. **135,** 1086–1103.

Bakketeig, L. S., Hoffman, H. J., Jacobsen, G., Hagen, J. A., and Storvik, B. E. (1997). Intrauterine growth pattern by the tendency to repeat small-for-gestational-age births in successive pregnancies. *Acta Obstet Gynecol Scand Suppl*. **165,** 3–7.

Balding, J., Healy, C. M., Livingstone, W. J., White, B., Mynett-Johnson, L., Cafferkey, M., and Smith, O. P. (2003). Genomic polymorphic profiles in an Irish population with meningococcaemia: Is it possible to predict severity and outcome of disease? *Genes and Immunity*. **4,** 533–540.

Balin, B. J., Gerard, H. C., Arking, E. J., Appelt, D. M., Branigan, P. J., Abrams, J. T., Whittum-Hudson, J. A., and Hudson, A. P. (1998). Identification and localization of *Chlamydia pneumoniae* in the Alzheimer's brain. *Med Microbiol Immunol (Berl)*. **187,** 23–42.

Balk, E. M., Lau, J., Goudas, L. C., Jordan, H. S., Kupelnick, B., Kim, L. U., Karas, R. H. (2003). Effects of statins on nonlipid serum markers associated with cardiovascular disease: a systematic review. *Ann Intern Med*. **139,** 670–682.

BalkBang, K., Lund, M., Wu, K., Mogensen, S. C., and Thestrup-Pedersen, K. (2001). CD4+ CD8+ (thymocyte-like) T lymphocytes present in blood and skin from patients with atopic dermatitis suggest immune dysregulation. *Br J Dermatology*. **144,** 1140–1147.

Barazzoni, R., Zanetti, M., Stebel, M., Biolo, G., Cattin, L., and Guarnieri, G. (2003). Hyperleptinemia prevents increased plasma ghrelin concentration during short-term moderate caloric restriction in rats. *Gastroenterology*. **124,** 1188–1192.

Barbieri, M., Bonafáe, M., Rizzo, M. R., Ragno, E., Olivieri, F., Marchegiani, F., Franceschi, C., and Paolisso, G. (2004). Gender specific association of genetic variation in peroxisome proliferator-activated receptor (PPAR) gamma-2 with longevity. *Exp Gerontol*. **39,** 1095–1100.

Barbieri, M., Bonafe, M., Franceschi, C., and Paolisso, G. (2003). Insulin/IGF-I-signaling pathway: An evolutionarily conserved mechanism of longevity from yeast to humans. *Am J Physiol Endocrinol Metab.* **285,** E1064–10671.

Barbouche, M. R., Levy-Soussan, P., Corcos, M., Poirier, M. F., Bourdel, M. C., Jeammet, P., and Avrameas, S. (1993). Anorexia nervosa and lower vulnerability to infections. *Am J psychiatry.* **150,** 169–70.

Barja, G. (2004). Aging in vertebrates, and the effect of caloric restriction: A mitochondrial free radical production-DNA damage mechanism? *Bio Rev Cambr Philos Soc.* **79,** 235–251.

Barker, D. J. (2002). Fetal programming of coronary heart disease. *Trends Endocrinol Metab.* **13,** 364–368.

Barker, D. J. (2004). The developmental origins of well-being. *Philos Tran Roy Soc London. Series B, Biol Sci.* **359,** 1359–1366.

Barker, D. J., Bull, A. R., Osmond, C., and Simmonds, S. J. (1990). Fetal and placental size and risk of hypertension in adult life. *Br Med J.* **301,** 259–262.

Barker, D. J., Forsen, T., Eriksson, J. G., and Osmond, C. (2002). Growth and living conditions in childhood and hypertension in adult life: A longitudinal study. *J Hypertens.* **20,** 1951–1956.

Barker, D. J., Martyn, C. N., Osmond, C., Hales, C. N., and Fall, C. H. (1993a). Growth in utero and serum cholesterol concentrations in adult life. *Br Med J.* **307,** 1524–1527.

Barker, D. J., and Osmond, C. (1986a). Infant mortality, childhood nutrition, and ischaemic heart disease in England and Wales. *Lancet.* **1,** 1077–1081.

Barker, D. J., Osmond, C., Forsén, T. J., Kajantie, E., and Eriksson, J. G. (2005). Trajectories of growth among children who have coronary events as adults. *New Engl J Med.* **353,** 1802–1809.

Barker, D. J., Osmond, C., and Law, C. M. (1989a). The intrauterine and early postnatal origins of cardiovascular disease and chronic bronchitis. *J Epidemiol Community Health.* **43,** 237–240.

Barker, D. J., Winter, P. D., Osmond, C., Margetts, B., and Simmonds, S. J. (1989b). Weight in infancy and death from ischaemic heart disease. *Lancet.* **2,** 577–580.

Barker, D. J. P., et al. (1993). Fetal nutrition and cardiovascular disease in adult life. *Lancet.* **341,** 938–940.

Barker, D. J. P., and Osmond, C. (1986). Infant mortality, childhood nutrition, and ischaemic heart disease: In England and Wales. *Lancet.* **1,** 1077–1081.

Barker, D. J. P., Osmond, C., and Golding, J.(1990). Height and mortality in the counties of England and Wales. *Ann Hum Biol.* **17,** 1–6.

Barker, D. J. P., Osmond, C., Simmonds, S. J., and Wield, G. A. (1993b). The relation of small head circumference and thinness at birth to death from cardiovascular disease in adult life. *Br Med J.* **306,** 422–426.

Barnea, A., and Nottebohm, F. (1994). Seasonal recruitment of hippocampal neurons in adult free-ranging black-capped chickadees. *Proc Natl Acad Sci USA.* **91,** 11217–11221.

Barnes, A. I., Boone, J. M., Jacobson, J., Partridge, L., and Chapman, T. (2006). No extension of lifespan by ablation of germ line in *Drosophila. Proc Biol Sci.* **273,** 939–947.

Barnoya, J., and Glantz, S. A. (2004). Secondhand smoke: The evidence of danger keeps growing. *Am J Medicine.* **116(3),** 201–202.

Baroldi, G., Oliveira, S. J., and Silver, M. D.(1997). Sudden and unexpected death in clinically 'silent' Chagas' disease. A hypothesis. *Int J Cardiol.* **58,** 263–268.

Baron, J. A. (2003). Epidemiology of non-steroidal anti-inflammatory drugs and cancer. *Progr Exp Tumor Res.* **37,** 1–24.

Barrett-Connor, E., Grady, D., and Stefanick, M. L. (2005). The rise and fall of menopausal hormone therapy. *Ann Rev Publ Health.* **26,** 115–140.

Barrett-Connor, E., and von Muhlen, D. (2003). The association of apolipoprotein E with sex hormones in a population-based sample of postmenopausal Caucasian women. *Eur J Endocrinol.* **148,** 487–488.

Barrett, L. A., Morris, J. G., Stensel, D. J., and Nevill, M. E. (2006). Effects of intermittent games activity on postprandial lipemia in young adults. *Med Sci Sports Exerc.* **38,** 1282–1287.

Barsoum, I., and Yao, H. H. (2006). The road to maleness: From testis to Wolffian duct. *Trends Endocrinol Metab.***17,** 223–228.

Barthel, A., and Schmoll, D. (2003). Novel concepts in insulin regulation of hepatic gluconeogenesis. *Am J Physiol Endocrinol Metab.* **285,** E685–692.

Bartke, A. (1998). Growth hormone and aging. *Endocrine Rev.* **8,** 103–108.

Bartke, A. (2003). Can growth hormone (GH) accelerate aging? Evidence from GH-transgenic mice. *Neuroendocrinology.* **78,** 210–216.

Bartke, A. (2005). Minireview: Role of the growth hormone/insulin-like growth factor system in mammalian aging. *Endocrinology.* **146,** 3718–3723.

Bartke, A. (2006). Long-lived Klotho mice: New insights into the roles of IGF-1 and insulin in aging. *Trends Endocrinol Metab.* **17,** 33–35.

Bartke, A., Wright, J. C., Mattison, J. A., Ingram, D. K., Miller, R. A., and Roth, G. S. (2001). Extending the lifespan of long-lived mice. *Nature.* **414,** 412.

Bartke, A., Wright, J. C., Mattison, J. A., Ingram, D. K., Miller, R. A., and Roth, G. S. (2002). Dietary restriction and life-span. *Science.* **296,** 2141–2142.

Bartolucci, A. A., and Howard, G. (2006). Meta-analysis of data from the six primary prevention trials of cardiovascular events using aspirin. *Am J Cardiol.* **98,** 746–750.

Bartzokis, G. (2004). Age-related myelin breakdown: A developmental model of cognitive decline and Alzheimer's disease. *Neurobiol Aging.* **25,** 5–18.

Bartzokis, G., Cummings, J. L., Sultzer, D., Henderson, V. W., Nuechterlein, K. H., and Mintz, J. (2003). White matter structural integrity in healthy aging adults and patients with Alzheimer disease: A magnetic resonance imaging study. *Arch Neurol.* **60,** 393–398.

Bartzokis, G., Lu, P. H., Geschwind, D. H., Edwards, N., Mintz, J., and Cummings, J. L. (2006). Apolipoprotein E genotype and age-related myelin breakdown in healthy individuals: Implications for cognitive decline and dementia. *Arch Gen Psychiatry.* **63,** 63–72.

Bartzokis, G., Lu, P. H., and Mintz, J. (2004a). Quantifying age-related myelin breakdown with MRI: Novel therapeutic targets for preventing cognitive decline and Alzheimer's disease. *J Alzheimers Dis.* **6(6 Suppl),** S53–59.

Barzilai, N., Atzmon, G., Schechter, C., Schaefer, E., Cupples, A., Lipton, R., Cheng, S., and Shuldiner, A. (2004). Unique lipoprotein phenotype and genotype associated with exceptional longevity. *JAMA.* **290,** 2030–2040.

Bashore, T. R. (1994). Some thoughts on cognitive slowing. *Acta Psychologia.* **86,** 295–325.

Bashore, T. R., and Ridderinkhof, K. R. (2002). Older age, traumatic brain injury, and cognitive slowing: Some convergent and divergent findings. *Psychol Bull.* **1228,** 151–198.

Bassuk, S. S., and Manson, J. E.(2005). Epidemiological evidence for the role of physical activity in reducing risk of type 2 diabetes and cardiovascular disease. *J Appl Physiol* **99,** 1193–1204.

Bassuk, S. S., and Manson, J. E. (2003). Physical activity and cardiovascular disease prevention in women: How much is good enough? *Exer Sport Sci Re.* **31,** 176–181.

Bastard, J.-P., Maachi, M., van Nhieu, J. T., Jardel, C., Bruckert, E., Grimaldi, A., Robert, J.-J., Capeau, J., and Hainque, B. (2002). Adipose tissue IL-6 content correlates with resistance to insulin activation of glucose uptake both *in vivo* and *in vitro.* *J Clin Endocrinol Metab.* **87,** 2084–2089.

Bateson, P. (2007) Developmental plasticity and evolutionary biology. *J Nutrit.* **137,** 1060–1062.

Bateson, P., Barker, D., Clutton-Brock, T., Deb, D., D'Udine, B., Foley, R. A., Gluckman, P., Godfrey, K., Kirkwood, T., Lahr, M. M., McNamara, J., Metcalfe, N. B., Monaghan, P., Spencer, H. G., Sultan, S. E. (2004). Developmental plasticity and human health. *Nature.* **430,** 419–421.

Bauer, J. H., and Helfand, S. L. (2006). New tricks of an old molecule: Lifespan regulation by p53. *Aging Cell.* **5,** 437–440.

Bauer, M., Hamm, A. C., Bonaus, M., Jacob, A., Jaekel, J., Schorle, H., Pankratz, M. J., and Katzenberger, J. D. (2004). Starvation response in mouse liver shows strong correlation with life-span-prolonging processes. *Physiol Genomics.* **17,** 230–244.

Bauman, A. E. (2004). Updating the evidence that physical activity is good for health: An epidemiological review 2000–2003. *J Sci Med Sport.* **7(1 Suppl),** 6–19.

Baumberger, J. P. (1954). James Rollin Slonaker, a worker in vision, nutrition, and activity. *Science.* **120,** 587–588.

Baur, J. A., and Sinclair, D. A. (2006). Therapeutic potential of resveratrol: The *in vivo* evidence. *Nat Rev Drug Discov.* **5,** 493–506.

Bayes-Genis, A., Conover, C. A., and Schwartz, R. S. (2000). The insulin-like growth factor axis: A review of atherosclerosis and restenosis. *Circulation Research.* **86,** 125–130.

Bayne, S., and Liu, J. P. (2005). Hormones and growth factors regulate telomerase activity in ageing and cancer. *Mol Cell Endocrinol.* **240,** 11–22.

Baynes, J. W. (2003). Chemical modification of proteins by lipids in diabetes. *Clin Chem Lab Med.* **41,** 1159–1165.

Bazzano, L. A., He, J., Muntner, P., Vupputuri, S., and Whelton, P. K. (2003). Relationship between cigarette smoking and novel risk factors for cardiovascular disease in the United States. *Ann Intern Med.* **138,** 891–897.

Beaton, G. H. (1989). Small but healthy? Are we asking the right question? *Eur J Clin Nutr.* **43,** 863–875.

Beauchamp, G. K., Keast, R. S., Morel, D., Lin, J., Pika, J., Han, Q., Lee, C. H., Smith, A. B., and Breslin, P. A. (2005). Phytochemistry: Ibuprofen-like activity in extra-virgin olive oil. *Nature.* **437,** 45–46.

Beaudeux, J. L., Burc, L., Imbert-Bismut, F., Giral, P., Bernard, M., Bruckert, E., and Chapman, M. J. (2003). Serum plasma pregnancy-associated protein A: A potential marker of echogenic carotid atherosclerotic plaques in asymptomatic hyperlipidemic subjects at high cardiovascular risk. *Arterioscler Thromb Vasc Biol.* **23,** e7–10.

Beck, J. D., Eke, P., Heiss, G., Madianos, P., Couper, D., Lin, D., Moss, K., Elter, J., and Offenbacher, S. (2005). Periodontal disease and coronary heart disease: A reappraisal of the exposure. *Circulation.* **112,** 19–24.

Beck, J. D., Elter, J. R., Heiss, G., Couper, D., Mauriello, S. M., and Offenbacher, S. (2001). Relationship of periodontal disease to carotid artery intima-media wall thickness: The atherosclerosis risk in communities (ARIC) study. *Arterioscler Thromb Vasc Biol.* **21,** 1816–1822.

Beck, J. D., and Offenbacher, S. (2001). The association between periodontal diseases and cardiovascular diseases: A state-of-the-science review. *Ann Periodontol.* **6,** 9–15.

Becker, K. J., Kindrick, D. L., Lester, M. P., Shea, C., and Ye, Z. C. (2005). Sensitization to brain antigens after stroke is augmented by lipopolysaccharide. *J Cereb Blood Flow Metab.* **25,** 1634–1644.

Beckman, K. B., Ames, B. N. (1998). The free radical theory of aging matures. *Physiol Rev.* **78,** 547–581.

Beckmann, N., Schuler, A., Mueggler, T., Meyer, E. P., Wiederhold, K. H., Staufenbiel, M., and Krucker, T. (2003). Age-dependent cerebrovascular abnormalities and blood flow disturbances in APP23 mice modeling Alzheimer's disease. *J Neurosci.* **23,** 8453–8459.

Beeri, M. S., Davidson, M., Silverman, J. M., Noy, S., Schmeidler, J., and Goldbourt, U.. (2005). Relationship between body height and dementia. *Am J Geriatr Psychiatry.* **13,** 116–123.

Beeson, J. G., and Duffy, P. E. (2005). The immunology and pathogenesis of malaria during pregnancy. *Curr Topics Microbiol Immunol.* **297,** 187–227.

Behl, C., Skutella, T., Lezoualc'h, F., Post, A., Widmann, M., Newton, C. J., and Holsboer, F. (1997). Neuroprotection against oxidative stress by estrogens: Structure-activity relationship. *Mol Pharmacol.* **51,** 535–541.

Beisel, W. R. (1982). Synergism and antagonism of parasitic diseases and malnutrition. *Rev Infect Diseases.* **4,** 746–750.

Beisel, W. R. (1995). Herman Award Lecture, 1995: Infection-induced malnutrition—From cholera to cytokines. *Am J Clin Nutr.* **62,** 813–819.

Belczewski, A. R., Ho, J., Taylor, F. B., Jr., Boffa, M. B., Jia, Z., and Koschinsky, M. L. (2005). Baboon lipoprotein(a) binds very weakly to lysine-agarose and fibrin despite the presence of a strong lysine-binding site in apolipoprotein(a) kringle IV type 10. *Biochemistry.* **44,** 555–564.

Belfer-Cohen, A.. (1991). The Natufian in the Levant. *Annu Rev Anthropol* **20,** 167–186.

Bell, C. (2004). Long term mortality after starvation during the Leningrad siege: No evidence that starvation around puberty causes later cardiovascular disease. *Br Med J* **328,** 346.

Bell, D. P., Elmes, P. C., and Wheeler, S. M. (1964). A colony of specific pathogen-free rats. *Nature.* **201,** 273–274.

Belland, R. J., Ouellette, S. P., Gieffers, J., and Byrne, G. I. (2004). *Chlamydia pneumoniae* and atherosclerosis. *Cell Microbiol.* **6,** 117–127.

Belmin, J., Corman, B., Merval, R., and Tedgui, A. (1993). Age-related changes in endothelial permeability and distribution volume of albumin in rat aorta. *Am J Physiol.* **264,** H679–685.

Beloosesky, R., Gayle, D. A., Amidi, F., Nunez, S. E., Babu, J., Desai, M., and Ross, M. G. (2006). N-acetyl-cysteine suppresses amniotic fluid and placenta inflammatory cytokine responses to lipopolysaccharide in rats. *Am J Obstet Gynecol.* **194,** 268–273.

Belqacem, Y. H., and Martin, J. R. (2006). Disruption of insulin pathways alters trehalose level and abolishes sexual dimorphism in locomotor activity in *Drosophila. J Neurobiol.* **66,** 19–32.

Benagiano, M., Azzurri, A., Ciervo, A., Amedei, A., Tamburini, C., Ferrari, M., Telford, J. L., Baldari, C. T., Romagnani, S., Cassone, A., D'Elios, M. M., and Del Prete, G. (2003). T helper type 1 lymphocytes drive inflammation in human atherosclerotic lesions. *Proc Natl Acad Sci USA.* **100,** 6658–6663.

Benetos, A., Gardner, J. P., Zureik, M., Labat, C., Xiaobin, L., Adamopoulos, C., Temmar, M., Bean, K. E., Thomas, F., and Aviv, A. (2004). Short telomeres are associated with increased carotid atherosclerosis in hypertensive subjects. *Hypertension.* **43,** 182–185.

Bengtsson, T., and Lindstrom, M. (2000). Childhood misery and disease in later life: The effects on mortality in old age of hazards experienced in early life, southern Sweden, 1760–1894. *Population Studies.* **54,** 263–277.

Bengtsson, T., and Lindstrom, M. (2003). Airborne infectious diseases during infancy and mortality in later life in southern Sweden, 1766–1894. *Int J Epidemiol.* **32,** 286–294.

Benito, M. J., Veale, D. J., Fitzgerald, O., van den Berg, W. B., and Bresnihan, B. (2005). Synovial tissue inflammation in early and late osteoarthritis. *Ann Rheum Dis.* **64,** 1263–1267.

Bennermo, M., Held, C., Stemme, S., Ericsson, C. G., Silveira, A., Green, F., and Tornvall, P. (2004). Genetic predisposition of the interleukin-6 response to inflammation: Implications for a variety of major diseases? *Clin Chem.* **50,** 2136–2140.

Bennett-Baker, P. E., Wilkowski, J., and Burke, D. T.(2003). Age-associated activation of epigenetically repressed genes in the mouse. *Genetics.* **165,** 2055–2062.

Berenson, G. S. (2004). Cardiovascular risk factors in youth with implications for aging: The Bogalusa Heart Study. *Neurobiol Aging.* **26,** 303–307.

Beresford, S. A., Johnson, K. C., Ritenbaugh, C., Lasser, N. L., Snetselaar, L. G., Black, H. R., Anderson, G. L., Assaf, A. R., Bassford, T., Bowen, D., Brunner, R. L., Brzyski, R. G., Caan, B., Chlebowski, R. T., Gass, M., Harrigan, R. C., Hays, J., Heber, D., Heiss, G., Hendrix, S. L., Howard, B. V., Hsia, J., Hubbell, F. A., Jackson, R. D., Kotchen, J. M., Kuller, L. H., LaCroix, A. Z., Lane, D. S., Langer, R. D., Lewis, C. E., Manson, J. E., Margolis, K. L., Mossavar-Rahmani, Y., Ockene, J. K., Parker, L. M., Perri, M. G., Phillips, L., Prentice, R. L., Robbins, J., Rossouw, J. E., Sarto, G. E., Stefanick, M. L., Van Horn, L., Vitolins, M. Z., Wactawski-Wende, J., Wallace, R. B., and Whitlock, E. (2006). Low-fat dietary pattern and risk of colorectal cancer: The Women's Health Initiative Randomized Controlled Dietary Modification Trial. *JAMA.* **295,** 643–654.

Berg, B. N. (1976). Pathology and aging. In *Hypothalamus, pituitary, and aging,* pp. 43–67. A.V. Everitt and J.A. Burgess, Eds., Springfield, IL: C.C. Thomas..

Berg, B. N., and Simms, H. S. (1960). Nutrition and longevity in the rat. II. Longevity and onset of disease with different levels of food intake. *J Nutr.* **71,** 255–263.

Berg, B. N., Wolf, A., and Simms, H. S. (1962). Nutrition and longevity in the rat. IV. Food restriction and the radiculoneuropathy of aging rats. *J Nutr.* **77,** 439–442.

Berg, H. F., Maraha, B., van der Zee, A., Gielis, S. K., Roholl, P. J., Scheffer, G. J., Peeters, M. F., and Kluytmans, J. A. (2005). Effect of clarithromycin treatment on *Chlamydia pneumoniae* in vascular tissue of patients with coronary artery disease: A randomized, double-blind, placebo-controlled trial. *J Clin Microbiol.* **43,** 1325–1329.

Berg, N. B. (1967). Longevity studies in rats: II. Pathology of ageing rats. In E. Cotchin and F. Roe, J. C., Eds., *Pathology of laboratory rats and mice,* Blackwell Scientific Publications: Oxford, pp. 749–786.

Berg, R. D., and Savage, D. C. (1975). Immune responses of specific pathogen-free and gnotobiotic mice to antigens of indigenous and nonindigenous microorganisms. *Infection and Immunity.* **11,** 320–329.

Berg, T., and Nilsson, B. A. (1969). The foetal development of serum levels of IgG and IgM. *Acta Paediatr Scand.* **58,** 577–583.

Berkman, L. F. (2005). Tracking social and biological experiences: The social etiology of cardiovascular disease. *Circulation.* **111,** 3022–3024.

Berkowitz, R. I., Stallings, V. A., Maislin, G., and Stunkard, A. J. (2005). Growth of children at high risk of obesity during the first 6 y of life: Implications for prevention. *Am J Clin Nutr.* **81,** 140–146.

Bernstein, L., Patel, A. V., Ursin, G., Sullivan-Halley, J., Press, M. F., Deapen, D., Berlin, J. A., Daling, J. R., McDonald, J. A., Norman, S. A., Malone, K. E., Strom, B. L., Liff, J., Folger, S. G., Simon, M. S., Burkman, R. T., Marchbanks, P. A., Weiss, L. K., and Spirtas, R. (2005). Lifetime recreational exercise activity and breast cancer risk among black women and white women. *J Natl Cancer Inst.* **97,** 1671–1679.

Bernstein, M. S., Costanza, M. C., James, R. W., Morris, M. A., Cambien, F., Raoux, S., and Morabia, A. (2002). Physical activity may modulate effects of ApoE genotype on lipid profile. *Arterioscler Thromb Vasc Biol.* **22,** 133–140.

Berrigan, D., Lavigne, J. A., Perkins, S. N., Nagy, T. R., Barrett, J. C., and Hursting, S. D. (2005). Phenotypic effects of calorie restriction and insulin-like growth factor-1 treatment on body composition and bone mineral density of C57BL/6 mice: Implications for cancer prevention. *In vivo.* **19,** 667–674.

Berrington de Gonzalez, A., Sweetland, S., and Spencer, E. (2003). A meta-analysis of obesity and the risk of pancreatic cancer. *Br J Cancer.* **89,** 519–523.

Bertram, L., McQueen, M. B., Mullin, K., Blacker, D., Tanzi, R. E. (2007). Systematic meta-analyses of Alzheimer disease genetic association studies: the AlzGene database. *Nat Genet* **39,** 17–23.

Bertrand, H. A., Lynd, F. T., Masoro, E. J., and Yu, B. P. (1980). Changes in adipose mass and cellularity through the adult life of rats fed ad libitum or a life-prolonging restricted diet. *J Gerontol.* **35,** 827–835.

Bertranpetit, J. and Calafell, F. (1996). Genetic and geographical variability in cystic fibrosis: evolutionary considerations. *Ciba Found Symp.* **197,** 97–114.

Besedovsky, H. O., and del Rey, A. (1996). Immune-neuro-endocrine interactions: Facts and hypotheses. *Endocr Rev.* **17,** 64–102.

Besson, A., Salemi, S., Gallati, S., Jenal, A., Horn, R., Mullis, P. S., and Mullis, P. E. (2003). Reduced longevity in untreated patients with isolated growth hormone deficiency. *J Clin Endocrinol Metab.* **88,** 3664–3667.

Bevilacqua, L., Ramsey, J. J., Hagopian, K., Weindruch, R., and Harper, M. E. (2005). Long-term caloric restriction increases UCP3 content but decreases proton leak and reactive oxygen species production in rat skeletal muscle mitochondria. *Am J Physiol. Endocrinol Metab.* **289,** E429–438.

Bhavnani, B. R. (1998). Pharmacokinetics and pharmacodynamics of conjugated equine estrogens: Chemistry and metabolism. *Proc Soc Exp Biol Med.* **217,** 6–16.

Bieler, S., Estrada, L., Lagos, R., Baeza, M., Castilla, J., and Soto, C. (2005). Amyloid formation modulates the biological activity of a bacterial protein. *J Biol Chem.* **280,** 26880–26885.

Biemel, K. M., Friedl, D. A., and Lederer, M. O. (2002). Identification and quantification of major Maillard cross-links in human serum albumin and lens protein. Evidence for glucosepane as the dominant compound. *J Biol Chem.* **277,** 24907–24915.

Billing, J., and Sherman, P. W. (1998). Antimicrobial functions of spices: Why some like it hot. *Q Rev Biol.* **73,** 3–49.

Birch, W. (2005). A possible case of shortness of breath at Çatalhöyük- black lungs. *Inhabiting Çatalhöyük: Reports from the 1995-1999 Seasons by Members of the Çatalhöyük Teams,* pp 593-596. London: McDonald Institute Monographs.

Birge, S. J., McEwen, B. S., and Wise, P. M. (2001). Effects of estrogen deficiency on brain function. Implications for the treatment of postmenopausal women. *Postgrad Med. Spec No,* 11–16.

Birmingham, C. L., Hodgson, D. M., Fung, J., Brown, R., Wakefield, A., Bartrop, R., and Beumont, P. (2003). Reduced febrile response to bacterial infection in anorexia nervosa patients. *Int J Eating Disord.* **34,** 269–272.

Bispo, A. L. (2000). Rheumatic fever. In L. A. B. Goldman, J. C., Ed., *Cecil textbook of medicine, 21st edition* pp. 1624–1630. Philadelphia: W.B. Saunders Company.

Biswas, S. K., McClure, D., Jimenez, L. A., Megson, I. L., and Rahman, I. (2005). Curcumin induces glutathione biosynthesis and inhibits NF-kappaB activation and interleukin-8 release in alveolar epithelial cells: Mechanism of free radical scavenging activity. *Antioxidants & Redox Signaling.* **7,** 32–41.

Bjorkbacka, H., Kunjathoor, V. V., Moore, K. J., Koehn, S., Ordija, C. M., Lee, M. A., Means, T., Halmen, K., Luster, A. D., Golenbock, D. T., and Freeman, M. W. (2004). Reduced atherosclerosis in MyD88–null mice links elevated serum cholesterol levels to activation of innate immunity signaling pathways. *Nature Med.* **10,** 416–421.

Bjorklund, H., Eriksdotter-Nilsson, M., Dahl, D., Rose, G., Hoffer, B., and Olson, L. (1985). Image analysis of GFA-positive astrocytes from adolescence to senescence. *Exp Brain Res.* **58,** 163–170.

Black, H. R. (2004). The paradigm has shifted to systolic blood pressure. J. *Human Hypertension.* **18(Suppl. 2),** S3–S7.

Black, P. H. (2002). Stress and the inflammatory response: A review of neurogenic inflammation. *Brain Behav Immun.* **16,** 622–653.

Black, P. H. (2003). The inflammatory response is an integral part of the stress response: Implications for atherosclerosis, insulin resistance, type II diabetes and metabolic syndrome X. *Brain Behav Immun.* **17,** 350–364.

Blacklock, C. J., Lawrence, J. R., Wiles, D., Malcolm, E. A., Gibson, I. H., Kelly, C. J., and Paterson, J. R. (2001). Salicylic acid in the serum of subjects not taking aspirin. Comparison of salicylic acid concentrations in the serum of vegetarians, non-vegetarians, and patients taking low dose aspirin. *J Clin Pathol.* **54,** 553–555

Blalock, E. M., Chen, K. C., Sharrow, K., Herman, J. P., Porter, N. M., Foster, T. C., and Landfield, P. W. (2003). Gene microarrays in hippocampal aging: Statistical profiling identifies novel processes correlated with cognitive impairment. *J Neurosci* **23,** 3807–3819.

Blalock, E. M., Geddes, J. W., Chen, K. C., Porter, N. M., Markesbery, W. R., and Landfield, P. W. (2004). Incipient Alzheimer's disease: Microarray correlation analyses reveal major transcriptional and tumor suppressor responses. *Proc Natl Acad Sci USA.* **101,** 2173–2178.

Blanc, P., Corsi, A. M., Gabbuti, A., Peduzzi, C., Meacci, F., Olivieri, F., Lauretani, F., Francesco, M., and Ferrucci, L. (2004). *Chlamydia pneumoniae* seropositivity and cardiovascular risk factors: The InCHIANTI Study. *J Am Geriatr Soc.* **52(10),** 1626–1631.

Blanchard, T. G., Drakes, M. L., and Czinn, S. J. (2004). Helicobacter infection: Pathogenesis. *Curr Opin Gastroenterol.* **20,** 10–15.

Blander, G., and Guarente, L. (2004). The Sir2 family of protein deacetylases. *Annu Rev Biochem.* **73,** 417–435.

Blanford, S., and Thomas, M. B. (1999). Host thermal biology: The key to understanding host–pathogen interactions and microbial pest control? *Agricult Forest Entomol.* **1,** 195–202.

Blank, J. L., and Desjardins, C. (1985). Differential effects of food restriction on pituitary-testicular function in mice. *Am J Physiol.* **248(2, Pt 2)**, R181–189.

Blom, A. B., van Lent, P. L., Holthuysen, A. E., van der Kraan, P. M., Roth, J., van Rooijen, N., and van den Berg, W. B. (2004). Synovial lining macrophages mediate osteophyte formation during experimental osteoarthritis. *Osteoarthritis Cartilage.* **12**, 627–635.

Bluher, M., Kahn, B. B., and Kahn, C. R. (2003). Extended longevity in mice lacking the insulin receptor in adipose tissue. *Science* **299**, 572–574.

Bluher, M., Michael, M. D., Peroni, O. D., Ueki, K., Carter, N., Kahn, B. B., and Kahn, C. R. (2002). Adipose tissue selective insulin receptor knockout protects against obesity and obesity-related glucose intolerance. *Developmental cell.* **3**, 25–38.

Blumenschine, R. J. and Pobiner, B. L. (2007). Zooarcheology and the ecology of Oldowan carnivory. *The evolution of human life history*, pp. 167–190. Sante Fe: School for American Research Press.

Blumenthal, H. T., Handler, F. P., and Blache, J. O. (1954). The histogenesis of arteriosclerosis of the larger cerebral arteries, with an analysis of the importance of mechanical factors. *Am J Medicine.* **17(3)**, 337–347.

Blumenthal, H. T., Lansing, A. I., and Wheeler, P. A. (1944). Calcification of the media of the human aorta and its relation to intimal arteriosclerosis, ageing and disease. *Am J Pathol.* **20**, 665–679.

Bodman-Smith, K. B., Melendez, A. J., Campbell, I., Harrison, P. T., Allen, J. M., and Raynes, J. G. (2002). C-reactive protein-mediated phagocytosis and phospholipase D signalling through the high-affinity receptor for immunoglobulin G (FcgammaRI). *Immunology.* **107**, 252–260.

Boerwinkle, E., Leffert, C. C., Lin, J., Lackner, C., Chiesa, G., Hobbs, H. H. (1992). Apolipoprotein(a) gene accounts for greater than 90% of the variation in plasma lipoprotein(a) concentrations. *J Clin Invest.* **90**, 52–60.

Boesch, C., and Boesch, H. (1989). Hunting behavior of wild chimpanzees in the Tai National Park. *Am J Phys Anthropol .* **78**, 547–573.

Bogin, B. (1999a). Evolutionary perspective on human growth. *Ann Rev Anthropol.* **28**, 109–156.

Bogin, B. (1999b). *Patterns of human growth.* Cambridge: Cambridge University Press.

Bogin, B. (2005). Prospects for secular trends in the growth of United States children and youth. In G. A. Toth, Ed., *Auxology: To the memory of Professor Otto G. Eiben*, pp. 17–21. Szombathely, Hungary: Savaria University Press.

Bogin, B., and Keep, R. (1999). Eight thousand years of economic and political history in Latin America revealed by anthropometry. *Ann Hum Biol.* **26(4)**, 333–351.

Bogin, B., Smith, P., Orden, A. B., Varela Silva, M. I., and Loucky, J. (2002). Rapid change in height and body proportions of Maya American children. *Am J Hum Biol.* **14**, 753–761.

Bokodi, G., Treszl, A., Derzbach, L., Balogh, A., and Vasarhelyi, B. (2005). The association of the carrier state of the tumor necrosis factor-alpha (TNFalpha)-308A allele with the duration of oxygen supplementation in preterm neonates. *Eur Cytokine Netw.* **16(1)**, 78–80.

Bokov, A., Chaudhuri, A., and Richardson, A. (2004). The role of oxidative damage and stress in aging. *Mech Ageing Dev.* **125**, 811–826.

Bolanowski, M. A., Jacobson, L. A., and Russell, R. L. (1983). Quantitative measures of aging in the nematode *Caenorhabditis elegans*. II. Lysosomal hydrolases as markers of senescence. *Mech Ageing Dev.* **21**, 295–319.

Bolanowski, M. A., Russell, R. L., and Jacobson, L. A. (1981). Quantitative measure of aging in the nematode *Caenorhabditis elegans*. I. Population and longitudinal studies of two behavioral parameters. *Mech. Aging Devel.* **15,** 279–295.

Bonafe, M., Barbieri, M., Marchegiani, F., Olivieri, F., Ragno, E., Giampieri, C., Mugianesi, E., Centurelli, M., Franceschi, C., and Paolisso, G. (2003). Polymorphic variants of insulin-like growth factor I (IGF-I) receptor and phosphoinositide 3-kinase genes affect IGF-I plasma levels and human longevity: Cues for an evolutionarily conserved mechanism of life span control. *J Clin Endocrinol Metab.* **88,** 3299–3304.

Bonafe, M., Olivieri, F., Cavallone, L., Giovagnetti, S., Mayegiani, F., Cardelli, M., Pieri, C., Marra, M., Antonicelli, R., Lisa, R., Rizzo, M. R., Paolisso, G., Monti, D., and Franceschi, C. (2001). A gender-dependent genetic predisposition to produce high levels of IL-6 is detrimental for longevity. *Eur J Immunol.* **31,** 2357–2361.

Bondolfi, L., Ermini, F., Long, J. M., Ingram, D. K., and Jucker, M. (2004). Impact of age and caloric restriction on neurogenesis in the dentate gyrus of C57BL/6 mice. *Neurobiol Aging.* **25(3),** 333–340.

Bondy, C. A., and Cheng, C. M. (2004). Signaling by insulin-like growth factor 1 in brain. *Eur J Pharmacol.* **490,** 25–31.

Boney, C. M., Verma, A., Tucker, R., and Vohr, B. R. (2005). Metabolic syndrome in childhood: Association with birth weight, maternal obesity, and gestational diabetes mellitus. *Pediatrics.* **115(3),** e290–296.

Bonkowski, M. S., Pamenter, R. W., Rocha, J. S., Masternak, M. M., Panici, J. A., and Bartke, A. (2006a). Long-lived growth hormone receptor knockout mice show a delay in age-related changes of body composition and bone characteristics. *J Gerontol. A Biol Sci Med Sci.* **61,** 562–567.

Bonkowski, M. S., Rocha, J. S., Masternak, M. M., Al Regaiey, K. A., and Bartke, A. (2006b). Targeted disruption of growth hormone receptor interferes with the beneficial actions of calorie restriction. *Proc Natl Acad Sci USA.* **103,** 7901–7905.

Bonnet, C. S., and Walsh, D. A. (2005). Osteoarthritis, angiogenesis and inflammation. *Rheumatology (Oxford).* **44,** 7–16.

Borenstein, A. R., Wu, Y., Mortimer, J. A., Schellenberg, G. D., McCormick, W. C., Bowen, J. D., McCurry, S., and Larson, E. B. (2005). Developmental and vascular risk factors for Alzheimer's disease. *Neurobiol Aging.* **26,** 325–334.

Borghans, J. A., Beltman, J. B., and De Boer, R. J. (2004). MHC polymorphism under host-pathogen coevolution. *Immunogenetics.* **55(11),** 732–739.

Borkow, G., Leng, Q., Weisman, Z., Stein, M., Galai, N., Kalinkovich, A., and Bentwich, Z. (2000). Chronic immune activation associated with intestinal helminth infections results in impaired signal transduction and anergy. *J Clin Invest.* **106,** 1053–1060.

Borra, M. T., Langer, M. R., Slama, J. T., and Denu, J. M. (2004). Substrate specificity and kinetic mechanism of the Sir2 family of NAD+-dependent histone/protein deacetylases. *Biochemistry.* **43,** 9877–9887.

Bos, J. L. (1989). Ras oncogenes in human cancer: A review. *Cancer Res.* **49,** 4682–4689.

Bosetti, C., Gallus, S., and La Vecchia, C. (2002). Aspirin and cancer risk: An update to 2001. *Eur J Cancer Prev.* **11,** 535–542.

Boston, P. F., Bennett, A., Horrobin, D. F., and Bennett, C. N. (2004). Ethyl-EPA in Alzheimer's disease—A pilot study. *Prostaglandins Leukotrienes & Essential Fatty Acids.* **71,** 341–346.

Botting, R. (2003). COX-1 and COX-3 inhibitors. *Thromb Res.* **110,** 269–272.

Botto, N., Berti, S., Manfredi, S., Al-Jabri, A., Federici, C., Clerico, A., Ciofini, E., Biagini, A., and Andreassi, M. G. (2005). Detection of mtDNA with 4977 bp deletion in blood cells and atherosclerotic lesions of patients with coronary artery disease. *Mutat Res.* **570**, 81–88.

Bouchard, C., Tremblay, A., Després, J. P., Nadeau, A., Lupien, P. J., Thériault, G., Dussault, J., Moorjani, S., Pinault, S., and Fournier, G. (1990). The response to long-term overfeeding in identical twins. *New Engl J Med.* **322**, 1477–1482.

Boulay, J. L., O'Shea, J. J., and Paul, W. E. (2003). Molecular phylogeny within type I cytokines and their cognate receptors. *Immunity.* **19**, 159–163.

Boulet, S. L., Alexander, G. R., Salihu, H. M., Kirby, R. S., and Carlo, W. A. (2006). Fetal growth risk curves: Defining levels of fetal growth restriction by neonatal death risk. *Am J Obstet Gynecol.* **195**, 1571–1577.

Bourcier, T., Sukhova, G., and Libby, P. (1997). The nuclear factor kappa-B signaling pathway participates in dysregulation of vascular smooth muscle cells *in vitro* and in human atherosclerosis. J. *Biol. Chem.* **272**, 15817–15824.

Bourne, G. H., and Sandler, M. (1973). Atherosclerosis in chimpanzees. The Chimpanzee **6**, 248–264.

Bourne, K. Z., Bourne, N., Reising, S. F., and Stanberry, L. R. (1999). Plant products as topical microbicide candidates: Assessment of *in vitro* and *in vivo* activity against herpes simplex virus type 2. *Antiviral Res.* **42**, 219–226.

Bowers, T. K., and Eckert, E. (1978). Leukopenia in anorexia nervosa. Lack of increased risk of infection. *Arch Int Med.* **138**, 1520–1523.

Bowman, B. H. (1993). *Hepatic Plasma Proteins*. San Diego: Academic Press.

Boyd-Kimball, D., Sultana, R., Mohmmad-Abdul, H., and Butterfield, D. A. (2004). Rodent Abeta(1–42) exhibits oxidative stress properties similar to those of human Abeta(1–42): Implications for proposed mechanisms of toxicity. *J Alzheimers Dis.* **6**, 515–525.

Boyd, D. B. (2003). Insulin and cancer. *Integr Cancer Ther.* **2**, 315–329.

Braak, H., and Braak, E. (1991). Neuropathological staging of Alzheimer-related changes. *Acta Neuropath.* **82**, 239–259.

Braak, H., Braak, E., Bohl, J., and Bratzke, H. (1998). Evolution of Alzheimer's disease related cortical lesions. *J Neural Transmission. Supplementum.* **54**, 97–106.

Brabin, B. J., Romagosa, C., Abdelgalil, S., Menendez, C., Verhoeff, F. H., McGready, R., Fletcher, K. A., Owens, S., D'Alessandro, U., Nosten, F., Fischer, P. R., and Ordi, J. (2004). The sick placenta—The role of malaria. *Placenta.* **25**, 359–378.

Braunwald, E. (1997). Shattuck lecture—Cardiovascular medicine at the turn of the millennium: Triumphs, concerns, and opportunities. *New Engl J Med.* **337**, 1360–1369.

Bray, G. A., and Bellanger, T.(2006). Epidemiology, trends, and morbidities of obesity and the metabolic syndrome. *Endocrine.* **29**, 109–117.

Breitner, J. C. (2003). NSAIDs and Alzheimer's disease: How far to generalise from trials? *Lancet Neurol.* **2**, 527.

Breitner, J. C., Gau, B. A., Welsh, K. A., Plassman, B. L., McDonald, W. M., Helms, M. J., and Anthony, J. C. (1994). Inverse association of anti-inflammatory treatments and Alzheimer's disease: Initial results of a co-twin control study. *Neurology.* **44**, 227–232.

Breitner, J. C., Wyse, B. W., Anthony, J. C., Welsh-Bohmer, K. A., Steffens, D. C., Norton, M. C., Tschanz, J. T., Plassman, B. L., Meyer, M. R., Skoog, I., Khachaturian, A. (1999). APOE-epsilon4 count predicts age when prevalence of AD increases, then declines: the Cache County Study. *Neurology.* **53**, 321–331.

Brennan, C. A., and Anderson, K. V. (2004). *Drosophila*: The genetics of innate immune recognition and response. *Annu Rev Immunol.* **22,** 457–483.

Brenner, B. M., Garcia, D. L., and Anderson, S. (1988). Glomeruli and blood pressure. Less of one, more the other? *Am J Hypertens.* **1(4, Pt 1),** 335–347.

Brenner, B. M., Meyer, T. W., and Hostetter, T. H. (1982). Dietary protein intake and the progressive nature of kidney disease: The role of hemodynamically mediated glomerular injury in the pathogenesis of progressive glomerular sclerosis in aging, renal ablation, and intrinsic renal disease. *New Engl J Med.* **307,** 652–659.

Brenner, S. (1974). The genetics of *Caenorhabditis elegans. Genetics.* **77,** 71–94.

Breslow, J. L. (2000). Genetics of lipoprotein abnormalities associated with coronary artery disease susceptibility. *Annu Rev Genet.* **34,** 233–254.

Bretsky, P., Guralnik, J. M., Launer, L., Albert, M., and Seeman, T. E. (2003). The role of APOE-epsilon4 in longitudinal cognitive decline: MacArthur Studies of Successful Aging. *Neurology.* **60,** 1077–1081.

Brierley, E. J., Johnson, M. A., Lightowlers, R. N., James, O. F., and Turnbull, D. M. (1998). Role of mitochondrial DNA mutations in human aging: Implications for the central nervous system and muscle. *Ann Neurol.* **43(2),** 217–223.

Brinton, R. D. (2004). Impact of estrogen therapy on Alzheimer's disease: A fork in the road? *CNS Drugs.* **18,** 405–422.

Brinton, R. D., and Nilsen, J. (2003). Effects of estrogen plus progestin on risk of dementia. [comment]. *JAMA.* **290,** 1706; author reply, 1707–1708.

Britten, R. J. (2002). Divergence between samples of chimpanzee and human DNA sequences is 5%, counting indels. *Proc Natl Acad Sci USA.* **99,** 13633–13635.

Broberger, C. (2005). Brain regulation of food intake and appetite: Molecules and networks. *J Intern Med.* **258,** 301–327.

Bronikowski, A. M., Carter, P. A., Morgan, T. J., Garland, T., Jr., Ung, N., Pugh, T. D., Weindruch, R., and Prolla, T. A. (2003). Lifelong voluntary exercise in the mouse prevents age-related alterations in gene expression in the heart. *Physiol Genomics.* **12,** 129–138.

Bronson, F. H. (2001). Puberty in female mice is not associated with increases in either body fat or leptin. *Endocrinology* **142,** 4758–4761.

Bronson, F. H., and Manning, J. M. (1991). The energetic regulation of ovulation: A realistic role for body fat. *Biol Reprod.* **44,** 945–990.

Bronson, R. T. (1990). Rate of occurrence of lesions in 20 inbred and hybrid genotypes of rats and mice sacrificed at 6 month intervals during the first years of life. In D. E. Harrison, Ed., *Genetic effects on aging II*, pp. 279–357. Caldwell, NJ: The Telford Press, Inc.

Brookes, P. S. (2004). Mitochondrial nitric oxide synthase. *Mitochondrion* **3,** 187–204.

Brookes, P. S., Land, J. M., Clark, J. B., and Heales, S. J. (1998). Peroxynitrite and brain mitochondria: Evidence for increased proton leak. *J Neurochem.* **70,** 2195–2202.

Brooks, W. W., and Conrad, C. H. (2000). Myocardial fibrosis in transforming growth factor beta(1)heterozygous mice. *J Mol Cell Cardiol.* **32(2),** 187–195.

Broughton, S. J., Piper, M. D., Ikeya, T., Bass, T. M., Jacobson, J., Driege, Y., Martinez, P., Hafen, E., Withers, D. J., Leevers, S. J., and Partridge, L. (2005). Longer lifespan, altered metabolism, and stress resistance in *Drosophila* from ablation of cells making insulin-like ligands. *Proc Natl Acad Sci USA.* **102,** 3105–10.

Brown-Borg, H. M., Borg, K. E., Meliska, C. J., and Bartke, A. (1996). Dwarf mice and the ageing process. *Nature.* **384,** 33.

Brown, B. G., Zhao, X. Q., Sacco, D. E., and Albers, J. J. (1993). Atherosclerosis regression, plaque disruption, and cardiovascular events: A rationale for lipid lowering in coronary artery disease. *Annual Review of Medicine.* **44,** 365–376.

Brown, D. C., Byrne, C. D., Clark, P. M., Cox, B. D., Day, N. E., Hales, C. N., Shackleton, J. R., Wang, T. W., and Williams, D. R. (1991). Height and glucose tolerance in adult subjects. *Diabetologia.* **34(7),** 531–533.

Brown, M. S., and Goldsteinn, J. L. (1974). Familial hypercholesterolemia: Defective binding of lipoproteins to cultured fibroblasts associated with impaired regulation of 3-hydroxy-3-methylglutaryl coenzyme A reductase activity. *Proc Natl Acad Sci USA.* **71,** 788–792.

Brown, S. M., Smith, D. M., Alt, N., Thorpe, S. R., and Baynes, J. W. (2005). Tissue-specific variation in glycation of proteins in diabetes: Evidence for a functional role of amadoriase enzymes. *Ann NY Acad Sci.* **1043,** 817–823.

Brownlee, M. (2001). Biochemistry and molecular cell biology of diabetic complications. *Nature.* **41,** 813–820.

Bruel-Jungerman, E., Laroche, S., Rampon, C. (2005). New neurons in the dentate gyrus are involved in the expression of enhanced long-term memory following environmental enrichment. *Eur J Neurosci.* **21,** 513–521.

Brull, D. J., Serrano, N., Zito, F., Jones, L., Montgomery, H. E., Rumley, A., Sharma, P., Lowe, G. D., World, M. J., Humphries, S. E., and Hingorani, A. D. (2003). Human CRP gene polymorphism influences CRP levels: Implications for the prediction and pathogenesis of coronary heart disease. *Arterioscler Thromb Vasc Biol.* **23(11),** 2063–2069.

Brummel, T., Ching, A., Seroude, L., Simon, A. F., and Benzer, S. (2004). *Drosophila* lifespan enhancement by exogenous bacteria. *Proc Natl Acad Sci USA.* **101(35),** 12974–12979.

Brunauer, L. S., and Clarke, S. (1986). Age-dependent accumulation of protein residues which can be hydrolyzed to D-aspartic acid in human erythrocytes. *J Biol Chem.* **261(27),** 12538–12543.

Brundage, S. C., and Fitzpatrick, A. N. (2006). Hepatitis A. *Am Fam Physician.* **73,** 2162–2168.

Brunet, M., Guy, F., Pilbeam, D., Mackaye, H. T., Likius, A., Ahounta, D., Beauvilain, A., Blondel, C., Bocherens, H., Boisserie, J. R., De Bonis, L., Coppens, Y., Dejax, J., Denys, C., Duringer, P., Eisenmann, V., Fanone, G., Fronty, P., Geraads, D., Lehmann, T., Lihoreau, F., Louchart, A., Mahamat, A., Merceron, G., Mouchelin, G., Otero, O., Pelaez Campomanes, P., Ponce De Leon, M., Rage, J. C., Sapanet, M., Schuster, M., Sudre, J., Tassy, P., Valentin, X., Vignaud, P., Viriot, L., Zazzo, A., and Zollikofer, C. (2002). A new hominid from the Upper Miocene of Chad, Central Africa. *Nature.* **418,** 145–151.

Bruun, J. M., Helge, J. W., Richelsen, B., and B., S. (2006). Diet and exercise reduce low-grade inflammation and macrophage infiltration in adipose tissue but not in skeletal muscle in severely obese subjects. *Am J Physiol Endocrinol Metab.* **290,** E961–967.

Bruunsgaard, H. (2005). Physical activity and modulation of systemic low-level inflammation. *J Leukocyte Biology.* **78,** 819–835.

Bruunsgaard, H., Andersen-Ranberg, K., Jeune, B., Pedersen, A. N., Skinhoj, P., and Pedersen, B. K. (1999a). A high plasma concentration of TNF-alpha is associated with dementia in centenarians. *J Gerontology, Sect A.0 Biol Sci Med Sci.* **54,** M357–364.

Bruunsgaard, H., Skinhj, P., Qvist, J., and Pedersen, B. K. (1999b). Elderly humans show prolonged *in vivo* inflammatory activity during pneumococcal infections. *J Infect Dis.* **180,** 551–554.

Bucala, R., Model, P., and Cerami, A. (1984). Modification of DNA by reducing sugars: A possible mechanism for nucleic acid aging and age-related dysfunction in gene expression. *PNAS*. **81,** 105–109.

Bucciantini, M., Giannoni, E., Chiti, F., Baroni, F., Formigli, L., Zurdo, J., Taddei, N., Ramponi, G., Dobson, C. M., and Stefani, M. (2002). Inherent toxicity of aggregates implies a common mechanism for protein misfolding diseases. [see comment]. *Nature*. **416,** 507–511.

Buchan, R. M., Rijal, P., Sandfort, D., and Keefe, T. (2002). Evaluation of airborne dust and endotoxin in corn storage and processing facilities in Colorado. *Int J Occ Med Env Health*. **15,** 57–64.

Bucher, N. L., Swaffield, M. N., and Ditroia, J. F. (1964). The influence of age upon the incorporation of thymidine-2-C14 into the DNA of regenerating rat liver. *Cancer Res.* **24,** 509–512.

Buck, C., and Simpson, H. (1982). Infant diarrhoea and subsequent mortality from heart disease and cancer. *J Epidemiol Comm Health*. **36,** 27–30.

Buckler, J. A. (1990). A longitudinal study of adolescent growth. London: Springer-Verlag.

Bull, I. D., Elhmmali, M. M., Perret, P., Matthew, W., Roberts, D. J., and Evershed, R. P. (2005). Biomarker evidence of fecal deposition in archeological sediments at Çatalhöyük. In *Inhabiting Çatalhöyük: reports from the 1995–1999 seasons*. pp. McDonald Insititute for Archeological Research/British Institute fof Archeology at Ankara Monograph., pp.415–420

Bullen, J. J., Rogers, H. J., Spalding, P. B., and Ward, C. G. (2005). Iron and infection: The heart of the matter. *FEMS Immunol Med Microbiol*. **43,** 325–330.

Bunn, H. T. (2007). Meat made us human. In: *Evolution of the Human Diet. The Known, Unknown, and the Unknowable*. (Ungar PS, ed), pp 191–211. New York: Oxford U Press.

Bunn, H. T., and Kroll, E. M. (1986). Systematic butchery by Plio/Pleistocene hominids at Oldvai Gorge, Tanzania. *Current Anthropology*. **27,** 431–452.

Burger, G. C. E., Drummond, J. C., and Sandstead, H. R. (1948). *Malnutrition and starvation in Western Netherlands.*" The Hague: General State Publishing Office.

Burgermeister, P., Calhoun, M. E., Winkler, D. T., and Jucker, M. (2000). Mechanisms of cerebrovascular amyloid deposition. Lessons from mouse models. *Ann NY Acad Sci.* **903,** 307–316.

Burns, J. M., Church, J. A., Johnson, D. K., Xiong, C., Marcus, D., Fotenos, A. F., Snyder, A. Z., Morris, J. C., and Buckner, R. L. (2005). White matter lesions are prevalent but differentially related with cognition in aging and early Alzheimer disease. *Arch Neurol.* **62,** 1870–1876.

Burrell, R. (1994). Human responses to bacterial endotoxin. *Circ Shock.* **43,** 137–153.

Bush, A. I., and Tanzi, R. E. (2002). The galvanization of beta-amyloid in Alzheimer's disease. *Proc Natl Acad Sci USA*. **99,** 7317–7319.

Butte, N. F., Wong, W. W., and Garza, C. (1989). Energy cost of growth during infancy. *Proc Nutrit Soc.* **48,** 303–312.

Butterfield, D. A. (2002). Amyloid beta-peptide (1–42)-induced oxidative stress and neurotoxicity: Implications for neurodegeneration in Alzheimer's disease brain. A review. *Free Rad Res.* **36,** 1307–1313.

Butterfield, D. A., Castegna, A., Lauderback, C. M., and Drake, J. (2002). Evidence that amyloid beta-peptide-induced lipid peroxidation and its sequelae in Alzheimer's disease brain contribute to neuronal death. *Neurobiol Aging*. **23,** 655–664.

Butterfield, D. A., and Lauderback, C. M. (2002). Lipid peroxidation and protein oxidation in Alzheimer's disease brain: Potential causes and consequences involving amyloid beta-peptide-associated free radical oxidative stress. *Free Radic Biol Med.* **32,** 1050–1060.

Buttgereit, F., and Brand, M. D. (1995). A hierarchy of ATP-consuming processes in mammalian cells. *Biochem J.* **312,** 163–167.

Buttgereit, F., Burmester, G. R., and Brand, M. D. (2000). Bioenergetics of immune functions: Fundamental and therapeutic aspects. *Immunol Today.* **21(4),** 192–199.

Buxbaum, J. D., Thinakaran, G., Koliatsos, V., O'Callahan, J., Slunt, H. H., Price, D. L., and Sisodia, S. S. (1998). Alzheimer amyloid protein precursor in the rat hippocampus: Transport and processing through the perforant path. *J Neurosci.* **18,** 9629–9637.

Buxbaum, J. N. (2004). The systemic amyloidoses. *Curr Opin Rheumatol.* **16,** 67–75.

Buxbaum, J. N., and Tagoe, C. E. (2000). The genetics of the amyloidoses. *Annual Review of Medicine.* **51,** 543–569.

Buyse, M., Bado, A., and Daugé, V. (2001). Leptin decreases feeding and exploratory behaviour via interactions with CCK(1) receptors in the rat. *Neuropharmacology.* **40,** 818–825.

Bygren, L.-O., Brostrom, G., and Edvinsson, S. (2000). Change in food availability during pregnancy: Is it related to adult sudden death from cerebro- and cardiovascular disease in offspring? *Am J Human Biology.* **12,** 447–453.

Cabanac, M. (1985). Influence of food and water deprivation on the behavior of the white rat foraging in a hostile environment. *Physiol Behav.* **35,** 701–709.

Cai, H. (2005). Hydrogen peroxide regulation of endothelial function: Origins, mechanisms, and consequences. *Cardiovasc. Res.* **68,** 26–36.

Cai, J. J., Woo, P. C., Lau, S. K., Smith, D. K., Yuen, K. Y. (2006). Accelerated evolutionary rate may be responsible for the emergence of lineage-specific genes in ascomycota. *J Mol Evol.* **63,** 1–11.

Cailliet, G. M., Andrews, A. H., Burton, E. J., Watters, D. L., Kline, D. E., and Ferry-Graham, L. A. (2001). Age determination and validation studies of marine fishes: Do deep-dwellers live longer? *Exp Gerontol.* **36,** 739–764.

Calder, W. A. I. (1984). *Size, function, and life history.* Cambridge: Harvard University Press.

Calhoun, M. E., Burgermeister, P., Phinney, A. L., Stalder, M., Tolnay, M., Wiederhold, K. H., Abramowski, D., Sturchler-Pierrat, C., Sommer, B., Staufenbiel, M., and Jucker, M. (1999). Neuronal overexpression of mutant amyloid precursor protein results in prominent deposition of cerebrovascular amyloid. *Proc Natl Acad Sci USA.* **96,** 14088–14093.

Callaghan, M. J., Ceradini, D. J., and Gurtner, G. C. (2005). Hyperglycemia-induced reactive oxygen species and impaired endothelial progenitor cell function. *Antioxid Redox Signal.* **7,** 1476–1482.

Calon, F., Lim, G. P., Morihara, T., Yang, F., Ubeda, O., Salem, N. J., Frautschy, S. A., and Cole, G. M. (2005). Dietary N-3 polyunsaturated fatty acid depletion activates caspases and decreases NMDA receptors in the brain of a transgenic mouse model of Alzheimer's disease. *Eur J Neurosci.* **22,** 617–626.

Calon, F., Lim, G. P., Yang, F., Morihara, T., Teter, B., Ubeda, O., Rostaing, P., Triller, A., Salem, N., Jr., Ashe, K. H., Frautschy, S. A., and Cole, G. M. (2004). Docosahexaenoic acid protects from dendritic pathology in an Alzheimer's disease mouse model. [see comment]. *Neuron.* **43,** 633–645.

Campagne, A., Pebayle, T., and Muzet, A. (2004). Correlation between driving errors and vigilance level: Influence of the driver's age. *Physiol Behav.* **80,** 515–524.

Campbell, D. I., Elia, M., and Lunn, P. G. (2003a). Growth faltering in rural Gambian infants is associated with impaired small intestinal barrier function, leading to endotoxemia and systemic inflammation. *J Nutr.* **133,** 1332–1338.

Campbell, D. I., Murch, S. H., Elia, M., Sullivan, P. B., Sanyang, M. S., Jobarteh, B., and Lunn, P. G. (2003b). Chronic T cell-mediated enteropathy in rural West African children: Relationship with nutritional status and small bowel function. *Pediatr Res.* **54**, 306–311.

Campbell, J. H., and Perkins, P. (1988). Transgenerational effects of drug and hormonal treatments in mammals: A review of observations and ideas. *Prog Brain Res.* **73**, 535–553.

Campbell, L. A., and Kuo, C. C. (2003). *Chlamydia pneumoniae* and atherosclerosis. *Sem Resp Infect.* **18**, 48–54.

Campbell, L. A., and Kuo, C. C. (2004). *Chlamydia pneumoniae*—An infectious risk factor for atherosclerosis? *Nature Rev. Microbiol.* **2**, 23–32.

Campisi, J. (2005). Aging, tumor suppression and cancer: High wire-act! *Mech Ageing Dev.* **126**, 51–58.

Carey, J. R., Harshman, L., Liedo, P., Muller, H. G., Wang, J. L., Zhang, Z. (2007). Interplay of calorie and yeast restriction underlies fertility-longevity tradeoffs in a tephrititid fly. *In Prep.*

Carey, J. R., Liedo, P., Harshman, L., Zhang, Y., Mèuller, H. G., Partridge, L., and Wang, J. L. (2002). Life history response of Mediterranean fruit flies to dietary restriction. *Aging cell.* **1**, 140–148.

Carey, J. R., Liedo, P., Orozco, D., and Vaupel, J. W. (1992). Slowing of mortality rates at older ages in large medfly cohorts. *Science.* **258**, 457–461.

Carlson, B. M., Dedkov, E. I., Borisov, A. B., and Faulkner, J. A. (2001). Skeletal muscle regeneration in very old rats. *J Gerontol. Series A, Biol Sci Med Sci.* **56(5)**, B224–233.

Carlsten, H. (2005). Immune responses and bone loss: The estrogen connection. *Immunol Rev.* **208**, 194–206.

Carmen, G. Y., and Victor, S. M. (2005). Signalling mechanisms regulating lipolysis. *Cell Signal.* **18**, 401–408.

Carr, K. D., Tsimberg, Y., Berman, Y., and Yamamoto, N. (2003). Evidence of increased dopamine receptor signaling in food-restricted rats. *Neuroscience.* **119**, 1157–1167.

Carrel, L., and Willard, H. F. (2005). X-inactivation profile reveals extensive variability in X-linked gene expression in females. *Nature.* **434**, 400–404.

Carrieri, G., Marzi, E., Olivieri, F., Marchegiani, F., Cavallone, L., Cardelli, M., Giovagnetti, S., Stecconi, R., Molendini, C., Trapassi, C., De Benedictis, G., Kletsas, D., and Franceschi, C. (2004). The G/C polymorphism of transforming growth factor beta1 is associated with human longevity: A study in Italian centenarians. *Aging cell.* **3**, 443–448.

Carro, E., Nunez, A., Busiguina, S., and Torres-Aleman, I. (2000). Circulating insulin-like growth factor I mediates effects of exercise on the brain. *J Neurosci.* **20**, 2926–2933.

Carro, E., and Torres-Aleman, I. (2004). The role of insulin and insulin-like growth factor I in the molecular and cellular mechanisms underlying the pathology of Alzheimer's disease. *Eur J Pharmacology.* **490**, 127–133.

Carroll, G. C., and Sebor, R. J. (1980). Dental flossing and its relationship to transient bacteremia. *J Periodontol.* **51**, 691–692.

Carroll, R. L. (1988). *Vertebrate Paleontology.* New York: Freeman Press.

Carulla, N., Caddy, G. L., Hall, D. R., Zurdo, J., Gairi, M., Feliz, M., Giralt, E., Robinson, C. V., and Dobson, C. M. (2005). Molecular recycling within amyloid fibrils. *Nature.* **436**, 554–558.

Caruso, C., Lio, D., Cavallone, L., and Franceschi, C. (2004). Aging, longevity, inflammation, and cancer. *Ann NY Acad Sci.* **1028**, 1–13.

Carvalho, G. B., Kapahi, P., and Benzer, S. (2005). Compensatory ingestion upon dietary restriction in *Drosophila melanogaster.* **2**, 813–815.

Casano-Sancho, P., Lopez-Bermejo, A., Fernandez-Real, J. M., Monros, E., Valls, C., Rodriguez-Gonzalez, F. X., Ricart, W., and Ibänez, L. (2006). The tumour necrosis factor (TNF)-alpha-308GA promoter polymorphism is related to prenatal growth and postnatal insulin resistance. *Clin Endocrinol (Oxf).* **64,** 129–135.

Caspari R, L. S. (2004). Older age becomes common late in human evolution. *Proc Natl Acad Sci USA.* **101,** 10895–10900.

Caspari, R. and Lee, S. H. (2006). Is human longevity a consequence of cultural change or modern biology? *Am J Phys Anthropol.* **129,** 512–517.

Cassano, P., Lezza, A. M., Leeuwenburgh, C., Cantatore, P., and Gadaleta, M. N. (2004). Measurement of the 4,834–bp mitochondrial DNA deletion level in aging rat liver and brain subjected or not to caloric restriction diet. *Ann NY Acad Sci.* **1019,** 269–273.

Cassell, G. H. (1982). Derrick Edward Award Lecture. The pathogenic potential of mycoplasmas: *Mycoplasma pulmonis* as a model. *Reviews of Infectious Diseases.* **4(Suppl),** S18–34.

Casserly, I., and Topol, E. (2004). Convergence of atherosclerosis and Alzheimer's disease: Inflammation, cholesterol, and misfolded proteins. *Lancet.* **363,** 1139–1146.

Castelli, W. P. (1996). Lipids, risk factors and ischaemic heart disease. *Atherosclerosis.* **124(Supp),** S1–S9.

Castrillo, A., Joseph, S. B., Vaidya, S. A., Haberland, M., Fogelman, A. M., Cheng, G., and Tontonoz, P. (2003). Crosstalk between LXR and Toll-like receptor signaling mediates bacterial and viral antagonism of cholesterol metabolism. *Mol Cell.* **12,** 805–816.

Cataldo, A. M., Barnett, J. L., Pieroni, C., and Nixon, R. A. (1997). Increased neuronal endocytosis and protease delivery to early endosomes in sporadic Alzheimer's disease: Neuropathologic evidence for a mechanism of increased beta-amyloidogenesis. *J Neurosci.* **17,** 6142–6151.

Cataldo, A. M., Petanceska, S., Terio, N. B., Peterhoff, C. M., Durham, R., Mercken, M., Mehta, P. D., Buxbaum, J., Haroutunian, V., and Nixon, R. A. (2004). Abeta localization in abnormal endosomes: Association with earliest Abeta elevations in AD and Down syndrome. *Neurobiol Aging.* **25,** 1263–1272.

Cavanagh, J. B. (1999). Corpora-amylacea and the family of polyglucosan diseases. *Brain Res. Brain Res Rev.* **29,** 265–295.

Cawthon, R. M., Smith, K. R., O'Brien, E., Sivatchenko, A., and Kerber, R. A. (2003). Association between telomere length in blood and mortality in people aged 60 years or older. *Lancet.* **361,** 393–395.

Cecim, M., Alvarez-Sanz, M., Van de Kar, L., Milton, S., Bartke, A. (1996). Increased plasma corticosterone levels in bovine growth hormone (bGH) transgenic mice: effects of ACTH, GH and IGF-I on in vitro adrenal corticosterone production. *Transgenic Res.* **5,** 187–192.

Cecim, M., Fadden, C., Kerr, J., Steger, R. W., Bartke, A. (1995). Infertility in transgenic mice overexpressing the bovine growth hormone gene: disruption of the neuroendocrine control of prolactin secretion during pregnancy. *Biol Reprod.* **52,** 1187–1192.

Ceddia, R. B., Bikopoulos, G. J., Hilliker, A. J., and Sweeney, G. (2003). Insulin stimulates glucose metabolism via the pentose phosphate pathway in *Drosophila* Kc cells. *FEBS Lett.* **555,** 307–310.

Ceesay, S. M., Prentice, A. M., Cole, T. J., Foord, F., Weaver, L. T., Poskitt, E. M., and Whitehead, R. G. (1997). Effects on birth weight and perinatal mortality of maternal dietary supplements in rural Gambia: 5 year randomised controlled trial. [erratum appears in *Br Med J,* 1997, Nov 1; 315(7116):1141]. *Br Med J.* **315,** 786–790.

Cela-Conde, C. J., and Ayala, F. J. (2003). Genera of the human lineage. *Proc Natl Acad Sci USA.* **100,** 7684–7689.

Cellini, E., Nacmias, B., Olivieri, F., Ortenzi, L., Tedde, A., Bagnoli, S., Petruzzi, C., Franceschi, C., and Sorbi, S. (2005). Cholesteryl ester transfer protein (CETP) I405V polymorphism and longevity in Italian centenarians. *Mech Ageing Dev.* **126,** 826–828.

Cerami, A. (1985). Hypothesis. Glucose as a mediator of aging. *J Am Geriatr Soc.* **33,** 626–634.

Cerhan, J. R., Anderson, K. E., Janney, C. A., Vachon, C. M., Witzig, T. E., and Habermann, T. M. (2003). Association of aspirin and other non-steroidal anti-inflammatory drug use with incidence of non-Hodgkin lymphoma. *Int J Cancer.* **106,** 784–788.

Cervenakova, L., Brown, P., Goldfarb, L. G., Nagle, J., Pettrone, K., Rubenstein, R., Dubnick, M., Gibbs CJ, et al. (1994). Infectious amyloid precursor gene sequences in primates used for experimental transmission of human spongiform encephalopathy. *Proc. Nat Acad Sci.* **91,** 12159–12162.

Cesari, M., Penninx, B. W., Pahor, M., Lauretani, F., Corsi, A. M., Rhys Williams, G., Guralnik, J. M., and Ferrucci, L. (2004). Inflammatory markers and physical performance in older persons: The InCHIANTI study. *J Gerontol. Series A, Biol Sci Med Sci.* **59,** 242–248.

Cetin, I., de Santis, M. S., Taricco, E., Radaelli, T., Teng, C., Ronzoni, S., Spada, E., Milani, S., and Pardi, G. (2005). Maternal and fetal amino acid concentrations in normal pregnancies and in pregnancies with gestational diabetes mellitus. *Am J Obstet Gynecol.* **192,** 610–617.

Cetin, I., Ronzoni, S., Marconi, A. M., Perugino, G., Corbetta, C., Battaglia, F. C., and Pardi, G. (1996). Maternal concentrations and fetal-maternal concentration differences of plasma amino acids in normal and intrauterine growth-restricted pregnancies. *Am J Obstet Gynecol* **174,** 1575–1583.

Chait, A., Han, C. Y., Oram, J. F., and Heinecke, J. W. (2005). Thematic review series: The immune system and atherogenesis. Lipoprotein-associated inflammatory proteins: Markers or mediators of cardiovascular disease? *J Lipid Res.* **46,** 389–403.

Chan, A. T., Giovannucci, E. L., Schernhammer, E. S., Colditz, G. A., Hunter, D. J., Willett, W. C., and Fuchs, C. S. (2004). A prospective study of aspirin use and the risk for colorectal adenoma. *Ann Intern Med.* **140,** 157–166.

Chan Carusone, S., Smieja, M., Molloy, W., Goldsmith, C. H., Mahony, J., Chernesky, M., Gnarpe, J., Standish, T., Smith, S., and Loeb, M. (2004). Lack of association between vascular dementia and *Chlamydia pneumoniae* infection: A case-control study. *BMC Neurol.* **4,** 15.

Chan, K. K., Oza, A. M., and Siu, L. L. (2003). The statins as anticancer agents. *Clin Cancer Res.* **9,** 10–19.

Chandra, H. R., Choudhary, N., O'Neill, C., Boura, J., Timmis, G. C., and O'Neill, W. W. (2001a). *Chlamydia pneumoniae* exposure and inflammatory markers in acute coronary syndrome (CIMACS). *Am J Cardiol.* **88,** 214–218.

Chandra, V., Pandav, R., Dodge, H. H., Johnston, J. M., Belle, S. H., DeKosky, S. T., and Ganguli, M. (2001). Incidence of Alzheimer's disease in a rural community in India: The Indo-US study. *Neurology.* **57(6),** 985–989.

Chandrasekhar, C. P., and Ghosh, J. (2003). The calorie consumption puzzle. In *The Hindu business line Feb. 11, 2003.* http://www.thehindubusinessline.com/2003/02/11/stories/2003021100210900.htm

Chandrashekar, V., and Bartke, A. (1993). Induction of endogenous insulin-like growth factor-I secretion alters the hypothalamic-pituitary-testicular function in growth hormone-deficient adult dwarf mice. *Biol Reprod.* **48,** 544–551.

Chandrruangphen, P., and Collins, P. (2002). Exercise-induced suppression of postprandial lipemia: A possible mechanism of endothelial protection? *Arterioscler Thromb Vasc Biol.* **22,** 1239.

Chang, E., and Harley, C. B. (1995). Telomere length and replicative aging in human vascular tissues. *Proc Natl Acad Sci USA.* **92,** 11190–11194.

Chapin, R. E., Gulati, D. K., Fail, P. A., Hope, E., Russell, S. R., Heindel, J. J., George, J. D., Grizzle, T. B., and Teague, J. L. (1993). The effects of feed restriction on reproductive function in Swiss CD-1 mice. *Fundam Appl Toxicol.* **20,** 15–22.

Chapman, H. A. (2004). Disorders of lung matrix remodeling. *J Clin Invest.* **113,** 148–157.

Chapman, T., Miyatake, T., Smith, H. K., and Partridge, L. (1998). Interactions of mating, egg production and death rates in females of the Mediterranean fruit fly, *Ceratitis capitata.* **265,** 1879–1894.

Chappel, C. I., and Howell, J. C. (1992). Caramel colours—A historical introduction. *Food Chem Toxicol.* **30,** 351–357.

Charakida, M., Donald, A. E., Terese, M., Leary, S., Halcox, J. P., Ness, A., Davey Smith, G., Golding, J., Friberg, P., Klein, N. J., and Deanfield, J. E. (2005). Endothelial dysfunction in childhood infection. *Circulation.* **111,** 1660–1665.

Charlesworth, B. (1996). Evolution of senescence: Alzheimer's disease and evolution. *Curr Biol.* **6,** 20–22.

Charlton, H. M., Clark, R. G., Robinson, I. C., Goff, A. E., Cox, B. S., Bugnon, C., and Bloch, B. A. (1988). Growth hormone-deficient dwarfism in the rat: A new mutation. *J Endocrinology.* **119,** 51–58.

Charnov, E. L. (1993). *Life history invariants: some explorations of symmetry in evolutionary biology.* New York: Oxford U. Press.

Che, W., Lerner-Marmarosh, N., Huang, Q., Osawa, M., Ohta, S., Yoshizumi, M., Glassman, M., Lee, J. D., Yan, C., Berk, B. C., Abe, J. (2002). Insulin-like growth factor-1 enhances inflammatory responses in endothelial cells: role of Gab1 and MEKK3 in TNF-alpha-induced c-Jun and NF-kappaB activation and adhesion molecule expression. *Circ Res.* **90,** 1222–1230.

Chen, B. J., Cui, X., Sempowski, G. D., and Chao, N. J. (2003a). Growth hormone accelerates immune recovery following allogeneic T-cell-depleted bone marrow transplantation in mice. *Exp Hematol.* **31,** 953–958.

Chen, F., Eriksson, P., Kimura, T., Herzfeld, I., and Valen, G. (2005). Apoptosis and angiogenesis are induced in the unstable coronary atherosclerotic plaque. *Coron Artery Dis.* **16,** 191–197.

Chen, F. C., and Li, W. H. (2001). Genomic divergences between humans and other hominoids and the effective population size of the common ancestor of humans and chimpanzees. *Am J Hum Genet.* **68,** 444–456.

Chen, H. W., Meier, H., Heiniger, H. J., and Huebner, R. J. (1972). Tumorigenesis in strain DW-J mice and induction by prolactin of the group-specific antigen of endogenous C-type RNA tumor virus. *J Natl Cancer Inst.* **49,** 1145–1154.

Chen, J., Astle, C. M., and Harrison, D. E. (2003b). Hematopoietic senescence is postponed and hematopoietic stem cell function is enhanced by dietary restriction. *Exp Hematol.* **31,** 1097–1103.

Chen, J. Z., Zhang, F. R., Tao, Q. M., Wang, X. X., and Zhu, J. H. (2004). Number and activity of endothelial progenitor cells from peripheral blood in patients with hypercholesterolaemia. *Clinical Science.* **107,** 273–280.

Chen, K., Li, F., Li, J., Cai, H., Strom, S., Bisello, A., Kelley, D.E., Friedman-Einat, M., Skibinski, G. A., McCrory, M. A., Szalai, A. J., Zhao, A. Z. (2006). Induction of leptin resistance through direct interaction of C-reactive protein with leptin. *Nat Med.* **12,** 425–432.

Chen, S., Averett, N. T., Manelli, A., Ladu, M. J., May, W., and Ard, M. D. (2005). Isoform-specific effects of apolipoprotein E on secretion of inflammatory mediators in adult rat microglia. *J Alzheimers Dis.* **7,** 25–35.

Chen, X. L., Varner, S. E., Rao, A. S., Grey, J. Y., Thomas, S., Cook, C. K., Wasserman, M. A., Medford, R. M., Jaiswal, A. K., and Kunsch, C. (2003). Laminar flow induction of antioxidant response element-mediated genes in endothelial cells. A novel anti-inflammatory mechanism. *J Biol Chem.* **278,** 703–711.

Cheng, T. O. (2006). Obesity, Hippocrates and Venus of Willendorf. *Int J Cardiol.* **113,** 257.

Chiappelli, M., Tampieri, C., Tumini, E., Porcellini, E., Caldarera, C. M., Nanni, S., Branzi, A., Lio, D., Caruso, M., Hoffmann, E., Caruso, C., and Licastro, F. (2005). Interleukin-6 gene polymorphism is an age-dependent risk factor for myocardial infarction in men. *Int J Immunogenet.* **32,** 349–353.

Chike-Obi, U., David, R. J., Coutinho, R., and Wu, S. Y. (1996). Birth weight has increased over a generation. *Am J Epidemiol.* **144,** 563–569.

Chiodi, H. (1940). The relationship between the thymus and the sexual organs. *Endocrinology.* **26,** 107–116.

Chiu, C. H., Lin, W. D., Huang, S. Y., and Lee, Y. H. (2004). Effect of a C/EBP gene replacement on mitochondrial biogenesis in fat cells. *Genes & Development.* **18,** 1970–1975.

Cho, H. Y., Zhang, L. Y., and Kleeberger, S. R. (2001). Ozone-induced lung inflammation and hyperreactivity are mediated via tumor necrosis factor-alpha receptors. *Am J Physiol. Lung Cell Mol Physiol.* **280,** L537–46.

Chobanian, A. V., Lichtenstein, A. H., Nilakhe, V., Haudenschild, C. C., Drago, R., and Nickerson, C. (1989). Influence of hypertension on aortic atherosclerosis in the Watanabe rabbit. *Hypertension.* **14,** 203–209.

Chockalingam, A., Gnanavelu, G., Elangovan, S., and Chockalingam, V. (2003). Current profile of acute rheumatic fever and valvulitis in southern India. *J Heart Valve Dis.* **12,** 573–576.

Choi, E. K., Park, S. A., Oh, W. M., Kang, H. C., Kuramitsu, H. K., Kim, B. G., and Kang, I. C. (2005a). Mechanisms of *Porphyromonas gingivalis*-induced monocyte chemoattractant protein-1 expression in endothelial cells. *FEMS Immunol Med Microbiol.* **44,** 51–58.

Choi, G. B., Dong, H. W., Murphy, A. J., Valenzuela, D. M., Yancopoulos, G. D., Swanson, L. W., and Anderson, D. J. (2005b). Lhx6 delineates a pathway mediating innate reproductive behaviors from the amygdala to the hypothalamus. *Neuron.* **46,** 647–660.

Chomyn, A., and Attardi, G. (2003). MtDNA mutations in aging and apoptosis. *Biochem Biophys Res Commun.* **304,** 519–529.

Chou, H. H., Hayakawa, T., Diaz, S., Krings, M., Indriati, E., Leakey, M., Paabo, S., Satta, Y., Takahata, N., and Varki, A. (2002). Inactivation of CMP-N-acetylneuraminic acid hydroxylase occurred prior to brain expansion during human evolution. *Proc Natl Acad Sci USA.* **99,** 11736–11741.

Chou, M. W., Kong, J., Chung, K. T., and Hart, R. W. (1993). Effect of caloric restriction on the metabolic activation of xenobiotics. *Mutat Res.* **295,** 223–235.

Chou, M. W., Pegram, R. A., Turturro, A., Holson, R., and Hart, R. W. (1993). Effect of caloric restriction on the induction of hepatic cytochrome P-450 and Ah receptor binding in C57BL/6N and DBA/2J mice. *Drug Chem Toxicol.* **16,** 1–19.

Chou, M. W., Shaddock, J. G., Kong, J., Hart, R. W., and Casciano, D. A. (1995). Effect of dietary restriction on partial hepatectomy-induced liver regeneration of aged F344 rats. *Cancer Lett.* **91(2),** 191–197.

Christensen, K., Johnson, T. E., and Vaupel, J. W. (2006). The quest for genetic determinants of human longevity: Challenges and insights. *Nature Rev Gene.* **7,** 436–448.

Christensen, K., Wienke, A., Skytthe, A., Holm, N. V., Vaupel, J. W., and Yashin, A. I. (2001). Cardiovascular mortality in twins and the fetal origins hypothesis. *Twin Res.* **4** 344–349.

Christiansen, L., Bathum, L., Andersen-Ranberg, K., Jeune, B., and Christensen, K. (2004). Modest implication of interleukin-6 promoter polymorphisms in longevity. *Mech Ageing Dev.* **125,** 391–395.

Chui, H. (2005). Neuropathology lessons in vascular dementia. *Alzheimer Dis Assoc Disord.* **19,** 45–52.

Chun, Y. H., Chun, K. R., Olguin, D., and Wang, H. L. (2005). Biological foundation for periodontitis as a potential risk factor for atherosclerosis. *J Periodontal Res.* **40,** 87–95.

Chung, H. Y., Kim, H. J., Kim, J. W., and Yu, B. P. (2001). The inflammation hypothesis of aging: Molecular modulation by calorie restriction. *Ann NY Acad Sci.* **928,** 327–335.

Clancy, D. J., Gems, D., Hafen, E., Leevers, S. J., and Partridge, L. (2002). Dietary restriction in long-lived dwarf flies. *Science.* **296,** 319.

Clancy, D. J., Gems, D., Harshman, L. G., Oldham, S., Stocker, H., Hafen, E., Leevers, S. J., and Partridge, L. (2001). Extension of life-span by loss of CHICO, a *Drosophila* insulin receptor substrate protein. *Science.* **292,** 104–106.

Clarke, C., and Haswell, M. (1970). *The economics of subsistence agriculture.* London: Macmillan.

Clarkson, T. B. (1998). Nonhuman primate models of atherosclerosis. *Lab An Sci.* **48,** 569–572.

Clarkson, T. B. (2002). The new conundrum: Do estrogens have any cardiovascular benefits? *Int J Ferild Women's Med.* **47,** 61–68.

Cleary, J. P., Walsh, D. M., Hofmeister, J. J., Shankar, G. M., Kuskowski, M. A., Selkoe, D. J., and Ashe, K. H. (2005). Natural oligomers of the amyloid-beta protein specifically disrupt cognitive function. *Nature Neurosci.* **8,** 79–84.

Clowes, J. A., Khosla, S., and Eastell, R. (2005). Potential role of pancreatic and enteric hormones in regulating bone turnover. *J Bone Min Res.* **20,** 1497–1506.

Coelho, M., Luiselli, D., Bertorelle, G., Lopes, A.I., Seixas, S., Destro-Bisol, G., et al (2005). Microsatellite variation and evolution of human lactase persistence. *Hum Genet.* **117,** 329–339.

Cohen, H. Y., Miller, C., Bitterman, K. J., Wall, N. R., Hekking, B., Kessler, B., Howitz, K. T., Gorospe, M., de Cabo, R., and Sinclair, D. A. (2004). Calorie restriction promotes mammalian cell survival by inducing the SIRT1 deacetylase. *Science.* **305,** 390–392.

Cohen, R. M., Szczepanik, J., McManus, M., Mirza, N., Putnam, K., Levy, J., and Sunderland, T. (2006). Hippocampal atrophy in the healthy is initially linear and independent of age. *Neurobiol Aging.* **27,** 1385–1394.

Coker, R., McKee, M., Atun, R., Dimitrova, B., Dodonova, E., Kuznetsov, S., and Drobniewski, F. (2006). Risk factors for pulmonary tuberculosis in Russia: Case-control study. *Br Med J.* **332,** 85–87.

Coker, R. H., and Kjaer, M. (2005). Glucoregulation during exercise: The role of the neuroendocrine system. *Sports Med* **35,** 575–583.

Col, N. F., Bowlby, L. A., and McGarry, K. (2005). The role of menopausal hormone therapy in preventing osteoporotic fractures: A critical review of the clinical evidence. *Minerva Medica.* **96,** 331–342.

Colcombe, S., and Kramer, A. F. (2003). Fitness effects on the cognitive function of older adults: A meta-analytic study. *Psychol Sci.,* **14,** 125–130.

Colcombe, S. J., Kramer, A. F., Erickson, K. I., Scalf, P., McAuley, E., Cohen, N. J., Webb, A., Jerome, G. J., Marquez, D. X., and Elavsky, S. (2004). Cardiovascular fitness, cortical plasticity, and aging. *Proc Natl Acad Sci USA.* **101,** 3316–3321.

Cole, G. M., Lim, G. P., Yang, F., Teter, B., Begum, A., Ma, Q., Harris-White, M. E., and Frautschy, S. A. (2005a). Prevention of Alzheimer's disease: Omega-3 fatty acid and phenolic anti-oxidant interventions. *Neurobiol Aging.* **Suppl 1,** 133–6.

Cole, S. L., Grudzien, A., Manhart, I. O., Kelly, B. L., Oakley, H., and Vassar, R. (2005b). Statins cause intracellular accumulation of amyloid precursor protein, beta-secretase-cleaved fragments, and amyloid beta-peptide via an isoprenoid-dependent mechanism. *J Biol Chem.* **280,** 18755–18770.

Collaboration, A. T. (2002). Collaborative meta-analysis of randomised trials of antiplatelet therapy for prevention of death, myocardial infarction, and stroke in high risk patients. *Brit Med J* **324,** 71–86.

Collett, G. D., and Canfield, A. E. (2005). Angiogenesis and pericytes in the initiation of ectopic calcification. *Circ Res.* **96,** 930–936.

Collinson, A. C., Moore, S. E., Cole, T. J., and Prentice, A. M. (2003). Birth season and environmental influences on patterns of thymic growth in rural Gambian infants. *Acta Paediatr.* **92,** 1014–1020.

Colman, P. D., Kaplan, B. B., Osterburg, H. H., and Finch, C. E. (1980). Brain poly(A)RNA during aging: Stability of yield and sequence complexity in two rat strains. *J Neurochem.* **34,** 335–345.

Colombani, J., Raisin, S., Pantalacci, S., Radimerski, T., Montagne, J., and Leopold, P. (2003). A nutrient sensor mechanism controls *Drosophila* growth. *Cell.* **114,** 739–749.

Colton, C. A., Needham, L. K., Brown, C., Cook, D., Rasheed, K., Burke, J. R., Strittmatter, W. J., Schmechel, D. E., and Vitek, M. P. (2004). APOE genotype-specific differences in human and mouse macrophage nitric oxide production. *J Neuroimmunol.* **147,** 62–67.

Congdon, J. D., Nagle, R. D., Kinney, O. M., van Loben Sels, R. C., Quinter, T., and Tinkle, D. W. (2003). Testing hypotheses of aging in long-lived painted turtles (*Chrysemys picta*). *Exp Gerontol.* **38,** 765–772.

Conklin-Brittain, N. L., Wrangham, R., and Smith, C. C. (2002). A two-stage model of increased dietary quality in early hominid evolution: The role of fiber. In P. S. Ungar and M. F. Teaford, Eds, *Human diet. Its origin and evolution* Chapter 6, pp. 61–76. Westport, CT: Bergin and Garvey.

Constancia, M., Angiolini, E., Sandovici, I., Smith, P., Smith, R., Kelsey, G., Dean, W., Ferguson-Smith, A., Sibley, C. P., Reik, W., and Fowden, A. (2005). Adaptation of nutrient supply to fetal demand in the mouse involves interaction between the Igf2 gene and placental transporter systems. *Proc Natl Acad Sci USA.* **102,** 19219–19224.

Conti, E., Carrozza, C., Capoluongo, E., Volpe, M., Crea, F., Zuppi, C., and Andreotti, F. (2004). Insulin-like growth factor-1 as a vascular protective factor. *Circulation.* **110,** 2260–2265.

Cook, N. R., Lee, I. M., Gaziano, J. M., Gordon, D., Ridker, P. M., Manson, J. E., Hennekens, C. H., and Buring, J. E. (2005). Low-dose aspirin in the primary prevention of cancer: The Women's Health Study: A randomized controlled trial. *JAMA.* **294,** 47–55.

Coombs, N. J., Taylor, R., Wilcken, N., Fiorica, J., and Boyages, J. (2005). Hormone replacement therapy and breast cancer risk in California. *Breast J.* **11,** 410–415.

Corbo, R. M., and Scacchi, R. (1999). Apolipoprotein E (APOE) allele distribution in the world. Is APOE*4 a 'thrifty' allele? *Ann Hum Genet.* **63,** 301–310.

Corbo, R. M., Scacchi, R., and Cresta, M. (2004a). Differential reproductive efficiency associated with common apolipoprotein e alleles in postreproductive-aged subjects. *Fertil Steril.* **81,** 104–107.

Corbo, R. M., Ulizzi, L., Scacchi, R., Martínez-Labarga, C., and De Stefano, G. F. (2004b). Apolipoprotein E polymorphism and fertility: A study in pre-industrial populations. *Mol Hum Reprod.* **10,** 617–620.

Cordain, L., Eaton, S. B., Miller, J. B., Mann, N., and Hill, K. (2002a). The paradoxical nature of hunter-gatherer diets: meat-based, yet non-atherogenic. *Eur J Clin Nutr* **56 Suppl 1,** S42–S52.

Cordain, L., Watkins, B. A., Florant, G. L., Kelher, M., Rogers, L., and Li, Y. (2002b). Fatty acid analysis of wild ruminant tissues: Evolutionary implications for reducing diet-related chronic disease. *Eur J Clin Nutr.* **56,** 181–191.

Cordain, L., Watkins, B. A., and Mann, N. J. (2001). Fatty acid composition and energy density of foods available to African hominids. Evolutionary implications for human brain development. *World Rev Nutrit Diet.* **90,** 144–161.

Corder, E. H., Basun, H., Fratiglioni, L., Guo, Z., Lannfelt, L., Viitanen, M., Corder, L. S., Manton, K. G., and Winblad, B. (2000). Inherited frailty. ApoE alleles determine survival after a diagnosis of heart disease or stroke at ages 85+. *Ann NY Acad Sci.* **908,** 295–298.

Corder, E. H., Saunders, A. M., Strittmatter, W. J., Schmechel, D. E., Gaskell, P. C., Small, G. W., Roses, A. D., Haines, J. L., and Pericak-Vance, M. A. (1993). Gene dose of apolipoprotein E type 4 allele and the risk of Alzheimer's disease in late onset families. *Science.* **261,** 921–923.

Corella, D., Tucker, K., Lahoz, C., Coltell, O., Cupples, L. A., Wilson, P. W., Schaefer, E. J., and Ordovas, J. M. (2001). Alcohol drinking determines the effect of the APOE locus on LDL-cholesterol concentrations in men: The Framingham Offspring Study. *Am J Clin Nutr.* **73,** 736–745.

Coria, F., Castäno, E., Prelli, F., Larrondo-Lillo, M., van Duinen, S., Shelanski, M. L., and Frangione, B. (1988). Isolation and characterization of amyloid P component from Alzheimer's disease and other types of cerebral amyloidosis. *Lab Invest.* **58,** 454–458.

Cornelius, C., Fastbom, J., Winblad, B., and Viitanen, M. (2004). Aspirin, NSAIDs, risk of dementia, and influence of the apolipoprotein E epsilon 4 allele in an elderly population. *Neuroepidemiology.* **23,** 135–143.

Corral-Debrinski, M., Shoffner, J. M., Lott, M. T., and Wallace, D. C. (1992). Association of mitochondrial DNA damage with aging and coronary atherosclerotic heart disease. *Mutat Res.* **275,** 169–180.

Corton, J. C., Apte, U., Anderson, S. P., Limaye, P., Yoon, L., Latendresse, J., Dunn, C., Everitt, J. I., Voss, K. A., Swanson, C., Kimbrough, C., Wong, J. S., Gill, S. S., Chandraratna, R. A., Kwak, M. K., Kensler, T. W., Stulnig, T. M., Steffensen, K. R., Gustafsson, J. A., and Mehendale, H. M. (2004). Mimetics of caloric restriction include agonists of lipid-activated nuclear receptors. *J Biol Chem.* **279,** 46204–46212.

Coschigano, K. T., Clemmons, D., Bellush, L. L., and Kopchick, J. J. (2000). Assessment of growth parameters and life span of GHR/BP gene-disrupted mice. *Endocrinology.* **141,** 2608–2613.

Coschigano, K. T., Holland, A. N., Riders, M. E., List, E. O., Flyvbjerg, A., and Kopchick, J. J. (2003). Deletion, but not antagonism, of the mouse growth hormone receptor results in severely decreased body weights, insulin, and insulin-like growth factor I levels and increased life span. *Endocrinology.* **144,** 3799–3810.

Cosman, F., Baz-Hecht, M., Cushman, M., Vardy, M. D., Cruz, J. D., Nieves, J. W., Zion, M., and Lindsay, R. (2005). Short-term effects of estrogen, tamoxifen and raloxifene on hemostasis: A randomized-controlled study and review of the literature. *Thrombosis Res.* **116,** 1–13.

Costa, D. L. (2000). Understanding the twentieth-century decline in chronic conditions among older men. *Demography.* **37,** 53–62.

Cotchin, E., and Roe, C. (1967). *Pathology of laboratory rats and mice.* Oxford, UK: Blackwell Scientific Publications.

Cotman, C. W., and Berchtold, N. C. (2002). Exercise: A behavioral intervention to enhance brain health and plasticity. *Trends Neurosci.* **25,** 295–301.

Coughlin, S. R., and Camerer, E. (2003). Participation in inflammation. *J Clin Invest.* **111,** 25–27.

Couillard, C., Ruel, G., Archer, W. R., Pomerleau, S., Bergeron, J., Couture, P., Lamarche, B., and Bergeron, N. (2005). Circulating levels of oxidative stress markers and endothelial adhesion molecules in men with abdominal obesity. *J Clin Endocrinol Metab.* **90,** 6454–6459.

Craft, S., and Watson, G. S. (2004). Insulin and neurodegenerative disease: Shared and specific mechanisms. *Lancet. Neurology.* **3,** 169–178.

Crawford, D. W., and Blankenhorn, D. H. (1979). Regression of atherosclerosis. *Annu Rev Med.* **30,** 289–300.

Crawford, F. C., Vanderploeg, R. D., Freeman, M. J., Singh, S., Waisman, M., Michaels, L., et al. (2002). APOE genotype influences acquisition and recall following traumatic brain injury. *Neurology.* **58,** 1115–1158.

Crawford, M., Galli, C., Visioli, F., Renaud, S., Simopoulos, A. P., and Spector, A. A. (2004). Role of plant-derived omega-3 fatty acids in human nutrition. *Ann Nutrit. Metab,* **44,** 263–265.

Crimmins, E., and Finch, C. E. (2006a). Infection, inflammation, height, and longevity. *PNAS.* **103,** 498–503.

Crimmins, E. M. and Finch, C. E. (2006b). Commentary: do older men and women gain equally from improving childhood conditions? *Int J Epidemiol.* **35,** 1270–1271.

Crisby, M., Carlson, L. A., and Winblad, B. (2002). Statins in the prevention and treatment of Alzheimer disease. *Alzheimer Dis Assoc Disord.* **16,** 131–136.

Cristofalo, V. J., Lorenzini, A., Allen, R. G., Torres, C., and Tresini, M. (2004). Replicative senescence: A critical review. *Mech Ageing Dev.* **125,** 827–848.

Crocker, I. P., Tanner, O. M., Myers, J. E., Bulmer, J. N., Walraven, G., and Baker, P. N. (2004). Syncytiotrophoblast degradation and the pathophysiology of the malaria-infected placenta. *Placenta.* **25,** 273–282.

Crocker, P. R. and Varki, A. (2001). Siglecs, sialic acids and innate immunity. *Trends in Immun.* **22,** 337–342.

Croll, N. A., Smith, J. M., and Zuckerman, B. M. (1977). The aging process of the nematode *Caenorhabditis elegans* in bacterial and axenic culture. *Exp Aging Res,* **3,** 175–189.

Cross, R., Bryson, J., and Roszman, T. (1992). Immunologic disparity in the hypopituitary dwarf mouse. *J Immunology.* **148,** 1347–1352.

Cryer, B., and Feldman, M. (1998). Cyclooxygenase-1 and cyclooxygenase-2 selectivity of widely used nonsteroidal anti-inflammatory drugs. *Am J Med.* **104,** 413–421.

Csiszar, A., Ungvari, Z., Edwards, J. G., Kaminski, P., Wolin, M. S., Koller, A., and Kaley, G. (2002). Aging-induced phenotypic changes and oxidative stress impair coronary arteriolar function. *Circ Res.* **90,** 1159–1166.

Csiszar, A., Ungvari, Z., Koller, A., Edwards, J. G., and Kaley, G. (2003). Aging-induced proinflammatory shift in cytokine expression profile in coronary arteries. *FASEB J.* **17,** 1183–1185.

Csiszar, A., Ungvari, Z., Koller, A., Edwards, J. G., and Kaley, G. (2004). Proinflammatory phenotype of coronary arteries promotes endothelial apoptosis in aging. *Physiol Genomics.* **17,** 21–30.

Cuevas, A. M., Guasch, V., Castillo, O., Irribarra, V., Mizon, C., San Martin, A., Strobel, P., Perez, D., Germain, A. M., and Leighton, F. (2000). A high-fat diet induces and red wine counteracts endothelial dysfunction in human volunteers. *Lipids.* **35,** 143–148.

Cunningham-Rundles, S., McNeeley, D. F., and Moon, A. (2005). Mechanisms of nutrient modulation of the immune response. *J Allergy Clin Immunol.* **115,** 1119–1128.

Cunningham, K. S., and Gotlieb, A. I. (2005). The role of shear stress in the pathogenesis of atherosclerosis. *Lab Invest.* **85,** 9–23.

Currat, M., Excoffier, L., Maddison, W., Otto, S. P., Ray, N., Whitlock, M. C., and Yeaman, S. (2006). Comment on "Ongoing adaptive evolution of ASPM, a brain size determinant in Homo sapiens" and "Microcephalin, a gene regulating brain size, continues to evolve adaptively in humans." *Science.* **313,** 172.

Cutler, R. G. (1975). Transcription of unique and reiterated DNA sequences in mouse liver and brain tissues as a function of age. *Exp Gerontol.* **10,** 37–59.

Cutler, R. G. (1984). Urate and ascorbate: Their possible roles as antioxidants in determining longevity of mammalian species. *Arch Gerontol Geriatr.* **3(4),** 321–348.

Cutler, R. G. (2005). Oxidative stress and aging: Catalase is a longevity determinant enzyme. *Rejuv Res* **8,** 138–140.

Cypser, J. R., and Johnson, T. E. (2003). Hormesis in *Caenorhabditis elegans* dauer-defective mutants. *Biogerontol.* **4,** 203–214.

Czarny, M., and Schnitzer, J. E. (2004). Neutral sphingomyelinase inhibitor scyphostatin prevents and ceramide mimics mechanotransduction in vascular endothelium. *Am J Physiol. Heart Circ Physiol.* **287,** H1344–1352.

D'Aiuto, F., Nibali, L., Parkar, M., Suvan, J., and Tonetti, M. S. (2005). Short-term effects of intensive periodontal therapy on serum inflammatory markers and cholesterol. *J Dent Res.* **84,** 269–273.

D'Aiuto, F., Parkar, M., Andreou, G., Suvan, J., Brett, P. M., Ready, D., and Tonetti, M. S. (2004). Periodontitis and systemic inflammation: Control of the local infection is associated with a reduction in serum inflammatory markers. *J Dent Res.* **83,** 156–160.

D'Amore, J. D., Kajdasz, S. T., McLellan, M. E., Bacskai, B. J., Stern, E. A., and Hyman, B. T. (2003). *In vivo* multiphoton imaging of a transgenic mouse model of Alzheimer disease reveals marked thioflavine-S-associated alterations in neurite trajectories. *J Neuropathol Exp Neurol.* **62,** 137–145.

D'Armiento, F. P., Bianchi, A., de Nigris, F., Capuzzi, D. M., D'Armiento, M. R., Crimi, G., Abete, P., Palinski, W., Condorelli, M., and Napoli, C. (2001). Age-related effects on atherogenesis and scavenger enzymes of intracranial and extracranial arteries in men without classic risk factors for atherosclerosis. *Stroke.* **32,** 2472–2479.

Dagon, Y., Avraham, Y., Magen, I., Gertler, A., Ben-Hur, T., and Berry, E. M. (2005). Nutritional status, cognition, and survival: A new role for leptin and AMP kinase. *J Biol Chem.* **280,** 42142–42148.

Dahlgren, J., Nilsson, C., Jennische, E., Ho, H. P., Eriksson, E., Niklasson, A., Bjëorntorp, P., Albertsson Wikland, K., and Holmang, A. (2001). Prenatal cytokine exposure results in obesity and gender-specific programming. *Am J Physiol Endocrinol Metab.* **281,** E326–334.

Dai, G., Kaazempur-Mofrad, M. R., Natarajan, S., Zhang, Y., Vaughn, S., Blackman, B. R., Kamm, R. D., Garcia-Cardena, G., and Gimbrone, M. A., Jr. (2004). Distinct endothelial phenotypes evoked by arterial waveforms derived from atherosclerosis-susceptible and resistant regions of human vasculature. *Proc Natl Acad Sci USA.* **101,** 14871–14876.

Daily, A., Nath, A., and Hersh, L. B. (2006). Tat peptides inhibit neprilysin. *J Neurovirol.* **12,** 153–160.

Daitoku, H., Hatta, M., Matsuzaki, H., Aratani, S., Ohshima, T., Miyagishi, M., Nakajima, T., Fukamizu, A., and Japan. (2004). Silent information regulator 2 potentiates FoxO1-mediated transcription through its deacetylase activity. *Proc Natl Acad Sci USA.* **101,** 10042–10047.

Dallinga-Thie, G. M., Groenendijk, M., Blom, R. N., De Bruin, T. W., and De Kant, E. (2001). Genetic heterogeneity in the apolipoprotein C-III promoter and effects of insulin. *J Lipid Res.* **42(9),** 1450–1456.

Dalpe, A., and Heeg, K. (2002). Signal integration following Toll-like receptor triggering. *Crit Rev Immunol.* **22,** 217–250.

Danesh, J. (1999). Coronary heart disease, *Helicobacter pylori*, dental disease, *Chlamydia pneumoniae*, and cytomegalovirus. *Am Heart J.* **138,** S434–S437.

Danesh, J., Wong, Y., Ward, M., and Muir, J. (1999). Chronic infection with *Helicobacter pylori*, *Chlamydia pneumoniae*, or cytomegalovirus: Population based study of coronary heart disease. *Heart.* **81,** 245–247.

Dao, H. H., Essalihi, R., Bouvet, C., and Moreau, P. (2005). Evolution and modulation of age-related medial elastocalcinosis: Impact on large artery stiffness and isolated systolic hypertension. *Cardiovasc Res.* **66,** 307–317.

Dart, R. (1953). The predatory transition from ape to man. *Int Anthrop Linguist Rev* **1,** 201–219.

Dasu, M. R. K., Herndon, D. N., Nesic, O., Perez-Polo, J. R. (2003). IGF-I gene transfer effects on inflammatory elements present after thermal trauma. *Am J Physiol Regul Integr Comp Physiol.* **285,** R741–746.

Davey Smith, G., and Ebrahim, S. (2002). Data dredging, bias, or confounding. *Br Med J.* **325,** 1437–1438.

Davey Smith, G., Hart, C., Upton, M., Hole, D., Gillis, C., Watt, G., and Hawthorne, V. (2000). Height and risk of death among men and women: Aetiological implications of associations with cardiorespiratory disease and cancer mortality. *J Epidemiology and Community Health.* **54,** 97–103.

Davey Smith, G., Timpson, N., Lawlor, D.A. (2006). C-reactive protein and cardiovascular disease risk: still an unknown quantity? *Ann Intern Med.* **145,** 70–72.

Davidson, E. H. (2006). *The regulatory genome.* San Diego: Academic Press.

Davidson, E. H., and Erwin, D. H. (2006). Gene regulatory networks and the evolution of animal body plans. *Science.* **311,** 796–800.

Davies, H. (1990). Atherogenesis and the coronary arteries of childhood. *Int J Cardiology.* **28,** 283–291.

Davies, M. J., Woolf, N., Rowles, P. M., and Pepper, J. (1988). Morphology of the endothelium over atherosclerotic plaques in human coronary arteries. *Br Heart J.* **60,** 459–464.

Davies, W., Isles, A. R., and Wilkinson, L. S. (2005). Imprinted gene expression in the brain. *Neurosci Biobehav Rev.* **29,** 421–430.

De Angelis, L., Millasseau, S. C., Smith, A., Viberti, G., Jones, R. H., Ritter, J. M., and Chowienczyk, P. J. (2004). Sex differences in age-related stiffening of the aorta in subjects with type 2 diabetes. *Hypertension.* **44,** 67–71.

de Beer, F. C., Nel, A. E., Gie, R. P., Donald, P. R., and Strachan, A. F. (1984). Serum amyloid A protein and C-reactive protein levels in pulmonary tuberculosis: Relationship to amyloidosis. *Thorax.* **39**, 196–200.

De Benedetti, F., Meazza, C., Martini, A. (2002). Role of interleukin-6 in growth failure: an animal model. *Horm Res.* **58**, 24–27.

De Boer, O. J., Teeling, P., Idu, M. M., Becker, A. E., Wal, A. C. (2006). Epstein Barr virus specific T-cells generated from unstable human atherosclerotic lesions: Implications for plaque inflammation. *Atherosclerosis.* **184**, 322–329.

de Boo, H. A., and Harding, J. E. (2006). The developmental origins of adult disease (Barker) hypothesis. *Aust N Z J Obstet Gynaecol.* **46**, 4–14.

de Bruin, J. P., Gosden, R. G., Finch, C. E., and Leaman, B. M. (2004). Ovarian aging in two species of long-lived rockfish, *Sebastes aleutianus* and *S. alutus. Biology of Reproduction.* **71**, 1036–1042.

De Bry, L. (1994). Anthropological implications of the Maillard reaction: An insight. In T. P. Labuza, G. A. Reineccius, V. M. Monnier, J. O'Brien, and J. W. Baynes, Eds., *Maillard reactions in chemistry, food, and health*, pp. 28–35. London:Royal Chemical Society.

de Cabo, R., Fèurer-Galban, S., Anson, R. M., Gilman, C., Gorospe, M., and Lane, M. A. (2003). An *in vitro* model of caloric restriction. *Exp Gerontol.* **38(6)**, 631–639.

DeChiara, T. M., Robertson, E. J., and Efstratiadis, A. (1991). Parental imprinting of the mouse insulin-like growth factor II gene. *Cell.* **64**, 849–859.

de Craen, A. J., Posthuma, D., Remarque, E. J., van den Biggelaar, A. H., Westendorp, R. G., and Boomsma, D. I. (2005). Heritability estimates of innate immunity: An extended twin study. *Genes Immu.* **6**, 167–170.

De Cuyper, C., and Vanfleteren, J. R. (1982). Nutritional alteration of life span in the nematode *Caenorhabditis elegans. Age.* **5**, 42–45.

Defleur, A., White, T., Valensi, P., Slimak, L., and Cregut-Bonnoure, E. (1999). Neanderthal cannibalism at Moula-Guercy, Ardeche, France. *Science.* **286**, 128–131.

de Geus, E. J., Posthuma, D., Ijzerman, R. G., and Boomsma, D. I. (2001). Comparing blood pressure of twins and their singleton siblings: Being a twin does not affect adult blood pressure. *Twin Res.* **4(5)**, 385–391.

de Grey, A. D. (2005). Reactive oxygen species production in the mitochondrial matrix: Implications for the mechanism of mitochondrial mutation accumulation. *Rejuvenation Res.* **8**, 13–17.

De Heinzelin, J., Clark, J. D., White, T., Hart, W., Renne, P., WoldeGabriel, G., et al. (1999). Environment and behavior of 2.5-million-year-old Bouri hominids. *Science.* **284**, 625–629.

De Jong, G., and Bochdanovits, Z. (2003). Latitudinal clines in *Drosophila melanogaster*: Body size, allozyme frequencies, inversion frequencies, and the insulin-signalling pathway. *J Genetics.* **82**, 207–223.

de Kruif, M. D., van Gorp, E. C., Keller, T. T., Ossewaarde, J. M., and ten Cate, H. (2005). *Chlamydia pneumoniae* infections in mouse models: Relevance for atherosclerosis research. *Cardiovasc Res.* **65**, 317–327.

De Lacalle, S., Cooper, J. D., Svendsen, C. N., Dunnett, S. B., and Sofroniew, M. V. (1996). Reduced retrograde labelling with fluorescent tracer accompanies neuronal atrophy of basal forebrain cholinergic neurons in aged rats. *Neuroscience.* **75**, 19–27.

Delaere, P., He, Y., Fayet, G., Duyckaerts, C., and Hauw, J. J. (1993). Beta A4 deposits are constant in the brain of the oldest old: An immunocytochemical study of 20 French centenarians. *Neurobiol Aging.* **14**, 191–194.

Del Bo, R., Comi, G. P., Bresolin, N., Castelli, E., Conti, E., Degiuli, A., Ausenda, C. D., and Scarlato, G. (1997). The apolipoprotein E epsilon4 allele causes a faster decline of cognitive performances in Down's syndrome subjects. *J Neurol Sci.* **145,** 87–91.

Deliargyris, E. N., Madianos, P. N., Kadoma, W., Marron, I., Smith, S. C., Jr., Beck, J. D., and Offenbacher, S. (2004). Periodontal disease in patients with acute myocardial infarction: Prevalence and contribution to elevated C-reactive protein levels. *Am Heart J.* **147,** 1005–1009.

Delorme, C., Brussow, H., Sidoti, J., Roche, N., Karlsson, K. A., Neeser, J. R., and Teneberg, S. (2001). Glycosphingolipid binding specificities of rotavirus: Identification of a sialic acid-binding epitope. *J Virol.* **75,** 2276–2287.

Del Valle, L., and Pina-Oviedo, S. (2006). HIV disorders of the brain: Pathology and pathogenesis. *Front Biosci.* **11,** 718–732.

de Magalhaes, J. P., Cabral, J., and Magalhaes, D. (2005). The influence of genes on the aging process of mice: a statistical assessment of the genetics of aging. *Genetics.* **169,** 265–274.

DeMar, J. C., Jr., Ma, K., Bell, J. M., Igarashi, M., Greenstein, D., and Rapoport, S. I. (2006). One generation of N-3 polyunsaturated fatty acid deprivation increases depression and aggression test scores in rats. *J Lipid Res.* **47,** 172–180.

Demarchi, D. A., Salzano, F. M., Altuna, M. E., Fiegenbaum, M., Hill, K., Hurtado, A. M., Tsunetto, L. T., Petzl-Erler, M. L., Hutz, M. H. (2005). APOE polymorphism distribution among Native Americans and related populations. *Ann Hum Biol.* **32,** 351–365.

De Meyer, G. R., De Cleen, D. M., Cooper, S., Knaapen, M. W., Jans, D. M., Martinet, W., Herman, A. G., Bult, H., and Kockx, M. M. (2002). Platelet phagocytosis and processing of beta-amyloid precursor protein as a mechanism of macrophage activation in atherosclerosis. [comment]. *Circ Res.* **90,** 1197–1204.

Demirovic, J., Prineas, R., Loewenstein, D., Bean, J., Duara, R., Sevush, S., and Szapocznik, J. (2003). Prevalence of dementia in three ethnic groups: The South Florida program on aging and health. *Ann Epidem.* **13,** 472–478.

Denley, A., Cosgrove, L. J., Booker, G. W., Wallace, J. C., and Forbes, B. E. (2005). Molecular interactions of the IGF system. *Cytokine & Growth Factor Rev.* **16,** 421–439.

de Nigris, F., Balestrieri, M. L., and Napoli, C. (2006a). Targeting c-Myc, Ras and IGF cascade to treat cancer and vascular disorders. *Cell Cycle.* **5,** 1621–1628.

de Nigris, F., Gallo, L., Sica, V., and Napoli, C., (2006b). Glycoxidation of low-density lipoprotein promotes multiple apoptotic pathways and NFkappaB activation in human coronary cells. *Basic Res Cardiol.* **101,** 101–108.

Densem, C. G., Hutchinson, I. V., Cooper, A., Yonan, N., and Brooks, N. H. (2000). Polymorphism of the transforming growth factor-beta 1 gene correlates with the development of coronary vasculopathy following cardiac transplantation. *J Heart Lung Transpl.* **19,** 551–556.

Densem, C. G., Hutchinson, I. V., Yonan, N., and Brooks, N. H. (2004). Donor and recipient-transforming growth factor-beta 1 polymorphism and cardiac transplant-related coronary artery disease. *Transpl Immunol.* **13,** 211–217.

Dentinger, C. M., Heinrich, N. L., Bell, B. P., Fox, L. M., Katz, D. J., Culver, D. H., and Shapiro, C. N. (2001). A prevalence study of hepatitis A virus infection in a migrant community: Is hepatitis A vaccine indicated? *J Pediatr.* **138(5),** 705–709.

De Palma, R., Del Galdo, F., Abbate, G., Chiariello, M., Calabró, R., Forte, L., Cimmino, G., Papa, M. F., Russo, M. G., Ambrosio, G., Giombolini, C., Tritto, I., Notaristefano, S., Berrino, L., Rossi, F., and Golino, P. (2006). Patients with acute coronary syndrome show oligoclonal T-cell recruitment within unstable plaque: Evidence for a local, intracoronary immunologic mechanism. *Circulation.* **113,** 640–646.

de Rooij, S. R., Painter, R. C., Phillips, D. I., Osmond, C., Tanck, M. W., Defesche, J. C., Bossuyt, P. M., Michels, R. P., Bleker, O. P., and Roseboom, T. J. (2006a). The effects of the Pro12Ala polymorphism of the peroxisome proliferator-activated receptor-{gamma}2 gene on glucose/insulin metabolism interact with prenatal exposure to famine. *Diabetes Care.* **29,** 1052–1057.

de Rooij, S. R., Painter, R. C., Roseboom, T. J., Phillips, D. I., Osmond, C., Barker, D. J., Tanck, M. W., Michels, R. P., Bossuyt, P. M., and Bleker, O. P. (2006b). Glucose tolerance at age 58 and the decline of glucose tolerance in comparison with age 50 in people prenatally exposed to the Dutch famine. *Diabetologia.* **10,** 1–7.

Despres, J. P. (2006). Intra-abdominal obesity: An untreated risk factor for type 2 diabetes and cardiovascular disease. *J Endocrinol Invest.* **29,** 77–82.

Devalapalli, A. P., Lesher, A., Shieh, K., Solow, J. S., Everett, M. L., Edala, A. S., Whitt, P., Long, R. R., Newton, N., and Parker, W. (2006). Increased levels of IgE and autoreactive, polyreactive IgG in wild rodents: Implications for the hygiene hypothesis. *Scand J Immunol.* **64(2),** 125–136.

DeVeale, B., Brummel, T., and Seroude, L. (2004). Immunity and aging: The enemy within? *Aging Cell.* **3,** 195–208.

Devillard, E., Burton, J. P., Hammond, J. A., Lam, D., and Reid, G. (2004). Novel insight into the vaginal microflora in postmenopausal women under hormone replacement therapy as analyzed by PCR-denaturing gradient gel electrophoresis. *Eur J Obstet Gynecol Reprod Biol.* **117(1),** 76–81.

Drevenstedt, G., Crimmins, E. M., Vasunilashorn, S., and Finch, C. E. (2007), *in prep.*

Devriendt, K. (2000). Genetic control of intra-uterine growth. *Eur J Obstet Gynecol Reprod Biol.* **92(1),** 29–34.

DeVry, C. G., Tsai, W., and Clarke, S. (1996). Structure of the human gene encoding the protein repair L-isoaspartyl (D-aspartyl) O-methyltransferase. *Arch Biochem Biophys.* **335,** 321–332.

Dey, M., Lyttle, C. R., and Pickar, J. H. (2000). Recent insights into the varying activity of estrogens. *Maturitas.* **34(Suppl 2),** S25–33.

Dhahbi, J. M., Cao, S. X., Mote, P. L., Rowley, B. C., Wingo, J. E., Spindler, S. R. (2002). Postprandial induction of chaperone gene expression is rapid in mice. *J Nutrit.* **132,** 31–37.

Dhahbi, J. M., Kim, H. J., Mote, P. L., Beaver, R. J., and Spindler, S. R. (2004). Temporal linkage between the phenotypic and genomic responses to caloric restriction. *Proc Natl Acad Sci USA.* **101,** 5524–5529.

Dhahbi, J. M., Mote, P. L., Wingo, J., Tillman, J. B., Walford, R. L., Spindler, S. R. (1999). Calories and aging alter gene expression for gluconeogenic, glycolytic, and nitrogen-metabolizing enzymes. *Am J phys.* **277,** E352–E360.

Dhahbi, J. M., Mote, P. L., Wingo, J., Rowley, B. C., Cao, S. X., Walford, R. L., and Spindler, S. R. (2001). Caloric restriction alters the feeding response of key metabolic enzyme genes. *Mech Ageing Dev.* **122,** 1033–1048.

Dhawan, S. (1995). Birth weights of infants of first generation Asian women in Britain compared with second generation Asian women. *Br Med J.* **311,** 86–88.

Dhurandhar, N. V., Israel, B. A., Kolesar, J. M., Mayhew, G. F., Cook, M. E., and Atkinson, R. L. (2000). Increased adiposity in animals due to a human virus. *Int J Obes Relat Metab Disord.* **24,** 989–996.

Diao, L. H., Bickford, P. C., Stevens, J. O., Cline, E. J., and Gerhardt, G. A. (1997). Caloric restriction enhances evoked DA overflow in striatum and nucleus accumbens of aged Fischer 344 rats. *Brain Res.* **763,** 276–280.

Diaz, J. V., Koff, J., Gotway, M. B., Nishimura, S., and Balmes, J. R. (2006). Case report: A case of wood-smoke-related pulmonary disease. *Environ Health Perspect.* **114,** 759–762.

Dietl, J. (2005). Maternal obesity and complications during pregnancy. J Perinat Med. **33,** 100–105

Dietrich, M. O., Mantese, C. E., Porciuncula, L. O., Ghisleni, G., Vinade, L., Souza, D. O., and Portela, L. V. (2005). Exercise affects glutamate receptors in postsynaptic densities from cortical mice brain. *Brain Res.* **1065,** 20–25.

Dik, M. G., Jonker, C., Hack, C. E., Smit, J. H., Comijs, H. C., and Eikelenboom, P. (2005). Serum inflammatory proteins and cognitive decline in older persons. *Neurology.* **64,** 1371–1377.

Ding, S. Z., O'Hara, A. M., Denning, T. L., Dirden-Kramer, B., Mifflin, R. C., Reyes, V. E., Ryan, K. A., Elliott, S. N., Izumi, T., Boldogh, I., Mitra, S., Ernst, P. B., and Crowe, S. E. (2004). *Helicobacter pylori* and H2O2 increase AP endonuclease-1/redox factor-1 expression in human gastric epithelial cells. *Gastroenterology.* **127,** 845–858.

DiPatre, P. L., and Gelman, B. B. (1997). Microglial cell activation in aging and Alzheimer disease: Partial linkage with neurofibrillary tangle burden in the hippocampus. *J Neuropathol Exp Neurol.* **56,** 143–149.

Dirx, M. J., van den Brandt, P. A., Goldbohm, R. A., and Lumey, L. H. (2001). Energy restriction in childhood and adolescence and risk of prostate cancer: Results from the Netherlands Cohort Study. *Am J Epidemiology.* **154,** 530–537.

Dirx, M. J., van den Brandt, P. A., Goldbohm, R. A., and Lumey, L. H. (2003a). Energy restriction early in life and colon carcinoma risk: Results of The Netherlands Cohort Study after 7.3 years of follow-up. *Cancer.* **97,** 46–55.

Dirx, M. J., Zeegers, M. P., Dagnelie, P. C., van den Bogaard, T., and van den Brandt, P. A. (2003b). Energy restriction and the risk of spontaneous mammary tumors in mice: A meta-analysis. *Int. J Cancer.* **106,** 766–770.

Djousse, L., Myers, R. H., Province, M. A., Hunt, S. C., Eckfeldt, J. H., Evans, G., Peacock, J. M., and Ellison, R. C. (2002). Influence of apolipoprotein E, smoking, and alcohol intake on carotid atherosclerosis: National Heart, Lung, and Blood Institute Family Heart Study. *Stroke.* **33,** 1357–1361.

Djousse, L., Pankow, J. S., Arnett, D. K., Eckfeldt, J. H., Myers, R. H., and Ellison, R. C. (2004). Apolipoprotein E polymorphism modifies the alcohol-HDL association observed in the National Heart, Lung, and Blood Institute Family Heart Study. *Am J Clin Nutr.* **80,** 1639–1644.

Doblhammer, G., and Vaupel, J. W. (2001). Lifespan depends on month of birth. *Proc Natl Acad Sci USA.* **98,** 2934–2939.

Dobrian, A. D., Schriver, S. D., Khraibi, A. A., and Prewitt, R. L. (2004). Pioglitazone prevents hypertension and reduces oxidative stress in diet-induced obesity. *Hypertension.* **43,** 48–56.

Dobrin, P. B., Littooy, F. N., and Endean, E. D. (1989). Mechanical factors predisposing to intimal hyperplasia and medial thickening in autogenous vein grafts. *Surgery.* **105,** 393–400.

Dobrovolskaia, M. A., and Kozlov, S. V. (2005). Inflammation and cancer: When NF-kappaB amalgamates the perilous partnership. *Curr Cancer Drug Targets.* **5,** 325–344.

Doherty, T. M., Asotra, K., Fitzpatrick, L. A., Qiao, J. H., Wilkin, D. J., Detrano, R. C., Dunstan, C. R., Shah, P. K., and Rajavashisth, T. B. (2003). Calcification in atherosclerosis: Bone biology and chronic inflammation at the arterial crossroads. *Proc Natl Acad Sci USA.* **100,** 11201–11206.

Doll, R., Peto, R., Boreham, J., and Sutherland, I. (2004). Mortality in relation to smoking: 50 years' observations on male British doctors. *Br Med J (Clinical Research Ed.).* **328,** 1519.

Doll, R., Peto, R., Boreham, J., and Sutherland, I. (2005). Mortality from cancer in relation to smoking: 50 years' observations on British doctors. *Br J Cancer.* **92,** 426–429.

Dominici, F. P., Hauck, S., Argentino, D. P., Bartke, A., and Turyn, D. (2002). Increased insulin sensitivity and upregulation of insulin receptor, insulin receptor substrate (IRS)-1 and IRS-2 in liver of Ames dwarf mice. *J Endocrinol.* **173,** 81–94.

Donato, F., Boffetta, P., and Puoti, M. (1998). A meta-analysis of epidemiological studies on the combined effect of hepatitis B and C virus infections in causing hepatocellular carcinoma. *Int J Cancer.* **75,** 347–354.

Dong, C., Crawford, L. E., and Goldschmidt-Clermont, P. J. (2005). Endothelial progenitor obsolescence and atherosclerotic inflammation. *J Am Coll Cardiol.* **45,** 1458–1460.

Dong, L. M., Wilson, C., Wardell, M. R., Simmons, T., Mahley, R. W., Weisgraber, K. H., and Agard, D. A. (1994). Human apolipoprotein E. Role of arginine 61 in mediating the lipoprotein preferences of the E3 and E4 isoforms. *J Biol Chem.* **269,** 22358–22365.

Dong, W., Kari, F. W., Selgrade, M. K., and Gilmour, M. I. (2000). Attenuated allergic responses to house dust mite antigen in feed-restricted rats. *Environ Health Perspect.* **108,** 1125–1131.

Dong, W., Selgrade, M. K., Gilmour, I. M., Lange, R. W., Park, P., Luster, M. I., and Kari, F. W. (1998). Altered alveolar macrophage function in calorie-restricted rats. *Am J Respir Cell Mol Biol.* **19,** 462–469.

Dore, S., Kar, S., and Quirion, R. (1997). Insulin-like growth factor I protects and rescues hippocampal neurons against beta-amyloid- and human amylin-induced toxicity. *Proc Natl Acad Sci USA.* **94,** 4772–4777.

Dorman, J. B., Albinder, B., Shroyer, T., and Kenyon, C. (1995). The age-1 and daf-2 genes function in a common pathway to control the lifespan of *Caenorhabditis elegans*. *Genetics.* **141,** 1399–1406.

Dorner, G. (1974). Environment dependent brain organization and neuroendocrine, neurovegetative, and neuronal behavioral functions. *Prog. Brain Res.* **41,** 221–237.

Dorner, G. (1976). *Hormones and brain differentiation.* Amsterdam: Elsevier.

Doucet, C., Huby, T., Chapman, J., and Thillet, J. (1994). Lipoprotein[a] in the chimpanezee: Relationship of apo[a] phenotype to elevated plasma Lp[a] levels. *J Lipid Res.* **35,** 263–270.

Doucet, C., Wickings, J., Chapman, J., and Thillet, J. (1998). Chimpanzee lipoprotein(A): Relationship between apolipoprotein(A) isoform size and the density profile of lipoprotein(A) in animals with different heterozygous apo(A) phenotypes. *J Medical Primatolgy.* **27,** 21–27.

Douek, D. C., and Koup, R. A. (2000). Evidence for thymic function in the elderly. *Vaccine.* **18,** 1638–1641.

Douglas, K. R., Brinkmeier, M. L., Kennell, J. A., Eswara, P., Harrison, T. A., Patrianakos, A. I., Sprecher, B. S., Potok, M. A., Lyons, R. H., Jr., MacDougald, O. A., and Camper, S. A. (2001). Identification of members of the Wnt signaling pathway in the embryonic pituitary gland. *Mamm Genome.* **12,** 843–851.

Douwes, J., Le Gros, G., Gibson, P., and Pearce, N. (2004). Can bacterial endotoxin exposure reverse atopy and atopic disease? *J Allergy Clin Immunol.* **114,** 1051–1054.

Doux, J. D., Bazar, K. A., Lee, P. Y., and Yun, A. J. (2005). Can chronic use of anti-inflammatory agents paradoxically promote chronic inflammation through compensatory host response? *Med Hypotheses.* **65,** 389–391.

Dow, D. E., Dennis, R. G., and Faulkner, J. A. (2005). Electrical stimulation attenuates denervation and age-related atrophy in extensor digitorum longus muscles of old rats. *J Gerontol. Series A, Biol Sci Med Sci.* **60,** 416–424.

Drabe, N., Zund, G., Grunenfelder, J., Sprenger, M., Hoerstrup, S. P., Bestmann, L., Maly, F. E., and Turina, M. (2001). Genetic predisposition in patients undergoing cardiopulmonary bypass surgery is associated with an increase of inflammatory cytokines. *Eur J Cardio-Thoracic Surgery.* **20,** 609–613.

Drenos, F., and Kirkwood, T. B. (2005). Modelling the disposable soma theory of ageing. *Mech Ageing Dev.* **126,** 99–103.

Dubois, L., and Girard, M. (2006). Determinants of birthweight inequalities: Population-based study. *Pediatr Int.* **48,** 470–478.

Dubos, R., Savage, D., and Schaedler, R. (1966). Biological Freudianism. Lasting effects of early environmental influences. *Pediatrics.* **38,** 789–800.

Dubos, R. J. (1955). Effect of metabolic factors on the susceptibility of albino mice to experimental tuberculosis. *J Exp Med.* **101,** 59–84.

Duca, L., Floquet, N., Alix, A. J., Haye, B., and Debelle, L. (2004). Elastin as a matrikine. *Critical Reviews in Oncology/Hematology.* **49,** 235–244.

Duclos, M., Bouchet, M., Vettier, A., and Richard, D. (2005). Genetic differences in hypothalamic-pituitary-adrenal axis activity and food restriction-induced hyperactivity in three inbred strains of rats. *J Neuroendocrinology.* **17,** 740–752.

Dudas, S. P., and Arking, R. (1995). A coordinate upregulation of antioxidant gene activities is associated with the delayed onset of senescence in a long-lived strain of *Drosophila. J Gerontol.* **50,** B117–127.

Duffy, P. E., and Fried, M. (2005). Malaria in the pregnant woman. *Curr Top Microbiol Immunol.* **295,** 169–200.

Dukic-Stefanovic, S., Gasic-Milenkovic, J., Deuther-Conrad, W., and Munch, G. (2003). Signal transduction pathways in mouse microglia N-11 cells activated by advanced glycation endproducts (AGEs). *J Neurochem.* **87,** 44–55.

Duncan, A. J., and Gordon, I. J. (1999). Habitat selection according to the ability of animals to eat, digest and detoxify foods. *Proc Nutr Soc.* **58,** 799–805.

Dunger, D. B., Ahmed, M. L., and Ong, K. K. (2005). Effects of obesity on growth and puberty. *Best Pract Res Clin Endocrinol Metab.* **19,** 375–390.

Dunn, T. B. (1954). Normal and pathological anatomy of the reticular tissue in laboratory mice, with a classification and discussion of neoplasms. J. *Natl. Canc. Inst.* **14,** 1281–1433.

Dunne, M. W. (2000). Rationale and design of a secondary prevention trial of antibiotic use in patients after myocardial infarction: The WIZARD (Weekly Intervention with Zithromax [Azithromycin] for Atherosclerosis and its Related Disorders) Trial. *J Infect Dis.* **181(Suppl 3),** S572–578.

Durand, E., Scoazec, A., Lafont, A., Boddaert, J., Al Hajzen, A., Addad, F., Mirshahi, M., Desnos, M., Tedgui, A., and Mallat, Z. (2004). *In vivo* induction of endothelial apoptosis leads to vessel thrombosis and endothelial denudation: A clue to the understanding of the mechanisms of thrombotic plaque erosion. *Circulation.* **109,** 2503–2506.

Dustman, R. E., Emmerson, R. Y., Ruhling, R. O., Shearer, D. E., Steinhaus, L. A., Johnson, S. C., Bonekat, H. W., and Shigeoka, J. W. (1990). Age and fitness effects on EEG, ERPs, visual sensitivity, and cognition. *Neurobiol Aging.* **11,** 193–200.

Duve, H., Thorpe, A., and Lazarus, N. R. (1979). Isolation of material displaying insulin-like immunological biological activity from the brain of the blowfly *Calliphora vomitoria. Biochem J.* **184,** 221–227.

Duve, H., Thorpe, A., Lazarus, N. R., and Lowry, P. J. (1982). A neuropeptide of the blowfly *Calliphora vomitoria* with an amino acid composition homologous with vertebrae pancreatic polypeptide. *Biochem J.* **201,** 429–432.

Duvernell, D. D., Schmidt, P. S., and Eanes, W. F. (2003). Clines and adaptive evolution in the Methuselah gene region in *Drosophila melanogaster. Molec Ecol.* **12,** 1277–1285.

Easterlin, R. A., and Crimmins, E. M. (1985). *The fertility revolution.* Chicago: University of Chicago.

Eaton, S. B., Eaton, S. B. I., and L., C. (2002). Evolution, diet, and health. In P. S. Ungar and M. F. Teaford, Eds *Human diet. Its origin and evolution*), pp. 7–18. Westport, CT: Bergin and Garvey, pp.7–18.

Eckburg, P. B., Bik, E. M., Bernstein, C. N., Purdom, E., Dethlefsen, L., Sargent, M., Gill, S. R., Nelson, K. E., and Relman, D. A. (2005). Diversity of the human intestinal microbial flora. *Science.* **308,** 1635–1638.

Economides, D. L., Nicolaides, K. H., Gahl, W. A., Bernardini, I., and Evans, M. I. (1989). Plasma amino acids in appropriate- and small-for-gestational-age fetuses. *Am J Obstet Gynecol.* **161,** 1219–1227.

Edney, E. B. and Gill, R. W. (1968). Evolution of senescence and specific longevity. *Nature.* **220,** 281–282.

Edo, M. D., and Andres, V. (2005). Aging, telomeres, and atherosclerosis. *Cardiovascular Research.* **66,** 213–221.

Effros, R. B. (2004). Replicative senescence of CD8 T cells: Effect on human ageing. *Exp Gerontol.* **39,** 517–524.

Effros, R. B., Allsopp, R., Chiu, C.P., Hausner, M.A., Hirji, K., Wang, L., Harley, C.B., Villeponteau, B., West, M.D., Giorgi, J.V. (1996). Shortened telomeres in the expanded CD28-CD8+ subset in HIV disease implicate replicative senescence in HIV pathogenesis. *AIDS.* **10,** F17–F22.

Effros, R. B., Boucher, N., Porter, V., Zhu, X., Spaulding, C., Walford, R.L., Kronenberg, M., Cohen, D., Schèachter, F. (1994). Decline in CD28+ T cells in centenarians and in long-term T cell cultures: a possible cause for both in vivo and in vitro immunosenescence. *Exp Gerontol.* **29,** 601–609.

Effros, R. B., Walford, R. L., Weindruch, R., Mitcheltree, C. (1991). Influences of dietary restriction on immunity to influenza in aged mice. *J Gerontol.* **46,** B142–B147.

Eggan, K., Jurga, S., Gosden, R. G., Min, I. M., and Wagers, A. J. (2006). Ovulated oocytes in adult mice derive from non-circulating germ cells. *Nature.* **441,** 1109–1114.

Ehehalt, R., Keller, P., Haass, C., Thiele, C., Simons, K. (2003). Amyloidogenic processing of the Alzheimer beta-amyloid precursor protein depends on lipid rafts. *J Cell Biol.* **160,** 113–123.

Eichner, J. E., Dunn, S. T., Perveen, G., Thompson, D. M., Stewart, K. E., and Stroehla, B. C. (2002). Apolipoprotein E polymorphism and cardiovascular disease: A HuGE review. *Am J Epidemiology.* **155,** 487–495.

Eide, M. G., Øyen, N., Skjaerven, R., Nilsen, S. T., Bjerkedal, T., and Tell, G. S. (2005). Size at birth and gestational age as predictors of adult height and weight. *Epidemiology.* **16(2),** 175–181.

Eidelman, R. S., Hebert, P. R., Weisman, S. M., and Hennekens, C. H. (2003). An update on aspirin in the primary prevention of cardiovascular disease. *Arch Int Med.* **163,** 2006–2010.

Eigenmann, J. E., Amador, A., and Patterson, D. F. (1988). Insulin-like growth factor I levels in proportionate dogs, chondrodystrophic dogs and in giant dogs. *Acta Endocrinol (Copenh).* **118,** 105–108.

Eigenmann, J. E., Patterson, D. F., Zapf, J., and Froesch, E. R. (1984). Insulin-like growth factor I in the dog: A study in different dog breeds and in dogs with growth hormone elevation. *Acta Endocrinologica.* **105,** 294–301.

Eikelenboom, P., and Stam, F. C. (1982). Immunoglobulins and complement factors in senile plaques. An immunoperoxidase study. *Acta Neuropathol (Berl).* **57,** 239–242.

Eilersen, P., and Faber, M. (1960). The human aorta. VI. The regression of atherosclerosis in pulmonary tuberculosis. *Archives of Pathology.* **70,** 103–107.

Eisenberg, L. M., and Eisenberg, C. A. (2006). Wnt signal transduction and the formation of the myocardium. *Dev Biol.* **293,** 305–315.

Ekdahl, C. T., Claasen, J. H., Bonde, S., Kokaia, Z., and Lindvall, O. (2003). Inflammation is detrimental for neurogenesis in adult brain. *Proc Natl Acad Sci USA.* **100,** 13632–13637.

Ekengren, S., and Hultmark, D. (2001a). A family of Turandot-related genes in the humoral stress response of *Drosophila. Biochem Biophys Res Comm.* **284,** 998–1003.

Ekengren, S., Tryselius, Y., Dushay, M. S., Liu, G., Steiner, H., and Hultmark, D. (2001b). A humoral stress response in *Drosophila. Curr Biol.* **11,** 1479.

Elenkov, I. J., and Chrousos, G. P. (2002). Stress hormones, proinflammatory and antiinflammatory cytokines, and autoimmunity. *Ann NY Acad Sci.* **966,** 290–303.

Elford, J., Whincup, P., and Shaper, A. G. (1991). Early life experience and adult cardiovascular disease: Longitudinal and case-control studies. *Int J Epidemiol.* **20,** 833–844.

Elias, S. G., Keinan-Boker, L., Peeters, P. H., Van Gils, C. H., Kaaks, R., Grobbee, D. E., and Van Noord, P. A. (2004). Long term consequences of the 1944–1945 Dutch famine on the insulin-like growth factor axis. *Int J Canc.* **108,** 628–630.

Elias, S. G., van Noord, P. A., Peeters, P. H., den Tonkelaar, I., and Grobbee, D. E. (2003). Caloric restriction reduces age at menopause: The effect of the 1944–1945 Dutch famine. *Menopause* **10,** 399–405.

Elias, S. G., van Noord, P. A., Peeters, P. H., den Tonkelaar, I., and Grobbee, D. E.(2005). Childhood exposure to the 1944–1945 Dutch famine and subsequent female reproductive function. *Hum Reprod.* **20,** 2483–2488.

Elloumi, M., El Elj, N., Zaouali, M., Maso, F., Filaire, E., Tabka, Z., and Lac, G. (2005). IGFBP-3, a sensitive marker of physical training and overtraining. *Br J Sports Medicine.* **39,** 604–610.

Elo, I. T., and Preston, S. H. (1992). Effects of early-life conditions on adult mortality: A review. *Pop Index.* **58,** 186–212.

Elosua, R., Demissie, S., Cupples, L. A., Meigs, J. B., Wilson, P. W., Schaefer, E. J., Corella, D., and Ordovas, J. M. (2003a). Obesity modulates the association among APOE genotype, insulin, and glucose in men. *Obes Res.* **11,** 1502–1508.

Elosua, R., Molina, L., Fito, M., Arquer, A., Sanchez-Quesada, J. L., Covas, M. I., Ordoänez-Llanos, J., and Marrugat, J. (2003b). Response of oxidative stress biomarkers to a 16-week aerobic physical activity program, and to acute physical activity, in healthy young men and women. *Atherosclerosis.* **167,** 327–334.

Elsayed, N. M. (2001). Diet restriction modulates lung response and survivability of rats exposed to ozone. *Toxicology.* **159,** 171–182.

Elton, S., Bishop, L. C., and Wood, B. (2001). Comparative context of Plio-Pleistocene hominin brain evolution. *J Hum Evol.* **41,** 1–27.

Emanuel, I., Filakti, H., Alberman, E., and Evans, S. J. (1992). Intergenerational studies of human birthweight from the 1958 birth cohort. 1. Evidence for a multigenerational effect. *Br J Obstetrics & Gynaecology.* **99,** 67–74.

Enard, W., Khaitovich, P., Klose, J., Zollner, S., Heissig, F., Giavalisco, P., Nieselt-Struwe, K., Muchmore, E., Varki, A., Ravid, R., Doxiadis, G. M., Bontrop, R. E., and Paabo, S. (2002a). Intra- and interspecific variation in primate gene expression patterns. *Science.* **296,** 340–343.

Enard, W., Przeworski, M., Fisher, S. E., Lai, C. S., Wiebe, V., Kitano, T., Monaco, A. P., and Paabo, S. (2002b). Molecular evolution of FOXP2, a gene involved in speech and language. *Nature.* **418,** 869–872.

Endres, M., and Laufs, U. (2006). Discontinuation of statin treatment in stroke patients. *Stroke.* **37,** 2640–2643.

Engelmann, M. G., Redl, C. V., Pelisek, J., Barz, C., Heesemann, J., and Nikol, S. (2006). Chronic perivascular inoculation with *Chlamydophila pneumoniae* results in plaque formation *in vivo. Lab Invest.* **86,** 467–476.

Enomoto, T. (1990). Social play and sexual behavior of the bonobo (*Pan paniscus*) with special reference to flexibility. *Primates.* **31,** 469–480.

Epel, E. S., Blackburn, E. H., Lin, J., Dhabhar, F. S., Adler, N. E., Morrow, J. D., and Cawthon, R. M. (2004). Accelerated telomere shortening in response to life stress. *Proc Natl Acad Sci USA.* **101,** 17312–17315.

Epstein, J., Himmelhoch, S., and Gershon, D. (1972). Studies on ageing in nematodes. III. Electron microscopical studies on age-associated cellular damage. *Mech Ageing Dev.* **1,** 245–255.

Epstein, S. E., Stabile, E., Kinnaird, T., Lee, C. W., Clavijo, L., and Burnett, M. S. (2004). Janus phenomenon: The interrelated tradeoffs inherent in therapies designed to enhance collateral formation and those designed to inhibit atherogenesis. *Circulation.* **109,** 2826–31.

Epstein, S. E., Zhou, Y. F., and Zhu, J. (1999). Infection and atherosclerosis: Emerging mechanistic paradigms. *Circulation.* **100,** e20–8.

Epstein, S. E., Zhu, J., Burnett, S., Zhou, Y. F., Vercellotti, G., and Hajjar, D. (2000). Infection and atherosclerosis. Potential roles of pathogen burden and molecular mimicry. *Arterioscler Thromb Vasc Biol.* **20,** 1417–1420.

Ercoli, L., Siddarth, P., Huang, S. C., Miller, K., Bookheimer, S. Y., Wright, B. C., Phelps, M. E., and Small, G., (2006). Perceived loss of memory ability and cerebral metabolic decline in persons with the apolipoprotein E-IV genetic risk for Alzheimer disease. *Arch Gen Psychiatry.* **63,** 442–448.

Eriksson, J. G. (2005). Early growth and adult health outcomes—lessons learned from the Helsinki Birth Cohort Study. *Matern Child Nutr.* **1,** 149–154.

Eriksson, J., Lindi, V., Uusitupa, M., Forsen, T., Laakso, M., Osmond, C., and Barker, D. (2003). The effects of the Pro12Ala polymorphism of the PPARgamma-2 gene on lipid metabolism interact with body size at birth. *Clinical Genetics.* **64,** 366–370.

Erlichman, J., Kerbey, A. L., and James, W. P. (2002). Physical activity and its impact on health outcomes. Paper 1: The impact of physical activity on cardiovascular disease and all-cause mortality: An historical perspective. *Obesity Rev.* **3,** 257–271.

Ershler, W. B., and Keller, E. T. (2000). Age-associated increased interleukin-6 gene expression, late-life diseases, and frailty. *Annu Rev Med.* **51**, 245–270.

Erwin, J. M., Hof, P. R., Ely, J. J., and Perl, D. P. (2002). On gerontology: Advancing understanding of aging through studies of the great apes and other primates. In J. M. Erwin and P. R. Hof, Eds., *Aging in nonhuman primates*, pp. 1–20. Basel: Karger.

Esiri, M. M., Biddolph, S. C., and Morris, C. S. (1998). Prevalence of Alzheimer plaques in AIDS. *J Neurol, Neurosurg Psychiat.* **65**, 29–33.

Eskdale, J., Gallagher, G., Verweij, C. L., Keijsers, V., Westendorp, R. G., and Huizinga, T. W. (1998). Interleukin 10 secretion in relation to human IL-10 locus haplotypes. *Proc Natl Acad Sci USA.* **95**, 9465–9470.

Espeland, M. A., Rapp, S. R., Shumaker, S. A., Brunner, R., Manson, J. E., Sherwin, B. B., Hsia, J., Margolis, K. L., Hogan, P. E., Wallace, R., Dailey, M., Freeman, R., Hays, J. and Women's Health Initiative Memory Study (2004). Conjugated equine estrogens and global cognitive function in postmenopausal women: Women's Health Initiative Memory Study. *JAMA.* **291**, 2959–2968.

Espinola-Klein, C., Rupprecht, H. J., Blankenberg, S., Bickel, C., Kopp, H., Rippin, G., Victor, A., Hafner, G., Schlumberger, W., and Meyer, J. (2002a). Impact of infectious burden on extent and long-term prognosis of atherosclerosis. *Circulation.* **105**, 15–21.

Espinola-Klein, C., Rupprecht, H. J., Blankenberg, S., Bickel, C., Kopp, H., Victor, A., Hafner, G., Prellwitz, W., Schlumberger, W., and Meyer, J. (2002b). Impact of infectious burden on progression of carotid atherosclerosis. *Stroke.* **33**, 2581–2586.

Esposito, K., Nappo, F., Marfella, R., Giugliano, G., Giugliano, F., Ciotola, M., Quagliaro, L., Ceriello, A., and Giugliano, D. (2002). Inflammatory cytokine concentrations are acutely increased by hyperglycemia in humans: Role of oxidative stress. *Circulation.* **106**, 2067–2072.

Esteve, E., Ricart, W., and Fernandez-Real, J. M. (2005). Dyslipidemia and inflammation: An evolutionary conserved mechanism. *Clin Nutrit* **24**, 16–31.

Etminan, M., Gill, S., and Samii, A. (2003). Effect of non-steroidal anti-inflammatory drugs on risk of Alzheimer's disease: Systematic review and meta-analysis of observational studies. *Br Med J.* **327**, 128–133.

Euler-Taimor, G., and Heger, J. (2006). The complex pattern of SMAD signaling in the cardiovascular system. *Cardiovasc Res.* **69**, 15–25.

Evans, J. D. (2004). Transcriptional immune responses by honey bee larvae during invasion by the bacterial pathogen, *Paenibacillus larvae. J Invertebr Pathol.* **85**, 105–111.

Evans, J. D., and Armstrong, T. N. (2006). Antagonistic interactions between honey bee bacterial symbionts and implications for disease. *BMC Ecol.* **21**, 1–9.

Evans, J. D., and Pettis, J. S. (2005). Colony-level impacts of immune responsiveness in honey bees, *Apis mellifera. Evol Int J Org Evol.* **59**, 2270–2274.

Evans, P. D., Gilbert, S. L., Mekel-Bobrov, N., Vallender, E. J., Anderson, J. R., Vaez-Azizi, L. M., Tishkoff, S. A., Hudson, R. R., and Lahn, B. T. (2005). Microcephalin, a gene regulating brain size, continues to evolve adaptively in humans. *Science.* **309**, 1717–1720.

Evason, K., Huang, C., Yamben, I., Covey, D. F., and Kornfeld, K. (2005). Anticonvulsant medications extend worm life-span. *Science.* **307**, 258–262.

Everitt, A. V., Seedsman, N. J., and Jones, F. (1980). The effects of hypophysectomy and continuous food restriction, begun at ages 70 and 400 days, on collagen aging, proteinuria, incidence of pathology and longevity in the male rat. *Mech Ageing Dev.* **12**, 161–172.

Ewaldsson, B., Fogelmark, B., Feinstein, R., Ewaldsson, L., and Rylander, R. (2002). Microbial cell wall product contamination of bedding may induce pulmonary inflammation in rats. *Lab Anim.* **36,** 282–290.

Ewbank, D. C. (2004). The APOE gene and differences in life expectancy in Europe. *J Gerontol Series A, Biol Sci Med Sci.* **59,** 16–20.

Exner, C., Hebebrand, J., Remschmidt, H., Wewetzer, C., Ziegler, A., Herpertz, S., Schweiger, U., Blum, W. F., Preibisch, G., Heldmaier, G., and Klingenspor, M. (2000). Leptin suppresses semi-starvation induced hyperactivity in rats: Implications for anorexia nervosa. *Molec Psychiat.* **5,** 476–481.

Exton, M. S. (1997). Infection-induced anorexia: Active host defence strategy. *Appetite.* **29,** 369–383.

Exton, M. S., Bull, D. F., and King, M. G. (1995a). Behavioral conditioning of lipopolysaccharide-induced anorexia. *Physiol Behav.* **57,** 401–405.

Exton, M. S., Bull, D. F., King, M. G., and Husband, A. J. (1995b). Behavioral conditioning of endotoxin-induced plasma iron alterations. *Pharmacol Biochem Behav.* **50,** 675–679.

Ezekowitz, R. A. B., and Hoffmann, J. A. (2003) *Innate immunity.* Totowa, NJ: Humana Press.

Faber, M., and Moller-Hou, G. (1952). The human aorta. V. Collagen and elastin in the normal and hypertensive aorta. *Acta Pathol Microbiol Scand.* **31,** 377–382.

Fabris, C., Toniutto, P., Bitetto, D., Minisini, R., Smirne, C., Caldato, M., and Pirisi, M. (2005). Low fibrosis progression of recurrent hepatitis C in apolipoprotein E epsilon4 carriers: Relationship with the blood lipid profile. *Liver Int.* **25,** 1128–1135.

Fabris, N., Mocchegiani, E., Muzzioli, M., and Provinciali, M. (1988). Neuroendocrine-thymus interactions: Perspectives for intervention in aging. *Ann NY Acad Sci.* **521,** 72–87.

Fabris, N., Pierpaoli, W., and Sorkin, E. (1971a). Hormones and the immunological capacity. 3. The immunodeficiency disease of the hypopituitary Snell-Bagg dwarf mouse. *Clin Exp Immunol.* **9,** 209–225.

Fabris, N., Pierpaoli, W., and Sorkin, E. (1971b). Hormones and the immunological capacity. IV. Restorative effects of developmental hormones or of lymphocytes on the immunodeficiency syndrome of the dwarf mouse. *Clin Exp Immunol.* **9,** 227–240.

Fabris, N., Pierpaoli, W., and Sorkin, E. (1972). Lymphocytes, hormones and ageing. *Nature.* **240,** 557–559.

Fabrizio, P., Battistella, L., Vardavas, R., Gattazzo, C., Liou, L. L., Diaspro, A., Dossen, J. W., Gralla, E. B., and Longo, V. D. (2004). Superoxide is a mediator of an altruistic aging program in *Saccharomyces cerevisiae. J Cell Biol* **166,** 1055–1067.

Fabrizio, P., Liou, L. L., Moy, V. N., Diaspro, A., SelverstoneValentine, J., Gralla, E. B., and Longo, V. D. (2003). SOD2 functions downstream of Sch9 to extend longevity in yeast. *Genetics.* **163,** 35–46.

Fabrizio, P., and Longo, V. D. (2003). The chronological life span of *Saccharomyces cerevisiae. Aging Cell.* **2(2),** 73–81.

Facchini, F. S., Hua, N., Abbasi, F., and Reaven, G. M. (2001). Insulin resistance as a predictor of age-related diseases. *J Clin Endocrinol Metab.* **86,** 3574–3578.

Faddy, M. J., Gosden, R. G., Gougeon, A., Richardson, S. J., and Nelson, J. F. (1992). Accelerated disappearance of ovarian follicles in mid-life: Implications for forecasting menopause. *Hum Repro.* **7,** 1342–1346.

Fairweather, F. A. (1967). Cardiovascular disease in rats. In E. Cotchin and F. J. C. Roe, Eds., *Pathology of laboratory rats and mice,* pp. 213–227. Oxford, UK: Blackwell Scientific Publishing.

Fakhrzadeh, L., Laskin, J. D., and Laskin, D. L. (2002). Deficiency in inducible nitric oxide synthase protects mice from ozone-induced lung inflammation and tissue injury. *Am J Resp Cell Mol Bio.* **26,** 413–419.

Falagas, M. E., and Kompoti, M. (2006). Obesity and infection. *Lancet Infect Dis.* **6,** 438–446.

Falcone, C., Emanuele, E., D'Angelo, A., Buzzi, M. P., Belvito, C., Cuccia, M., and Geroldi, D. (2005). Plasma levels of soluble receptor for advanced glycation end products and coronary artery disease in nondiabetic men. *Arterioscler Thromb Vasc Biol.* **25,** 1032–1037.

Falconer, D. S., and Mackay, T. F. C. (1996). *Introduction to quantitative genetics.* London: Longman.

Fan, R. and Tenner, A. J. (2004). Complement C1q expression induced by Abeta in rat hippocampal organotypic slice cultures. *Exp neurol.* **185,** 241–253.

Fang, J., Wylie-Rosett, J., Cohen, H.W., Kaplan, R.C., Alderman, M.H. (2003). Exercise, body mass index, caloric intake, and cardiovascular mortality. *Am J Prev Med.* **25,** 283–289.

FAO. (2006). *Water, a shared responsibility. The 2nd UN World Water Development Report.* Paris: UNESCO.

Farinati, F., Cardin, R., Russo, V. M., Busatto, G., Franco, M., Falda, A., Mescoli, C., and Rugge, M. (2004). Differential effects of *Helicobacter pylori* eradication on oxidative DNA damage at the gastroesophageal junction and at the gastric antrum. *Cancer Epidemiol Biomarkers Prev.* **13,** 1722–1728.

Farinati, F., Cardin, R., Russo, V. M., Busatto, G., Franco, M., and Rugge, M. (2003). *Helicobacter pylori* CagA status, mucosal oxidative damage and gastritis phenotype: A potential pathway to cancer? *Helicobacter.* **8,** 227–234.

Farkas, E., Donka, G., de Vos, R. A., Mihaly, A., Bari, F., and Luiten, P. G. (2004). Experimental cerebral hypoperfusion induces white matter injury and microglial activation in the rat brain. *Acta Neuropath.* **108,** 57–64.

Farkas, M. H., Weisgraber, K. H., Shepherd, V. L., Linton, M. F., Fazio, S., and Swift, L. L. (2004). The recycling of apolipoprotein E and its amino-terminal 22 kDa fragment: Evidence for multiple redundant pathways. *J Lipid Res.* **45,** 1546–1554.

Farlow, M. R., He, Y., Tekin, S., Xu, J., Lane, R., Charles, H. C. (2004). Impact of APOE in mild cognitive impairment. *Neurology.* **63,** 1898–1901.

Farris, W., Mansourian, S., Leissring, M. A., Eckman, E. A., Bertram, L., Eckman, C. B., Tanzi, R. E., and Selkoe, D. J. (2004). Partial loss-of-function mutations in insulin-degrading enzyme that induce diabetes also impair degradation of amyloid beta-protein. *Am J Pathol.* **164,** 1425–1434.

Felblinger, D. M. (2003). Malnutrition, infection, and sepsis in acute and chronic illness. *Critl Care Nursing Clin North Am.* **15,** 71–78.

Feng, L., Matsumoto, C., Schwartz, A., Schmidt, A. M., Stern, D. M., and Pile-Spellman, J. (2005). Chronic vascular inflammation in patients with type 2 diabetes: Endothelial biopsy and RT-PCR analysis. *Diabetes Care.* **28,** 379–384.

Fernandes, G., Yunis, E. J., and Good, R. A. (1976). Influence of diet on survival of mice. *Proc Natl Acad Sci USA.* **73,** 1279–1283.

Fernandez-Real, J. M. (2006). Genetic predispositions to low-grade inflammation and type 2 diabetes. *Diabetes Technol Ther.* **8,** 55–66.

Fernandez-Real, J. M., López-Bermejo, A., Vendrell, J., Ferri, M. J., Recasens, M., and Ricart, W. (2006). Burden of infection and insulin resistance in healthy middle-aged men. *Diabetes Care.* **29,** 1058–1064.

Ferrari, S. L., Ahn-Luong, L., Garnero, P., Humphries, S. E., and Greenspan, S. L. (2003). Two promoter polymorphisms regulating interleukin-6 gene expression are associated with circulating levels of C-reactive protein and markers of bone resorption in postmenopausal women. *J Clin Endocrinol Metab.* **88,** 255–9.

Ferrucci, L., Corsi, A., Lauretani, F., Bandinelli, S., Bartali, B., Taub, D. D., Guralnik, J. M., and Longo, D. L. (2005). The origins of age-related proinflammatory state. *Blood.* **105,** 2294–2299.

Ferrucci, L., Harris, T. B., Guralnik, J. M., Tracy, R. P., Corti, M. C., Cohen, H. J., Penninx, B., Pahor, M., Wallace, R., and Havlik, R. J. (1999). Serum IL-6 level and the development of disability in older persons. *J Am Geriatr Soc.* **47,** 639–646.

Fiala, M., Zhang, L., Gan, X., Sherry, B., Taub, D., Graves, M. C., Hama, S., Way, D., Weinand, M., Witte, M., Lorton, D., Kuo, Y. M., and Roher, A. E. (1998). Amyloid-beta induces chemokine secretion and monocyte migration across a human blood-brain barrier model. *Molecular Medicine (Cambridge, MA.)* **4,** 480–489.

Figueiredo, C., Machado, J. C., Pharoah, P., Seruca, R., Sousa, S., Carvalho, R., Capelinha, A. F., Quint, W., Caldas, C., van Doorn, L. J., and Carneiro, F. (2002). *Helicobacter pylori* and interleukin 1 genotyping: An opportunity to identify high-risk individuals for gastric carcinoma. *J National Cancer Institute.* **94,** 1680–1687.

Filteau, S. M., Morris, S. S., Raynes, J. G., Arthur, P., Ross, D. A., Kirkwood, B. R., Tomkins, A. M., and Gyapong, J. O. (1995). Vitamin A supplementation, morbidity, and serum acute-phase proteins in young Ghanaian children. *Am J Clin Nutr.* **62,** 434–438.

Finch, C., Morgan, T., Rozovsky, I., Xie, Z., Weindruch, R., and Prolla, T. (2002). Microglia and aging in the brain. In W. Streit, Ed., *Microglia in the regenerating and degenerating central nervous system,* pp. 275–305. New York: Springer-Verlag.

Finch, C. E. (1969). Cell activities during aging in mammals. (Ph.D. Dissertation. Rockefeller University, New York City.) Published by MSS Information Systems, 1970.

Finch, C. E. (1972a). Comparative biology of senescence: Evolutionary and developmental considerations. In *Animal models for biomedical research, IV,* pp. 47–67. Washington D.C.: National Academy of Sciences.

Finch, C. E. (1972b). Enzyme activities, gene function, and aging in mammals (review). *Exp Gerontol.* **7,** 53–67.

Finch, C. E. (1973a). Catecholamine metabolism in the brains of ageing male mice. *Brain Res.* **52,** 261–276.

Finch, C. E. (1973b). Retardation of hair regrowth, a phenomenon of senescence in C57B/6J male mice. *J Gerontol.* **28,** 13–17.

Finch, C. E. (1976a). Alfred Ezra Mirsky, October 17, 1900–June 19, 1974. *Genetics.* **83(3, Pt. 1 Suppl),** S124–125.

Finch, C. E. (1976b). The regulation of physiological changes during mammalian aging. *Q Rev Biol.* **51,** 49–83.

Finch, C. E. (1976c). Supracentenarians. Review of *The Centenarians of the Andes,* by D. Davies. *Bioscience.* **27,** 54.

Finch, C. E. (1977). Response to comments by HT Blumenthal (editorial response). *J Gerontol.* **32,** 642.

Finch, C. E. (1988). Neural and endocrine approaches to the resolution of time as a dependent variable in the aging processes of mammals. Kleemeier Award Lecture, 1985. *Gerontologist.* **28,** 29–42.

Finch, C. E. (1990). *Longevity, senescence, and the genome.* Chicago: University of Chicago Press.

Finch, C. E. (1996). Biological bases for plasticity during aging of individual life histories. In D. Magnusson, Ed., *The lifespan development of individuals: A synthesis of biological and psychosocial perspectives, Nobel Symposium*, pp. 488–501. New York: Cambridge University Press.

Finch, C. E. (1998). Variations in senescence and longevity include the possibility of negligible senescence. *J Gerontol.* **53A**, B235–B239.

Finch, C. E. (1999). Clusterin in normal brain functions and during neurodegeneration. In *Neuroscience intelligence unit.* Austin, TX: R.G. Landes.

Finch, C. E. (2002). Evolution and the plasticity of aging in the reproductive schedules in long-lived animals. The importance of genetic variation in neuroendocrine mechanisms. In D. W. Pfaff, Ed., *Hormones, bran, and behavior*, Vol. 4, pp. 799–820. New York: Elsevier.

Finch, C. E. (2004a). Dining with Roy. *Exp Aging Res.* **39**, 893–894.

Finch, C. E. (2004b). The neurotoxicology of hard foraging and fat-melts. *Proc Natl Acad Sci USA.* **101**, 17887–17888.

Finch, C. E. (2005). Developmental origins of aging in brain and blood vessels: An overview. *Neurobiol Aging.* **26**, 281–292.

Finch, C. E., and Cohen, D. M. (1997). Aging, metabolism, and Alzheimer disease: Review and hypotheses. *Exp Neurol.* **143**, 82–102.

Finch, C. E., and Crimmins, E. M. (2004). Inflammatory exposure and historical changes in human life spans. *Science.* **305**, 1736–1739.

Finch, C. E., and Crimmins, E. M. (2005). Response to comment on "Inflammatory exposure and historical changes in human life-spans." *Science.* **308**, 1743.

Finch, C. E., Felicio, L. S., Mobbs, C. V., and Nelson, J. F. (1984). Ovarian and steroidal influences on neuroendocrine aging processes in female rodents. *Endocr Rev* **5**, 467–497.

Finch, C. E., and Flurkey, K. (1977). The molecular biology of estrogen replacement. *Contemp Ob Gyn.* **9**, 97–107.

Finch, C. E., and Foster, J. R. (1973). Hematologic and serum electrolyte values of the C57BL-6J male mouse in maturity and senescence. *Lab Anim Sci.* **23**, 339–349.

Finch, C. E., Foster, J. R., and Mirsky, A. E. (1969a). Ageing and the regulation of cell activities during exposure to cold. *J General Physiology.* **54**, 690–712.

Finch, C. E., Huberman, H. S., and Mirsky, A. E. (1969b). Regulation of liver tyrosine aminotransferase by endogenous factors in the mouse. *J General Physiology.* **54**, 675–689.

Finch, C. E., Jonec, V., Wisner, J. R., Jr., Sinha, Y. N., de Vellis, J. S., and Swerdloff, R. S. (1977). Hormone production by the pituitary and testes of male C57BL/6J mice during aging. *Endocrinology.* **101**, 1310–1317.

Finch, C. E., and Kirkwood, T. B. (2000). *Chance, development, and aging.* New York: Oxford University Press.

Finch, C. E., Laping, N. J., Morgan, T. E., Nichols, N. R., and Pasinetti, G. M. (1993). TGF-beta 1 is an organizer of responses to neurodegeneration. *J Cell Biochem.* **53**, 314–322.

Finch, C. E., and Loehlin, J. C. (1998). Environmental influences that may precede fertilization: A first examination of the prezygotic hypothesis from maternal age influences on twins. *Behavior Genetics.* **28**, 101–106.

Finch, C. E., and Longo, V. D. (2001a). The gero-inflammatory manifold. In J. Rogers, Ed., *Neuroinflammatory mechanisms in Alzheimer disease basic and clinical research*, pp. 238–258. Boston, MA: Birkhauser Verlag.

Finch, C. E., and Marchalonis, J. J. (1996). Evolutionary perspectives on amyloid and inflammatory features of Alzheimer disease. *Neurobiol Aging.* **17**, 809–815.

Finch, C. E. (1993). Neuron atrophy during aging: programmed or sporadic? *Trends in Neurosciences*. **16**, 104–110.

Finch, C. E., and Pike, M. C. (1996). Maximum life span predictions from the Gompertz mortality model. *J Gerontol. A Biol Sci Med Sci*. **51**, B183–194.

Finch, C. E., Pike, M. C., and Witten, M. (1990). Slow mortality rate accelerations during aging in some animals approximate that of humans. *Science*. **249**, 902–905.

Finch, C. E., and Rose, M. R. (1995). Hormones and the physiological architecture of life history evolution. *Q Rev Biol* **70**, 1–52.

Finch, C. E., and Ruvkun, G. (2001). The genetics of aging. *Annu Rev Genomics Hum Genet*. **2**, 435–462.

Finch, C. E., and Sapolsky, R. M. (1999). The evolution of Alzheimer disease, the reproductive schedule, and apoE isoforms. *Neurobiol Aging*. **20**, 407–428.

Finch, C. E., and Stanford, C. B. (2004). Meat-adaptive genes and the evolution of slower aging in humans. *Q Rev Biol* **79**, 3–50.

Finch, C. E., and Tanzi, R. E. (1997). Genetics of aging. *Science*. **278**, 407–411.

Finkel, S. E., and Kolter, R. (1999). Evolution of microbial diversity during prolonged starvation. *Proc Natl Acad Sci USA*. **96**, 4023–4027.

Finkelstein, M. M., Jerrett, M., and Sears, M. R. (2005). Environmental inequality and circulatory disease mortality gradients. *J Epidemiol Comm Health*. **59**, 481–487.

Finot, P. A. (2005). Historical perspective of the Maillard reaction in food science. *Ann N Y Acad Sci*. **1043**, 1–8.

Fishel, M. A., Watson, G. S., Montine, T. J., Wang, Q., Green, P. S., Kulstad, J. J., Cook, D. G., Peskind, E. R., Baker, L. D., Goldgaber, D., Nie, W., Asthana, S., Plymate, S. R., Schwartz, M. W., and Craft, S. (2005). Hyperinsulinemia provokes synchronous increases in central inflammation and {beta}-amyloid in normal adults. *Arch Neurol*. **62**, 1539–1544.

Fitzpatrick, A. L., Kuller, L. H., Ives, D. G., Lopez, O. L., Jagust, W., Breitner, J. C., Jones, B., Lyketsos, C., and Dulberg, C. (2004). Incidence and prevalence of dementia in the Cardiovascular Health Study. *J Am Geriatr Soc*. **52**, 195–204.

Flatt, T., and Kawecki, T. J. (2004). Pleiotropic effects of Methoprene-tolerant (Met), a gene involved in juvenile hormone metabolism, on life history traits in *Drosophila melanogaster*. *Genetica*. **122**, 141–160.

Flatt, T., Tu, M. P., and Tatar, M. (2005). Hormonal pleiotropy and the juvenile hormone regulation of *Drosophila* development and life history. *Bioessays*. **27**, 999–1010.

Flegal, K. M., Carroll, M. D., Ogden, C. L., and Johnson, C. L. (2002). Prevalence and trends in obesity among US adults, 1999–2000. *JAMA*. **288**, 1723–1727.

Flegal, K. M., Graubard, B. I., Williamson, D. F., and Gail, M. H. (2005). Excess deaths associated with underweight, overweight, and obesity. *JAMA*. **293**, 1861–1867.

Fleisher, A., Grundman, M., Jack, C. R., Jr., Petersen, R. C., Taylor, C., Kim, H. T., Schiller, D. H., Bagwell, V., Sencakova, D., Weiner, M. F., DeCarli, C., DeKosky, S. T., van Dyck, C. H., and Thal, L. J. (2005). Sex, apolipoprotein E epsilon 4 status, and hippocampal volume in mild cognitive impairment. *Arch Neurol*. **62**, 953–957.

Fletcher, J. M., Vukmanovic-Stejic, M., Dunne, P. J., Birch, K. E., Cook, J. E., Jackson, S. E., Salmon, M., Rustin, M. H., and Akbar., A. N. (2005). Cytomegalovirus-specific CD4+ T cells in healthy carriers are continuously driven to replicative exhaustion. *J Immunol*. **175**, 8218–8225.

Flores-Villanueva, P. O., Ruiz-Morales, J. A., Song, C. H., Flores, L. M., Jo, E. K., Montano, M., Barnes, P. F., Selman, M., and Granados, J. (2005). A functional promoter polymorphism in monocyte chemoattractant protein-1 is associated with increased susceptibility to pulmonary tuberculosis. *J Exp Med.* **202,** 1649–1658.

Florez, J. C., Hirschhorn, J., and Altshuler, D. (2003). The inherited basis of diabetes mellitus: Implications for the genetic analysis of complex traits. *Annu Rev Genomics Hum Genet* **4,** 257–291.

Florez, J. C., Jablonski, K. A., Bayley, N., Pollin, T. I., de Bakker, P. I., Shuldiner, A. R., Knowler, W. C., Nathan, D. M., and Altshuler, D. (2006). TCF7L2 polymorphisms and progression to diabetes in the Diabetes Prevention Program. *New Engl J Med.* **355,** 241–250.

Florini, J. R. (1989). Limitations of interpretation of age-related changes in hormone levels: Illustration by effects of thyroid hormones on cardiac and skeletal muscle. *J Gerontol.* **44,** B107–109.

Floud, R., Wachter, K., and Gregory, A. (1990). *Height, health, and history.* New York: Cambridge University Press.

Floyd, K., Hutubessy, R., Samyshkin, Y., Korobitsyn, A., Fedorin, I., Volchenkov, G., Kazeonny, B., Coker, R., Drobniewski, F., Jakubowiak, W., Shilova, M., and Atun, R. A. (2006). Health-systems efficiency in the Russian Federation: Tuberculosis control. *Bull World Health Organ.* **84,** 43–51.

Flurkey, K., and Currer, J. M. (2004). Pitfalls of animal model systems in ageing research. *Best Practice & Research. Clinical Endo Metab.* **18,** 407–421.

Flurkey, K., and Harrison, D. E. (1990). Use of genetic models to invetigate the hypophyseal regulation of senescence. In D. E. Harrison, Ed., *Genetic effects on aging II*, pp. 437–430. Caldwell, NJ: The Telford Press.

Flurkey, K., Papaconstantinou, J., and Harrison, D. E. (2002). The Snell dwarf mutation Pit1(dw) can increase life span in mice. *Mech Ageing Dev.* **123,** 121–130.

Flurkey, K., Papaconstantinou, J., Miller, R. A., and Harrison, D. E. (2001). Lifespan extension and delayed immune and collagen aging in mutant mice with defects in growth hormone production. *Proc Natl Acad Sci USA.* **98,** 6736–6741.

Flyg, C., and Boman, H. G. (1988). Drosophila genes *cut* and *miniature* are associated with the susceptibility to infection by Serratia marcescens *Genet. Res. Cambridge.* **52,** 51.

Flynn, R. J., Brennan, P. C., and Fritz, T. E. (1965). Pathogen status of commercially produced labroatory mice. *Lab Anim Care.* **15,** 440–447.

Flyvbjerg, A., Dorup, I., Everts, M. E., and Orskov, H. (1991). Evidence that potassium deficiency induces growth retardation through reduced circulating levels of growth hormone and insulin-like growth factor I. *Metabolism.* **40,** 769–775.

Fogel, R. W. (2004). *The escape from hunger and premature death, 1700–2100: Europe, America, and the Third World.* New York: Cambridge University Press.

Fogel, R. W., and Costa, D. L. (1997). A theory of technophysio evolution, with some implications for forecasting population, health care costs, and pension costs. *Demography.* **34,** 49–66.

Foley, R. N. (2005). Myocardial disease, anemia, and erythrocyte-stimulating proteins in chronic kidney disease. *Rev Cardiovasc Med.* **6,** S27–34.

Foley, R. N., Wang, C., and Collins, A. J. (2005). Cardiovascular risk factor profiles and kidney function stage in the US general population: The NHANES III Study. *Mayo Clin Proc.* **80,** 1270–1277.

Fonarow, G. C., and Watson, K. E. (2003). Effective strategies for long-term statin use. *Am J Cardiol.* **92,** 27i–34i.

Fontana, L. (2006). Excessive adiposity, calorie restriction, and aging. *JAMA.* **295,** 1577–1578.

Fontana, L., Klein, S., Holloszy, J. O., and Premachandra, B. N. (2006). Effect of long-term calorie restriction with adequate protein and micronutrients on thyroid hormones. *J Clin Endocrinol Metab.* **91**, 3232–3235.

Fontana, L., Meyer, T. E., Klein, S., and Holloszy, J. O. (2004a). Long-term calorie restriction is highly effective in reducing the risk for atherosclerosis in humans. *Proc Natl Acad Sci USA.* **101**, 6659–6663.

Fontana, R., Mendes, M. A., de Souza, B. M., Konno, K., César, L. M., Malaspina, O., and Palma, M. S. (2004b). Jelleines: A family of antimicrobial peptides from the Royal Jelly of honeybees (*Apis mellifera*). *Peptides.* **25**, 919–928.

Formenty, P., Boesch, C., Wyers, M., Steiner, C., Donati, F., Dind, F., Walker, F., and Le Guenno, B. (1999). Ebola virus outbreak among wild chimpanzees living in a rain forest of Cote d'Ivoire. *J Infect Dis.* **179**, S120–126.

Formicola, V. (2003). More is not always better: Trotter and Gleser's equations and stature estimates of Upper Paleolithic European samples. *J Hum Evol.* **45**, 239–243.

Fornieri, C., Quaglino, D., Jr., and Mori, G. (1992). Role of the extracellular matrix in age-related modifications of the rat aorta. Ultrastructural, morphometric, and enzymatic evaluations. *Arteriosclerosis and Thrombosis.* **12**, 1008–1016.

Forsdahl, A. (1977). Are poor living conditions in childhood and adolescence an important risk factor for arteriosclerotic heart disease? *Br J Prev Soc Med.* **31**, 91–95.

Forster, M. J., Morris, P., and Sohal, R. S. (2003). Genotype and age influence the effect of caloric intake on mortality in mice. *FASEB J.* **17(6)**, 690–692.

Forster, M. J., Sohal, B. H., and Sohal, R. S. (2000). Reversible effects of long-term caloric restriction on protein oxidative damage. *J Gerontol. Series A, Biol Sci Med Sci.* **55**, B522–529.

Forster, T., Roy, D., and Ghazal, P. (2003). Experiments using microarray technology: Limitations and standard operating procedures. *J Endocrinol.* **178**, 195–204.

Foster, M. P., Jensen, E. R., Montecino-Rodriguez, E., Leathers, H., Horseman, N., and Dorshkind, K. (2000). Humoral and cell-mediated immunity in mice with genetic deficiencies of prolactin, growth hormone, insulin-like growth factor-I, and thyroid hormone. *Clin Immunol.* **96**, 140–149.

Fotenos, A. F., Snyder, A. Z., Girton, L. E., Morris, J. C., and Buckner, R. L. (2005). Normative estimates of cross-sectional and longitudinal brain volume decline in aging and AD. *Neurology.* **64**, 1032–1039.

Fowler, K., and Partridge, L. (1989). A cost of mating in female fruitflies. *Nature.* **338**, 760–761.

Fox, C. J., Hammerman, P. S., and Thompson, C. B. (2005). Fuel feeds function: Energy metabolism and the T-cell response. *Nat Rev Immunol.* **5**, 844–852.

Fraga, M. F., Ballestar, E., Paz, M. F., Ropero, S., Setien, F., Ballestar, M. L., Heine-Suäner, D., Cigudosa, J. C., Urioste, M., Benitez, J., Boix-Chornet, M., Sanchez-Aguilera, A., Ling, C., Carlsson, E., Poulsen, P., Vaag, A., Stephan, Z., Spector, T. D., Wu, Y. Z., Plass, C., and Esteller, M. (2005). Epigenetic differences arise during the lifetime of monozygotic twins. *Proc Natl Acad Sci USA.* **102**, 10604–10609.

Frahm, T., Mohamed, S. A., Bruse, P., Gemund, C., Oehmichen, M., and Meissner, C. (2005). Lack of age-related increase of mitochondrial DNA amount in brain, skeletal muscle and human heart. *Mech Ageing Dev.* **126**, 1192–1200.

Franceschi, C., Olivieri, F., Marchegiani, F., Cardelli, M., Cavallone, L., Capri, M., Salvioli, S., Valensin, S., De Benedictis, G., Di Iorio, A., Caruso, C., Paolisso, G., and Monti, D. (2005). Genes involved in immune response/inflammation, IGF1/insulin pathway and response to oxidative stress play a major role in the genetics of human longevity: The lesson of centenarians. *Mech Ageing Dev.* **126**, 351–361.

Franchimont, D., Kino, T., Galon, J., Meduri, G. U., and Chrousos, G. (2003). Glucocorticoids and inflammation revisited: The state of the art. NIH Clinical Staff Conference. *Neuroimmunomodulation.* **10**, 247–260.

Francia, P., delli Gatti, C., Bachschmid, M., Martin-Padura, I., Savoia, C., Migliaccio, E., Pelicci, P. G., Schiavoni, M., Lèuscher, T. F., Volpe, M., and Cosentino, F. (2004). Deletion of p66shc gene protects against age-related endothelial dysfunction. *Circulation.* **110**, 2889–2895.

Franklin, S. S. (2005a). Arterial stiffness and hypertension: A two-way street? *Hypertension.* **45**, 349–351.

Franklin, S. S., Pio, J. R., Wong, N. D., Larson, M. G., Leip, E. P., Vasan, R. S., and Levy, D. (2005b). Predictors of new-onset diastolic and systolic hypertension: the Framingham Heart Study. *Circulation.* **111**, 1121–1127.

Fraser, H. B., Khaitovich, P., Plotkin, J. B., Pèaèabo, S., and Eisen, M. B. (2005). Aging and gene expression in the primate brain. *PLoS Biol.* **3**, e274.

Frayn, K. N. (2000). Visceral fat and insulin resistance—causative or correlative. *Br J Nutr.* **83**, S71–S77.

Friedland, R. P., Fritsch, T., Smyth, K. A., Koss, E., Lerner, A. J., Chen, C. H., Petot, G. J., and Debanne, S. M. (2001). Patients with Alzheimer's disease have reduced activities in midlife compared with healthy control-group members. Proc Natl Acad Sci USA. **98**, 3440–3445.

Friedrich, U., Griese, E., Schwab, M., Fritz, P., Thon, K., and Klotz, U. (2000). Telomere length in different tissues of elderly patients. *Mech Ageing Dev.* **119**, 89–99.

Frikke-Schmidt, R., Sing, C. F., Nordestgaard, B. G., and Tybjaerg-Hansen, A. (2004a). Gender- and age-specific contributions of additional DNA sequence variation in the 5' regulatory region of the APOE gene to prediction of measures of lipid metabolism. *Human Genetics.* **115**, 331–345.

Frikke-Schmidt, R., Sing, C. F., Nordestgaard, B. G., and Tybjaerg-Hansen, A. (2004b). Gender- and age-specific contributions of additional DNA sequence variation in the 5' regulatory region of the APOE gene to prediction of measures of lipid metabolism. *Hum Genet.* **115(4)**, 331–345.

Frisch, R. E., and Revelle, R. (1970). Height and weight at menarche and a hypothesis of critical body weights and adolescent events. *Science.* **169**, 397–399.

Frohlich, M., Muhlberger, N., Hanke, H., Imhof, A., Doring, A., Pepys, M. B., and Koenig, W. (2003). Markers of inflammation in women on different hormone replacement therapies. *Ann Med.* **35**, 253–261.

Frolkis, V. V., Tanin, S. A., Marcinko, V. I., Kulchitsky, O. K., and Yasechko, A. V. (1985). Axoplasmic transport of substances in motoneuronal axons of the spinal cord in old age. *Mech Ageing Dev.* **29**, 19–28.

Frost, R. A., Lang, C. H., and Gelato, M. C. (1997). Transient exposure of human myoblasts to tumor necrosis factor-alpha inhibits serum and insulin-like growth factor-I stimulated protein synthesis. *Endocrinology.* **138**, 4153–4159.

Frothingham, C. (1911). The relationship between acute infectious diseases and arterial lesions. *Arch Intern Med.* **8**, 153–162.

Fry, A. J., and Rand, D. M. (2002). Wolbachia interactions that determine *Drosophila melanogaster* survival. *Evolution Int J Org Evolution.* **56**, 1976–1981.

Fryer, L. G., and Carling, D. (2005). AMP-activated protein kinase and the metabolic syndrome. *Biochem Soc Trans.* **33(Pt2)**, 362–366.

Fu, T., and Borensztajn, J. (2002). Macrophage uptake of low-density lipoprotein bound to aggregated C-reactive protein: Possible mechanism of foam-cell formation in atherosclerotic lesions. *Biochem J.* **366(Pt) 1,** 195–201.

Fujishima, M., and Kiyohara, Y. (2002). Incidence and risk factors of dementia in a defined elderly Japanese population: The Hisayama study. *Ann NY Acad Sci.* **977,** 1–8.

Fukagawa, N. K., Li, M., Liang, P., Russell, J. C., Sobel, B. E., and Absher, P. M. (1999). Aging and high concentrations of glucose potentiate injury to mitochondrial DNA. *Free Radic Biol Med.* **27,** 1437–1443.

Fullerton, S. M., Clark, A. G., Weiss, K. M., Nickerson, D. A., Taylor, S. L., Stengãard, J. H., Salomaa, V., Vartiainen, E., Perola, M., Boerwinkle, E., and Sing, C. F. (2000). Apolipoprotein E variation at the sequence haplotype level: Implications for the origin and maintenance of a major human polymorphism. *Am J Hum Genet.* **67,** 881–900.

Furst, A. (1987). Hormetic effects in pharmacology: Pharmacological inversions as prototypes for hormesis. *Health Physics.* **52,** 527–530.

Furukawa, S., Fujita, T., Shimabukuro, M., Iwaki, M., Yamada, Y., Nakajima, Y., Nakayama, O., Makishima, M., Matsuda, M., and Shimomura, I. (2004). Increased oxidative stress in obesity and its impact on metabolic syndrome. *J Clin Invest.* **114,** 1752–1761.

Furuyama, T., Yamashita, H., Kitayama, K., Higami, Y., Shimokawa, I., and Mori, N. (2002). Effects of aging and caloric restriction on the gene expression of FoxO1, 3, and 4 (FKHR, FKHRL1, and AFX) in the rat skeletal muscles. *Microsc Res Tech.* **59,** 331–334.

Fuster, V., Fayad, Z. A., Moreno, P. R., Poon, M., Corti, R., and Badimon, J. J. (2005a). Atherothrombosis and high-risk plaque: Part II: Approaches by noninvasive computed tomographic/magnetic resonance imaging. *J Am Coll Cardiol.* **46,** 1209–1218.

Fuster, V., Moreno, P. R., Fayad, Z. A., Corti, R., and Badimon, J. J. (2005b). Atherothrombosis and high-risk plaque: Part I: Evolving concepts. *J Am Coll Cardiol.* **46,** 937–954.

Gabriel, S. E., Brigman K. N., Koller, B. H., Boucher, R. C., Stutts, M. J. (1994). Cystic fibrosis heterozygote resistance to cholera toxin in the cystic fibrosis mouse model. *Science.* **266,** 107–109.

Gaenzer, H., Sturm, W., Neumayr, G., Kirchmair, R., Ebenbichler, C., Ritsch, A., Fèoger, B., Weiss, G., and Patsch, J. R. (2001). Pronounced postprandial lipemia impairs endothelium-dependent dilation of the brachial artery in men. *Cardiovasc Res.* **52,** 509–516.

Galdzicki, Z., and Siarey, R. J. (2003). Understanding mental retardation in Down's syndrome using trisomy 16 mouse models. *Genes Brain Behav.* **2,** 167–178.

Galetta, F., Franzoni, F., Cupisti, A., Morelli, E., Santoro, G., and Pentimone, F. (2005). Early detection of cardiac dysfunction in patients with anorexia nervosa by tissue Doppler imaging. *Int J Cardiol.* **101,** 33–37.

Gallagher, M., P. W. Landfield, McEwen, B., Meaney, M. J., Rapp, P. R., Sapolsky, R. M., West, M. J. (1996). Hippocampal neurodegeneration in again. *Science* **274,** 484–485.

Gamba, M., and Pralong, F. P. (2006). Control of GnRH neuronal activity by metabolic factors: The role of leptin and insulin. *Mol Cell Endocrinol.* **254–255,** 133–139.

Gamble, C. N. (1986). The pathogenesis of hyaline arteriolosclerosis. *Am J Pathol.* **122,** 410–420.

Gao, Y., Qian, W. P., Dark, K., Toraldo, G., Lin, A. S., Guldberg, R. E., Flavell, R. A., Weitzmann, M. N., and Pacifici, R. (2004). Estrogen prevents bone loss through transforming growth factor beta signaling in T cells. *Proc Natl Acad Sci USA.* **101,** 16618–16623.

Garces, C., Benavente, M., Ortega, H., Rubio, R., Lasuncion, M. A., Rodriguez Artalejo, F., Fernandez Pardo, J., and de Oya, M. (2002). Influence of birth weight on the apo E genetic determinants of plasma lipid levels in children. *Pediatr Res.* **52,** 873–878.

Garcia-Cruz, D., Figuera, L., and Cantu, J. (2002). Inherited hypertrichoses. *Clinical Genetics.* **61,** 321–329.

Garcia-Touchard, A., Henry, T. D., Sangiorgi, G., Spagnoli, L. G., Mauriello, A., Conover, C., and Schwartz, R. S. (2005). Extracellular proteases in atherosclerosis and restenosis. *Arterioscler Thromb Vasc Biol.* **25,** 1119–1127.

Gardiner, K., Davisson, M. T., Pritchard, M., Patterson, D., Groner, Y., Crnic, L. S., Antonarakis, S., and Mobley, W. (2005). Report on the 'Expert Workshop on the Biology of Chromosome 21: Towards gene-phenotype correlations in Down syndrome', held June 11–14, 2004, Washington D.C. *Cytogenet Genome Res.* **108,** 269–277.

Gardner, E. M. (2005). Caloric restriction decreases survival of aged mice in response to primary influenza infection. *J Gerontol Series A, Biol Sci Med Sci.* **60,** 688–694.

Gardner, M. P., Fowler, K., Barton, N. H., and Partridge, L. (2005). Genetic variation for total fitness in *Drosophila melanogaster*: Complex yet replicable patterns. *Genetics.* **169,** 1553–1571.

Gariepy, J., Denarie, N., Chironi, G., Salomon, J., Levenson, J., and Simon, A. (2000). Gender difference in the influence of smoking on arterial wall thickness. *Atherosclerosis.* **153,** 139–145.

Garigan, D., Hsu, A. L., Fraser, A. G., Kamath, R. S., Ahringer, J., and Kenyon, C. (2002). Genetic analysis of tissue aging in *Caenorhabditis elegans*: A role for heat-shock factor and bacterial proliferation. *Genetics.* **161,** 1101–1112.

Garn, S., M., Shaw, H. A., and McCabe, K. D. (1978). Dose-response effect of maternal smoking. *Pediatrics.* **62,** 861–863.

Garsin, D. A., Villanueva, J. M., Begun, J., Kim, D. H., Sifri, C. D., Calderwood, S. B., Ruvkun, G., and Ausubel, F. M. (2003). Long-lived *C. elegans* daf-2 mutants are resistant to bacterial pathogens. *Science.* **300,** 1921.

Gasic-Milenkovic, J., Dukic-Stefanovic, S., Deuther-Conrad, W., Gartner, U., and Munch, G. (2003). Beta-amyloid peptide potentiates inflammatory responses induced by lipopolysaccharide, interferon -gamma and 'advanced glycation endproducts' in a murine microglia cell line. *Eur J Neurosci.* **17,** 813–821.

Gaspari, L., Pedotti, P., Bonafáe, M., Franceschi, C., Marinelli, D., Mari, D., Garte, S., and Taioli, E. (2003). Metabolic gene polymorphisms and p53 mutations in healthy centenarians and younger controls. *Biomarkers.* **8,** 522–528.

Gasparini, L., and Xu, H. (2003). Potential roles of insulin and IGF-1 in Alzheimer's disease. *Trends in Neurosciences.* **26,** 404–406.

Gatz, M., Mortimer, J. A., Fratiglioni, L., Johansson, B., Berg, S., Reynolds, C. A., and Pedersen, N. L. (2006). Potentially modifiable risk factors for dementia in identical twins. *Alzheim Dementia.* **2,** 110–117.

Gatz, M., Pedersen, N. L., Berg, S., Johansson, B., Johansson, K., Mortimer, J. A., Posner, S. F., Viitanen, M., Winblad, B., and Ahlbom, A. (1997). Heritability for Alzheimer's disease: The study of dementia in Swedish twins. *J Gerontol. Series A, Biol Sci Med Sci.* **52,** M117–125.

Gaudzinski, S., and Roebroeks, W. (2000). Adults only. Reindeer hunting at the middle Palaeolithic site Salzgitter Lebenstedt, Northern Germany. *J Hum Evol.* **38,** 497–521.

Gay, F. W., Maguire, M. E., and Baskerville, A. (1972). Etiology of chronic pneumonia in rats and a study of the experimental disease in mice. *Infect Immun.* **6,** 83–91.

Gearing, M., Tigges, J., Mori, H., and Mirra, S. S. (1997). Beta-amyloid (A beta) deposition in the brains of aged orangutans. *Neurobiol Aging.* **18,** 139–146.

Geary, N., Asarian, L., Sheahan, J., and Langhans, W. (2004). Estradiol-mediated increases in the anorexia induced by intraperitoneal injection of bacterial lipopolysaccharide in female rats. *Physiol Behav.* **82,** 251–261.

Gebbink, M. F., Claessen, D., Bouma, B., Dijkhuizen, L., and Wosten, H. A. (2005). Amyloids—A functional coat for microorganisms. *Nature Rev. Microbiol.* **3,** 333–341.

Geiger-Thornsberry, G. L., and Mackay, T. F. (2004). Quantitative trait loci affecting natural variation in *Drosophila* longevity. *Mech Ageing Dev.* **125,** 179–189.

Geinisman, Y., Bondareff, W., and Telser, A. (1977). Diminished axonal transport of glycoproteins in the senescent rat brain. *Mech Ageing Dev.* **6,** 363–378.

Gems, D., and Partridge, L. (2001). Insulin/IGF signalling and ageing: Seeing the bigger picture. *Cur Opin Genet Dev.* **11,** 287–292.

Gems, D., and Riddle, D. L. (2000). Genetic, behavioral and environmental determinants of male longevity in *Caenorhabditis elegans. Genetics.* **154,** 1597–1610.

George, D. M. (1984). *London life in the eighteenth century.* Chicago: Academy Chicago Publishers.

George, J., Goldstein, E., Abashidze, S., Deutsch, V., Shmilovich, H., Finkelstein, A., Herz, I., Miller, H., and Keren, G. (2004). Circulating endothelial progenitor cells in patients with unstable angina: Association with systemic inflammation. *Eur Heart J.* **25,** 1003–1008.

Georges, J. L., Rupprecht, H. J., Blankenberg, S., Poirier, O., Bickel, C., Hafner, G., Nicaud, V., Meyer, J., Cambien, F., and Tiret, L. (2003). Impact of pathogen burden in patients with coronary artery disease in relation to systemic inflammation and variation in genes encoding cytokines. *Am J Cardiol.* **92,** 515–521.

Gerard, H. C., Wildt, K. L., Whittum-Hudson, J. A., Lai, Z., Ager, J., and Hudson, A. P. (2005). The load of *Chlamydia pneumoniae* in the Alzheimer's brain varies with APOE genotype. *Microb Pathog.* **39,** 19–26.

Gerdes, L. U., Gerdes, C., Hansen, P. S., Klausen, I. C., and Faergeman, O. (1996). Are men carrying the apolipoprotein epsilon 4- or epsilon 2 allele less fertile than epsilon 3 epsilon 3 genotypes? *Hum Genet.* **98,** 239–242.

Gerdes, L. U., Jeune, B., Ranberg, K. A., Nybo, H., and Vaupel, J. W. (2000). Estimation of apolipoprotein E genotype-specific relative mortality risks from the distribution of genotypes in centenarians and middle-aged men: Apolipoprotein E gene is a "frailty gene," not a "longevity gene." *Genet Epidemiol.* **19,** 202–210.

Gerdes, L. U., Klausen, I. C., Sihm, I., and Faergeman, O. (1992). Apolipoprotein E polymorphism in a Danish population compared to findings in 45 other study populations around the world. *Genet Epidemiol.* **9,** 155–167.

Gerisch, B., and Antebi, A. (2004). Hormonal signals produced by DAF-9/cytochrome P450 regulate *C. elegans* dauer diapause in response to environmental cues. *Development.* **131,** 1765–1776.

Gerisch, B., Weitzel, C., Kober-Eisermann, C., Rottiers, V., and Antebi, A. (2001). A hormonal signaling pathway influencing *C. elegans* metabolism, reproductive development, and life span. *Devel Cell.* **1,** 841–851.

Gerven, M., Kaplan, H., Montecino, M. E., Finch, C. E., and Crimmins, E. (2007). Inflammation levels in two epidemiological worlds., in prep.

Getliffe, K. M., Al Dulaimi, D., Martin-Ruiz, C., Holder, R. L., von Zglinicki, T., Morris, A., and Nwokolo, C. U. (2005). Lymphocyte telomere dynamics and telomerase activity in inflammatory bowel disease: Effect of drugs and smoking. *Aliment Pharmacol Therap.* **21,** 121–131.

Getz, G. S., and Reardon, C. A. (2004). Paraoxonase, a cardioprotective enzyme: Continuing issues. *Curr Opin Lipidol* **15,** 261–267.

Geuerin, J. C. (2004). Emerging area of aging research: Long-lived animals with "negligible senescence." *Ann NY Acad Sci.* **1019,** 518–520.

Ghebremedhin, E., Schultz, C., Braak, E., and Braak, H. (1998). High frequency of apolipoprotein E epsilon4 allele in young individuals with very mild Alzheimer's disease-related neurofibrillary changes. *Exp Neurol.* **153,** 152–155.

Ghio, A. J., Silbajoris, R., Carson, J. L., and Samet, J. M. (2002a). Biologic effects of oil fly ash. *Environ Health Persp.* **110,** 89–94.

Ghio, A. J., Suliman, H. B., Carter, J. D., Abushamaa, A. M., and Folz, R. J. (2002b). Overexpression of extracellular superoxide dismutase decreases lung injury after exposure to oil fly ash. *Am J Physiol. Lung Cell Mol Physiol.* **283,** L211–218.

Gieffers, J., Reusche, E., Solbach, W., and Maass, M. (2000). Failure to detect *Chlamydia pneumoniae* in brain sections of Alzheimer's disease patients. *J Clin Microbiol.* **38,** 881–882.

Gilani, G. S., Cockell, K. A., and Sepehr, E. (2005). Effects of antinutritional factors on protein digestibility and amino acid availability in foods. *J AOAC Int.* **88,** 967–987.

Gill, R., Kemp, J. A., Sabin, C., and Pepys, M. B. (2004). Human C-reactive protein increases cerebral infarct size after middle cerebral artery occlusion in adult rats. *J Cereb Blood Flow Metab.* **24,** 1214–1218.

Gilliland, F. D., Li, Y. F., Dubeau, L., Berhane, K., Avol, E., McConnell, R., Gauderman, W. J., and Peters, J. M. (2002). Effects of glutathione S-transferase M1, maternal smoking during pregnancy, and environmental tobacco smoke on asthma and wheezing in children. *Am J Respir Crit Care Med.* **166,** 457–463.

Gillman, T., and Hathorn, M. (1959). Sex incidence of vascular lesions in aging rats in relation to previous pregnancies. *Nature.* **183,** 1139–1140.

Gimbutas, M. (1982). *The goddesses and gods of old Europe. 6500–3500 BC. Myths and cult images.* Berkeley: University of California Press.

Ginaldi, L., Di Benedetto, M. C., and De Martinis, M. (2005). Osteoporosis, inflammation and ageing. *Immun. Ageing.* **2,** 14.

Giovannucci, E. (2001). Insulin, insulin-like growth factors and colon cancer: A review of the evidence. *J Nutr* **131,** 3109S–320S.

Giri, R. K., Rajagopal, V., Shahi, S., Zlokovic, B. V., and Kalra, V. K. (2005). Mechanism of amyloid peptide induced CCR5 expression in monocytes and its inhibition by siRNA for Egr-1. *Am J Physiol. Cell Physio.* **289,** C264–276.

Girones, X., Guimera, A., Cruz-Sanchez, C. Z., Ortega, A., Sasaki, N., Makita, Z., Lafuente, J. V., Kalaria, R., and Cruz-Sanchez, F. F. (2004). N epsilon-carboxymethyllysine in brain aging, diabetes mellitus, and Alzheimer's disease. *Free Radic Biol Med.* **36,** 1241–1247.

Giudice, G. (2001). Conserved cellular and molecular mechanisms in development. *Cell Biol Int.* **25,** 1081–1090.

Giulian, D., Baker, T. J., Shih, L. C., and Lachman, L. B. (1986). Interleukin 1 of the central nervous system is produced by ameboid microglia. *J Exp Med.* **164,** 594–604.

Glenner, G. G., and Wong, C. W. (1984). Alzheimer's disease: Initial report of the purification and characterization of a novel cerebrovascular amyloid protein. *Biochem Biophys Res Comm.* **120,** 885–890.

Gluckman, P. D., Cutfield, W., Hofman, P., and Hanson, M. A. (2005). The fetal, neonatal, and infant environments—The long-term consequences for disease risk. *Early Hum Dev.* **81,** 51–59.

Gluckman, P. D., and Hanson, M. A. (2005). *The fetal matrix: Evolution, development, and disease.* Cambridge UK: Cambridge University Press.

Go, Y. M., Gipp, J. J., Mulcahy, R. T., and Jones, D. P. (2004). H2O2-dependent activation of GCLC-ARE4 reporter occurs by mitogen-activated protein kinase pathways without oxidation of cellular glutathione or thioredoxin-1. *J Biol Chem.* **279,** 5837–5845.

Godbout, J. P., Chen, J., Abraham, J., Richwine, A. F., Berg, B. M., Kelley, K. W., and Johnson, R. W. (2005). Exaggerated neuroinflammation and sickness behavior in aged mice following activation of the peripheral innate immune system. *FASEB J.* **19,** 1329–1331.

Godbout, J. P., and Johnson, R. W. (2004). Interleukin-6 in the aging brain. *J Neuroimmunol.* **147,** 141–144.

Godfrey, P., Rahal, J. O., Beamer, W. G., Copeland, N. G., Jenkins, N. A., and Mayo, K. E. (1993). GHRH receptor of little mice contains a missense mutation in the extracellular domain that disrupts receptor function. *Nat Genet.* **4,** 227–232.

Godoy, R. A., Leonard, W. R., Reyes-García, V., Goodman, E., McDade, T., Huanca, T., Tanner, S., and Vadez, V. (2006). Physical stature of adult Tsimane' Amerindians, Bolivian Amazon in the 20th century. *Econ Hum Biol.* **4,** 184–205.

Godsland, I. F. (2001). Effects of postmenopausal hormone replacement therapy on lipid, lipoprotein, and apolipoprotein (a) concentrations: Analysis of studies published from 1974–2000. *Fertil Steril.* **75,** 898–915.

Goemaere-Vanneste, J., Couraud, J. Y., Hassig, R., Di Giamberardino, L., and van den Bosch de Aguilar, P. (1988). Reduced axonal transport of the G4 molecular form of acetylcholinesterase in the rat sciatic nerve during aging. *J Neurochem.* **51,** 1746–1754.

Goff, S. A., and Klee, H. J. (2006). Plant volatile compounds: Sensory cues for health and nutritional value? *Science.* **311,** 815–819.

Gognies, S., Barka, E. A., Gainvors-Claisse, A., and Belarbi, A. (2006). Interactions between yeasts and grapevines: Filamentous growth, endopolygalacturonase and phytopathogenicity of colonizing yeasts. *Microb Ecol.* **51,** 109–116.

Gold, J. A., Jagirdar, J., Hay, J. G., Addrizzo-Harris, D. J., Naidich, D. P., and Rom, W. N. A. (2000). Hut lung. A domestically acquired particulate lung disease. *Medicine.* **79,** 310–317.

Goldberg, T., Cai, W., Peppa, M., Dardaine, V., Baliga, B. S., Uribarri, J., and Vlassara, H. (2004). Advanced glycoxidation end products in commonly consumed foods. *J Am Diet Assoc.* **104,** 1287–1291.

Golden, T. R., and Melov, S. (2004). Microarray analysis of gene expression with age in individual nematodes. *Aging cell.* **3,** 111–124.

Goldhammer, E., Tanchilevitch, A., Maor, I., Beniamini, Y., Rosenschein, U., and Sagiv, M. (2005). Exercise training modulates cytokines activity in coronary heart disease patients. *Int J Cardiol.* **100,** 93–99.

Goldstein, S., Moerman, E. J., Soeldner, J. S., Gleason, R. E., and Barnett, D. M. (1978). Chronologic and physiologic age affect replicative life-span of fibroblasts from diabetic, prediabetic, and normal donors. *Science.* **199,** 781–782.

Goldstein, S., Moerman, E. J., Soeldner, J. S., Gleason, R. E., and Barnett, D. M. (1979). Diabetes mellitus and genetic prediabetes. Decreased replicative capacity of cultured skin fibroblasts. *J Clin Invest.* **63,** 358–370.

Gong, Y., Chang, L., Viola, K. L., Lacor, P. N., Lambert, M. P., Finch, C. E., Krafft, G. A., and Klein, W. L. (2003). Alzheimer's disease-affected brain: Presence of oligomeric A beta ligands (ADDLs) suggests a molecular basis for reversible memory loss. *Proc Natl Acad Sci USA.* **100,** 10417–10422.

Gonzalez, A. A., Kumar, R., Mulligan, J. D., Davis, A. J., Weindruch, R., and Saupe, K. W. (2004a). Metabolic adaptations to fasting and chronic caloric restriction in heart, muscle, and liver do not include changes in AMPK activity. *Am J Physiol Endocrinol Metab.* **287,** E1032–1037.

Gonzales, C., Voirol, M. J., Giacomini, M., Gaillard, R. C., Pedrazzini, T., and Pralong, F. P. (2004b). The neuropeptide Y Y1 receptor mediates NPY-induced inhibition of the gonadotrope axis under poor metabolic conditions. *FASEB J.* **18,** 137–139.

Gonzalez, B., Lamas, S., and Melian, E. M. (2001). Cooperation between low density lipoproteins and IGF-I in the promotion of mitogenesis in vascular smooth muscle cells. *Endocrinology.* **142,** 4852–4860.

Goodall, J. (1983). Population dynamics during a 15 year period in one community of free-living chimpanzees in the Gombe National Park, Tanzania. *Z fur Tierpsychol.* **61,** 1–60.

Goodall, J. (1986). *The chimpanzees of Gombe: Patterns of behavior.* Cambridge MA: Harvard University Press.

Goodrick, C. L., Ingram, D. K., Reynolds, M. A., Freeman, J. R., and Cider, N. (1990). Effects of intermittent feeding upon body weight and lifespan in inbred mice: Interaction of genotype and age. *Mech Ageing Dev.* **55,** 69–87.

Goodrick, C. L., Ingram, D. K., Reynolds, M. A., Freeman, J. R., and Cider, N. L. (1983a). Differential effects of intermittent feeding and voluntary exercise on body weight and lifespan in adult rats. *J Gerontol.* **38,** 36–45.

Goodrick, C. L., Ingram, D. K., Reynolds, M. A., Freeman, J. R., and Cider, N. L. (1983b). Effects of intermittent feeding upon growth, activity, and lifespan in rats allowed voluntary exercise. *Exp Aging Res.* **9,** 203–209.

Gordon, H. A., Bruckner-Kardoss, E., and Wostman, B. S. (1966). Ageing in germ-free mice: Life tables and lesions observed at death. *J Gerontol.* **21,** 380–387.

Gordon, S. (2003). Do macrophage innate immunity receptors enhance atherogenesis? *Devel. Cell.* **5,** 666–668.

Gordon, S. M., and Finch, C. E. (1974). An electrophoretic study of protein synthesis in brain regions of senescent male mice. *Exp Gerontol.* **9,** 269–273.

Goren-Inbar, N., Alperson, N., Kislev, M. E., Simchoni, O., Melamed, Y., Ben-Nun, A., and Werker, E. (2004). Evidence of hominin control of fire at Gesher Benot Ya'aqov, Israel. *Science.* **304,** 725–727.

Gosden, R. G. (1985). The biology of menopause: The causes and consequences of ovarian aging. San Diego: Academic Press.

Gosden, R. G., Laing, S. C., Felicio, L. S., Nelson, J. F., and Finch, C. E. (1983). Imminent oocyte exhaustion and reduced follicular recruitment mark the transition to acyclicity in aging C57BL/6J mice. *Biol Reprod.* **28,** 255–260.

Goto, S., Radak, Z., Nyakas, C., Chung, H. Y., Naito, H., Takahashi, R., Nakamoto, H., and Abea, R. (2004). Regular exercise: An effective means to reduce oxidative stress in old rats. *Ann NY Acad Sci.* **1019,** 471–474.

Goto, S., Takahashi, R., Kumiyama, A. A., Radak, Z., Hayashi, T., Takenouchi, M., and Abe, R. (2001). Implications of protein degradation in aging. *Ann NY Acad Sci.* **928,** 54–64.

Gould, K. G., Flint, M., and Graham, C. E. (1981). Chimpanzee reproductive senescence: A possible model for evolution of the menopause. *Maturitas.* **3,** 157–166.

Grady, D., Rubin, S. M., Petitti, D. B., Fox, C. S., Black, D., Ettinger, B., Ernster, V. L., and Cummings, S. R. (1992). Hormone therapy to prevent disease and prolong life in post-menopausal women. *Ann Intern Med.* **117,** 1016–1037.

Graham, C. E. (1979). Reproductive function in aged female chimpanzees. *Am J Phys Anthropol.* **50,** 291–300.

Graham, C. E., Kling, O. R., and Steiner, R. A. (1979). Reproductive senescence in female nonhuman primates. In D. Bowden, Ed., *Aging in nonhuman primates,* pp. 183–202. New York: Van Nostrand.

Grahn, D. (1970). Biological effects of protracted low dose radiation exposure of man and animals. In R. J. M. Fry, D. Grahn, M. L. Griem, and J. H. Rust, Eds., *Colloquium on late effects of radiation, Chicago, 1969.* London: Taylor & Francis, pp. 101–111.

Grandjean, P., Weihe, P., Burse, V. W., Needham, L. L., Storr-Hansen, E., Heinzow, B., Debes, F., Murata, K., Simonsen, H., Ellefsen, P., Budtz-Jørgensen, E., Keiding, N., and White, R. F. (2001). Neurobehavioral deficits associated with PCB in 7-year-old children prenatally exposed to seafood neurotoxicants. *Neurotoxicol Teratol.* **23,** 305–317.

Grant, B. D., and Wilkinson, H. A. (2003). Functional genomic maps in *Caenorhabditis elegans. Curr Opin Cell Biol.* **5,** 206–212.

Grant, S. F., Thorleifsson, G., Reynisdottir, I., Benediktsson, R., Manolescu, A., Sainz, J., Helgason, A., Stefansson, H., Emilsson, V., Helgadottir, A., Styrkarsdottir, U., Magnusson, K. P., Walters, G. B., Palsdottir, E., Jonsdottir, T., Gudmundsdottir, T., Gylfason, A., Saemundsdottir, J., Wilensky, R. L., Reilly, M. P., Rader, D. J., Bagger, Y., Christiansen, C., Gudnason, V., Sigurdsson, G., Thorsteinsdottir, U., Gulcher, J. R., Kong, A., and Stefansson, K. (2006). Variant of transcription factor 7-like 2 (TCF7L2) gene confers risk of type 2 diabetes. *Nat Genet.* **38,** 320–323.

Grant, W. D. (2003). Diet and risk of dementia: Does fat matter? The Rotterdam Study. *Neurology.* **60,** 2020–2021.

Gray, J. V., Petsko, G. A., Johnston, G. C., Ringe, D., Singer, R. A., and Werner-Washburne, M. (2004). "Sleeping beauty": Quiescence in *Saccharomyces cerevisiae. Microbiol Mol Biol Rev.* **68,** 187–206.

Grayston, J. T. (2000). Background and current knowledge of *Chlamydia pneumoniae* and atherosclerosis. *J Infect Dis.* **181,** S402–410.

Green, D. A., Masliah, E., Vinters, H. V., Beizai, P., Moore, D. J., and Achim, C. L. (2005). Brain deposition of beta-amyloid is a common pathologic feature in HIV positive patients. *AIDS.* **19,** 407–411.

Green, R. C., Cupples, L. A., Go, R., Benke, K. S., Edeki, T., Griffith, P. A., Williams, M., Hipps, Y., Graff-Radford, N., Bachman, D., and Farrer, L. A. (2002). Risk of dementia among white and African American relatives of patients with Alzheimer disease. *JAMA.* **287,** 329–336.

Grehan, J. R. (2006). Mona Lisa smile: The morphological enigma of human and great ape evolution. *Anat Rec B New Anat.* **289,** 139–157.

Griffin, W. S., Stanley, L. C., Ling, C., White, L., MacLeod, V., Perrot, L. J., White, C. L., 3rd, and Araoz, C. (1989). Brain interleukin 1 and S-100 immunoreactivity are elevated in Down syndrome and Alzheimer disease. *Proc Natl Acad Sci USA.* **86,** 7611–7615.

Griffin, W. S. T. (2005). Glia and their cytokines in progression of neurodegenerative disease. *Neurobiol Aging.* **26,** 349–354.

Grine, F. E., Bailey, R. M., Nathan, R. P., Morris, A. G., Henderson, G. M., Ribot, I., et al. (2007). Late Pleistocene human skull from Hofmeyr, South Africa, and modern human origins. *Science.* **315,** 226–229.

Grobbee, D. E., and Bots, M. L. (2003). Statin treatment and progression of atherosclerotic plaque burden. *Drugs.* **63,** 893–911.

Grodstein, F., Stampfer, M. J., Colditz, G. A., Willett, W. C., Manson, J. E., Joffe, M., Rosner, B., Fuchs, C., Hankinson, S. E., Hunter, D. J., Hennekens, C. H., and Speizer, F. E. (1997). Postmenopausal hormone therapy and mortality. *New Engl J Med.* **336,** 1769–1775.

Gronbaek, M. (2006). Factors influencing the relation between alcohol and cardiovascular disease. *Curr Opin Lipidol.* **17,** 17–21.

Grove, K. L., Grayson, B. E., Glavas, M. M., Xiao, X. Q., and Smith, M. S. (2005). Development of metabolic systems. *Physiol Behav.* **86,** 646–660.

Grunenfelder, J., Umbehr, M., Plass, A., Bestmann, L., Maly, F. E., Zèund, G., and Turina, M. (2004). Genetic polymorphisms of apolipoprotein E4 and tumor necrosis factor beta as predisposing factors for increased inflammatory cytokines after cardiopulmonary bypass. *J Thorac Cardiovasc Surgery.* **128,** 92–97.

Guerrant, R. L., Oria, R., Bushen, O. Y., Patrick, P. D., Houpt, E., and Lima, A. A., (2005). Global impact of diarrheal diseases that are sampled by travelers: The rest of the hippopotamus. *Clin Infect Dis.* **41,** S524–530.

Guerrant, R. L., Schorling, J. B., McAuliffe, J. F., and de Souza, M. A. (1992). Diarrhea as a cause and an effect of malnutrition: Diarrhea prevents catch-up growth and malnutrition increases diarrhea frequency and duration. *Am J Trop Med Hyg.* **47,** 28–35.

Gunnell, D. J., Davey Smith, G., Frankel, S., Nanchahal, K., Braddon, F. E., Pemberton, J., and Peters, T. J. (1998). Childhood leg length and adult mortality: Follow up of the Carnegie (Boyd Orr) Survey of Diet and Health in pre-war Britain. *J Epidemiol Comm Health.* **52,** 142–152.

Guo, L., LaDu, M. J., and Van Eldik, L. J. (2004). A dual role for apolipoprotein E in neuroinflammation: Anti- and pro-inflammatory activity. *J Mol Neurosci:* **23,** 205–212.

Guo, Z., Mitchell-Raymundo, F., Yang, H., Ikeno, Y., Nelson, J., Diaz, V., Richardson, A., and Reddick, R. (2002). Dietary restriction reduces atherosclerosis and oxidative stress in the aorta of apolipoprotein E-deficient mice. *Mech Ageing Dev.* **123,** 1121–1131.

Gurven, M., and Kaplan, H. (2007). Longevity among hunter-gatherers: A cross cultural examination. *Pop Devel Rev.*, in press.

Gurven, M., Kaplan, H., and Gutierrez, M. (2006). How long does it take to become a proficient hunter? Implications for the evolution of extended development and long life span. *J Hum Evol.* **51,** 454–470.

Gurven, M., Kaplan, H., Montecinos, M. E., Wiking, J., Finch, C. E., and Crimmins, E. M. (2007). Inflammation levels in two epidemiological worlds, *J Gerontol, Biol Med Sci.*

Gustafson, D., Rothenberg, E., Blennow, K., Steen, B., and Skoog, I. (2003). An 18-year follow-up of overweight and risk of Alzheimer disease. *Arch Intern Med.* **163,** 1524–1528.

Gutierrez, E., Vazquez, R., and Boakes, R. A. (2002). Activity-based anorexia: Ambient temperature has been a neglected factor. *Psychonom Bull Review.* **9,** 239–249.

Guy, F., Lieberman, D. E., Pilbeam, D., de León, M. P., Likius, A., Mackaye, H. T., Vignaud, P., Zollikofer, C., and Brunet, M. (2005). Morphological affinities of the *Sahelanthropus tchadensis* (Late Miocene hominid from Chad) cranium. *Proc Natl Acad Sci USA.* **102,** 18836–18841.

Guzik, T. J., Sadowski, J., Guzik, B., Jopek, A., Kapelak, B., Przybylowski, P., Wierzbicki, K., Korbut, R., Harrison, D. G., and Channon, K. M. (2006). Coronary artery superoxide production and nox isoform expression in human coronary artery disease. *Arterioscler Thromb Vasc Biol.* **26,** 333–339.

Haan, M. N., Shemanski, L., Jagust, W. J., Manolio, T. A., and Kuller, L. (1999). The role of APOE epsilon4 in modulating effects of other risk factors for cognitive decline in elderly persons. *JAMA.* **282,** 40–46.

Haberny, S. L., Berman, Y., Meller, E., and Carr, K. D. (2004). Chronic food restriction increases D-1 dopamine receptor agonist-induced phosphorylation of extracellular signal-regulated kinase 1/2 and cyclic AMP response element-binding protein in caudate-putamen and nucleus accumbens. *Neuroscience.* **125**, 289–298.

Haddad, E. H., Berk, L. S., Kettering, J. D., Hubbard, R. W., Peters, W. R. (1999). Dietary intake and biochemical, hematologic, and immune status of vegans compared with nonvegetarians. *Amer J Clin Nut.* **70**, 586S–593S.

Hadsell, D. L., Murphy, K. L., Bonnette, S. G., Reece, N., Laucirica, R., and Rosen, J. M. (2000). Cooperative interaction between mutant p53 and des(1–3)IGF-I accelerates mammary tumorigenesis. *Oncogene.* **19**, 889–898.

Hagberg, J. M., Wilund, K. R., and Ferrell, R. E. (2000). APO E gene and gene-environment effects on plasma lipoprotein-lipid levels. *Physiol Genomics.* **4**, 101–108.

Hagopian, K., Harper, M. E., Ram, J. J., Humble, S. J., Weindruch, R., and Ramsey, J. J. (2005). Long-term calorie restriction reduces proton leak and hydrogen peroxide production in liver mitochondria. *Am J Physiol. Endocrinology and Metabolism.* **288**, E674–684.

Hagopian, K., Ramsey, J. J., and Weindruch, R. (2004). Krebs cycle enzymes from livers of old mice are differentially regulated by caloric restriction. *Exp Gerontol.* **39**, 1145–1154.

Hahn-Windgassen, A., Nogueira, V., Chen, C. C., Skeen, J. E., Sonenberg, N., and Hay, N. (2005). Akt activates the mammalian target of rapamycin by regulating cellular ATP level and AMPK activity. *J Biol Chem.* **280**, 32081–32089.

Haig, D. (1993). Genetic conflicts in human pregnancy. *Q Rev Biol.* **68**, 495–532.

Haig, D. (1996). Gestational drive and the green-bearded placenta. *Proc Natl Acad Sci USA.* **93**, 6547–6551.

Hajishengallis, G., Sojar, H., Genco, R. J., and DeNardin, E. (2004). Intracellular signaling and cytokine induction upon interactions of *Porphyromonas gingivalis* fimbriae with pattern-recognition receptors. *Immunol Invest.* **33**, 157–172.

Hajjar, D. P. (2000). Oxidized lipoproteins and infectious agents: Are they in collusion to accelerate atherogenesis? *Arterioscler Thromb Vasc Biol.* **20**, 1421–1422.

Hajjar, D. P., and Haberland, M. E. (1997). Lipoprotein trafficking in vascular cells. Molecular Trojan horses and cellular saboteurs. *J Biol Chem.* **272**, 22975–22978.

Hajra, L., Evans, A. I., Chen, M., Hyduk, S. J., Collins, T., and Cybulsky, M. I. (2000). The NF-kappa B signal transduction pathway in aortic endothelial cells is primed for activation in regions predisposed to atherosclerotic lesion formation. *Proc Natl Acad Sci USA.* **97**, 9052–9057.

Hakim, F. T., Memon, S. A., Cepeda, R., Jones, E. C., Chow, C. K., Kasten-Sportes, C., Odom, J., Vance, B. A., Christensen, B. L., Mackall, C. L., and Gress, R. E. (2005). Age-dependent incidence, time course, and consequences of thymic renewal in adults. *J Clin Invest.* **115**, 930–939.

Hakkinen, A. (1992). On attitudes and living strategies in the Finnish countryside in the years of the famine 1867–1868. In A. Hakkinen, Ed., *Just a sack of potatoes? Crisis experiences in European societies, past and present*, Vol. Studia Historia 44, pp. 149–166. Helinsinki: Societas Historica Finlandia.

Häkkinen, T., Karkola, K., and Ylä-Herttuala, S. (2000). Macrophages, smooth muscle cells, endothelial cells, and T-cells express CD40 and CD40L in fatty streaks and more advanced human atherosclerotic lesions. *Virchows Archiv.* **437**, 396–405.

Halcox, J. P., and Deanfield, J. E. (2004). Beyond the laboratory: Clinical implications for statin pleiotropy. *Circulation.* **109**, 1142–1148.

Hales, C. N., and Barker, D. J. (2001). The thrifty phenotype hypothesis. *Br Med Bull.* **60,** 5–20.

Hales, C. N., Barker, D. J., Clark, P. M., Cox, L. J., Fall, C., Osmond, C., and Winter, P. D. (1991). Fetal and infant growth and impaired glucose tolerance at age 64. *Br Med J.* **303,** 1019–1022.

Hales, C. N., and Ozanne, S. E. (2003). The dangerous road of catch-up growth. *J Physiol.* **547,** 5–10.

Hall, M. A., Bartke, A., and Martinko, J. M. (2002). Humoral immune response in mice over-expressing or deficient in growth hormone. *Exp Biol Med.* **227,** 535–544.

Hallemeesch, M. M., Cobben, D. C., Dejong, C. H., Soeters, P. B., and Deutz, N. E. (2000). Renal amino acid metabolism during endotoxemia in the rat. *J Surg Res.* **92,** 193–200.

Hamilton, C. A., Brosnan, M. J., McIntyre, M., Graham, D., and Dominiczak, A. F. (2001). Superoxide excess in hypertension and aging: A common cause of endothelial dysfunction. *Hypertension.* **37,** 529–534.

Hamilton, M. L., Van Remmen, H., Drake, J. A., Yang, H., Guo, Z. M., Kewitt, K., Walter, C. A., and Richardson, A. (2001). Does oxidative damage to DNA increase with age? *Proc Natl Acad Sci USA.* **98,** 10469–10474.

Hamilton, W. D. (1966). The moulding of senescence by natual selection. *J Theor Biol.* **12,** 12–45.

Hamlin, C. R., and Kohn, R. R. (1971). Evidence for progressive, age-related structural changes in post-mature human collagen. *Biochim Biophys Acta.* **236,** 458–467.

Hampel, B., Wagner, M., Teis, D., Zwerschke, W., Huber, L. A., and Jansen-Durr, P. (2005). Apoptosis resistance of senescent human fibroblasts is correlated with the absence of nuclear IGFBP-3. *Aging Cell.* **4,** 325–330.

Han, B. H., DeMattos, R. B., Dugan, L. L., Kim-Han, J. S., Brendza, R. P., Fryer, J. D., Kierson, M., Cirrito, J., Quick, K., Harmony, J. A., Aronow, B. J., and Holtzman, D. M. (2001). Clusterin contributes to caspase-3–independent brain injury following neonatal hypoxia-ischemia. *Nat Med.* **7,** 338–343.

Han, E. S., Evans, T. R., Shu, J. H., Lee, S., and Nelson, J. F. (2001). Food restriction enhances endogenous and corticotropin-induced plasma elevations of free but not total corticosterone throughout life in rats. *J Gerontol. Series A, Biol Sci Med Sci.* **56,** B391–397.

Han, J. H., Roh, M. S., Park, C. H., Park, K. C., Cho, K. H., Kim, K. H., Eun, H. C., and Chung, J. H. (2004). Selective COX-2 inhibitor, NS-398, inhibits the replicative senescence of cultured dermal fibroblasts. *Mech Ageing Dev.* **125,** 359–366.

Han, Z., Yi, P., Li, X., and Olson, E. N. (2006). Hand, an evolutionarily conserved bHLH transcription factor required for *Drosophila* cardiogenesis and hematopoiesis. *Development.* **133,** 1175–1182.

Hanlon, C. S., and Rubinsztein, D. C. (1995). Arginine residues at codons 112 and 158 in the apolipoprotein E gene correspond to the ancestral state in humans. *Atherosclerosis.* **112,** 85–90.

Hansen, E., Buecher, E. J., and Yarwood, E. A. (1964). Development and maturation of *Caenorhabditis briggsae* in response to growth factor. *Nematologica.* **10,** 623–630.

Hansen, L. A., Armstrong, D. M., and Terry, R. D. (1987). An immunohistochemical quantification of fibrous astrocytes in the aging human cerebral cortex. *Neurobiol Aging.* **8(1),** 1–6.

Haraszthy, V. I., Zambon, J. J., Trevisan, M., Zeid, M., and Genco, R. J. (2000). Identification of periodontal pathogens in atheromatous plaques. *J Periodontology.* **71,** 1554–1560.

Harding, J. R. (1976). Certain Upper Palaeolithic 'Venus' statuettes considered in relation to the pathological condition known as massive hypertrophy of the breasts. *Man.* **11,** 271–272.

Hardman, J. G., and Limbird, L. E., Eds. (2001). *Goodman & Gilman's The pharmacological basis of therapeutics* (10th ed.). New York: McGraw Hill.

Hardy-Smith, T., and Edwards, P. C. (2004). The garbage crisis in prehistory: Artifact discard patterns at the Early Natufian site of Wadi Hammeh 27 and the origins of household refuse disposal strategies. *J. Anthropl. Archeol.* **23,** 253–289.

Hardy, J., and Selkoe, D. J. (2002). The amyloid hypothesis of Alzheimer's disease: Progress and problems on the road to therapeutics. *Science.* **297,** 353–356.

Hare, L. G., Woodside, J. V., and Young, I. S. (2003). Dietary salicylates. [comment]. *J Clin Pathol.* **56,** 649–650.

Harman, D. (1956). Ageing: A theory based on free radical and radiation chemistry. *J Gerontol.* **11,** 298–300.

Harman, D. (2003). The free radical theory of aging. *Antioxid Redox Signal.* **5,** 557–561.

Harman, D., and Harman, H. (2003). "I thought, thought, thought for four months in vain and suddenly the idea came"—an interview with Denham and Helen Harman. Interview by K. Kitani and G.O. Ivy. *Biogerontology.* **4,** 401–412.

Harman, S. M. (2005). Testosterone in older men after the Institute of Medicine Report: Where do we go from here? *Climacteric.* **8,** 124–135.

Harper, J. M., Leathers, C. W., and Austad, S. N. (2006a). Does caloric restriction extend life in wild mice? *Aging Cell.* **5,** 441–449.

Harper, J. M., Salmon, A. B., Chang, Y., Bonkowski, M., Bartke, A., and Miller, R. A. (2006b). Stress resistance and aging: Influence of genes and nutrition. *Mech Ageing Dev.* **127,** 687–694.

Harper, J. M., Wolf, N., Galecki, A. T., Pinkosky, S. L., and Miller, R. A. (2003). Hormone levels and cataract scores as sex-specific, mid-life predictors of longevity in genetically heterogeneous mice. *Mech Ageing Dev.* **124,** 801–810.

Harper, M. E., Bevilacqua, L., Hagopian, K., Weindruch, R., and Ramsey, J. J. (2004). Ageing, oxidative stress, and mitochondrial uncoupling. *Acta Physiol Scand.* **182,** 321–331.

Harris, C. L., and Fraser, C. (2004). Malnutrition in the institutionalized elderly: The effects on wound healing. *Ostomy Wound Manage,* **50,** 54–63.

Harris, F. M., Tesseur, I., Brecht, W. J., Xu, Q., Mullendorff, K., Chang, S., Wyss-Coray, T., Mahley, R. W., and Huang, Y. (2004). Astroglial regulation of apolipoprotein E expression in neuronal cells. Implications for Alzheimer's disease. *J Biol Chem.* **279,** 3862–3868.

Harris, S. L., and Levine, A. J. (2005). The p53 pathway: Positive and negative feedback loops. *Oncogene.* **24,** 2899–2908.

Harris, T. B., Ferrucci, L., Tracy, R. P., Corti, M. C., Wacholder, S., Ettinger, W. H., Jr., Heimovitz, H., Cohen, H. J., and Wallace, R. (1999). Associations of elevated interleukin-6 and C-reactive protein levels with mortality in the elderly. *Am J Med.* **106,** 506–512.

Harris, W. S. (2005). Alpha-linolenic acid: A gift from the land? *Circulation.* **111,** 2872–2874.

Harrison, D. E., and Archer, J. R. (1987). Genetic influences in effects of food restriction on aging in mice. *J Nutrition.* **117,** 376–382.

Harrison, D. E., and Archer, J. R. (1989). Natural selection for extended longevity from food restriction. *Growth Dev Aging.* **53,** 3.

Harrison, D. E., Archer, J. R., and Astle, C. M. (1984). Effects of food restriction on aging: Separation of food intake and adiposity. *Proc Natl Acad Sci USA.* **81,** 1835–1838.

Hart, B. L. (1990). Behavioral adaptations to pathogens and parasites: Five strategies. *Neuroscience & Biobehavioral Reviews.* **14,** 273–294.

Harvey, R. F., Spence, R. W., Lane, J. A., Nair, P., Murray, L. J., Harvey, I. M., and Donovan, J. (2002). Relationship between the birth cohort pattern of *Helicobacter pylori* infection and the epidemiology of duodenal ulcer. *Quarterly J Medicine.* **95,** 519–525.

Hathcock, K. S., Jeffrey Chiang, Y., and Hodes, R. J. (2005). *In vivo* regulation of telomerase activity and telomere length. *Immunol Rev.* **205,** 104–113.

Hava, D. L., Brigl, M., van den Elzen, P., Zajonc, D. M., Wilson, I. A., and Brenner, M. B. (2005). CD1 assembly and the formation of CD1-antigen complexes. *Curr Opin Immunol.* **17,** 88–94.

Hawkes, K. (2003). Grandmothers and the evolution of human longevity. *Am J Human Biol.* **15,** 380–400.

Hawkes, K. (2006). Slow life histories and human evolution. *The Evolution of human life history.* pp 95–126. Sante Fe: School for American Research Press.

Hawkes, K. and O'Connell, J. F. (2005). How old is human longevity?. *J Hum Evol.* **49,** 650–653.

Hawkes, K., O'Connell, J. F., Jones, N. G., Alvarez, H., and Charnov, E. L. (1998). Grandmothering, menopause, and the evolution of human life histories. *Proc Natl Acad Sci USA.* **95,** 1336–1339.

Hayakawa, T., Aki, I., Varki, A., Satta, Y., and Takahata, N. (2006). Fixation of the human-specific CMP-N-acetylneuraminic acid hydroxylase pseudogene and implications of haplotype diversity for human evolution. *Genetics* **172,** 1139–1146.

Hayakawa, T., Angata, T., Lewis, A. L., Mikkelsen, T. S., Varki, N. M., and Varki, A., (2005). A human-specific gene in microglia. *Science.* **309,** 1693.

Hayflick, L. (2000). The illusion of cell immortality. *Br Med J.* **83,** 841–846.

Hayflick, L., and Moorhead, P. S. (1961). The serial cultivation of human diploid cell strains. *Exp Cell Res.* **25,** 585–621.

Haynes, L. (2005). The effect of aging on cognate function and development of immune memory. *Curr Opin Immunol.* **17,** 476–479.

He, L., Chinnery, P. F., Durham, S. E., Blakely, E. L., Wardell, T. M., Borthwick, G. M., Taylor, R. W., and Turnbull, D. M. (2002). Detection and quantification of mitochondrial DNA deletions in individual cells by real-time PCR. *Nucl Acids Res.* **30,** e68.

He, T., Peterson, T. E., Holmuhamedov, E. L., Terzic, A., Caplice, N. M., Oberley, L. W., and Katusic, Z. S. (2004). Human endothelial progenitor cells tolerate oxidative stress due to intrinsically high expression of manganese superoxide dismutase. *Arterioscler Thromb Vasc Biol.* **24,** 2021–2027.

Heart Protection Study Collaborative Group. (2002). MRC/BHF Heart Protection Study of cholesterol lowering with simvastatin in 20,536 high-risk individuals: A randomised placebo-controlled trial. *Lancet.* **360,** 7–22.

Hebebrand, J., Exner, C., Hebebrand, K., Holtkamp, C., Casper, R. C., Remschmidt, H., Herpertz-Dahlmann, B., and Klingenspor, M. (2003). Hyperactivity in patients with anorexia nervosa and in semistarved rats: Evidence for a pivotal role of hypoleptinemia. *Physiol Behav.* **79,** 25–37.

Hebert, P. R., Rich-Edwards, J. W., Manson, J. E., Ridker, P. M., Cook, N. R., O'Connor, G. T., Buring, J. E., and Hennekens, C. H. (1993). Height and incidence of cardiovascular disease in male physicians. *Circulation.* **88,** 1437–1443.

Heck, D. E., Kagan, V. E., Shvedova, A. A., and Laskin, J. D. (2005). An epigrammatic (abridged) recounting of the myriad tales of astonishing deeds and dire consequences pertaining to nitric oxide and reactive oxygen species in mitochondria with an ancillary missive concerning the origins of apoptosis. *Toxicology.* **208,** 259–271.

Heikkinen, S. (1996). *Finnish Food consumption 1860–1890*, pp. 1–27. Helsinki: National Consuer Research Center.

Heilbronn, L. K. (2006). Effect of 6-month caloric restriction on biomarkers of longevity. *JAMA.* **295,** 1539–1548.

Heinemann, C., and Reid, G., C. (2005). Vaginal microbial diversity among post-menopausal women with and without hormone replacement therapy. *Can J Microbiol* **51,** 777–781.

Heiss, C., Keymel, S., Niesler, U., Ziemann, J., Kelm, M., and Kalka, C. (2005). Impaired progenitor cell activity in age-related endothelial dysfunction. *J Am Coll Cardiol.* **45,** 1441–1448.

Hekimi, S., and Guarente, L. (2003). Genetics and the specificity of the aging process. *Science.* **299,** 1351–1354.

Helfman, P. M., and Bada, J. L. (1975). Aspartic acid racemization in tooth enamel from living humans. *Proc Natl Acad Sci USA.* **72,** 2891–2894.

Helge, J. W., Stallknecht, B., Pedersen, B. K., Galbo, H., Kiens, B., and Richter, E. A. (2003). The effect of graded exercise on IL-6 release and glucose uptake in human skeletal muscle. *J Physiol.* **546,** 299–305.

Helin-Salmivaara, A., Virtanen, A., Vesalainen, R., Gronroos, J. M., Klaukka, T., Idanpaan-Heikkila, J. E., and Huupponen, R. (2006). NSAID use and the risk of hospitalization for first myocardial infarction in the general population: A nationwide case-control study from Finland. *Eur Heart J.* **27,** 1657–1663.

Heller, S., R. (2002). Abnormalities of the electrocardiogram during hypoglycaemia: The cause of the dead in bed syndrome? *Int J Clin Pract Suppl.* **129,** 27–32.

Hellmig, S., Mascheretti, S., Renz, J., Frenzel, H., Jelschen, F., Rehbein, J. K., Fèolsch, U., Hampe, J., and Schreiber, S. (2005a). Haplotype analysis of the CD11 gene cluster in patients with chronic *Helicobacter pylori* infection and gastric ulcer disease. *Tissue Antigens.* **65,** 271–274.

Hellmig, S., Titz, A., Steinel, S., Ott, S., Folsch, U. R., Hampe, J., and Schreiber, S. (2005b). Influence of IL-1 gene cluster polymorphisms on the development of *H. pylori* associated gastric ulcer. *Immunol. Lett.* **100,** 107–112.

Hemmes, G. D. (1945). Besmettelijke Ziekten. Epidemiologie en praeventieve maatregelen. In I. Boerma, Ed., *Medische Ervaringen in Nederland Tijdens de Bezetting 1940–1945*, pp. 105–129. Groningen, Netherlands: J.B. Wolters.

Henderson, B. E., Pike, M. C., and Ross, R. K. (1984). Epidemiology and risk factors. In G. Bonodonna, Ed., *Breast cancer: Diagnosis and management*, pp. 15–33. New York: Wiley.

Henderson, S. T., and Johnson, T. E. (2001). DAF-16 integrates developmental and environmental inputs to mediate aging in the nematode *Caenorhabditis elegans. Curr Biol.* **11,** 1975–1980.

Hendrie, H. C., Ogunniyi, A., Hall, K. S., Baiyewu, O., Unverzagt, F. W., Gureje, O., Gao, S., Evans, R. M., Ogunseyinde, A. O., Adeyinka, A. O., Musick, B., and Hui, S. L. (2001). Incidence of dementia and Alzheimer disease in 2 communities: Yoruba residing in Ibadan, Nigeria, and African Americans residing in Indianapolis, Indiana. *JAMA.* **285,** 739–747.

Hennig, B., Meerarani, P., Slim, R., Toborek, M., Daugherty, A., Silverstone, A. E., and Robertson, L. W. (2002). Proinflammatory properties of coplanar PCBs: *in vitro* and *in vivo* evidence. *Toxicol Appl Pharmacol.* **181,** 174–183.

Hennig, B., Reiterer, G., Majkova, Z., Oesterling, E., Meerarani, P., and Toborek, M. (2005). Modification of environmental toxicity by nutrients: Implications in atherosclerosis. *Cardiovasc Toxicol* **5,** 153–160.

Henriques de Gouveia, R., van der Wal, A., C., van der Loos, C. M., and Becker, A. E. (2002). Sudden unexpected death in young adults. Discrepancies between initiation of acute plaque complications and the onset of acute coronary death. *Euro Heart J,* **23,** 1433–1440.

Henry, J. P., Liu, Y. Y., Nadra, W. E., Qian, C. G., Mormede, P., Lemaire, V., Ely, D., and Hendley, E. D. (1993). Psychosocial stress can induce chronic hypertension in normotensive strains of rats. *Hypertension.* **21,** 714–723.

Henry, P. F. (2003). The eastern box turtle at the Patuxent Wildlife Research Center 1940s to the present: Another view. *Exp Gerontol.* **38,** 773–776.

Herbert, A., Gerry, N. P., McQueen, M. B., Heid, I. M., Pfeufer, A., Illig, T., Wichmann, H. E., Meitinger, T., Hunter, D., Hu, F. B., Colditz, G., Hinney, A., Hebebrand, J., Koberwitz, K., Zhu, X., Cooper, R., Ardlie, K., Lyon, H., Hirschhorn, J. N., Laird, N. M., Lenburg, M. E., Lange, C., and Christman, M. F. (2006). A common genetic variant is associated with adult and childhood obesity. *Science.* **213,** 279–283.

Hercus, M. J., Loeschcke, V., and Rattan, S. I. (2003). Lifespan extension of *Drosophila melanogaster* through hormesis by repeated mild heat stress. *Biogerontology.* **4,** 149–156.

Herendeen, J. M., and Lindley, C. (2003). Use of NSAIDs for the chemoprevention of colorectal cancer. *Annals Pharmacother.* **37,** 1664–1674.

Herndon, L. A., Schmeissner, P. J., Dudaronek, J. M., Brown, P. A., Listner, K. M., Sakano, Y., Paupard, M. C., Hall, D. H., and Driscoll, M. (2002). Stochastic and genetic factors influence tissue-specific decline in ageing *C. elegans. Nature.* **419,** 808–814.

Herrera, E., Amusquivar, E., López-Soldado, I., and Ortega, H. (2006). Maternal lipid metabolism and placental lipid transfer. *Horm Res.* **65,** 59–64.

Herrera, L. A., Benítez-Bribiesca, L., Mohar, A., and Ostrosky-Wegman, P. (2005). Role of infectious diseases in human carcinogenesis. *Env Mol Mutagen.* **45,** 284–303.

Herskind, A. M., McGue, M., Holm, N. V., Sørensen, T. I., Harvald, B., and Vaupel, J. W. (1996). The heritability of human longevity: A population-based study of 2872 Danish twin pairs born 1870–1900. *Hum Genet.* **97,** 319–323.

Hertweck, M., Gèobel, C., and Baumeister, R. (2004). *C. elegans* SGK-1 is the critical component in the Akt/PKB kinase complex to control stress response and life span. *Developmental Cell.* **6,** 577–588.

Heude, B., Ducimetiere, P., and Berr, C. (2003). Cognitive decline and fatty acid composition of erythrocyte membranes—The EVA Study. *Am J Clin Nutr.* **77,** 803–808.

Hickey, M., Davis, S. R., and Sturdee, D. W. (2005). Treatment of menopausal symptoms: What shall we do now? *Lancet.* **366,** 409–421.

Higami, Y., Pugh, T. D., Page, G. P., Allison, D. B., Prolla, T. A., and Weindruch, R. (2004). Adipose tissue energy metabolism: Altered gene expression profile of mice subjected to long-term caloric restriction. *FASEB J.* **18,** 415–417.

Hill, A. V., Allsopp, C. E., Kwiatkowski, D., Anstey, N. M., Twumasi, P., Rowe, P. A., et al. (1991). Common west African HLA antigens are associated with protection from severe malaria. *Nature.* **352,** 595–600.

Hill, A. V., Jepson, A., Plebanski, M., and Gilbert, S. C. (1997). Genetic analysis of host-parasite coevolution in human malaria. *Phil Trans Roy Soc London, Series B, Biol Sci.* **352,** 1317–1325.

Hill, K., Boesch, C., Goodall, J., Pusey, A., Williams, J., and Wrangham, R. (2001). Mortality rates among wild chimpanzees. *J Hum Evol.* **40,** 437–450.

Hill, K., and Hurtado, A. M. (1996). *Ache life history: The ecology and demography of a foraging people.* Hawthorne, NY: Aldine.

Himes, C. L. (1994). Age patterns of mortality and cause-of-death structures in Sweden, Japan, and the United States. *Demography* **31,** 633–650.

Hino, A., Adachi, H., Toyomasu, K., Yoshida, N., Enomoto, M., Hiratsuka, A., Hirai, Y., Satoh, A., and Imaizumi, T. (2004). Very long chain N-3 fatty acids intake and carotid atherosclerosis: An epidemiological study evaluated by ultrasonography. *Atherosclerosis.* **176,** 145–149.

Hinz, B., and Brune, K. (2004). Pain and osteoarthritis: New drugs and mechanisms. *Curr Opin Rheumatol.* **16,** 628–633.

Hippisley-Cox, J., and Coupland, C. (2005). Risk of myocardial infarction in patients taking cyclo-oxygenase-2 inhibitors or conventional non-steroidal anti-inflammatory drugs: Population based nested case-control analysis. *Br Med J.* **330,** 1366.

Hirayama, A., Horikoshi, Y., Maeda, M., Ito, M., and Takashima, S. (2003). Characteristic developmental expression of amyloid beta40, 42 and 43 in patients with Down syndrome. *Brain Devel.* **25,** 180–185.

Hirokawa, K., Kubo, S., Utsuyama, M., Kurashima, C., and Sado, T. (1986). Age-related change in the potential of bone marrow cells to repopulate the thymus and splenic T cells in mice. *Cell Immunol.* **100,** 443–451.

Hiroki, M., Miyashita, K., and Oda, M. (2002). Tortuosity of the white matter medullary arterioles is related to the severity of hypertension. *Cerebrovasc Dis.* **13,** 242–250.

Hirsch, S. (1941). L'atheroma aortique des enfants. *Cardiologia.* **5,** 122.

Hirvonen, J., Ylèa-Herttuala, S., Laaksonen, H., Mèottèonen, M., Nikkari, T., Pesonen, E., Raekallio, J., and Akerblom, H. K. (1985). Coronary intimal thickenings and lipids in Finnish children who died violently. *Acta Paed Scand—Suppl.* **318,** 221–224.

Hoberg, E. (2002). *Taenia* tapeworms: Their biology, evolution and socioeconomic significance. *Microbes Infect.* **4,** 859–866.

Hodder, I. (2005). *Inhabiting Çatalhöyük.: reports from the 1995-1999 seasons by members of the Çatalhöyük teams.* London: McDonald Institute Monographs.

Hodder, I. (2006). *The leopard's tale. Revealing the mysteries of Çatalhöyük.* London: Thames and Hudson.

Hodis, H. N., Mack, W. J. (2007a). Postmenopausal hormone therapy and cardiovascular disease: making sense of the evidence. *Curr Cardiovasc Risk Rep.* **1,** in press.

Hodis, H. N., Mack, W. J. (2007b). Postmenopausal hormone therapy in clinical perspective. *Menopause.* **14,** 1–14.

Hodis, H. N., Mack, W. J., Azen, S. P., Lobo, R. A., Shoupe, D., Mahrer, P. R., Faxon, D. P., Cashin-Hemphill, L., Sanmarco, M. E., French, W. J., Shook, T. L., Gaarder, T. D., Mehra, A. O., Rabbani, R., Sevanian, A., Shil, A. B., Torres, M., Vogelbach, K. H., and Selzer, R. H. (2003a). Hormone therapy and the progression of coronary-artery atherosclerosis in postmenopausal women. [see comment]. *New Engl J Med.* **349,** 535–455.

Hodis, H. N., Mack, W. J., and Lobo, R. A. (2003b). Randomized controlled trial evidence that estrogen replacement therapy reduces the progression of subclinical atherosclerosis in healthy postmenopausal women without preexisting cardiovascular disease. [comment]. *Circulation*. **108**, e5.

Hodis, H. N., Mack, W. J., Lobo, R. A., Shoupe, D., Sevanian, A., Mahrer, P. R., Selzer, R. H., Liu Cr, C. R., Liu Ch, C. H., and Azen, S. P. (2001). Estrogen in the prevention of atherosclerosis. A randomized, double-blind, placebo-controlled trial. *Ann Intern Med*. **135**, 939–953.

Hoffmann, H. J., Iversen, M., Brandslund, I., Sigsgaard, T., Omland, O., Oxvig, C., Holmskov, U., Bjermer, L., Jensenius, J. C., and Dahl, R. (2003). Plasma C3d levels of young farmers correlate with respirable dust exposure levels during normal work in swine confinement buildings. *Ann Agricult Environ Med*. **10**, 53–60.

Hokanson, J. E., Kinney, G. L., Cheng, S., Erlich, H. A., Kretowski, A., and Rewers, M. (2006). Susceptibility to type 1 diabetes is associated with ApoCIII gene haplotypes. *Diabetes*. **55**, 834–838.

Holcomb, L., Gordon, M. N., McGowan, E., Yu, X., Benkovic, S., Jantzen, P., Wright, K., Saad, I., Mueller, R., Morgan, D., Sanders, S., Zehr, C., O'Campo, K., Hardy, J., Prada, C. M., Eckman, C., Younkin, S., Hsiao, K., and Duff, K. (1998). Accelerated Alzheimer-type phenotype in transgenic mice carrying both mutant amyloid precursor protein and presenilin 1 transgenes. *Nat Med*. **4**, 97–100.

Holehan, A. M., and Merry, B. J. (1985a). Lifetime breeding studies in fully fed and dietary restricted female CFY Sprague-Dawley rats. 1. Effect of age, housing conditions and diet on fecundity. *Mech Ageing Dev*. **33**, 19–28.

Holehan, A. M., and Merry, B. J. (1985b). Modification of the oestrous cycle hormonal profile by dietary restriction. *Mech Ageing Dev*. **32**, 63–76.

Holliday, R. (1989). Food, reproduction and longevity: Is the extended lifespan of calorie-restricted animals an evolutionary adaptation? *BioEssays*. **10**, 125–127.

Holloszy, J. O. (1992). Exercise and food restriction in rats. *J Nutr*. **122**, 774–777.

Holloszy, J. O. (1997). Mortality rate and longevity of food-restricted exercising male rats: A reevaluation. *J Appl. Physiol*. **82**, 399–403.

Holloszy, J. O. (2005). Exercise-induced increase in muscle insulin sensitivity. *J Appl Physiol*. **99**, 338–343.

Holloszy, J. O., and Schechtman, K. B. (1991). Interaction between exercise and food restriciton: Effects on longeivty of male rats. *J Applied Physiol*. **70**, 1529–1535.

Holloszy, J. O., and Smith, E. K. (1986). Longevity of cold-exposed rats: A reevaluation of the "rate-of-living theory.". *J Appl Physiol*. **61**, 1656–1660.

Holloszy, J. O., Smith, E. K., Vining, M., and Adams, S. (1985). Effect of voluntary exercise on longevity of rats. *J Appl Physiol*. **59**, 826–831.

Holmen, C., Elsheikh, E., Stenvinkel, P., Qureshi, A. R., Pettersson, E., Jalkanen, S., and Sumitran-Holgersson, S. (2005). Circulating inflammatory endothelial cells contribute to endothelial progenitor cell dysfunction in patients with vasculitis and kidney involvement. *J Am Soc Nephro*. **16**, 3110–3120.

Holtkamp, K., Herpertz-Dahlmann, B., Hebebrand, K., Mika, C., Kratzsch, J., and Hebebrand, J. (2006). Physical activity and restlessness correlate with leptin levels in patients with adolescent anorexia nervosa. *Biol Psychiatr*. **60**, 311–313.

Holub, D. J., and Holub, B. J. (2004). Omega-3 fatty acids from fish oils and cardiovascular disease. *Mol Cell Biochem*. **263**, 217–225.

Holzenberger, M., Dupont, J., Ducos, B., Leneuve, P., Géloèen, A., Even, P. C., Cervera, P., and Le Bouc, Y. (2003). IGF-1 receptor regulates lifespan and resistance to oxidative stress in mice. *Nature.* **421,** 182–187.

Hoogerbrugge, N., Zillikens, M. C., Jansen, H., Meeter, K., Deckers, J. W., and Birkenhager, J. C. (1998). Estrogen replacement decreases the level of antibodies against oxidized low-density lipoprotein in postmenopausal women with coronary heart disease. *Metabolism: Clin Expl.* **47,** 675–680.

Hoppa, R. D., and Vaupel, J. W. (2002). Eds, *Paleodemography: age distributions from skeletal samples.* In *Cambridge studies in biological and evolutionary anthropology,* Vol. 31, pp. 258. New York: Cambridge University Press.

Horbury, S. R., Mercer, J. G., and Chappell, L. H. (1995). Anorexia induced by the parasitic nematode, *Nippostrongylus brasiliensis*: Effects on NPY and CRF gene expression in the rat hypothalamus. *J Neuroendocrinol.* **7,** 867–873.

Horiuchi, S. (1997). Postmenopausal acceleration of age-related mortality increase. *J Gerontol Series A–Biol Sci Med Sci.* **52,** B78–92.

Horiuchi, S. (1999). Epidemiological transitions in human history. In *Health and mortality: Issues of global concern,* pp. 54–71. New York: United Nations Population Division, Dept Economic and Social Affairs.

Horiuchi, S., Finch, C. E., Meslé, F., and Vallin, J. (2003). Differential patterns of age-related mortality increase in middle age and old age. *J Gerontol. Series A, Biol Sci Med Sci.* **58,** 495–507.

Horvath, B. (2006). *Beyond absolute brain size? The allure of allometry and of the encephalization quotient.* M.S. Thesis, Dept. Anthropology. George Washington University.

Horvath, T. L. (2005). The hardship of obesity: A soft-wired hypothalamus. *Nature Neuroscience.* **8,** 561–565.

Horvath, T. L., and Bruning, J. C. (2006). Developmental programming of the hypothalamus: A matter of fat. *Nat Med.* **12,** 52–53.

Hoshi, A., and Inaba, Y. (1995). Risk factors for mortality and mortality rate of sumo wrestlers. *Nippon Eiseigaku Zasshi. Japanese J Hygiene.* **50,** 730–736.

Hostetter, T. H., Meyer, T. W., Rennke, H. G., and Brenner, B. M. (1986). Chronic effects of dietary protein in the rat with intact and reduced renal mass. *Kidney Int.* **30,** 509–517.

Houthoofd, K., Braeckman, B. P., Johnson, T. E., and Vanfleteren, J. R. (2003). Life extension via dietary restriction is independent of the Ins/IGF-1 signalling pathway in *Caenorhabditis elegans. Exp Gerontol.* **38,** 947–954.

Houthoofd, K., Braeckman, B. P., Lenaerts, I., Brys, K., De Vreese, A., Van Eygen, S., and Vanfleteren, J. R. (2002). Axenic growth up-regulates mass-specific metabolic rate, stress resistance, and extends life span in *Caenorhabditis elegans. Exp Gerontol.* **37,** 1371–1378.

Houthoofd, K., Braeckman, B. P., Lenaerts, I., Brys, K., Matthijssens, F., De Vreese, A., Van Eygen, S., and Vanfleteren, J. R. (2005). DAF-2 pathway mutations and food restriction in aging *Caenorhabditis elegans* differentially affect metabolism. *Neurobiol Aging.* **26,** 689–696.

Houthoofd, K., Braeckman, B. P., and Vanfleteren, J. R. (2004). The hunt for the record life span in *Caenorhabditis elegans. J Gerontol. Series A, Biol Sci Med Sci.* **59,** 408–410.

Houthoofd, K., Gems, D., Johnson, T.E.,and Vanfleteren, J. R. (2007). Dietary restriction in the nematode *Caenorhabditis elegans.* Interdisc Top *Gerontol.* **35,** 98–114.

Howard, B. V., Van Horn, L., Hsia, J., Manson, J. E., Stefanick, M. L., Wassertheil-Smoller, S., Kuller, L. H., LaCroix, A. Z., Langer, R. D., Lasser, N. L., Lewis, C. E., Limacher, M. C., Margolis, K. L., Mysiw, W. J., Ockene, J. K., Parker, L. M., Perri, M. G., Phillips, L., Prentice,

R. L., Robbins, J., Rossouw, J. E., Sarto, G. E., Schatz, I. J., Snetselaar, L. G., Stevens, V. J., Tinker, L. F., Trevisan, M., Vitolins, M. Z., Anderson, G. L., Assaf, A. R., Bassford, T., Beresford, S. A., Black, H. R., Brunner, R. L., Brzyski, R. G., Caan, B., Chlebowski, R. T., Gass, M., Granek, I., Greenland, P., Hays, J., Heber, D., Heiss, G., Hendrix, S. L., Hubbell, F. A., Johnson, K. C., and Kotchen, J. M. (2006). Low-fat dietary pattern and risk of cardiovascular disease: The Women's Health Initiative Randomized Controlled Dietary Modification Trial. *JAMA*. **295,** 655–666.

Howard, M. L., and Davidson, E. H. (2004). cis-Regulatory control circuits in development. *Dev. Biol*. **271,** 108–118.

Howland, B. E., and Ibrahim, E. A. (1973). Increased LH-suppressing effect of oestrogen in ovariectomized rate as a result of underfeeding. *J Repro Ferti*. **35,** 545–548.

Hoyert, D. L., Mathews, T. J., Menacker, F., Strobino, D. M., and Guyer, B. (2006). Annual summary of vital statistics: 2004. *Pediatrics*. **117,** 168–183.

Hoyle, B., Yunus, M., and Chen, L. C. (1980). Breast-feeding and food intake among children with acute diarrheal disease. *Am J Clin Nutr*. **33,** 2365–2371.

Hrdy, S. B. (2000). The optimal number of fathers. Evolution, demography, and history in the shaping of female mate preferences. *Ann NY Acad Sci*. **907,** 75–96.

Hrdy, S.B. (2005). Comes the child before man: how cooperative breeding and prolonged post-weaning dependence shaped human potentials. In: *Culture and ecology of hunter-gatherer children*. B.S. Hewlett and E. Lamb (Eds.). New York, Aldine: 65–91.

Hsieh, E. A., Chai, C. M., de Lumen, B. O., Neese, R. A., and Hellerstein, M. K. (2004a). Dynamics of keratinocytes *in vivo* using HO labeling: A sensitive marker of epidermal proliferation state. *J Invest Dermatol*. **123,** 530–536.

Hsieh, E. A., Chai, C. M., de Lumen, B. O., Neese, R. A., Hellerstein, M. K., Department of Nutritional, S., and Toxicology, U. o. C.-B. B. C. A. U. S. A. (2004b). Dynamics of keratinocytes *in vivo* using HO labeling: a sensitive marker of epidermal proliferation state. *J Invest Dermatol*. **123,** 530–6.

Hsieh, E. A., Chai, C. M., and Hellerstein, M. K. (2005). Effects of caloric restriction on cell proliferation in several tissues in mice: Role of intermittent feeding. *Am J Physiol Endocrinol Metab*. **288,** E965–972.

Hsin, H., and Kenyon, C. (1999). Signals from the reproductive system regulate the lifespan of *C. elegans. Nature*. **399,** 362–366.

Hsu, A. L., Murphy, C. T., and Kenyon, C. (2003). Regulation of aging and age-related disease by DAF-16 and heat-shock factor. *Science*. **300,** 1142–1145.

Hsueh, S. F., Lu, C. Y., Chao, C. S., Tan, P. H., Huang, Y. W., Hsieh, S. W., Hsiao, H. T., Chung, N. C., Lin, S. H., Huang, P. L., Lyu, P. C., and Yang, L. C. (2004). Nonsteroidal anti-inflammatory drugs increase expression of inducible COX-2 isoform of cyclooxygenase in spinal cord of rats with adjuvant induced inflammation. *Brain Res. Mol Brain Res*. **125,** 113–119.

Hu, D., Serrano, F., Oury, T. D., and Klann, E. (2006a). Aging-dependent alterations in synaptic plasticity and memory in mice that overexpress extracellular superoxide dismutase. *J Neurosci*. **26,** 3933–3941.

Hu, P., Bretsky, P., Crimmins, E. M., Guralnik, J. M., Reuben, D. B., and Seeman, T. E. (2006b). Association between serum beta-carotene levels and decline of cognitive function in high-functioning older persons with or without apolipoprotein E4 alleles: MacArthur Studies of Successful Aging. *J Gerontol. A Biol Sci Med Sci*. **61,** 616–620.

Hu, P., Greendale, G. A., Palla, S. L., Reboussin, B. A., Herrington, D. M., E., B.-C., and Reuben, D. B. (2005). The effects of hormone therapy on the markers of inflammation and endothelial function and plasma matrix metalloproteinase-9 level in post-menopausal women: The postmenopausal estrogen progestin intervention (PEPI) trial. *Atherosclerosis.* **185,** 347–352.

Hu, T., Grosberg, A. Y., Shklovskii, B. I. (2006). How proteins search for their specific sites on DNA: the role of DNA conformation. *Biophys J.* **90,** 2731–2744.

Huang, A., and Kaley, G. (2004). Gender-specific regulation of cardiovascular function: Estrogen as key player. *Microcirculation (New York: 1994).* **11(1),** 9–38.

Huang, C., Xiong, C., and Kornfeld, K. (2004a). Measurements of age-related changes of physiological processes that predict lifespan of *Caenorhabditis elegans. Proc Natl Acad Sci USA.* **101,** 8084–8089.

Huang, Q., Raya, A., DeJesus, P., Chao, S. H., Quon, K. C., Caldwell, J. S., Chanda, S. K., Izpisua-Belmonte, J. C., and Schultz, P. G. (2004b). Identification of p53 regulators by genome-wide functional analysis. *Proc Natl Acad Sci USA.* **101,** 3456–3461.

Huang, X., Atwood, C. S., Moir, R. D., Hartshorn, M. A., Tanzi, R. E., and Bush, A. I. (2004c). Trace metal contamination initiates the apparent auto-aggregation, amyloidosis, and oligomerization of Alzheimer's Abeta peptides. *J Biol Inorg Chem.* **9,** 954–960.

Hublin, J. J., Spoor, F., Braun, M., Zonneveld, F., and Condemi, S. (1996). A late Neanderthal associated with Upper Palaeolithic artefacts. *Nature.* **381,** 224–226.

Huby, T., Dachet, C., Lawn, R. M., Wickings, J., Chapman, M. J., and Thillet, J. (2001). Functional analysis of the chimpanzee and human apo(a) promoter sequences: Identification of sequence variations responsible for elevated transcriptional activity in chimpanzee. *J Biol Chem.* **276,** 22209–22214.

Hudson, B. I., Harja, E., Moser, B., and Schmidt, A. M. (2005). Soluble levels of receptor for advanced glycation endproducts (sRAGE) and coronary artery disease: The next C-reactive protein? *Arterioscler Thromb Vasc Biol.* **25,** 879–882.

Hughes, J. F., Skaletsky, H., Pyntikova, T., Minx, P. J., Graves, T., Rozen, S., Wilson, R. K., and Page, D. C. (2005). Conservation of Y-linked genes during human evolution revealed by comparative sequencing in chimpanzee. *Nature.* **437,** 100–103.

Hujoel, P., Drangsholt, M., Spiekerman, C., and DeRouen, T. (2000). Periodontitis: Systemic disease associations in the presence of smoking: Causal or coincidental? *Periodontology.* **30,** 51–60.

Hukshorn, C. J., Lindeman, J. H., Toet, K. H., Saris, W. H., Eilers, P. H., Westerterp-Plantenga, M. S., and Kooistra, T. (2004). Leptin and the proinflammatory state associated with human obesity. *J Clin Endocrinol Metab.* **89,** 1773–1778.

Hulbert, A. J., Faulks, S. C., Buffenstein, R. (2006). Oxidation-resistant membrane phospholipids can explain longevity differences among the longest-living rodents and similarly-sized mice. *J Gerontol A Biol Sci Med Sci.* **61,** 1009–1018.

Hummel, K. P., and Barnes, L. L. (1938). Calcification of the aorta, heart and kidneys of the albino rat. *Am J Pathol.* **14,** 121.

Humphreys, E. M. (1957). The occurrence of atheromatous lesions in the coronary arteries of rats. *Quarterly J Exp Physiol Cognate Med Sci.* **42,** 96–103.

Hunt, N. H., Manduci, N., and Thumwood, C. M. (1993). Amelioration of murine cerebral malaria by dietary restriction. *Parasitology.* **107,** 471–476.

Hunter, R. J., Patel, V. B., Miell, J. P., Wong, H. J., Marway, J. S., Richardson, P. J., and Preedy, V. R. (2001). Diarrhea reduces the rates of cardiac protein synthesis in myofibrillar protein fractions in rats *in vivo. J Nutr.* **131,** 1513–1519.

Hunter, W. S., Croson, W. B., Bartke, A., Gentry, M. V., Meliska, C. J. (1999). Low body temperature in long-lived Ames dwarf mice at rest and during stress. *Physiol Behav.* **67,** 433–437.

Huppert, F. A., Pinto, E. M., Morgan, K., and Brayne, C. (2003). Survival in a population sample is predicted by proportions of lymphocyte subsets. *Mech Ageing Dev.* **124,** 449–451.

Hurme, M., Lehtimaki, T., Jylha, M., Karhunen, P. J., and Hervonen, A. (2005). Interleukin-6-174G/C polymorphism and longevity: A follow-up study. *Mech Ageing Dev.* **126,** 417–418.

Hurst, G. D., Johnson, A. P., Schulenburg, J. H., Fuyama, Y. (2000). Male-killing Wolbachia in Drosophila: a temperature-sensitive trait with a threshold bacterial density. *Genetics.* **156,** 699–709.

Huxley, R., Owen, C. G., Whincup, P. H., Cook, D. G., Colman, S., and Collins, R. (2004). Birth weight and subsequent cholesterol levels: Exploration of the "fetal origins" hypothesis. *JAMA.* **292,** 2755–2764.

Huxley, R. R., Shiell, A. W., and Law, C. M. (2000). The role of size at birth and postnatal catch-up growth in determining systolic blood pressure: A systematic review of the literature. *J Hypertens.* **18,** 815–831.

Hwangbo, D. S., Gersham, B., Tu, M. P., Palmer, M., and Tatar, M. (2004). *Drosophila* dFoxO controls lifespan and regulates insulin signalling in brain and fat body. *Nature.* **429,** 562–566.

Ibrahim, Y. H., and Yee, D. (2005). Insulin-like growth factor-I and breast cancer therapy. *Clin Cancer Res.* **11,** 944s–950s.

Igarashi, A., Kikuchi, S., Konno, S., and Olmarker, K. (2004). Inflammatory cytokines released from the facet joint tissue in degenerative lumbar spinal disorders. *Spine.* **29,** 2091–2095.

Ikeno, Y., Bronson, R. T., Hubbard, G. B., Lee, S., and Bartke, A. (2003). Delayed occurrence of fatal neoplastic diseases in Ames dwarf mice: Correlation to extended longevity. *J Gerontol. Series A, Biol Sci Med Sci.* **58,** 291–296.

Ikeya, T., Galic, M., Belawat, P., Nairz, K., and Hafen, E. (2002). Nutrient-dependent expression of insulin-like peptides from neuroendocrine cells in the CNS contributes to growth regulation in *Drosophila. Curr Biol.* **12(15),** 1293–1300.

Ikonen, V. (1990). Kahden kotitalouden kulutus: 1860–Iuvlla. In M. Peltonen, Ed., *Arki Ja Murros*, pp. 35–50. Helsinki, Suomen Historiallinen Seura.

Imae, M., Fu, Z., Yoshida, A., Noguchi, T., and Kato, H. (2003). Nutritional and hormonal factors control the gene expression of FoxOs, the mammalian homologues of DAF-16. *J Mol Endocrinol.* **30,** 253–262.

Imanishi, T., Hano, T., and Nishio, I. (2005a). Angiotensin II accelerates endothelial progenitor cell senescence through induction of oxidative stress. *J Hypertension.* **23,** 97–104.

Imanishi, T., Hano, T., and Nishio, I. (2005b). Estrogen reduces endothelial progenitor cell senescence through augmentation of telomerase activity. *J Hypertension.* **23,** 1699–1706.

Imbimbo, B. P. (2004). The potential role of non-steroidal anti-inflammatory drugs in treating Alzheimer's disease. *Expert Opin Investig Drugs.* **13,** 1469–1481.

Imperial, J. C. (1999). Natural history of chronic hepatitis B and C. *J Gastroenterol Hepatol.* **14,** S1–5.

in t' Veld, B. A., Ruitenberg, A., Hofman, A., Launer, L. J., van Duijn, C. M., Stijnen, T., Breteler, M. M., and Stricker, B. H. (2001). Nonsteroidal antiinflammatory drugs and the risk of Alzheimer's disease. *New Engl J Med.* **345,** 1515–1521.

Infante-Rivard, C., Levy, E., Rivard, G. E., Guiguet, M., and Feoli-Fonseca, J. C. (2003). Small babies receive the cardiovascular protective apolipoprotein epsilon 2 allele less frequently than expected. *J Med Genet.* **40,** 626–629.

Lizarralde, G., and Veldhuis, J. D. (1991). Age and relative adiposity are specific negative determinants of the frequency and amplitude of growth hormone secretory bursts and half life of endogenous GH in healthy men. *J. Clin. Endocrinol. Metab.* **73,** 1081–1088.

Isacson, O., Seo, H., Lin, L., Albeck, D., and Granholm, A. C. (2002). Alzheimer's disease and Down's syndrome: Roles of APP, trophic factors and ACh. *Trends Neurosci.* **25,** 79–84.

Isenovic, E. R., Meng, Y., Divald, A., Milivojevic, N., Sowers, J. R. (2002). Role of phosphatidylinositol 3-kinase/Akt pathway in angiotensin II and insulin-like growth factor-1 modulation of nitric oxide synthase in vascular smooth muscle cells. *Endocrine.* **19,** 287–292.

Isenovic, E. R., Meng, Y., Jamali, N., Milivojevic, N., Sowers, J. R. (2004). Ang II attenuates IGF-1-stimulated Na+, K(+)-ATPase activity via PI3K/Akt pathway in vascular smooth muscle cells. *Int J Mol Med.* **13,** 915–922.

Ishihara, K., and Hirano, T. (2002). IL-6 in autoimmune disease and chronic inflammatory proliferative disease. *Cytokine Growth Factor Rev.* **13,** 357–368.

Ishii, T. (1958). Histochemistry of the senile changes of the brain of the senile dementia. *Psychiatr Neurol Jpn.* **60,** 768–781.

Isles, A. R., and Holland, A. J. (2005). Imprinted genes and mother-offspring interactions. *Early Hum Dev.* **81,** 73–77.

Itzhaki, R. (2004). Herpes simplex virus type 1, apolipoprotein E and Alzheimer' disease. *Herpes.* **11,** 77A–82A.

Itzhaki, R. F., Lin, W. R., Shang, D., Wilcock, G. K., Faragher, B., and Jamieson, G. A. (1997). Herpes simplex virus type 1 in brain and risk of Alzheimer's disease. *Lancet.* **349,** 241–244.

Itzkowitz, S. H., and Yio, X. (2004). Inflammation and cancer IV. Colorectal cancer in inflammatory bowel disease: The role of inflammation. *Am J Physiol—Gastrointes Liver Physiol.* **287,** G7–17.

Iwasa, M., Iwata, K., Kaito, M., Ikoma, J., Yamamoto, M., Takeo, M., Kuroda, M., Fujita, N., Kobayashi, Y., and Adachi, Y. (2004). Efficacy of long-term dietary restriction of total calories, fat, iron, and protein in patients with chronic hepatitis C virus. *Nutrition.* **20,** 368–371.

Iwasaki, K., Gleiser, C. A., Masoro, E. J., McMahan, C. A., Seo, E. J., and Yu, B. P. (1988a). The influence of dietary protein source on longevity and age-related disease processes of Fischer rats. *J Gerontol.* **43,** B5–12.

Iwasaki, K., Gleiser, C. A., Masoro, E. J., McMahan, C. A., Seo, E. J., and Yu, B. P. (1988b). Influence of the restriction of individual dietary components on longevity and age-related disease of Fischer rats: The fat component and the mineral component. *J Gerontol.* **43,** B13–21.

Izycka-Swieszewska, E., Zóltowska, A., Rzepko, R., Gross, M., and Borowska-Lehman, J. (2000). Vasculopathy and amyloid beta reactivity in brains of patients with acquired immune deficiency (AIDS). *Folia Neuropathol.* **38,** 172–182.

Jabs, W. J., Theissing, E., Nitschke, M., Bechtel, J. F., Duchrow, M., Mohamed, S., Jahrbeck, B., Sievers, H. H., Steinhoff, J., and Bartels, C. (2003). Local generation of C-reactive protein in diseased coronary artery venous bypass grafts and normal vascular tissue. *Circulation.* **108,** 1428–1431.

Jackman, R. W., and Kandarian, S. C. (2004). The molecular basis of skeletal muscle atrophy. *Am J Physiol. Cell Physiology.* **287,** C834–843.

Jackson, A. U., Galecki, A. T., Burke, D. T., and Miller, R. A. (2002). Mouse loci associated with life span exhibit sex-specific and epistatic effects. *J Gerontol. Series A, Biol Sci Med Sci.* **57,** B9–B15.

Jackson, G. S., Beck, J. A., Navarrete, C., Brown, J., Sutton, P. M., Contreras, M., et al. (2001). HLA-DQ7 antigen and resistance to variant CJD. *Nature.* **15,** 269–270.

Jacoby, R. O., and Lindsey, J. R. (1997). Health care for research animals is essential and affordable. *FASEB J.* **11,** 609–614.

Jagielo, P. J., Thorne, P. S., Watt, J. L., Frees, K. L., Quinn, T. J., and Schwartz, D. A. (1996). Grain dust and endotoxin inhalation challenges produce similar inflammatory responses in normal subjects. *Chest.* **110,** 263–270.

Jagust, W. (2001). Untangling vascular dementia. *Lancet.* **358,** 2097–2098.

Jain, A., Batista, E. L. J., Serhan, C., Stahl, G. L., and Van Dyke, T. E. (2003). Role for periodontitis in the progression of lipid deposition in an animal model. *Infect Immun.* **71,** 6012–6018.

Jankowsky, J. L., Fadale, D. J., Anderson, J., Xu, G. M., Gonzales, V., Jenkins, N. A., Copeland, N. G., Lee, M. K., Younkin, L. H., Wagner, S. L., Younkin, S. G., and Borchelt, D. R. (2004). Mutant presenilins specifically elevate the levels of the 42 residue beta-amyloid peptide *in vivo*: Evidence for augmentation of a 42-specific gamma secretase. *Human Molecular Genetics.* **13(2),** 159–170.

Jankowsky, J. L., Melnikova, T., Fadale, D. J., Xu, G. M., Slunt, H. H., Gonzales, V., Younkin, L. H., Younkin, S. G., Borchelt, D. R., and Savonenko, A. V. (2005a). Environmental enrichment mitigates cognitive deficits in a mouse model of Alzheimer's disease. *J Neurosci.* **25(21),** 5217–5224.

Jankowsky, J. L., Melnikova, T., Fadale, D. J., Xu, G. M., Slunt, H. H., Gonzales, V., Younkin, L. H., Younkin, S. G., Borchelt, D. R., Savonenko, A. V. (2005b). Environmental enrichment mitigates cognitive deficits in a mouse model of Alzheimer's disease. *J Neurosci.* **25,** 5217–24.

Jankowsky, J. L., Xu, G., Fromholt, D., Gonzales, V., and Borchelt, D. R (2003). Environmental enrichment exacerbates amyloid plaque formation in a transgenic mouse model of Alzheimer disease. *J Neuropathol Exp Neurol.* **62,** 1220–1227.

Jans, D. M., Martinet, W., Fillet, M., Kockx, M. M., Merville, M. P., Bult, H., Herman, A. G., and De Meyer, G. R. (2004). Effect of non-steroidal anti-inflammatory drugs on amyloid-beta formation and macrophage activation after platelet phagocytosis. *J Cardiovascular Pharmacology.* **43,** 462–470.

Janssens, J. P., and Krause, K. H. (2004). Pneumonia in the very old. *Lancet Infect Dis.* **4,** 112–124.

Jansson, T., Cetin, I., Powell, T. L., Desoye, G., Radaelli, T., Ericsson, A., and Sibley, C. P. (2006a). Placental transport and metabolism in fetal overgrowth—A workshop report. *Placenta.* **27(Suppl A),** S109–113.

Jansson, T., and Powell, T. L. (2006b). IFPA 2005 Award in Placentology Lecture. Human placental transport in altered fetal growth: Does the placenta function as a nutrient sensor? A review. *Placenta.* **27(Suppl A),** S91–97.

Jauniaux, E., Poston, L., and Burton, G. J. (2006). Placental-related diseases of pregnancy: Involvement of oxidative stress and implications in human evolution. *Hum Reprod Update*. **12**, 747–755.

Jazwinski, S. M., Egilmez, N. K., Chen, J. B. (1989). Replication control and cellular life span. *Exp Gerontol*. **24**, 423–436.

Jenkins, N. L., McColl, G., and Lithgow, G. J. (2004). Fitness cost of extended lifespan in *Caenorhabditis elegans*. *Proc Biol Sci*. **271**, 2523–2526.

Jenkinson, M. L., Bliss, M. R., Brain, A. T., and Scott, D. L. (1989). Rheumatoid arthritis and senile dementia of the Alzheimer's type. *Br J Rheumatology*. **28**, 86–88.

Jezek, P., and Hlavata, L. (2005). Mitochondria in homeostasis of reactive oxygen species in cell, tissues, and organism. *Int J Biochem Cell Biol*. **37**, 2478–2503.

Jeziorska, M., McCollum, C., and Woolley, D. E. (1998). Calcification in atherosclerotic plaque of human carotid arteries: Associations with mast cells and macrophages. *J Pathol*. **185(1)**, 10–17.

Ji, Y., Gong, Y., Gan, W., Beach, T., Holtzman, D. M., and Wisniewski, T. (2003). Apolipoprotein E isoform-specific regulation of dendritic spine morphology in apolipoprotein E transgenic mice and Alzheimer's disease patients. *Neuroscience*. **122**, 305–315.

Ji, Z. S., Mèullendorff, K., Cheng, I. H., Miranda, R. D., Huang, Y., and Mahley, R. W. (2006). Reactivity of apolipoprotein E4 and amyloid beta peptide: Lysosomal stability and neurodegeneration. *J Biol Chem*. **281**, 2683–2692.

Jia, K., Albert, P. S., and Riddle, D. L. (2002). DAF-9, a cytochrome P450 regulating *C. elegans* larval development and adult longevity. *Development*. **129**, 221–231.

Jia, K., Chen, D., and Riddle, D. L. (2004). The TOR pathway interacts with the insulin signaling pathway to regulate *C. elegans* larval development, metabolism and life span. *Development*. **131**, 3897–906.

Jiang, B., Godfrey, K. M., Martyn, C. N., and Gale, C. R. (2006). Birth weight and cardiac structure in children. *Pediatrics*. **117**, e257–61.

Jiang, Q., Lykkesfeldt, J., Shigenaga, M. K., Shigeno, E. T., Christen, S., and Ames, B. N. (2002). Gamma-tocopherol supplementation inhibits protein nitration and ascorbate oxidation in rats with inflammation. *Free Radic Biol Med*. **33**, 1534–1542.

Jiang, W., Zhu, Z., Bhatia, N., Agarwal, R., and Thompson, H. J. (2002b). Mechanisms of energy restriction: Effects of corticosterone on cell growth, cell cycle machinery, and apoptosis. *Cancer Res*. **62**, 5280–5287.

Jick, H., Zornberg, G. L., Jick, S. S., Seshadri, S., and Drachman, D. A. (2000). Statins and the risk of dementia. *Lancet*. **356**, 1627–1631.

Jilka, R. L., Hangoc, G., Girasole, G., Passeri, G., Williams, D. C., Abrams, J. S., Boyce, B., Broxmeyer, H., and Manolagas, S. C. (1992). Increased osteoclast development after estrogen loss: Mediation by interleukin-6. *Science*. **257**, 88–91.

Jing, H., and Kitts, D. D. (2002). Chemical and biochemical properties of casein-sugar Maillard reaction products. *Food Chem Toxicol*. **40**, 1007–1015.

Johnson, J., Bagley, J., Skaznik-Wikiel, M., Lee, H. J., Adams, G. B., Niikura, Y., Tschudy, K. S., Tilly, J. C., Cortes, M. L., Forkert, R., Spitzer, T., Iacomini, J., Scadden, D. T., and Tilly, J. L. (2005). Oocyte generation in adult mammalian ovaries by putative germ cells in bone marrow and peripheral blood. *Cell*. **122**, 303–315.

Johnson, R. W. (1998). Immune and endocrine regulation of food intake in sick animals. *Domest Anim Endocrinol*. **15**, 309–319.

Johnson, S. A., Lampert-Etchells, M., Pasinetti, G. M., Rozovsky, I., and Finch, C. E. (1992a). Complement mRNA in the mammalian brain: Responses to Alzheimer's disease and experimental brain lesioning. *Neurobiol Aging.* **13,** 641–648.

Johnson, S. A., Lampert-Etchells, M., Pasinetti, G. M., Rozovsky, I., Finch, C. E (1992b). Complement mRNA in the mammalian brain: responses to Alzheimer's disease and experimental brain lesioning. *Neurobiol Aging.* **13,** 641–8.

Johnson, T. E. (1987). Aging can be genetically dissected into component processes using long-lived lines of *Caenorhabditis elegans. Proc Natl Acad Sci USA.* **84,** 3777–3781.

Johnson, T. E. (1990). Increased life-span of age-1 mutants in *Caenorhabditis elegans* and lower Gompertz rate of aging. *Science.* **249,** 908–12.

Johnson, T. E. (2005). Genes, phenes, and dreams of immortality. The Kleeimeier Award Lecture. *J Gerontol A Biol Sci Med Sci.* **60,** 680–687.

Johnson, T. E., de Castro, E., Hegi de Castro, S., Cypser, J., Henderson, S., and Tedesco, P. (2001a). Relationship between increased longevity and stress resistance as assessed through gerontogene mutations in *Caenorhabditis elegans. Exp Gerontol.* **36,** 1609–1617.

Johnson, T. E., Wu, D., Tedesco, P., Dames, S., and Vaupel, J. W. (2001b). Age-specific demographic profiles of longevity mutants in *Caenorhabditis elegans* show segmental effects. *J Geronto. Series A, Biol Sci Med Sci.* **56,** B331–339.

Johnston, F. E., Malina, R. M., Galbraith, M. A., Frisch, R. E., Revelle, R., and Cook, S. (1971). Height, weight and age at menarche and the "critical weight" hypothesis. *Science.* **174,** 1148–1149.

Johnstone, E. M., Chaney, M. O., Norris, F. H., Pascual, R., and Little, S. P. (1991). Conservation of the sequence of the Alzheimer's disease amyloid peptide in dog, polar bear and five other mammals by cross-species polymerase chain reaction analysis. *Brain Res. Mol Brain Res.* **10,** 299–305.

Joint National Committee on Prevention, Detection, Evaluation, and Treatment of High Blood Pressure. (1997b). The sixth report of the Joint National Committee on Prevention, Detection, Evaluation, And Treatment of High Blood Pressure. *Arch Intern Med.* **157,** 2413–2446.

Jolly, M. C., Sebire, N. J., Harris, J. P., Regan, L., and Robinson, S. (2003). Risk factors for macrosomia and its clinical consequences: A study of 350,311 pregnancies. *Eur J Obstet Gynecol Reprod Biol.* **111,** 9–14.

Jonassen, T., Davis, D. E., Larsen, P. L., and Clarke, C. F. (2003). Reproductive fitness and quinone content of *Caenorhabditis elegans* clk-1 mutants fed coenzyme Q isoforms of varying length. *J Biol Chem.* **278,** 51735–51742.

Jones, H., B. (1956). A special consideration of the aging process, disease, and life expectancy. *Adv Biol Med Physics* **4,** 281–337.

Jones, R. D., Nettleship, J. E., Kapoor, D., Jones, H. T., and Channer, K. S. (2005). Testosterone and atherosclerosis in aging men: Purported association and clinical implications. *Am J Cardiovascular Drugs: Drugs, Devices, Other Interventions.* **5,** 141–154.

Jonsson, Y., Rubáer, M., Matthiesen, L., Berg, G., Nieminen, K., Sharma, S., Ernerudh, J., and Ekerfelt, C. (2006). Cytokine mapping of sera from women with preeclampsia and normal pregnancies. *J Reprod Immunol.* **70,** 83–91.

Jorm, A. F., and Jolley, D. (1998). The incidence of dementia: A meta-analysis. *Neurology.* **61,** 728–733.

Joseph, A., Ackerman, D., Talley, J. D., Johnstone, J., and Kupersmith, J. (1993). Manifestations of coronary atherosclerosis in young trauma victims—An autopsy study. *J Am Coll Cardiol.* **22,** 459–467.

Jukema, J. W., and Simoons, M. L. l. (1999). Treatment and prevention of coronary heart disease by lowering serum cholesterol levels; from the pioneer work of C.D. de Langen to the third "Dutch Consensus on Cholesterol." *Acta Cardiologica.* **54,** 163–168.

Jung, H. J., Hwang, I. A., Sung, W. S., Kang, H., Kang, B. S., Seu, Y. B., and Lee, D. G. (2005). Fungicidal effect of resveratrol on human infectious fungi. *Arch Pharm Res.* **28,** 557–560.

Juni, P., Nartey, L., Reichenbach, S., Sterchi, R., Dieppe, P. A., and Egger, M. (2004). Risk of cardiovascular events and rofecoxib: Cumulative meta-analysis. *Lancet.* **364,** 2021–2029.

Juvonen, J., Juvonen, T., Laurila, A., Kuusisto, J., Alarakkola, E., Sarkioja, T., Bodian, C. A., Kairaluoma, M. I., and Saikku, P. (1998). Can degenerative aortic valve stenosis be related to persistent *Chlamydia pneumoniae* infection? *Ann Intern Med.* **128,** 741–744.

Jylha, M., Volpato, S., and Guralnik, J. M. (2006). Self-rated health showed a graded association with frequently used biomarkers in a large population sample. *J Clin Epidemiol.* **59,** 465–471.

Kaaks, R., Lukanova, A., and Kurzer, M. S., (2002). Obesity, endogenous hormones, and endometrial cancer risk: A synthetic review. *Cancer Epidemiol Biomarkers Prev.* **11,** 1531–1543.

Kaati, G., Bygren, L. O., and Edvinsson, S. (2002). Cardiovascular and diabetes mortality determined by nutrition during parents' and grandparents' slow growth period. *Eur J Hum Genet.* **10(11),** 682–688.

Kabir, M., Catalano, K. J., Ananthnarayan, S., Kim, S. P., Van Citters, G. W., Dea, M. K., and Bergman, R. N. (2005). Molecular evidence supporting the portal theory: A causative link between visceral adiposity and hepatic insulin resistance. *Am J Physiol. Endocrinol Metab.* **288,** E454–461.

Kahn, B. B., Alquier, T., Carling, D., and Hardie, D. G. (2005). AMP-activated protein kinase: anCient energy gauge provides clues to modern understanding of metabolism. *Cell Metab.* **1,** 15–25.

Kakisis, J. D., Liapis, C. D., and Sumpio, B. E. (2005). Effects of cyclic strain on vascular cells. *Endothelium.* **11,** 17–28.

Kalanda, B. F., van Buuren, S., Verhoeff, F. H., and Brabin, B. J. (2005). Anthropometry of fetal growth in rural Malawi in relation to maternal malaria and HIV status. *Archives of Disease in Childhood Fetal & Neonatal Edition.* **90,** F161–165.

Kalayoglu, M. V., Libby, P., and Byrne, G. I. (2002). *Chlamydia pneumoniae* as an emerging risk factor in cardiovascular disease. *JAMA.* **288,** 2724–2731.

Kalback, W., Esh, C., Castaño, E. M., Rahman, A., Kokjohn, T., Luehrs, D. C., Sue, L., Cisneros, R., Gerber, F., Richardson, C., Bohrmann, B., Walker, D. G., Beach, T. G., and Roher, A. E. (2004). Atherosclerosis, vascular amyloidosis and brain hypoperfusion in the pathogenesis of sporadic Alzheimer's disease. *Neurol Res.* **26,** 525–539.

Kalinkovich, A., Borkow, G., Weisman, Z., Tsimanis, A., Stein, M., and Bentwich, Z. (2001). Increased CCR5 and CXCR4 expression in Ethiopians living in Israel: Environmental and constitutive factors. *Clin Immunol.* **100,** 107–117.

Kalinkovich, A., Weisman, Z., Greenberg, Z., Nahmias, J., Eitan, S., Stein, M., and Bentwich, Z. (1998). Decreased CD4 and increased CD8 counts with T cell activation is associated with chronic helminth infection. *Clin Exp Immunol.* **114,** 414–21.

Kalm, L. M., and Semba, R. D. (2005). They starved so that others be better fed: Remembering Ancel Keys and the Minnesota experiment. *J Nutr.* **135,** 1347–1352.

Kalu, D. N., Masoro, E. J., Yu, B. P., Hardin, R. R., and Hollis, B. W. (1988). Modulation of age-related hyperparathyroidism and senile bone loss in Fischer rats by soy protein and food restriction. *Endocrinology.* **122,** 1847–1854.

Kamal, A., Stokin, G. B., Yang, Z., Xia, C. H., and Goldstein, L. S. (2000). Axonal transport of amyloid precursor protein is mediated by direct binding to the kinesin light chain subunit of kinesin-I. *Neuron.* **28,** 449–459.

Kamalvand, G., and Ali-Khan, Z. (2004). Immunolocalization of lipid peroxidation/advanced glycation end products in amyloid A amyloidosis. *Free Radic Biol Med.* **36,** 657–664.

Kamenetz, F., Tomita, T., Hsieh, H., Seabrook, G., Borchelt, D., Iwatsubo, T., Sisodia, S., and Malinow, R. (2003). APP processing and synaptic function. *Neuron.* **37,** 925–937.

Kamiyama, M., Utsunomiya, K., Taniguchi, K., Yokota, T., Kurata, H., Tajima, N., and Kondo, K. (2003). Contribution of Rho A and Rho kinase to platelet-derived growth factor-BB-induced proliferation of vascular smooth muscle cells. *J Atheroscl Thromb.* **10,** 117–123.

Kaneda, A., and Feinberg, A. P. (2005). Loss of imprinting of IGF2: A common epigenetic modifier of intestinal tumor risk. *Cancer Res.* **65,** 11236–11240.

Kang, I., Hong, M. S., Nolasco, H., Park, S. H., Dan, J. M., Choi, J. Y., and Craft, J. (2004). Age-associated change in the frequency of memory CD4+ T cells impairs long term CD4+ T cell responses to influenza vaccine. *J Immunol.* **173,** 673–681.

Kang, S., Bader, A. G., Zhao, L., and Vogt, P. K. (2005). Mutated PI 3-kinases: Cancer targets on a silver platter. *Cell Cycle.* **4,** 578–581.

Kannisto, V., Christensen, K., and Vaupel, J. W. (1997). No increased mortality in later life for cohorts born during famine. *Am J Epidemiol.* **145,** 987–994.

Kapahi, P., Boulton, M. E., and Kirkwood, T. B. (1999). Positive correlation between mammalian life span and cellular resistance to stress. *Free Radic Biol Med.* **26,** 495–500.

Kapahi, P., Zid, B. M., Harper, T., Koslover, D., Sapin, V., and Benzer, S. (2004). Regulation of lifespan in *Drosophila* by modulation of genes in the TOR signaling pathway. *Curr Biol.* **14(10),** 885–890.

Kaplan, H., Hill, K., Lancaster, J., and Hurtado, A. M. (2000). A theory of human life hsitory evolution. Diet, intelligence, and longevity. *Evol Anthropol.* **9,** 165–185.

Kaplan, H. S., and Robson, A. J. (2002). The emergence of humans: The coevolution of intelligence and longevity with intergenerational transfers. *Proc Natl Acad Sci USA.* **99,** 10221–10226.

Kaplanski, G., Marin, V., Montero-Julian, F., Mantovani, A., and Farnarier, C. (2003). IL-6: A regulator of the transition from neutrophil to monocyte recruitment during inflammation. *Trends Immunol.* **24,** 25–29.

Kappelman, J. (1997). They might have been giants. *Nature.* **387,** 126–127.

Karam, J. H. (1996). Reversible insulin resistance in non-insulin-dependent diabetes mellitus. *Hormone Metab Res.* **28,** 440–444.

Karaman, M. W., Houck, M. L., Chemnick, L. G., Nagpal, S., Chawannakul, D., Sudano, D. et al. (2003). Comparative analysis of gene-expression patterns in human and African great ape cultured fibroblasts. *Genome Res.* **13,** 1619–1630.

Karasik, D., Demissie, S., Cupples, L. A., and Kiel, D. P. (2005). Disentangling the genetic determinants of human aging: Biological age as an alternative to the use of survival measures. *J Gerontol. Series A, Biol Sci Med Sci.* **60,** 574–587.

Kari, F., Hatch, G., Slade, R., Crissman, K., Simeonova, P. P., and Luster, M. (1997). Dietary restriction mitigates ozone-induced lung inflammation in rats: A role for endogenous antioxidants. *Am J Respir Cell Mol Biol.* **17,** 740–747.

Kari, F. W., Dunn, S. E., French, J. E., and Barrett, J. C. (1999). Roles for insulin-like growth factor-1 in mediating the anti-carcinogenic effects of caloric restriction. *J Nutr Health Aging.* **3,** 92–101.

Karim, R., Mack, W. J., Lobo, R. A., Hwang, J., Liu, C. R., Liu, C. H., Sevanian, A., and Hodis, H. N. (2005). Determinants of the effect of estrogen on the progression of subclinical atherosclerosis: Estrogen in the Prevention of Atherosclerosis Trial. *Menopause.* **12,** 366–373.

Karn, M. N., and Penrose, L. S. (1952). Birth weight and gestation time in relation to maternal age, parity and infant survival. *Ann Eugen.* **16,** 147–164.

Karra, R., Vemullapalli, S., Dong, C., Herderick, E. E., Song, X., Slosek, K., Nevins, J. R., West, M., Goldschmidt-Clermont, P. J., and Seo, D. (2005). Molecular evidence for arterial repair in atherosclerosis. *PNAS.* **102,** 16789–16794.

Kass, D. H., Batzer, M. A., and Deininger, P. L. (1995). Gene conversion as a secondary mechanism of short interspersed element (SINE) evolution. *Mol Cell Biol.* **15,** 19–25.

Kass, D. H., Knight, A., and Deininger, P. L. (2004). Evolution of a hypervariable region of the low density lipoprotein receptor (LDLR) gene in humans and other hominoids. *Genetica.* **121,** 187–193.

Kastrati, A., Dibra, A., Mehilli, J., Mayer, S., Pinieck, S., Pache, J., Dirschinger, J., and Schomig, A. (2006). Predictive factors of restenosis after coronary implantation of sirolimus- or paclitaxel-Eluting stents. *Circulation.* **113,** 2293–3000.

Katic, M., and Kahn, C. R. (2005). The role of insulin and IGF-1 signaling in longevity. *Cell Mol Life Sci.* **62,** 320–343.

Katzel, L. I., Fleg, J. L., Paidi, M., Ragoobarsingh, N., and Goldberg, A. P. (1993). ApoE4 polymorphism increases the risk for exercise-induced silent myocardial ischemia in older men. *Arterioscler Thromb.* **13,** 1495–1500.

Kaushik, C. P., Ravindra, K., Yadav, K., Mehta, S., and Haritash, A. K. (2006). Assessment of ambient air quality in urban centres of Haryana (India) in relation to different anthropogenic activities and health risks. *Environ Monit Assess.* **122,** 27–40.

Kawai, M., Kalaria, R. N., Harik, S. I., and Perry, G. (1990). The relationship of amyloid plaques to cerebral capillaries in Alzheimer's disease. *Am J Pathol.* **137,** 1435–1446.

Kawamura, S., Takahashi, M., Ishihara, T., and Uchino, F. (1995). Incidence and distribution of isolated atrial amyloid: Histologic and immunohistochemical studies of 100 aging hearts. *Pathol Internat.* **45,** 335–342.

Kawas, C. H., and Katzman, R. (1999). Epidemiology of dementia and Alzheimer disease. In J. Morris, R. Terry, R. Katzman, K. Bick, and S. Sisodia, Eds., *Alzheimer disease,* pp. 95–116. Philadelphia: Lippincott Williams & Wilkins.

Kay, M. M., Mendoza, J., Hausman, S., and Dorsey, B. (1979). Age-related changes in the immune system of mice of eight medium and long-lived strains and hybrids. II. Short- and long-term effects of natural infection with parainfluenza type 1 virus (*Sendai*). *Mech Ageing Dev.* **11,** 347–362.

Kayed, R., Head, E., Thompson, J. L., McIntire, T. M., Milton, S. C., Cotman, C. W., and Glabe, C. G. (2003). Common structure of soluble amyloid oligomers implies common mechanism of pathogenesis. [see comment]. *Science.* **300,** 486–489.

Kazui, H., and Fujisawa, K. (1988). Radiculoneuropathy of ageing rats: A quantitative study. *Neuropath Appl Neurobiol.* **14,** 137–156.

Keaney, J. F., Jr., Larson, M. G., Vasan, R. S., Wilson, P. W., Lipinska, I., Corey, D., Massaro, J. M., Sutherland, P., Vita, J. A., and Benjamin, E. J. (2003). Obesity and systemic oxidative stress: Clinical correlates of oxidative stress in the Framingham Study. *Arterioscler Thromb Vasc Biol.* **23,** 434–439.

Kearney, P. M., Baigent, C., Godwin, J., Halls, H., Emberson, J. R., and Patrono, C., (2006). Do selective cyclo-oxygenase-2 inhibitors and traditional non-steroidal anti-inflammatory drugs increase the risk of atherothrombosis? Meta-analysis of randomised trials. *Br Med J.* **332,** 1302–1308.

Keith, S. W., Redden, D. T., Katzmarzyk, P. T., Boggiano, M. M., Hanlon, E. C., Benca, R. M., Ruden, D., Pietrobelli, A., Barger, J. L., Fontaine, K. R., Wang, C., Aronne, L. J., Wright, S. M., Baskin, M., Dhurandhar, N. V., Lijoi, M. C., Grilo, C. M., DeLuca, M., Westfall, A. O., and Allison, D. B. (2006). Putative contributors to the secular increase in obesity: Exploring the roads less traveled. *Int J Obes.* **30,** 1585–1594.

Kelberman, D., Fife, M., Rockman, M. V., Brull, D. J., Woo, P., and Humphries, S. E. K. (2004). Analysis of common IL-6 promoter SNP variants and the AnTn tract in humans and primates and effects on plasma IL-6 levels following coronary artery bypass graft surgery. *Biochim Biophys Acta.* **1688,** 160–167.

Kelley, J. L., Chi, D. S., Abou-Auda, W., Smith, J. K., Krishnaswamy, G. (2000). The molecular role of mast cells in atherosclerotic cardiovascular disease. *Molec Med Today.* **6,** 304–308.

Kemna, E., Pickkers, P., Nemeth, E., van der Hoeven, H., and Swinkels, D. (2005). Time-course analysis of hepcidin, serum iron, and plasma cytokine levels in humans injected with LPS. *Blood* **106(5),** 1864–1866.

Kemper, T. (1984). Neuroanatomical and neuropathological changes in normal aging and in dementia. In M. L. Albert, Ed., *Clinical neurology of aging,* pp. 9–52. New York: Oxford University Press.

Kempermann, G., Gast, D., Gage, F. H. (2002). Neuroplasticity in old age: sustained five-fold induction of hippocampal neurogenesis by long-term environmental enrichment. *Anal Neurol.* **52,** 135–143.

Kennedy, G. E. (2005). From the ape's dilemma to the weanling's dilemma: early weaning and its evolutionary context. *J Hum Biol.* **48,** 123–145.

Kennedy, B. K., Austriaco, N. R., Zhang, J., Guarente, L. (1995). Mutation in the silencing gene SIR4 can delay aging in S. cerevisiae. *Cell.* **80,** 485–496.

Kenyon, C. (2001). A conserved regulatory system for aging. *Cell.* **105,** 165–168.

Kenyon, C. (2005). The plasticity of aging: Insights from long-lived mutants. *Cell.* **120,** 449–460.

Kermack, W. O., McKendrick, A. G., and McKinlay, P. L. (1934). Death-rates in Great Britain and Sweden. Some general regularities and their significance. *Lancet.* **30,** 698–703.

Kety, S. S. (1956). Human cerebral blood flow and oxygen consumption as related to aging. *Chronic Dis.* **3,** 478–486.

Keyes, W. M., and Mills, A. A. (2006). p63: A new link between senescence and aging. *Cell Cycle.* **5(3),** 260–265.

Keyes, W. M., Wu, Y., Vogel, H., Guo, X., Lowe, S. W., and Mills, A. A. (2005). p63 deficiency activates a program of cellular senescence and leads to accelerated aging. *Genes Dev.* **19(17),** 1986–1999.

Keys, A. (1994). 1944 symposium on convalescence and rehabilitation. *FASEB J.* **8,** 1201–1202.

Keys, A., Brozek, J., Henschel, A., Mickelson, O., and Taylor, H. L. (1950). *The biology of human starvation.* Minneapolis: University of Minnesota Press.

Khachaturian, A. S., Corcoran, C. D., Mayer, L. S., Zandi, P. P., and Breitner, J. C. (2004). Apolipoprotein E epsilon4 count affects age at onset of Alzheimer disease, but not life-time susceptibility: The Cache County Study. *Arch Gen Psychiatry.* **61,** 518–524.

Khachaturian, Z. S. (1985). Diagnosis of Alzheimer's disease. *Arch Neurol.* **42,** 1097–1105.

Khan, A. S., Sane, D. C., Wannenburg, T., and Sonntag, W. E. (2002a). Growth hormone, insulin-like growth factor-1 and the aging cardiovascular system. *Cardiovasc Res.* **54,** 25–35.

Khan, N., Hislop, A., Gudgeon, N., Cobbold, M., Khanna, R., Nayak, L., Rickinson, A. B., and Moss, P. A. (2004). Herpesvirus-specific CD8 T cell immunity in old age: Cytomegalovirus impairs the response to a coresident EBV infection. *J Immunol.* **173,** 7481–7489.

Khan, N., Shariff, N., Cobbold, M., Bruton, R., Ainsworth, J. A., Sinclair, A. J., Nayak, L., and Moss, P. A. (2002b). Cytomegalovirus seropositivity drives the CD8 T cell repertoire toward greater clonality in healthy elderly individuals. *J Immunol.* **169,** 1984–1992.

Khazaeli, A. A., Tatar, M., Pletcher, S. D., and Curtsinger, J. W. (1997). Heat-induced longevity extension in *Drosophila*. I. Heat treatment, mortality, and thermotolerance. *J Gerontol. A Biol Sci Med Sci.* **52,** B48–B52.

Khazaeli, A. A., Xiu, L., and Curtsinger, J. W. (1995). Effect of adult cohort density on age-specific mortality in *Drosophila melanogaster. J Gerontol. A Biol Sci Med Sci.* **50,** B262–269.

Khovidhunkit, W., Kim, M. S., Memon, R. A., Shigenaga, J. K., Moser, A. H., Feingold, K. R., and Grunfeld, C. (2004). Effects of infection and inflammation on lipid and lipopro-tein metabolism: Mechanisms and consequences to the host. *J Lipid Res.* **45,** 1169–1196.

Khurad, A. M., Mahulikar, A., Rathod, M. K., Rai, M. M., Kanginakudru, S., and Nagaraju, J. (2004). Vertical transmission of nucleopolyhedrovirus in the silkworm, *Bombyx mori L. J Invertebr Pathol.* **87,** 8–15.

Kidd, M. (1964). Alzheimer's disease—An electron microscopical study. *Brain.* **87,** 307–320.

Kieper, W. C., Troy, A., Burghardt, J. T., Ramsey, C., Lee, J. Y., Jiang, H. Q., Dummer, W., Shen, H., Cebra, J. J., and Surh, C. D. (2005). Recent immune status determines the source of antigens that drive homeostatic T cell expansion. *J Immunol.* **174,** 3158–3163.

Kikafunda, J. K., Walker, A. F., Collett, D., and Tumwine, J. K. (1998). Risk factors for early childhood malnutrition in Uganda. *Pediatrics.* **102,** E45.

Kikugawa, K. (2004). Prevention of mutagen formation in heated meats and model systems. *Mutagenesis.* **19,** 431–439.

Kim, D. H., and Ausubel, F. M. (2005). Evolutionary perspectives on innate immunity from the study of *Caenorhabditis elegans. Curr Opin Immunol.* **17,** 4–10.

Kim, D. H., Feinbaum, R., Alloing, G., Emerson, F. E., Garsin, D. A., Inoue, H., Tanaka-Hino, M., Hisamoto, N., Matsumoto, K., Tan, M. W., and Ausubel, F. M. (2002). A conserved p38 MAP kinase pathway in *Caenorhabditis elegans* innate immunity. *Science.* **297,** 623–626.

Kim, H., Kadowaki, H., Sakura, H., Odawara, M., Momomura, K., Takahashi, Y., Miyazaki, Y., Ohtani, T., Akanuma, Y., Yazaki, Y., Kasuga, M., Taylor, S.I., and Kadowaki, T. (1992). Detection of mutations in the insulin receptor gene in patients with insulin resistance by analysis of single-stranded conformational polymorphisms. *Diabetologia.* **35,** 261–266.

Kim, H. J., Jung, K. J., Yu, B. P., Cho, C. G., Choi, J. S., and Chung, H. Y. (2002). Modulation of redox-sensitive transcription factors by calorie restriction during aging. *Mech Ageing Dev.* **123,** 1589–1595.

Kim, J. D., Yu, B. P., McCarter, R. J., Lee, S. Y., and Herlihy, J. T., (1996). Exercise and diet modulate cardiac lipid peroxidation and antioxidant defenses. *Free Radic Biol Med.* **20(1),** 83–88.

Kim, S., H, and Reaven, G. M. (2004). The metabolic syndrome: One step forward, two steps back. *Diab Vasc Dis Res.* **1,** 68–75.

Kim, S. K., and Rulifson, E. J. (2004). Conserved mechanisms of glucose sensing and regulation by *Drosophila corpora cardiaca* cells. *Nature.* **431,** 316–320.

Kim, Y. P., Kim, H., Shin, M. S., Chang, H. K., Jang, M. H., Shin, M. C., Lee, S. J., Lee, H. H., Yoon, J. H., Jeong, I. G., and Kim, C. J. (2004). Age-dependence of the effect of treadmill exercise on cell proliferation in the dentate gyrus of rats. *Neuroscience Lett.* **355,** 152–154.

Kim, Y. S., Nam, H. J., Chung, H. Y., Kim, N. D., Ryu, J. H., Lee, W. J., Arking, R., and Yoo, M. A. (2001). Role of xanthine dehydrogenase and aging on the innate immune response of *Drosophila. J Am Aging Assoc.* **24,** 187–193.

Kimberly, W. T., Zheng, J. B., Town, T., Flavell, R. A., and Selkoe, D. J. (2005). Physiological regulation of the beta-amyloid precursor protein signaling domain by c-Jun N-terminal kinase JNK3 during neuronal differentiation. *J Neurosci.* **25,** 5533–5543.

Kimura, K. D., Tissenbaum, H. A., Liu, Y., and Ruvkun, G. (1997). *daf-2,* an insulin receptor-like gene that regulates longevity and diapause in *Caenorhabditis elegans. Science.* **277,** 942–946.

King, A. E., Fleming, D. C., Critchley, H. O., and Kelly, R. W. (2003). Differential expression of the natural antimicrobials, beta-defensins 3 and 4, in human endometrium. *J Reprod Immunol.* **59(1),** 1–16.

King, J. C. (2006). Maternal obesity, metabolism, and pregnancy outcomes. *Annu Rev Nutr.* **26,** 271–291.

King, V., and Tower, J. (1999). Aging-specific expression of Drosophila hsp22. Developmental Biology. **207(1),** 107–118.

Kirk, K. L. (2000). New paradigms of CFTR chloride channel regulation. *Cell Mol Life Sci.* **57,** 623–634.

Kirkwood, T. B., Feder, M., Finch, C. E., Franceschi, C., Globerson, A., Klingenberg, C. P., LaMarco, K., Omholt, S., and Westendorp, R. G. (2005). What accounts for the wide variation in life span of genetically identical organisms reared in a constant environment? *Mech Ageing Dev.* **126,** 439–443.

Kirkwood, T. B., and Finch, C. E. (2002). Ageing: The old worm turns more slowly. *Nature.* **419,** 794–795.

Kirkwood, T. B., and Holliday, R. (1979). The evolution of ageing and longevity. *Proc R Soc Lond B Biol Sci.* **205,** 531–546.

Kirkwood, T. B. L. (2001). Sex and ageing. *Exp Gerontol.* **36,** 413–418.

Kirschning, C. J., Au-Young, J., Lamping, N., Reuter, D., Pfeil, D., Seilhamer, J. J., and Schumann, R. R. (1997). Similar organization of the lipopolysaccharide-binding protein (LBP) and phospholipid transfer protein (PLTP) genes suggests a common gene family of lipid-binding proteins. *Genomics.* **46,** 416–425.

Kirwan, J. P., Krishnan, R. K., Weaver, J. A., Del Aguila, L. F., and Evans, W. J. (2001). Human aging is associated with altered TNF-alpha production during hyperglycemia and hyperinsulinemia. *Am J Physiol Endocrinol Metab.* **281,** E1137–1143.

Kisilevsky, R. (2000). Review: Amyloidogenesis—Unquestioned answers and unanswered questions. *J Struct Biol.* **130,** 99–108.

Kitazawa, M., Oddo, S., Yamasaki, T. R., Green, K. N., and LaFerla, F. M. (2005). Lipopolysaccharide-induced inflammation exacerbates tau pathology by a cyclin-dependent kinase 5-mediated pathway in a transgenic model of Alzheimer's disease. J Neurosci. **25,** 8843–8853.

Kivipelto, M., Ngandu, T., Fratiglioni, L., Viitanen, M., Kêareholt, I., Winblad, B., Helkala, E. L., Tuomilehto, J., Soininen, H., and Nissinen, A. (2005). Obesity and vascular risk factors at midlife and the risk of dementia and Alzheimer disease. *Arch Neurol.* **62,** 1556–1560.

Kiyotaki, C., Peisach, J., and Bloom, B. R. (1984). Oxygen metabolism in cloned macrophage cell lines: Glucose dependence of superoxide production, metabolic and spectral analysis. *J Immunol.* **132,** 857–866.

Klass, M. R. (1977). Aging in the nematode *Caenorhabditis elegans*: Major biological and environmental factors influencing life span. *Mech Ageing Dev.* **6,** 413–429.

Klass, M. R. (1983). A method for the isolation of longevity mutants in the nematode *Caenorhabditis elegans* and initial results. *Mech Ageing Dev.* **22,** 279–286.

Klebanoff, M. A., Schulsinger, C., Mednick, B. R., and Secher, N. J. (1997). Preterm and small-for-gestational-age birth across generations. *Am J Obstet Gynecol.* **176,** 521–526.

Klebanov, S. (2007). Can short-term dietary restriction and fasting have a long-term anti-carcinogenic effect? *Interdiscip Top Gerontol.* **25,** 176–192.

Klebanov, S., Diais, S., Stavinoha, W. B., Suh, Y., and Nelson, J. F. (1995). Hyperadrenocorticism, attenuated inflammation, and the life-prolonging action of food restriction in mice. *J Gerontol. A Biol Sci Med Sci.* **50,** B79–82.

Klegeris, A., Singh, E. A., and McGeer, P. L. (2002). Effects of C-reactive protein and pentosan polysulphate on human complement activation. *Immunology.* **106,** 381–388.

Klein, J. (1986). *Natural history of the major histocompatibility complex.* New York: John Wiley and Sons.

Klein, W. L., Krafft, G. A., and Finch, C. E. (2001). Targeting small Abeta oligomers: The solution to an Alzheimer's disease conundrum? *Trends Neurosci.* **24,** 219–224.

Klouche, M., Peri, G., Knabbe, C., Eckstein, H. H., Schmid, F. X., Schmitz, G., and Mantovani, A. (2004). Modified atherogenic lipoproteins induce expression of pentraxin-3 by human vascular smooth muscle cells. *Atherosclerosis.* **175,** 221–228.

Knight, B., Shields, B. M., Turner, M., Powell, R. J., Yajnik, C. S., and Hattersley, A. T. (2005). Evidence of genetic regulation of fetal longitudinal growth. *Early Hum Dev.* **81(10),** 823–831.

Knight, J. C. (2004). Regulatory polymorphisms underlying complex disease traits. *J Mol Med.* **83,** 97–109.

Knoblauch, H., Bauerfeind, A., Toliat, M. R., Becker, C., Luganskaja, T., Gunther, U. P., Rohde, K., Schuster, H., Junghans, C., Luft, F. C., Nurnberg, P., and Reich, J. G. (2004). Haplotypes and SNPs in 13 lipid-relevant genes explain most of the genetic variance in high-density lipoprotein and low-density lipoprotein cholesterol. *Hum Mol Genet.* **13,** 993–1004.

Knowles, R. B., Wyart, C., Buldyrev, S. V., Cruz, L., Urbanc, B., Hasselmo, M. E., Stanley, H. E., and Hyman, B. T. (1999). Plaque-induced neurite abnormalities: Implications for disruption of neural networks in Alzheimer's disease. *Proc Natl Acad Sci USA.* **96,** 5274–5279.

Koch, S., Solana, R., Dela Rosa, O., Pawelec, G. (2006). Human cytomegalovirus infection and T cell immunosenescence: a mini review. *Mech Ageing Dev.* **127,** 538–543.

Kodama, M., Fujioka, T., Murakami, K., Okimoto, T., Sato, R., Watanabe, K., and Nasu, M. (2005). Eradication of *Helicobacter pylori* reduced the immunohistochemical detection of p53 and MDM2 in gastric mucosa. *J Gastroenterol Hepatol.* **20,** 941–946.

Koga, M., Hirano, K., Hirano, M., Nishimura, J., Nakano, H., and Kanaide, H. (2004). Akt plays a central role in the anti-apoptotic effect of estrogen in endothelial cells. *Biochem Biophys Res Comm.* **324,** 321–325.

Koike, T., Vernon, R. B., Gooden, M. D., Sadoun, E., and Reed, M. J. (2003). Inhibited angiogenesis in aging: a role for TIMP-2. *J Gerontol. Series A, Biol Sci Med Sci.* **58,** B798–805.

Koizumi, A., Tsukada, M., Wada, Y., Masuda, H., and Weindruch, R. (1992). Mitotic activity in mice is suppressed by energy restriction-induced torpor. *J Nutr.* **122,** 1446–1453.

Kojro, E., Gimpl, G., Lammich, S., Marz, W., and Fahrenholz, F. (2001). Low cholesterol stimulates the nonamyloidogenic pathway by its effect on the alpha-secretase ADAM 10. *Proc Natl Acad Sci USA.* **98,** 5815–5820.

Kolltveit, K. M., and Eriksen, H. M. (2001). Is the observed association between periodontitis and atherosclerosis causal? *Eur J Oral Sci.* **109,** 2–7.

Kolodgie, F. D., Gold, H. K., Burke, A. P., Fowler, D. R., Kruth, H. S., Weber, D. K., Farb, A., Guerrero, L. J., Hayase, M., Kutys, R., Narula, J., Finn, A. V., Virmani, R. (2003). Intraplaque hemorrhage and progression of coronary atheroma. *N Engl J Med.* **349,** 2316–2325.

Konigsberg, L. W. and Herrmann, N.P. (2006). The osteological evidence for human longevity in the recent past. In K. Hawkes and R. R. Paine, Eds., *The evolution of human life history.* Santa Fe, NM: School for American Research Press, pp.267–306.

Konova, E., Baydanoff, S., Atanasova, M., and Velkova, A. (2004). Age-related changes in the glycation of human aortic elastin. *Exp Gerontol.* **39,** 249–254.

Konsman, J. P., Vigues, S., Mackerlova, L., Bristow, A., and Blomqvist, A. (2004). Rat brain vascular distribution of interleukin-1 type-1 receptor immunoreactivity: Relationship to patterns of inducible cyclooxygenase expression by peripheral inflammatory stimuli. *J Comp Neurol.* **472,** 113–129.

Kontush, A., Chantepie, S., and Chapman, M. J. (2003). Small, dense HDL particles exert potent protection of atherogenic LDL against oxidative stress. *Arterioscler Thromb Vasc Biol.* **23,** 1881–1888.

Koochmeshgi, J. (2004a). Reproductive switch and aging: The case of leptin change in dietary restriction. *Ann NY Acad Sci.* **1019,** 436–438.

Koochmeshgi, J., Hosseini-Mazinani, S. M., Morteza Seifati, S., Hosein-Pur-Nobari, N., and Teimoori-Toolabi, L. (2004b). Apolipoprotein E genotype and age at menopause. *Ann NY Acad Sci.* **1019,** 564–567.

Kopchick, J. J., and Laron, Z. (1999). Is the Laron mouse an accurate model of Laron syndrome? *Mol Genet Metab.* **68,** 232–236.

Kopsidas, G., Zhang, C., Yarovaya, N., Kovalenko, S., Graves, S., Richardson, M., and Linnane, A. W. (2002). Stochastic mitochondrial DNA changes: Bioenergy decline in type I skeletal muscle fibres correlates with a decline in the amount of amplifiable full-length mtDNA. *Biogerontology.* **3,** 29–36.

Kornfeld, K., and Evason, K. (2006). Effects of anticonvulsant drugs on life span. *Arch Neurol.* **63,** 491–496.

Koschinsky, T., Bunting, C. E., Rutter, R., and Gries, F. A. (1985). Vascular growth factors and the development of macrovascular disease in diabetes mellitus. *Hormone Metabol Res. Supplement Series.* **15,** 23–27.

Koschinsky, T., He, C. J., Mitsuhashi, T., Bucala, R., Liu, C., Buenting, C., Heitmann, K., and Vlassara, H. (1997). Orally absorbed reactive glycation products (glycotoxins): An environmental risk factor in diabetic nephropathy. *Proc Natl Acad Sci USA.* **94,** 6474–6479.

Koster, A., Bosma, H., Penninx, B. W., Newman, A. B., Harris, T. B., van Eijk, J. T., Kempen, G. I., Simonsick, E. M., Johnson, K. C., Rooks, R. N., Ayonayon, H. N., Rubin, S. M., and Kritchevsky, S. B. (2006). Association of inflammatory markers with socioeconomic status. *J Gerontol. A Biol Sci Med Sci.* **61,** 284–290.

Kougias, P., Chai, H., Lin, P. H., Yao, Q., Lumsden, A. B., and Chen, C. (2005). Effects of adipocyte-derived cytokines on endothelial functions: Implication of vascular disease. *J Surg Res.* **126,** 121–129.

Kovacs, A., Green, F., Hansson, L. O., Lundman, P., Samnegard, A., Boquist, S., Ericsson, C. G., Watkins, H., Hamsten, A., and Tornvall, P. (2005). A novel common single nucleotide polymorphism in the promoter region of the C-reactive protein gene associated with the plasma concentration of C-reactive protein. *Atherosclerosis.* **178,** 193–198.

Koza, R. A., Nikonova, L., Hogan, J., Rim, J. S., Mendoza, T., Faulk, C., Skaf, J., Kozak, L. P. (2006). Changes in gene expression foreshadow diet-induced obesity in genetically identical mice. *PLoS Genet.* **2,** e81.

Koziris, L. P., Hickson, R. C., Chatterton, R. T., Jr., Groseth, R. T., Christie, J. M., Goldflies, D. G., and Unterman, T. G. (1999). Serum levels of total and free IGF-I and IGFBP-3 are increased and maintained in long-term training. *J Appl Physiol.* **86,** 1436–1442.

Kraaijeveld, A. R., and Godfray, H. C. (1997). Trade-off between parasitoid resistance and larval competitive ability in *Drosophila melanogaster. Nature.* **389,** 278–280.

Kraaijeveld, A. R., Limentani, E. C., and Godfray, H. C. (2001). Basis of the trade-off between parasitoid resistance and larval competitive ability in *Drosophila melanogaster. Proc Biol Sci.* **268,** 259–261.

Kraemer, W. J., and Ratamess, N. A. (2005). Hormonal responses and adaptations to resistance exercise and training. *Sports Med.* **35,** 339–361.

Kramer, B. K., Kammerl, M. C., and Komhoff, M. (2004a). Renal cyclooxygenase-2 (COX-2). Physiological, pathophysiological, and clinical implications. *Kidney Blood Press Res.* **27,** 43–62.

Kramer, H. J., Stevens, J., Grimminger, F., and Seeger, W. (1996). Fish oil fatty acids and human platelets: Dose-dependent decrease in dienoic and increase in trienoic thromboxane generation. *Biochem Pharmacol.* **52,** 1211–1217.

Kramer, M. S. (1987). Intrauterine growth and gestational duration determinants. *Pediatrics.* **80,** 502–511.

Kramer, M. S. (1993). Effects of energy and protein intakes on pregnancy outcome: An overview of the research evidence from controlled clinical trials. *Am J Clin Nutr.* **58,** 627–635.

Kramer, M. S., and Joseph, K. S. (1996). Enigma of fetal/infant-origins hypothesis. *Lancet.* **348,** 1254–1255.

Kramer, M. S. (2004). Commentary: Maternal nutrition, body proportions at birth, and adult chronic disease. *Int J Epidemiol* **33,** 837–838.

Kranzler, J. H., Rosenbloom, A. L., Martinez, V., and Guevara-Aguirre, J. (1998). Normal intelligence with severe insulin-like growth factor I deficiency due to growth hormone receptor deficiency: A controlled study in a genetically homogeneous population. *J Clin Endocrinol Metab.* **83,** 1953–1958.

Kreier, F., Kap, Y. S., Mettenleiter, T. C., van Heijningen, C., van der Vliet, J., Kalsbeek, A., Sauerwein, H. P., Fliers, E., Romijn, J. A., and Buijs, R. M. (2005). Tracing from fat tissue, liver and pancreas: A neuroanatomical framework for the role of the brain in type 2 diabetes. *Endocrinology.* **147,** 1140–1147.

Krinke, G. (1983). Spinal radiculoneuropathy in aging rats: demyelination secondary to neuronal dwindling? *Acta Neuropathol.* **59,** 63–69.

Kritchevsky, D. (1995). The effect of over- and undernutrition on cancer. *Eur J Cancer Prevention.* **4,** 445–451.

Kritchevsky, D. (2003). Diet and cancer: What's next? *Am Soc Nutritional Sciences.* **133,** 3827S–3829S.

Krohn, K., Rozovsky, I., Wals, P., Teter, B., Anderson, C. P., and Finch, C. E. (1999). Glial fibrillary acidic protein transcription responses to transforming growth factor-beta1 and interleukin-1beta are mediated by a nuclear factor-1–like site in the near-upstream promoter. *J Neurochem.* **72(4),** 1353–1361.

Kronenberg, G., Bick-Sander, A., Bunk, E., Wolf, C., Ehninger, D., and Kempermann, G. (2005). Physical exercise prevents age-related decline in precursor cell activity in the mouse dentate gyrus. *Neurobiol Aging.* **27,** 1505–1513.

Krucker, T., Schuler, A., Meyer, E. P., Staufenbiel, M., and Beckmann, N. (2004). Magnetic resonance angiography and vascular corrosion casting as tools in biomedical research: Application to transgenic mice modeling Alzheimer's disease. *Neurological Research.* **26,** 507–516.

Krumbahr, E. R. (1939). Lymphatic tissue. In E. V. Cowdry, Ed. *Problems of aging. Biological and medical aspects*, pp. 149–198. Williams and Wilkins Co. Reprinted 1979 by ARNO Press, New York, Baltimore.

Krupitsky, E. M., Zvartau, E. E., Lioznov, D. A., Tsoy, M. V., Egorova, V. Y., Belyaeva, T. V., Antonova, T. V., Brazhenko, N. A., Zagdyn, Z. M., Verbitskaya, E. V., Zorina, Y., Karandashova, G. F., Slavina, T. Y., Grinenko, A. Y., Samet, J. H., and Woody, G. E. (2006). Co-morbidity of infectious and addictive diseases in St. Petersburg and the Leningrad Region, Russia. *Eur Addict Res.* **12,** 12–19.

Kubaszek, A., Pihlajamèaki, J., Komarovski, V., Lindi, V., Lindstrèom, J., Eriksson, J., Valle, T. T., Hèamèalèainen, H., Ilanne-Parikka, P., Keinèanen-Kiukaanniemi, S., Tuomilehto, J., Uusitupa, M., and Laakso, M. (2003a). Promoter polymorphisms of the TNF-alpha (G-308A) and IL-6 (C-174G) genes predict the conversion from impaired glucose tolerance to type 2 diabetes: The Finnish Diabetes Prevention Study. *Diabetes.* **52(7),** 1872–1876.

Kubaszek, A., Pihlajamaki, J., Punnonen, K., Karhapaa, P., Vauhkonen, I., and Laakso, M. (2003b). The C-174G promoter polymorphism of the IL-6 gene affects energy expenditure and insulin sensitivity. *Diabetes.* **52,** 558–561.

Kuhnke, A., Burmester, G. R., Krauss, S., and Buttgereit, F. (2003). Bioenergetics of immune cells to assess rheumatic disease activity and efficacy of glucocorticoid treatment. *Ann Rheum Dis.* **62,** 133–139.

Kuk, J. L., Katzmarzyk, P. T., Nichaman, M. Z., Church, T. S., Blair, S. N., and Ross, R. (2006). Visceral fat is an independent predictor of all-cause mortality in men. *Obesity.* **14,** 336–341.

Kukar, T., Murphy, M. P., Eriksen, J. L., Sagi, S. A., Weggen, S., Smith, T. E., Ladd, T., Khan, M. A., Kache, R., Beard, J., Dodson, M., Merit, S., Ozols, V. V., Anastasiadis, P. Z., Das, P., Fauq, A., Koo, E. H., and Golde, T. E. (2005). Diverse compounds mimic Alzheimer disease-causing mutations by augmenting Abeta42 production. *Nature Med.* **11,** 545–550.

Kumar, S., Filipski, A., Swarna, V., Walker, A., and Hedges, S. B. (2005). Placing confidence limits on the molecular age of the human-chimpanzee divergence. *Proc Natl Acad Sci USA.* **102,** 18842–18847.

Kuniyasu, H., Kitadai, Y., Mieno, H., and Yasui, W. (2003). *Helicobacter pylori* infection is closely associated with telomere reduction in gastric mucosa. *Oncology.* **65,** 275–282.

Kunstyr, I., and Leuenberger, H. G. (1975). Gerontological data of C57BL/6J mice. I. Sex differences in survival curves. *J Gerontol.* 157–162.

Kurapati, R., Passananti, H. B., Rose, M. R., and Tower, J. (2000). Increased hsp22 RNA levels in *Drosophila* lines genetically selected for increased longevity. *J Gerontol. Series A, Biol Sci Med Sci.* **55,** B552–559.

Kuro-o, M., Matsumura, Y., Aizawa, H., Kawaguchi, H., Suga, T., Utsugi, T., Ohyama, Y., Kurabayashi, M., Kaname, T., Kume, E., Iwasaki, H., Iida, A., Shiraki-Iida, T., Nishikawa, S., Nagai, R., and Nabeshima, Y. I. (1997). Mutation of the mouse Klotho gene leads to a syndrome resembling ageing. *Nature.* **390,** 45–51.

Kuroki, Y., Toyoda, A., Noguchi, H., Taylor, T. D., Itoh, T., Kim, D. S., Kim, D. W., Choi, S. H., Kim, I. C., Choi, H. H., Kim, Y. S., Satta, Y., Saitou, N., Yamada, T., Morishita, S., Hattori, M., Sakaki, Y., Park, H. S., and Fujiyama, A. (2006). Comparative analysis of chimpanzee and human Y chromosomes unveils complex evolutionary pathway. *Nat Genet.* **38,** 158–167.

Kurosu, H., Yamamoto, M., Clark, J. D., Pastor, J. V., Nandi, A., Gurnani, P., McGuinness, O. P., Chikuda, H., Yamaguchi, M., Kawaguchi, H., Shimomura, I., Takayama, Y., Herz, J., Kahn, C. R., Rosenblatt, K. P., and Kuro-o, M. (2005). Suppression of aging in mice by the hormone Klotho. *Science* **309,** 1829–1833.

Kurz, C. L., Chauvet, S., Andráes, E., Aurouze, M., Vallet, I., Michel, G. P., Uh, M., Celli, J., Filloux, A., De Bentzmann, S., Steinmetz, I., Hoffmann, J. A., Finlay, B. B., Gorvel, J. P., Ferrandon, D., and Ewbank, J. J. (2003). Virulence factors of the human opportunistic pathogen *Serratia marcescens* identified by *in vivo* screening. *Embo J.* **22,** 1451–1460.

Kurz, C. L., and Tan, M. W. (2004). Regulation of aging and innate immunity in *C. elegans. Aging cell.* **3(4),** 185–193.

Kurz, D. J., Decary, S., Hong, Y., Trivier, E., Akhmedov, A., and Erusalimsky, J. D. (2004). Chronic oxidative stress compromises telomere integrity and accelerates the onset of senescence in human endothelial cells. *J Cell Sci.* **117,** 2417–2426.

Kuzawa, C. W. (1998). Adipose tissue in human infancy and childhood: An evolutionary perspective. *Yearb Phys Anthropol.* **41,** 177–209.

Kwak, B. R., Mulhaupt, F., and Mach, F. (2003). Atherosclerosis: Anti-inflammatory and immunomodulatory activities of statins. *Autoimmune Rev.* **2,** 332–338.

Laberge, M. A., Moore, K. J., and Freeman, M. W. (2005). Atherosclerosis and innate immune signaling. *Ann Med.* **37,** 130–140.

Lacor, P. N., Buniel, M. C., Chang, L., Fernandez, S. J., Gong, Y., Viola, K. L., Lambert, M. P., Velasco, P. T., Bigio, E. H., Finch, C. E., Krafft, G. A., and Klein, W. L. (2004). Synaptic targeting by Alzheimer's-related amyloid beta oligomers. *J Neurosci.* **24,** 10191–10200.

Lacut, K., Oger, E., Le Gal, G., Blouch, M. T., Abgrall, J. F., Kerlan, V., Scarabin, P. Y., Mottier, D. (2003). Differential effects of oral and transdermal postmenopausal estrogen replacement therapies on C-reactive protein. *Thromb Haemost.* **90,** 124–131.

LaFerla, F. M., and Oddo, S. (2005). Alzheimer's disease: Abeta, tau and synaptic dysfunction. *Trends Mol Med.* **11,** 170–176.

Laine, L., Cominelli, F., Sloane, R., Casini-Raggi, V., Marin-Sorensen, M., and Weinstein, W. M. (1995). Interaction of NSAIDs and *Helicobacter pylori* on gastrointestinal injury and prostaglandin production: A controlled double-blind trial. *Aliment Pharmacol Therap.* **9,** 127–135.

Lakatta, E. G. (2003). Arterial and cardiac aging: Major shareholders in cardiovascular disease enterprises: Part III: Cellular and molecular clues to heart and arterial aging. *Circulation.* **107,** 490–497.

Lakatta, E. G., and Levy, D. (2003b). Arterial and cardiac aging: Major shareholders in cardiovascular disease enterprises: Part I: Aging arteries: a "set up" for vascular disease. *Circulation.* **107,** 139–146.

Lakatta, E. G., and Levy, D. (2003c). Arterial and cardiac aging: Major shareholders in cardiovascular disease enterprises: Part II: The aging heart in health: Links to heart disease. *Circulation.* **107,** 346–354.

Lakowski, B., and Hekimi, S. (1998). The genetics of caloric restriction in *Caenorhabditis elegans. Proc Natl Acad Sci USA.* **95,** 13091–13096.

Lam, W., Park, S. Y., Leung, C. H., and Cheng, Y. C. (2006). APE-1 protein level is associated with the cytotoxicity of L-configuration deoxycytidine analogs (L-OddC, LFd4C) but not D-configuration deoxycytidine analogs (dFdC, AraC). *Mol Pharmacol.* **69,** 1607–1614.

Lamas, O., Martínez, J. A., and Marti, A. (2004). Energy restriction restores the impaired immune response in overweight (cafeteria) rats. *J Nutr Biochem* **15,** 418–425.

Lamb, D. (1975). Rat lung pathology and quality of laboratory animals: The user's view. *Lab Anim.* **9,** 1–8.

Lambers, D. S., and Clark, K. E. (1996). The maternal and fetal physiologic effects of nicotine. *Semin Perinatol.* **20,** 115–126.

Lambert, A. J., Wang, B., and Merry, B. J. (2004). Exogenous insulin can reverse the effects of caloric restriction on mitochondria. *Biochem Biophys Res Comm.* **316,** 1196–1201.

Lambert, J. C., Brousseau, T., Defosse, V., Evans, A., Arveiler, D., Ruidavets, J. B., Haas, B., Cambou, J. P., Luc, G., Ducimetiáere, P., Cambien, F., Chartier-Harlin, M. C., and Amouyel, P. (2000). Independent association of an APOE gene promoter polymorphism with increased risk of myocardial infarction and decreased APOE plasma concentrations-the ECTIM study. *Hum Mol Genet.* **9,** 57–61.

Lambert, M., Delvin, E. E., Paradis, G., O'Loughlin, J., Hanley, J. A., and Levy, E. (2004b). C-reactive protein and features of the metabolic syndrome in a population-based sample of children and adolescents. *Clin Chem.* **50,** 1762–1768.

Lamming, D. W., Wood, J. G., and Sinclair, D. A. (2004). Small molecules that regulate lifespan: Evidence for xenohormesis. *Molec Microbiol.* **53,** 1003–1009.

Lampl, M., and Jeanty, P. (2004). Exposure to maternal diabetes is associated with altered fetal growth patterns: A hypothesis regarding metabolic allocation to growth under hyperglycemic-hypoxemic conditions. *Am J Hum Biol.* **16,** 237–263.

Landfield, P.W., Blalock, E.M., Chen, K.C., and Porter, N.M. (2007). A new glucocorticoid hypothesis of brain aging: implications for Alzheimer's disease. *Curr Alzheimer Res.* **4,** 205–212.

Landfield, P. W., Braun, L. D., Pitler, T. A., Lindsey, J. D., Lynch, G. (1981). Hippocampal aging in rats: a morphometric study of multiple variables in semithin sections. *Neurobiol Aging.* **2,** 265–275.

Landfield, P. W., Rose, G., McEwen, B., Meaney, M. J., Rapp, P. R., Sapolsky, R., West, M. J. (1977). Patterns of astroglial hypertrophy and neuronal degeneration in the hippocampus of ages, memory-deficient rats. *J Gerontol.* **32,** 3–12.

Landis, G. N., Abdueva, D., Skvortsov, D., Yang, J., Rabin, B. E., Carrick, J., Tavaré, S., and Tower, J. (2004). Similar gene expression patterns characterize aging and oxidative stress in *Drosophila melanogaster*. *Proc Natl Acad Sci USA*. **101,** 7663–7668.

Landis, G. N., and Tower, J. (2005). Superoxide dismutase evolution and life span regulation. *Mech Ageing Dev*. **126,** 365–379.

Lane-Petter, W., Olds, R. J., Hacking, M. R., and Lane-Petter, M. E. (1970). Respiratory disease in a colony of rats. I. The natural disease. *J Hygiene*. **68,** 655–662.

Lane, J. A., Harvey, R. F., Murray, L. J., Harvey, I. M., Donovan, J. L., Nair, P., and Egger, M. (2002). A placebo-controlled randomized trial of eradication of *Helicobacter pylori* in the general population: Study design and response rates of the Bristol Helicobacter Project. *Controlled Clinical Trials*. **23,** 321–332.

Lane, M. A., Baer, D. J., Rumpler, W. V., Weindruch, R., Ingram, D. K., Tilmont, E. M., Cutler, R. G., and Roth, G. S. (1996). Calorie restriction lowers body temperature in rhesus monkeys, consistent with a postulated anti-aging mechanism in rodents. *Proc Natl Acad Sci USA*. **93,** 4159–4164.

Lang, C. A., Mills, B. J., Mastropaolo, W., and Liu, M. C. (2000). Blood glutathione decreases in chronic diseases. *J Lab Clin Med*. **135,** 402–405.

Lang, C. A., Wu, W. K., Chen, T., and Mills, B. J. (1989). Blood glutathione: A biochemical index of life span enhancement in the diet restricted Lobund-Wistar rat. *Prog Clin Biol Res*. **287,** 241–246.

Lang, C. H., Chen, T. S., and Mills, B. J. (1990). Glutathione status and longevity are enhanced by dietary retriction. *FASEB J*. **4,** Abstract 601.

Langa, K. M., Foster, N. L., and Larson, E. B. (2004). Mixed dementia: Emerging concepts and therapeutic implications. *JAMA*. **292,** 2901–2908.

Langenberg, C., Shipley, M. J., Batty, G. D., and Marmot, M. G. (2005). Adult socioeconomic position and the association between height and coronary heart disease mortality: Findings from 33 years of follow-up in the Whitehall Study. *Am J Public Health*. **95,** 628–632.

Langheinrich, A. C., and Bohle, R. M. (2005). Atherosclerosis: Humoral and cellular factors of inflammation. *Virchows Archiv*. **446,** 101–111.

Lanner, R. M., and Connor, K. F. (2001). Does bristlecone pine senesce? *Exp Gerontol*. **36,** 675–685.

Lantz, R. C., Chen, G. J., Solyom, A. M., Jolad, S. D., and Timmermann, B. N. (2005). The effect of turmeric extracts on inflammatory mediator production. *Phytomedicine*. **12,** 445–452.

Lara-Pezzi, E., Gomez-Gaviro, M. V., Galvez, B. G., Mira, E., Iniguez, M. A., Fresno, M., Martinez-A, C., Arroyo, A. G., and Lopez-Cabrera, M. (2002). The hepatitis B virus X protein promotes tumor cell invasion by inducing membrane-type matrix metalloproteinase-1 and cyclooxygenase-2 expression. J Clin Invest. **110,** 1831–1838.

Larke, A., and Crews, D. E. (2006). Parental investment, late reproduction, and increased reserve capacity are associated with longevity in humans. *J Physiol Anthropol*. **25,** 119–131.

Laron, Z. (1999). The essential role of IGF-I: Lessons from the long-term study and treatment of children and adults with Laron syndrome. *J Clin Endocrinol Metab*. **84,** 4397–4404.

Laron, Z. (2005). Do deficiencies in growth hormone and insulin-like growth factor-1 (IGF-1) shorten or prolong longevity? *Mech Ageing Dev*. **126,** 307–307.

Larsen, P. L., and Clarke, C. F. (2002). Extension of life-span in *Caenorhabditis elegans* by a diet lacking coenzyme Q. *Science*. **295,** 120–123.

Larson-Meyer, D. E., Heilbronn, L. K., Redman, L. M., Newcomer, B. R., Frisard, M. I., Anton, S., Smith, S. R., Alfonso, A., and Ravussin, E. (2006). Effect of calorie restriction with or without exercise on insulin sensitivity, beta-cell function, fat cell size, and ectopic lipid in overweight subjects. *Diabetes Care.* **29,** 1337–1344.

Lassinger, B. K., Kwak, C., Walford, R. L., and Jankovic, J. (2004). Atypical Parkinsonism and motor neuron syndrome in a Biosphere 2 participant: A possible complication of chronic hypoxia and carbon monoxide toxicity? *Mov Disord.* **19,** 465–469.

Latkovskis, G., Licis, N., and Kalnins, U. (2004). C-reactive protein levels and common polymorphisms of the interleukin-1 gene cluster and interleukin-6 gene in patients with coronary heart disease. *Eur J Immunogenet.* **31,** 207–213.

Launer, L. J., Scheltens, P., Lindeboom, J., Barkhof, F., Weinstein, H. C., and Jonker, C. (1995). Medial temporal lobe atrophy in an open population of very old persons: Cognitive, brain atrophy, and sociomedical correlates. *Neurology.* **45,** 747–752.

Laurin, D., Verreault, R., Lindsay, J., MacPherson, K., and Rockwood, K. (2001). Physical activity and risk of cognitive impairment and dementia in elderly persons. *Arch Neurol.* **58,** 498–504.

Lavie, L., Reznick, A. Z., and Gershon, D. (1982). Decreased protein and puromycinyl-peptide degradation in livers of senescent mice. *Biochem J.* **202,** 47–51.

Law, M. R., Wald, N. J., and Rudnicka, A. R. (2003). Quantifying effect of statins on low density lipoprotein cholesterol, ischaemic heart disease, and stroke: Systematic review and meta-analysis. *Br Med J.* **326,** 1423.

Lawrence, M., Coward, W. A., Lawrence, F., Cole, T. J., and Whitehead, R. G. (1987a). Fat gain during pregnancy in rural African women: The effect of season and dietary status. *Am J Clin Nutr.* **45,** 1442–1450.

Lawrence, M., Lawrence, F., Coward, W. A., Cole, T. J., and Whitehead, R. G. (1987b). Energy requirements of pregnancy in The Gambia. *Lancet.* **2,** 1072–1076.

Laws, T. R., Harding, S. V., Smith, M. P., Atkins, T. P., and Titball, R. W. (2004). Age influences resistance of *Caenorhabditis elegans* to killing by pathogenic bacteria. *FEMS Microbiol Lett.* **234(2),** 281–287.

Lazarov, O., Lee, M., Peterson, D. A., and Sisodia, S. S. (2002). Evidence that synaptically released beta-amyloid accumulates as extracellular deposits in the hippocampus of transgenic mice. *J Neurosci.* **22,** 9785–9793.

Lazarov, O., Robinson, J., Tang, Y. P., Hairston, I. S., Korade-Mirnics, Z., Lee, V. M., Hersh, L. B., Sapolsky, R. M., Mirnics, K., and Sisodia, S. S., (2005). Environmental enrichment reduces Abeta levels and amyloid deposition in transgenic mice. *Cell.* **120,** 701–713.

Leach, C. T. (2004). Hepatitis A in the United States. *Pediatr Infect Dis J.* **23,** 551–552.

Leaf, A. (1990). Long-lived populations (extreme old age). In W. R. Hazzard, R. Andres, E. L. Bierman, and J. P. Blass, Eds., *Principles of geriatric medicine*, pp. 142–145. New York: McGraw-Hill.

Lechtig, A., and Mata, L. J. (1971a). Cord IgM levels in Latin American neonates. *J Pediatr.* **78,** 909–910.

Lechtig, A., and Mata, L. J. (1971b). Levels of IgG, IgA and IgM in cord blood of Latin American newborns from different ecosystems. *Rev Latinoam Microbiol.* **13,** 173–179.

Lechtig, A., and Mata, L. J. (1972). Levels in C3 in newborns and mothers from different ecosystems. *Rev Latinoam Microbiol.* **14,** 73–76.

Lee, A. T., and Cerami, A. (1990). *In vitro* and *in vivo* reactions of nucleic acids with reducing sugars. *Mut Res.* **238,** 185–191.

Lee, C. K., Weindruch, R., Prolla, T. A. (2000). Gene-expression profile of the ageing brain in mice. *Nat Genet.* **25,** 294–297.

Lee, D. W., and Opanashuk, L. A. (2004). Polychlorinated biphenyl mixture aroclor 1254-induced oxidative stress plays a role in dopaminergic cell injury. *Neurotoxicology.* **25,** 925–939.

Lee, H. G., Castellani, R. J., Zhu, X., Perry, G., and Smith, M. A. (2005). Amyloid-beta in Alzheimer's disease: The horse or the cart? Pathogenic or protective? *Int J Exp Pathology.* **86,** 133–138.

Lee, I. M., Hsieh, C., and Paffenbarger, R. S., Jr. (1995). Exercise intensity and longevity in men: The Harvard Alumni Health Study. *JAMA.* **273,** 1179–1184.

Lee, I. M., Sesso, H. D., Oguma, Y., and Paffenberger, R. S. (2004). The "Weekend Warrior" and risk of mortality. *Am J Epidemiol.* **160,** 636–641.

Lee, S. K., Posthauer, M. E., Dorner, B., Redovian, V., and Maloney, M. J. (2006). Pressure ulcer healing with a concentrated, fortified, collagen protein hydrolysate supplement: A randomized controlled trial. *Adv Skin Wound Care.* **19,** 92–96.

Lee, S. S., Kennedy, S., Tolonen, A. C., and Ruvkun, G. (2003). DAF-16 target genes that control *C. elegans* life-span and metabolism. *Science.* **300,** 644–647.

Lee, Y. H., and Pratley, R. E. (2005b). The evolving role of inflammation in obesity and the metabolic syndrome. *Curr Diabetes Rep.* **5,** 70–75.

Leeuwenburgh, C., Wagner, P., Holloszy, J. O., Sohal, R. S., and Heinecke, J. W. (1997). Caloric restriction attenuates dityrosine cross-linking of cardiac and skeletal muscle proteins in aging mice. *Arch Biochem Biophys.* **346,** 74–80.

Leger, J., Levy-Marchal, C., Bloch, J., Pinet, A., Chevenne, D., Porquet, D., Collin, D., and Czernichow, P., (1997). Reduced final height and indications for insulin resistance in 20 year olds born small for gestational age: Regional cohort study. *Br Med J.* **315,** 341–347.

Lehtimaki, T., Ojala, P., Rontu, R., Goebeler, S., Karhunen, P. J., Jylhèa, M., Mattila, K., Metso, S., Jokela, H., Nikkilèa, M., Wuolijoki, E., Hervonen, A., and Hurme, M. (2005). Interleukin-6 modulates plasma cholesterol and C-reactive protein concentrations in nonagenarians. *J Am Geriatr Soc.* **53,** 1552–1558.

Leissring, M. A., Farris, W., Chang, A. Y., Walsh, D. M., Wu, X., Sun, X., Frosch, M. P., and Selkoe, D. J. (2003). Enhanced proteolysis of beta-amyloid in APP transgenic mice prevents plaque formation, secondary pathology, and premature death. *Neuron.* **40,** 1087–1093.

Leistikow, E. A. (1998). Is coronary artery disease initiated perinatally? *Semin Thromb Hemost.* **24,** 139–143.

Leon, A. S., Togashi, K., Rankinen, T., Després, J. P., Rao, D. C., Skinner, J. S., Wilmore, J. H., and Bouchard, C. (2004). Association of apolipoprotein E polymorphism with blood lipids and maximal oxygen uptake in the sedentary state and after exercise training in the HERITAGE family study. *Metabolism.* **53,** 108–116.

Leon, D. A. (2001). The foetal origins of adult disease: Interpreting the evidence from twin studies. *Twin Res.* **4(5),** 321–326.

Lerman, L. O., Chade, A. R., Sica, V., and Napoli, C. (2005). Animal models of hypertension: An overview. *J Lab Clin Medicine.* **146,** 160–173.

Lerner, S. P., Anderson, C. P., Harrison, D. E., Walford, R. L., and Finch, C. E. (1992). Polygenic influences on the length of oestrous cycles in inbred mice involve MHC alleles. *Eur J Immunogenet.* **19,** 361–371.

Lerner, S. P., Anderson, C. P., Walford, R. L., and Finch, C. E. (1988). Genotypic influences on reproductive aging of inbred female mice: Effects of H-2 and non-H-2 alleles. *Biol Repro.* **38,** 1035–1043.

Lerner, S. P., and Finch, C. E. (1991). The major histocompatibility complex and reproductive functions. *Endocr Rev.* **12,** 78–90.

Leroi, A. M., Chippendale, A. K., and Rose, M. R. (1994). Long-term labarotory evolution of a genetic life history trade-off in *Drosophila melanogaster*:I. The role of genotype-by-environment interaction. *Evolution*. **48,** 1244–1257.

Leslie, K. O., Schwarz, J., Simpson, K., and Huber, S. A. (1990). Progressive interstitial collagen deposition in Coxsackievirus B3-induced murine myocarditis. *Am J Pathol.* **136,** 683–693.

Lesne, S., Koh, M. T., Kotilinek, L., Kayed, R., Glabe, C. G., Yang, A., Gallagher, M., and Ashe, K. H. (2006). A specific amyloid-beta protein assembly in the brain impairs memory. *Nature.* **440,** 352–357.

Lesser, G. T., Deutsch, S., and Markofsky, J. (1973). Aging in the rat: Longitudinal and cross-sectional studies of body composition. *Am J Physiol.* **225,** 1472–1478.

Letenneur, L., Larrieu, S., and Barberger-Gateau, P. (2004). Alcohol and tobacco consumption as risk factors of dementia: A review of epidemiological studies. *Biomed Pharmacother.* **58,** 95–99.

Lev-Ari, S., Strier, L., Kazanov, D., Elkayam, O., Lichtenberg, D., Caspi, D., and Arber, N. (2006). Curcumin synergistically potentiates the growth-inhibitory and pro-apoptotic effects of celecoxib in osteoarthritis synovial adherent cells. *Rheumatolog.* **45,** 171–177.

Levels, J. H., Marquart, J. A., Abraham, P. R., van den Ende, A. E., Molhuizen, H. O., van Deventer, S. J., and Meijers, J. C. (2005). Lipopolysaccharide is transferred from high-density to low-density lipoproteins by lipopolysaccharide-binding protein and phospholipid transfer protein. *Infect Immun.* **73,** 2321–2326.

Levesque, L. E., Brophy, J. M., and Zhang, B. (2005). The risk for myocardial infarction with cyclooxygenase-2 inhibitors: A population study of elderly adults. *Ann Intern Med.* **142,** 481–489.

Levin-Allerhand, J. A., Lominska, C. E., and Smith, J. D. (2002). Increased amyloid-levels in APPSWE transgenic mice treated chronically with a physiological high-fat high-cholesterol diet. *J Nutr Health Aging* **6,** 315–319.

Levin, B. E., and Dunn-Meynell, A. A. (2002). Reduced central leptin sensitivity in rats with diet-induced obesity. *Am J Physiol Regul Integr Comp Physiol.* **283,** R941–948.

Levin, B. E., and Dunn-Meynell, A. A. (2004). Chronic exercise lowers the defended body weight gain and adiposity in diet-induced obese rats. *Am J Physiol Regul Integr Comp Physiol.* **286,** R771–778.

Levine, M. M., Rennels, M. B., Cisneros, L., Hughes, T. P., Nalin, D. R., and Young, C. R. (1980). Lack of person-to-person transmission of enterotoxigenic *Escherichia coli* despite close contact. *Am J Epidemiology.* **111,** 347–355.

Levrero, M., De Laurenzi, V., Costanzo, A., Gong, J., Wang, J. Y., and Melino, G. (2000). The p53/p63/p73 family of transcription factors: Overlapping and distinct functions. *J Cell Sci.* **113,** 1661–1670.

Levy-Marchal, C., and Czernichow, P. (2006). Small for gestational age and the metabolic syndrome: Which mechanism is suggested by epidemiological and clinical studies? *Horm Res.* **65(Suppl 3),** 123–130.

Lewin, E., and Olgaard, K. (2006). Klotho, an important new factor for the activity of Ca2+ channels, connecting calcium homeostasis, ageing and uraemia. *Nephrol Dial Transplant.* **21,** 1770–1772.

Lewington, S., Clarke, R., Qizilbash, N., Peto, R., and Collins, R. (2002). Age-specific relevance of usual blood pressure to vascular mortality: A meta-analysis of individual data for one million adults in 61 prospective studies. *Lancet.* **360,** 1903–1913.

Ley, R. E., Peterson, D. A., and Gordon, J. I. (2006). Ecological and evolutionary forces shaping microbial diversity in the human intestine. *Cell.* **12,** 837–848.

Li, D., Ng, A., Mann, N. J., and Sinclair, A. J. (1998). Contribution of meat fat to dietary arachidonic acid. [erratum appears in *Lipids* 1998, 33(8):837]. *Lipids.* **33,** 437–440.

Li, G., Shofer, J. B., Kukull, W. A., Peskind, E. R., Tsuang, D. W., Breitner, J. C., McCormick, W., Bowen, J. D., Teri, L., Schellenberg, G. D., and Larson, E. B. (2005a). Serum cholesterol and risk of Alzheimer disease: A community-based cohort study. *Neurology.* **65,** 1045–1050.

Li, H., Stein, A. D., Barnhart, H. X., Ramakrishnan, U., and Martorell, R. , Division of, B., Biomedical Sciences, N., and Health Sciences Program, (2003a). Associations between prenatal and postnatal growth and adult body size and composition. *Am J Clin Nutr.* **77,** 1498–1505.

Li, K. Z., Lindenberger, U., Freund, A. M., and Baltes, P. B. (2001). Walking while memorizing: Age-related differences in compensatory behavior. *Psychol Sci.* **12,** 230–237.

Li, L., Cao, D., Garber, D. W., Kim, H., and Fukuchi, K. (2003b). Association of aortic atherosclerosis with cerebral beta-amyloidosis and learning deficits in a mouse model of Alzheimer's disease. *Am J Pathol.* **163,** 2155–2164.

Li, L., Roumeliotis, N., Sawamura, T., Renier, G. (2004). C-reactive protein enhances LOX-1 expression in human aortic endothelial cells: relevance of LOX-1 to C-reactive protein-induced endothelial dysfunction. *Circ Res.* **95,** 877–883.

Li, Q., Withoff, S., and Verma, I. M. (2005b). Inflammation-associated cancer: NF-kappaB is the lynchpin. *Trends Immunol.* **26,** 318–325.

Li, S., Chen, W., Srinivasan, S. R., Bond, M. G., Tang, R., Urbina, E. M., and Berenson, G. S. (2003). Childhood cardiovascular risk factors and carotid vascular changes in adulthood: The Bogalusa Heart Study. [see comment][erratum appears in *JAMA* 2003; 290(22):2943]. *JAMA.* **290,** 2271–2276.

Li, S., Huang, N. F., and Hsu, S. (2005c). Mechanotransduction in endothelial cell migration. *J Cell Biochem.* **96,** 1110–1126.

Li, W., Hellsten, A., Xu, L. H., Zhuang, D. M., Jansson, K., Brunk, U. T., and Yuan, X. M. (2005d). Foam cell death induced by 7beta-hydroxycholesterol is mediated by labile iron-driven oxidative injury: Mechanisms underlying induction of ferritin in human atheroma. *Free Radic Biol Med.* **39,** 864–875.

Li, X., and Stark, G. R. (2002). NFkappaB-dependent signaling pathways. *Exp Hematol.* **30,** 285–296.

Li, X. A., Hatanaka, K., Ishibashi-Ueda, H., Yutani, C., and Yamamoto, A. (1995). Characterization of serum amyloid P component from human aortic atherosclerotic lesions. *Arterioscler Thromb Vasc Biol.* **15,** 252–257.

Li, Y. F., Langholz, B., Salam, M. T., and Gilliland, F. D. (2005e). Maternal and grandmaternal smoking patterns are associated with early childhood asthma. *Chest.* **127,** 1232–1241.

Li, Z., Froehlich, J., Galis, Z. S., and Lakatta, E. G. (1999). Increased expression of matrix metalloproteinase-2 in the thickened intima of aged rats. *Hypertension.* **33,** 116–123.

Liang, H., Masoro, E. J., Nelson, J. F., Strong, R., McMahan, C. A., and Richardson, A. (2003). Genetic mouse models of extended lifespan. *Exp Gerontol.* **38,** 1353–1364.

Liang, P., Hughes, V., Fukagawa, N. K. (1997). Increased prevalence of mitochondrial DNA deletions in skeletal muscle of older individuals with impaired glucose tolerance: possible marker of glycemic stress. *Diabetes.* **46,** 920–923.

Liao, D., Arnett, D. K., Tyroler, H. A., Riley, W. A., Chambless, L. E., Szklo, M., and Heiss, G. (1999). Arterial stiffness and the development of hypertension. The ARIC Study. *Hypertension.* **34,** 201–206.

Libby, P. (2003). Vascular biology of atherosclerosis: Overview and state of the art. *Am J Cardiol.* **91,** 3A–6A.

Libby, P., and Ridker, P. M. (2004). Inflammation and atherosclerosis: Role of C-reactive protein in risk assessment. *Am J Med.* **116(Suppl 6A),** 9S–16S.

Liberman, J. N., Stewart, W. F., Wesnes, K., Troncoso, J. (2002). Apolipoprotein E epsilon 4 and short-term recovery from predominantly mild brain injury. *Neurology.* **58,** 1038–1044.

Liberski, P. P., and Gajdusek, D. C. (1997). Kuru: Forty years later, a historical note. *Brain Pathology.* **7,** 555–560.

Libert, S., Chao, Y. J., Chu, X., and Pletcher, S. D. (2007). Trade-offs between longevity and pathogen resistance in Drosophila melanogaster are mediated by NFkB signaling. Aging Cell.**5,** 533–543

Libina, N., Berman, J. R., and Kenyon, C. (2003). Tisssue-specific activities of C. elegans DAF-16 in the regulation of lifespan. Cell. **115,** 489–502.

Licastro, F., Porcellini, E., Caruso, C., Lio, D., and Corder, E. H. (2006). Genetic risk profiles for Alzheimer's disease: Integration of APOE genotype and variants that up-regulate inflammation. *Neurobiol Aging.* In press.

Lichtenwalner, R. J., Forbes, M. E., Sonntag, W. E., and Riddle, D. R. (2006). Adult-onset deficiency in growth hormone and insulin-like growth factor-I decreases survival of dentate granule neurons: Insights into the regulation of adult hippocampal neurogenesis. *J Neurosci Res.* **83,** 199–210.

Lieber, C. S. (2004). Alcoholic fatty liver: Its pathogenesis and mechanism of progression to inflammation and fibrosis. *Alcohol.* **34,** 9–19.

Lieberman, E., Gremy, I., Lang, J. M., and Cohen, A. P. (1994). Low birthweight at term and the timing of fetal exposure to maternal smoking. *Am J Public Health.* **84,** 1127–1131.

Lieskovska, J., Guo, D., and Derman, E. (2003). Growth impairment in IL-6–overexpressing transgenic mice is associated with induction of SOCS3 mRNA. *Growth Horm IGF Res.* **13,** 26–35.

Lim, G. P., Chu, T., Yang, F., Beech, W., Frautschy, S. A., and Cole, G. M. (2001a). The curry spice curcumin reduces oxidative damage and amyloid pathology in an Alzheimer transgenic mouse. *J Neurosci.* **21,** 8370–8377.

Lim, G. P., Yang, F., Chu, T., Gahtan, E., Ubeda, O., Beech, W., Overmier, J. B., Hsiao-Ashec, K., Frautschy, S. A., and Cole, G. M. (2001b). Ibuprofen effects on Alzheimer pathology and open field activity in APPsw transgenic mice. *Neurobiol Aging.* **22,** 983–991.

Lin, H. C. (2004). Small intestinal bacterial overgrowth: A framework for understanding irritable bowel syndrome. *JAMA.* **292,** 852–858.

Lin, R. Y., Choudhury, R. P., Cai, W., Lu, M., Fallon, J. T., Fisher, E. A., and Vlassara, H. (2003). Dietary glycotoxins promote diabetic atherosclerosis in apolipoprotein E-deficient mice. *Atherosclerosis.* **168,** 213–220.

Lin, S. J., and Guarente, L. (2003). Nicotinamide adenine dinucleotide, a metabolic regulator of transcription, longevity and disease. *Curr Opin Cell Biol.* **15,** 241–246.

Lin, W. R., Jennings, R., Smith, T. L., Wozniak, M. A., and Itzhaki, R. F. (2001). Vaccination prevents latent HSV1 infection of mouse brain. *Neurobiol Aging.* **22,** 699–703.

Lin, W. R., Wozniak, M. A., Wilcock, G. K., and Itzhaki, R. F. (2002). Cytomegalovirus is present in a very high proportion of brains from vascular dementia patients. *Neurobiol Dis.* **9(1),** 82–87.

Lin, Y., Berg, A. H., Iyengar, P., Lam, T. K., Giacca, A., Combs, T. P., Rajala, M. W., Du, X., Rollman, B., Li, W., Hawkins, M., Barzilai, N., Rhodes, C. J., Fantus, I. G., Brownlee, M., and Scherer, P. E. (2005). The hyperglycemia-induced inflammatory response in adipocytes: The role of reactive oxygen species. *J Biol Chem.* **280,** 4617–4626.

Lin, Y., Rajala, M. W., Berger, J. P., Moller, D. E., Barzilai, N., and Scherer, P. E. (2001). Hyperglycemia-induced production of acute phase reactants in adipose tissue. *J Biol Chem.* **276,** 42077–42083.

Lin, Y. J., Seroude, L., and Benzer, S. (1998). Extended life-span and stress resistance in the *Drosophila* mutant Methuselah. *Science.* **282,** 943–946.

Lindsberg, P. J., and Grau, A. J. (2003). Inflammation and infections as risk factors for ischemic stroke. *Stroke.* **34,** 2518–2532.

Lindsey, J. R. (1998). Pathogen status in the 1990s: Abused terminology and compromised principles. *Lab An Sci.* **48,** 557–558.

Lindsey, J. R., Davidson, M. K., Schoeb, T. R., and Cassell, G. H. (1985). *Mycoplasma pulmonis*-host relationships in a breeding colony of Sprague-Dawley rats with enzootic murine respiratory mycoplasmosis. *Lab An Sci.* **35,** 597–608.

Lindsley, J. E., and Rutter, J. (2004). Nutrient sensing and metabolic decisions. *Comp Biochem Physiol B Biochem Mol Biol.* **139,** 543–559.

Lindstedt, K. A., and Kovanen, P. T. (2004). Mast cells in vulnerable coronary plaques: Potential mechanisms linking mast cell activation to plaque erosion and rupture. *Curr Opin Lipidol.* **15,** 567–573.

Ling, P. R., Mueller, C., Smith, R. J., and Bistrian, B. R. (2003). Hyperglycemia induced by glucose infusion causes hepatic oxidative stress and systemic inflammation, but not STAT3 or MAP kinase activation in liver in rats. *Metabolism.* **52,** 868–874.

Linke, A., Mèuller, P., Nurzynska, D., Casarsa, C., Torella, D., Nascimbene, A., Castaldo, C., Cascapera, S., Bèohm, M., Quaini, F., Urbanek, K., Leri, A., Hintze, T. H., Kajstura, J., Anversa, P. (2005). Stem cells in the dog heart are self-renewing, clonogenic, and multipotent and regenerate infarcted myocardium, improving cardiac function. *Proc Natl Acad Sci U S A.* **102,** 8966–8971.

Linnamo, V., Pakarinen, A., Komi, P. V., Kraemer, W. J., and Hèakkinen, K. (2005). Acute hormonal responses to submaximal and maximal heavy resistance and explosive exercises in men and women. *J Strength Cond Res.* **19,** 566–571.

Linton, P. J., and Dorshkind, K. (2004). Age-related changes in lymphocyte development and function. *Nature Immunol.* **5,** 133–139.

Lio, D., Candore, G., Crivello, A., Scola, L., Colonna-Romano, G., Cavallone, L., Hoffmann, E., Caruso, M., Licastro, F., Caldarera, C. M., Branzi, A., Franceschi, C., and Caruso, C. (2004). Opposite effects of interleukin 10 common gene polymorphisms in cardiovascular diseases and in successful ageing: Genetic background of male centenarians is protective against coronary heart disease. *J Med Genet.* **41,** 790–794.

Lipman, R. D., Dallal, G. E., and Bronson, R. T. (1999a). Effects of genotype and diet on age-related lesions in *ad libitum* fed and calorie-restricted F344, BN, and BNF3F1 rats. *J Gerontol. A Biol Sci Med Sci.* **54,** B478–491.

Lipman, R. D., Dallal, G. E., and Bronson, R. T. (1999b). Lesion biomarkers of aging in B6C3F1 hybrid mice. *J Gerontol. A Biol Sci Med Sci.* **54,** B466–477.

Lipman, R. D., Gaillard, E. T., Harrison, D. E., and Bronson, R. T. (1993). Husbandry factors and the prevalence of age-related amyloidosis in mice. *Lab An Sci.* **43,** 439–444.

Lithell, H. O., McKeigue, P. M., Berglund, L., Mohsen, R., Lithell, U. B., and Leon, D. A. (1996). Relation of size at birth to non-insulin dependent diabetes and insulin concentrations in men aged 50–60 years. *Br Med J.* **312**, 406–410.

Lithgow, G. J. (2003). Does anti-aging equal anti-microbial? *Science of Aging Knowledge Environment [electronic resource]: SAGE KE.* **2003**, PE16.

Little, C. S., Hammond, C. J., MacIntyre, A., Balin, B. J., and Appelt, D. M. (2004). *Chlamydia pneumoniae* induces Alzheimer-like amyloid plaques in brains of BALB/c mice. *Neurobiol Aging.* **25**, 419–429.

Liu, H., Bravata, D. M., Olkin, I., Nayak, S., Roberts, B., Garber, A. M., Hoffman, A. R. (2007). Systematic review: the safety and efficacy of growth hormone in the healthy elderly. *Ann Intern Med.* **146**, 104–115.

Liu, J., Yang, G., Thompson-Lanza, J. A., Glassman, A., Hayes, K., Patterson, A., Marquez, R. T., Auersperg, N., Yu, Y., Hahn, W. C., Mills, G. B., and Bast, R. C. J. (2004). A genetically defined model for human ovarian cancer. *Cancer Res.* **64**, 1655–63.

Liu, L. J., Yang, Y. J., Kuo, P. H., Wang, S. M., and Liu, C. C. (2005). Diagnostic value of bacterial stool cultures and viral antigen tests based on clinical manifestations of acute gastroenteritis in pediatric patients. *Eur J Clin Microbiol Infect Dis.* **24**, 559–561.

Liu, P. Y., Swerdloff, R. S., and Veldhuis, J. D. (2004). Clinical review 171: The rationale, efficacy and safety of androgen therapy in older men: Future research and current practice recommendations. *J Clin Endocrinol Metab.* **89**, 4789–4796.

Liu, Y., Zhu, Y., Rannou, F., Lee, T. S., Formentin, K., Zeng, L., Yuan, X., Wang, N., Chien, S., Forman, B. M., and Shyy, J. Y. (2004). Laminar flow activates peroxisome proliferator-activated receptor-gamma in vascular endothelial cells. *Circulation.* **110**, 1128–1133.

Liuba, P., Karnani, P., Pesonen, E., Paakkari, I., Forslid, A., Johansson, L., Persson, K., Wadstrom, T., and Laurini, R. (2000). Endothelial dysfunction after repeated *Chlamydia pneumoniae* infection in apolipoprotein E-knockout mice. *Circulation.* **102**, 1039–1044.

Liuba, P., Persson, J., Luoma, J., Ylèa-Herttuala, S., and Pesonen, E. (2003a). Acute infections in children are accompanied by oxidative modification of LDL and decrease of HDL cholesterol, and are followed by thickening of carotid intima-media. *Eur Heart J.* **24**, 515–521.

Liuba, P., Pesonen, E., Paakkari, I., Batra, S., Andersen, L., Forslid, A., Ylèa-Herttuala, S., Persson, K., Wadstrom, T., Wang, X., and Laurini, R. (2003b). Co-infection with *Chlamydia pneumoniae* and *Helicobacter pylori* results in vascular endothelial dysfunction and enhanced VCAM-1 expression in apoE-knockout mice. *J Vascular Res.* **40**, 115–122.

Liuba, P., Pesonen, E., Paakkari, I., Batra, S., Forslid, A., Kovanen, P., Pentikainen, M., Persson, K., and Sandstrom, S. (2003c). Acute *Chlamydia pneumoniae* infection causes coronary endothelial dysfunction in pigs. *Atherosclerosis.* **167**, 215–222.

Livingstone, F. B. (1985). *Frequencies of hemoglobin variants: Thalassemia, the glucose-6 phosphate dehydrigenase deficiency, g6pd variants, and ovalocytosis in human populations.* New York: Oxford University Press.

Lochmiller, R. L., and Deerenberg, C. (2000). Trade-offs in evolutionary immunology: Just what is the cost of immunity? *Oikos* **88**, 87–98.

Lockie, P., Harley, G., Walland, M., and Officer, K. (1992). Lacrimal probing. *Australian and New Zealand J Ophthalmology.* **20**, 351–352.

Loeb, M. B., Molloy, D. W., Smieja, M., Standish, T., Goldsmith, C. H., Mahony, J., Smith, S., Borrie, M., Decoteau, E., Davidson, W., McDougall, A., Gnarpe, J., O'D, O. M., and

Chernesky, M. (2004). A randomized, controlled trial of doxycycline and rifampin for patients with Alzheimer's disease. *J Am Geriatr Soc.* **52,** 381–387.

Loeser, R., F. Jr. (2004). Aging cartilage and osteoarthritis—What's the link? *Sci Aging Knowledge Environ.* **2004,** pe31.

Lof, M., and Forsum, E. (2006). Activity pattern and energy expenditure due to physical activity before and during pregnancy in healthy Swedish women. *Br J Nutr.* **95,** 296–302.

Lof, M., Olausson, H., Bostrom, K., Janerot-Sjèoberg, B., Sohlstrom, A., and Forsum, E. (2005). Changes in basal metabolic rate during pregnancy in relation to changes in body weight and composition, cardiac output, insulin-like growth factor I, and thyroid hormones and in relation to fetal growth. *Am J Clin Nutr.* **81,** 678–685.

Loffreda, S., Yang, S. Q., Lin, H. Z., Karp, C. L., Brengman, M. L., Wang, D. J., Klein, A. S., Bulkley, G. B., Bao, C., Noble, P. W., Lane, M. D., and Diehl, A. M. (1998). Leptin regulates proinflammatory immune responses. *FASEB J* **12,** 57–65.

Loftus, I. M., Naylor, A. R., Goodall, S., Crowther, M., Jones, L., Bell, P. R., and Thompson, M. M. (2000). Increased matrix metalloproteinase-9 activity in unstable carotid plaques. A potential role in acute plaque disruption. *Stroke.* **31,** 40–47.

Lombard, M. (2005). Evidence of hunting and hafting during the Middle Stone Age at Sibidu Cave, KwaZulu-Natal, South Africa: A multianalytical approach. *J Hum Evol.* **48,** 279–300.

Long, E. R. (1933). The development of our knowledge of arteriosclerosis. In E. V. Cowdry, Ed., *Arteriosclerosis. A survey of the problem*, pp. 19–52. New York: Macmillan.

Long, J. M., Kalehua, A. N., Muth, N. J., Calhoun, M. E., Jucker, M., Hengemihle, J. M., Ingram, D. K., and Mouton, P. R. (1998). Stereological analysis of astrocyte and microglia in aging mouse hippocampus. *Neurobiol Aging.* **19,** 497–503.

Long, X., Muller, F., and Avruch, J. (2004). TOR action in mammalian cells and in *Caenorhabditis elegans. Curr Top Microbiol Immunol.* **279,** 115–138.

Long, X., Spycher, C., Han, Z. S., Rose, A. M., Mèuller, F., and Avruch, J. (2002). TOR deficiency in *C. elegans* causes developmental arrest and intestinal atrophy by inhibition of mRNA translation. *Curr Biol.* **12,** 1448–1461.

Longo, V. D., and Finch, C. E. (2003). Evolutionary medicine: From starvation and dwarf model systems to healthy centenarians? *Science.* **299,** 1342–1346.

Longo, V. D., and Kennedy, B. K. (2006). Sirtuins in aging and age-related disease. *Cell.* **126,** 257–268.

Longo, V. D., Mitteldorf, J., and Skulachev, V. P. (2005). Opinion: Programmed and altruistic ageing. *Nat Rev Genet.* **6,** 866–872.

Longo, V. D., Viola, K. L., Klein, W. L., and Finch, C. E. (2000). Reversible inactivation of superoxide-sensitive aconitase in Abeta1-42-treated neuronal cell lines. *J Neurochem.* **75(5),** 1977–1985.

Lopez-Miranda, J., Ordovas, J. M., Mata, P., Lichtenstein, A. H., Clevidence, B., Judd, J. T., and Schaefer, E. J. (1994). Effect of apolipoprotein E phenotype on diet-induced lowering of plasma low density lipoprotein cholesterol. *J Lipid Res.* **35,** 1965–1975.

Lopez-Quesada, E., Vilaseca, M. A., Artuch, R., Gomez, E., and Lailla, J. M. (2003). Homocysteine and other plasma amino acids in preeclampsia and in pregnancies without complications. *Clin Biochem.* **36,** 185–192.

Lopez-Torres, M., Gredilla, R., Sanz, A., and Barja, G. (2002). Influence of aging and long-term caloric restriction on oxygen radical generation and oxidative DNA damage in rat liver mitochondria. *Free Radic Biol Med.* **32,** 882–889.

Lopez-Torres, M., Perez-Campo, R., Rojas, C., Cadenas, S., and Barja, G. (1993). Maximum life span in vertebrates: Relationship with liver antioxidant enzymes, glutathione system, ascorbate, urate, sensitivity to peroxidation, true malondialdehyde, *in vivo* H2O2, and basal and maximum aerobic capacity. *Mech Ageing Dev.* **70**, 177–199.

Lopez, N. J., Jara, L., and Valenzuela, C. Y. (2005). Association of interleukin-1 polymorphisms with periodontal disease. *J Periodontology.* **76**, 234–243.

Lopuhaa, C. E., Roseboom, T. J., Osmond, C., Barker, D. J., Ravelli, A. C., Bleker, O. P., van der Zee, J. S., and van der Meulen, J. H. (2000). Atopy, lung function, and obstructive airways disease after prenatal exposure to famine. *Thorax.* **55**, 555–561.

Lorberg, A., and Hall, M. N. (2004). TOR: The first 10 years. *Curr Top Microbiol Immunol.* **279**, 1–18.

Lord, G. M., Matarese, G., Howard, J. K., Baker, R. J., Bloom, S. R., and Lechler, R. I. (1998). Leptin modulates the T-cell immune response and reverses starvation-induced immunosuppression. *Nature.* **394**, 897–901.

Lordkipanidze, D., Vekua, A., Ferring, R., Rightmire, G. P., Agusti, J., Kiladze, G., Mouskhelishvili, A., Nioradze, M., Ponce de León, M. S., Tappen, M., and Zollikofer, C. P. (2005). Anthropology: The earliest toothless hominin skull. *Nature.* **434**, 717–718.

Lorenzini, A., McCarter, R., Ikeno, Y., Masoro, E., Liu, M., Cristofalo, V. J., and Sell, C. (2004). Longevity in mice hypomorphic for the Igf1 allele. *Gerontologist* (Abstr).

Lorenzini, A., Tresini, M., Austad, S. N., and Cristofalo, V. J. (2005). Cellular replicative capacity correlates primarily with species body mass not longevity. *Mech Ageing Dev.* **126**, 1130–1133.

Losito, A., Kalidas, K., Santoni, S., and Jeffery, S. (2003). Association of interleukin-6 -174G/C promoter polymorphism with hypertension and left ventricular hypertrophy in dialysis patients. *Kidney Int.* **64**, 616–622.

Lott, I. T. (2005). Alzheimer disease and Down Syndrome: Factors in pathogenesis. *Neurobiol Aging.* **26**, 383–389.

Loucks, E. B., Berkman, L. F., Gruenewald, T. L., and Seeman, T. E. (2006). Relation of social integration to inflammatory marker concentrations in men and women 70 to 79 years. *Am J Cardiol.* **97**, 1010–1016.

Louwman, M. W., van Dusseldorp, M., van de Vijver, F. J., Thomas, C. M., Schneede, J., Ueland, P. M., Refsum, H., and van Staveren, W. A. (2000). Signs of impaired cognitive function in adolescents with marginal cobalamin status. *Am J Clin Nutr.* **72**, 762–769.

Lovell, M. A., Robertson, J. D., Buchholz, B. A., Xie, C., and Markesbery, W. R. (2002). Use of bomb pulse carbon-14 to age senile plaques and neurofibrillary tangles in Alzheimer's disease. *Neurobiol Aging.* **23**, 179–186.

Lovell, M. A., Robertson, J. D., Teesdale, W. J., Campbell, J. L., and Markesbery, W. R. (1998). Copper, iron and zinc in Alzheimer's disease senile plaques. *J Neural Sci.* **158**, 47–52.

Lovell, N. C. (2000). Skeletal evidence of systemic inflammatory disease in free-ranging chimpanzees and gorillas. *Primates.* **41**, 275–290.

Lu, C., He, J. C., Cai, W., Liu, H., Zhu, L., and Vlassara, H. (2004a). Advanced glycation endproduct (AGE) receptor 1 is a negative regulator of the inflammatory response to AGE in mesangial cells. *Proc Natl Acad Sci USA.* **101**, 11767–11772.

Lu, T., Pan, Y., Kao, S.-Y., Li, C., Kohane, I. S., Chan, J., and Yankner, B. A. (2004b). Gene regulation and DNA damage in the ageing human brain. *Nature.* **429**, 883-891.

Luc, G., Bard, J. M., Juhan-Vague, I., Ferrieres, J., Evans, A., Amouyel, P., Arveiler, D., Fruchart, J. C., and Ducimetiere, P. (2003). C-reactive protein, interleukin-6, and fibrinogen as predictors of coronary heart disease: The PRIME Study. *Arterioscler Thromb Vasc Biol.* **23,** 1255–1261.

Luchsinger, J. A., and Mayeux, R. (2004a). Cardiovascular risk factors and Alzheimer's disease. *Curr Atheroscler Rep.* **6,** 261–266.

Luchsinger, J. A., and Mayeux, R. (2004b). Dietary factors and Alzheimer's disease. *Lancet Neuro.* **3,** 579–587.

Luchsinger, J. A., Patel, B., Tang, M. X., Shupf, N., and Mayeux, R. (2006). Measures of adiposity and dementia risk in the elderly. In prep.

Luchsinger, J. A., Tang, M. X., Shea, S., and Mayeux, R. (2002). Caloric intake and the risk of Alzheimer disease. *Archives of Neurology.* **59,** 1258–63.

Luckinbill, L. S., Arking, R., Clare, M. J., Cirocco, W. C., and Buck, S. A. (1984). Selection for lifespan in *Drosophila melanogaster. Heredity.* **55,** 9–18.

Lucotte, G., and Mercier, G. (2005). The population distribution of the Met allele at the PRNP129 polymorphism (a high risk factor for Creutzfeldt-Jakob disease) in various regions of France and in West Europe. *Infect Genet Evol.* **5(2),** 141–144.

Lumey, L. H., and Stein, A. D., and Academic Medical Center, A. T. N. (1997a). In utero exposure to famine and subsequent fertility: The Dutch Famine Birth Cohort Study. *Am J Public Health.* **87,** 1962–1966.

Lumey, L. H., and Stein, A. D. (1997). Offspring birth weights after maternal intrauterine undernutrition: A comparison within sibships. *Am J Epidemiol.* **146,** 810–819.

Lumey, L. H., Stein, A. D., and Ravelli, A. C. (1995). Timing of prenatal starvation in women and birth weight in their first and second born offspring: The Dutch Famine Birth Cohort Study. *Eur J Obstet Gynecol Reprod Biol.* **61,** 23–30.

Lutter, C. K., Mora, J. O., Habicht, J. P., Rasmussen, K. M., Robson, D. S., Sellers, S. G., Super, C. M., and Herrera, M. G. (1989). Nutritional supplementation: Effects on child stunting because of diarrhea. *Am J Clin Nutr.* **50,** 1–8.

Lynch, J. R., Tang, W., Wang, H., Vitek, M. P., Bennett, E. R., Sullivan, P. M., Warner, D. S., and Laskowitz, D. T. (2003). APOE genotype and an ApoE-mimetic peptide modify the systemic and central nervous system inflammatory response. *J Biol Chem.* **278,** 48529–48533.

Lynch, N. J., Willis, C. L., Nolan, C. C., Roscher, S., Fowler, M. J., Weihe, E., Ray, D. E., and Schwaeble, W. J., (2004). Microglial activation and increased synthesis of complement component C1q precedes blood-brain barrier dysfunction in rats. *Molecular Immunology.* **40,** 709–716.

Lyon, C. J., Law, R. E., and Hsueh, W. A. (2003). Minireview: Adiposity, inflammation, and atherogenesis. *Endocrinology.* **144,** 2195–2200.

Lyons, M. J., Faust, I. M., Hemmes, R. B., Buskirk, D. R., Hirsch, J., and Zabriskie, J. B. (1982). A virally induced obesity syndrome in mice. *Science.* **216,** 82–85.

Lyons, M. J., Nagashima, K., and Zabriskie, J. B. (2002). Animal models of postinfectious obesity: Hypothesis and review. *J Neurovirol.* **8,** 1–5.

Ma, H., Bernstein, L., Pike, M. C., and Ursin, G. (2006). Reproductive factors and breast cancer risk according to joint estrogen and progesterone receptor status: A meta-analysis of epidemiological studies. *Breast Cancer Res.* **8,** R43.

Ma, J., Giovannucci, E., Pollak, M., Leavitt, A., Tao, Y., Gaziano, J. M., and Stampfer, M. J. (2004). A prospective study of plasma C-peptide and colorectal cancer risk in men. *J Natl Cancer Inst.* **96,** 546–553.

Macinnis, R. J., and English, D. R. (2006). Body size and composition and prostate cancer risk: Systematic review and meta-regression analysis. *Cancer Causes Control.* **17,** 989–1003.

MacIntyre, A., Abramov, R., Hammond, C. J., Hudson, A. P., Arking, E. J., Little, C. S., Appelt, D. M., and Balin, B. J. (2003). *Chlamydia pneumoniae* infection promotes the transmigration of monocytes through human brain endothelial cells. *J Neurosci Res.* **71,** 740–750.

MacIntyre, A., Hammond, C. J., Little, C. S., Appelt, D. M., and Balin, B. J. (2002). *Chlamydia pneumoniae* infection alters the junctional complex proteins of human brain microvascular endothelial cells. *FEMS Microbiology Lett.* **217(2),** 167–172.

Mack, W. J., Slater, C. C., Xiang, M., Shoupe, D., Lobo, R. A., and Hodis, H. N. (2004). Elevated subclinical atherosclerosis associated with oophorectomy is related to time since menopause rather than type of menopause. *Fertil Steril.* **82,** 391–397.

Maclean, C. H., Issa, A. M., Newberry, S. J., Mojica, W. A., Morton, S. C., Garland, R. H., Hilton, L. G., Traina, S. B., and Shekelle, P. G. (2005). Effects of omega-3 fatty acids on cognitive function with aging, dementia, and neurological diseases. *Evid Rep Technol Assess (Summ).* **114,** 1–3.

MacNee, W. (2001). Oxidative stress and lung inflammation in airways disease. *Eur J Pharmacol.* **429(1–3),** 195–207.

Madden, D. J. (2001). Speed and timing of behavioral processes. In J. E. B. K. W. Schaie, Ed., *Handbook of the psychology of aging,* pp. 288–369. San Diego: Academic Press.

Madsen, C., Dagnaes-Hansen, F., Møller, J., and Falk, E. (2003). Hypercholesterolemia in pregnant mice does not affect atherosclerosis in adult offspring. *Atherosclerosis.* **168,** 221–228.

Maeda, H., Gleiser, C. A., Masoro, E. J., Murata, I., McMahan, C. A., and Yu, B. P. (1985). Nutritional influences on aging of Fischer 344 rats: II. Pathology. *J Gerontol.* **40,** 671–688.

Maeshima, S., Okita, R., Yamaga, H., Ozaki, F., and Moriwaki, H. (2003). Relationships between event-related potentials and neuropsychological tests in neurologically healthy adults. *J Clin Neurosci.* **10,** 60–62.

Magee, D. M. (1998). Arterial disease in antiquity. *Med J Austral.* **169,** 663–666.

Magnuson, B. A., South, E. H., Exon, J. H., Dashwood, R. H., Xu, M., Hendrix, K., and Hubele, S. (2000). Increased susceptibility of adult rats to azoxymethane-induced aberrant crypt foci. *Cancer Lett.* **161,** 185–193.

Magwere, T., Chapman, T., and Partridge, L. (2004). Sex differences in the effect of dietary restriction on life span and mortality rates in female and male *Drosophila melanogaster. J Gerontol. A Biol Sci Med Sci.* **59,** 3–9.

Magwere, T., Pamplona, R., Miwa, S., Martinez-Diaz, P., Portero-Otin, M., Brand, M. D., and Partridge, L. (2006). Flight activity, mortality rates, and lipoxidative damage in *Drosophila. J Gerontol. A Biol Sci Med Sci.* **61(2),** 136–145.

Mahley, R. W. (1988). Apolipoprotein E: Cholesterol transport protein with expanding role in cell biology. *Science.* **240,** 622–630.

Mahley, R. W., and Rall, S. C., Jr. (2000). Apolipoprotein E: Far more than a lipid transport protein. *Annu Rev Genomics Hum Genet.* **1,** 507–537.

Mai, V., Colbert, L. H., Berrigan, D., Perkins, S. N., Pfeiffer, R., Lavigne, J. A., Lanza, E., Haines, D. C., Schatzkin, A., and Hursting, S. D. (2003). Calorie restriction and diet composition modulate spontaneous intestinal tumorigenesis in Apc(Min) mice through different mechanisms. *Cancer Res.* **63,** 1752–1755.

Maier, B., Gluba, W., Bernier, B., Turner, T., Mohammad, K., Guise, T., Sutherland, A., Thorner, M., and Scrable, H. (2004). Modulation of mammalian life span by the short isoform of p53. *Genes Devel.* **18,** 306–319.

Maillard, L. C. (1912). Action des acides amines sur les sucre: formation des melanoides par voie methodique. *CR Acad Sci.* **154,** 66–68.

Main, A. J. (1979). Eastern equine encephalomyelitis virus in experimentally infected bats. *J Wildlife Diseases.* **15,** 467–477.

Mair, W., Goymer, P., Pletcher, S. D., and Partridge, L. (2003). Demography of dietary restriction and death in *Drosophila. Science.* **301,** 1731–1733.

Mair, W., Sgro, C. M., Johnson, A. P., Chapman, T., and Partridge, L., (2004). Lifespan extension by dietary restriction in female *Drosophila melanogaster* is not caused by a reduction in vitellogenesis or ovarian activity. *Exp Gerontol.* **39,** 1011–1019.

Mak, H. Y., and Ruvkun, G. (2004). Intercellular signaling of reproductive development by the *C. elegans* DAF-9 cytochrome P450. *Development.* **131,** 1777–1786.

Makimura, H., Mizuno, T. M., Isoda, F., Beasley, J., Silverstein, J. H., and Mobbs, C. V. (2003). Role of glucocorticoids in mediating effects of fasting and diabetes on hypothalamic gene expression. *BMC Physiology.* **3,** 5.

Makimura, H., Mizuno, T. M., Mastaitis, J. W., Agami, R., and Mobbs, C. V. (2002). Reducing hypothalamic AGRP by RNA interference increases metabolic rate and decreases body weight without influencing food intake. *BMC Neuroscience.* **3,** 18.

Malandro, M. S., Beveridge, M. J., Kilberg, M. S., and Novak, D. A. (1996). Effect of low-protein diet-induced intrauterine growth retardation on rat placental amino acid transport. *Am J Physiol.* **271(Pt 1),** C295–303.

Malcolm, J. C., Lawson, M. L., Gaboury, I., Lough, G., and Keely, E. (2006). Glucose tolerance of offspring of mother with gestational diabetes mellitus in a low-risk population. *Diabet Med.* **23,** 565–570.

Malide, D., Davies-Hill, T. M., Levine, M., and Simpson, I. A. (1998). Distinct localization of GLUT-1, -3, and -5 in human monocyte-derived macrophages: Effects of cell activation. *Am J Physiol.* **274,** E516–526.

Malik, S., Wong, N. D., Franklin, S. S., Kamath, T. V., L'Italien, G. J., Pio, J. R., and Williams, G. R. (2004). Impact of the metabolic syndrome on mortality from coronary heart disease, cardiovascular disease, and all causes in United States adults. *Circulation.* **110,** 1245–1250.

Mallo, G. V., Kurz, C. L., Couillault, C., Pujol, N., Granjeaud, S., Kohara, Y., and Ewbank, J. J. (2002). Inducible antibacterial defense system in *C. elegans. Curr Biol.* **12,** 1209–1214.

Maloney, C. A., and Rees, W. D. (2005). Gene-nutrient interactions during fetal development. *Reproduction.* **130,** 401–410.

Mancini-Dinardo, D., Steele, S. J., Levorse, J. M., Ingram, R. S., and Tilghman, S. M. (2006). Elongation of the Kcnq1ot1 transcript is required for genomic imprinting of neighboring genes. *Genes Dev.* **20,** 1268–1282.

Mancuso, P., Huffnagle, G. B., Olszewski, M. A., Phipps, J., and Peters-Golden, M. (2006). Leptin corrects host defense defects after acute starvation in murine pneumococcal pneumonia. *Am J Respir Crit Care Med.* **173,** 212–218.

Mandal, A. (2006). Do malnutrition and nutritional supplementation have an effect on the wound healing process? *J Wound Care.* **15,** 254–257.

Manfras, B. J., Weidenbach, H., Beckh, K. H., Kern, P., Mèoller, P., Adler, G., Mertens, T., and Boehm, B. O. (2004). Oligoclonal CD8+ T-cell expansion in patients with chronic hepatitis C is associated with liver pathology and poor response to interferon-alpha therapy. *J Clin Immunol.* **24(3),** 258–271.

Mangel, M., and Abrahams, M. V. (2001). Age and longevity in fish, with consideration of the ferox trout. *Exp Gero.* **36,** 765–790.

Maniero, G. D. (2002). Classical pathway serum complement activity throughout various stages of the annual cycle of a mammalian hibernator, the golden-mantled ground squirrel, *Spermophilus lateralis. Dev Comp Immunol.* **26,** 563–574.

Mann, N., Sinclair, A., Pille, M., Johnson, L., Warrick, G., Reder, E., and Lorenz, R. (1997). The effect of short-term diets rich in fish, red meat, or white meat on thromboxane and prostacyclin synthesis in humans. *Lipids.* **32,** 635–644.

Marcellin, P., Castelnau, C., Martinot-Peignoux, M., and Boyer, N. (2005). Natural history of hepatitis B. *Minerva Gastroenterol Dietol.* **51,** 63–75.

Marchalonis, J. J., Kaveri, S., Lacroix-Desmazes, S., and Kazatchkine, M. D. (2002). Natural recognition repertoire and the evolutionary emergence of the combinatorial immune system. *FASEB J.* **16,** 842–848.

Marchegiani, F., Marra, M., Spazzafumo, L., James, R. W., Boemi, M., Olivieri, F., Cardelli, M., Cavallone, L., Bonfigli, A. R., and Franceschi, C. (2006). Paraoxonase activity and genotype predispose to successful aging. *J Gerontol. A Biol Sci Med Sci.* **61,** 541–546.

Marcovecchio, M., Mohn, A., and Chiarelli, F. (2005). Type 2 diabetes mellitus in children and adolescents. *J Endocrinol Invest.* **28,** 853–863.

Markowski, B. (1945). Some experiences of a medical prisoner of war. *Br Med J ,* 361–363.

Markus, H. S., Labrum, R., Bevan, S., Reindl, M., Egger, G., Wiedermann, C. J., Xu, Q., Kiechl, S., and Willeit, J., (2006). Genetic and acquired inflammatory conditions are synergistically associated with early carotid atherosclerosis. *Stroke.* **37,** 2253–2259.

Marlowe, F. (2000) Paternal investment and the human mating system. *Behav. Processes* **51,** 45–61.

Marmorstein, R. (2004). Structure and chemistry of the Sir2 family of NAD(+)-dependent histone/protein deactylases. *Biochem Soc Trans.* **32,** 904–909.

Marmot, M. G. (2006). Status syndrome: A challenge to medicine. *JAMA.* **295,** 1304–1307.

Marmot, M. G., Adelstein, A. M., Robinson, N., and Rose, G. A. (1978). Changing social-class distribution of heart disease. *Br Med J.* **2,** 1109–1112.

Marsland, A. L., Bachen, E. A., Cohen, S., Rabin, B., and Manuck, S. B. (2002). Stress, immune reactivity and susceptibility to infectious disease. *Physiol Behav.* **77,** 711–716.

Martin-Ruiz, C., Saretzki, G., Petrie, J., Ladhoff, J., Jeyapalan, J., Wei, W., Sedivy, J., and von Zglinicki, T. (2004). Stochastic variation in telomere shortening rate causes heterogeneity of human fibroblast replicative life span. *J Biol Chem.* **279,** 17826–17833.

Martin-Ruiz, C. M., Gussekloo, J., van Heems, D., von Zglinicki, T., and Westendorp, R. G. (2005). Telomere length in white blood cells is not associated with morbidity or mortality in the oldest old: A population-based study. *Aging Cell.* **4,** 287–290.

Martin, G. M. (1999). APOE alleles and lipophylic pathogens. *Neurobiol Aging* **20,** 441–3.

Martin, G. M. (2005). Epigenetic drift in aging identical twins. *PNAS.* **102,** 10413–10414.

Martin, G. M., Sprague, C. A., and Epstein, C. J. (1970). Replicative life-span of cultivated human cells. Effects of donor's age, tissue, and genotype. *Lab Invest* **23,** 86–92.

Martin, K., and Kirkwood, T. B. L. (1998). Age changes in stem cells of murine small intestinal crypts. *Exp. Cell Res.* **241,** 316–323.

Martin, K., Potten, C. S., Roberts, S. A., and Kirkwood, T. B. (1998). Altered stem cell regeneration in irradiated intestinal crypts of senescent mice. *J Cell Sci.* **111,** 2297–2303.

Martin, L. B. I., Navara, K. J., Weil, Z. M., and Nelson, R. J. (2007). Immunological memory is compromised by food restriction in deer mice. *Am J Physiol, Reg. Comp, Integ.* **292,** R316–320.

Martin, R. D. (1981). Relative brain size and basaql metabolic rate interrestrial vertebrates. *Nature*. **293**, 57–60.

Martinelli, C., and Reichhart, J. M. (2005). Evolution and integration of innate immune systems from fruit flies to man: Lessons and questions. *J Endotoxin Res*. **11**, 243–248.

Martorell, R., Habicht, J. P., and Rivera, J. A. (1995). History and design of the INCAP longitudinal study (1969–77) and its follow-up (1988–89). *J Nutr*. **125 (Suppl)**, 1027S–1041S.

Martorell, R., Habicht, J. P., Yarbrough, C., Lechtig, A., Klein, R. E., and Western, K. A. (1975). Acute morbidity and physical growth in rural Guatemalan children. *Am J Dis Child*. **129**, 1296–1301.

Martorell, R., Schroeder, D. G., Rivera, J. A., and Kaplowitz, H. J. (1995). Patterns of linear growth in rural Guatemalan adolescents and children. *J Nutr*. **125(4 Suppl)**, 1060S–1067S.

Martorell, R., Yarbrough, C., Lechtig, A., Habicht, J. P., and Klein, R. E. (1975b). Diarrheal diseases and growth retardation in preschool Guatemalan children. *Am J Phys Anthropol*. **43(3)**, 341–346.

Martorell, R., Yarbrough, C., Yarbrough, S., and Klein, R. E. (1980). The impact of ordinary illnesses on the dietary intakes of malnourished children. *Am J Clin Nutr*. **33(2)**, 345–350.

Martyn, C. N., Barker, D. J., Jespersen, S., Greenwald, S., Osmond, C., and Berry, C. (1995). Growth in utero, adult blood pressure, and arterial compliance. *Brit Heart Jl* **73**, 116–121.

Martyn, C. N., and Greenwald, S. E. (1997). Impaired synthesis of elastin in walls of aorta and large conduit arteries during early development as an initiating event in pathogenesis of systemic hypertension. *Lancet*. **350**, 953–955.

Martyn, C. N., and Greenwald, S. E. (2001). A hypothesis about a mechanism for the programming of blood pressure and vascular disease in early life. *Clin Exp Pharmacol & Physiol*. **28**, 948–951.

Martyn, C. N., Meade, T. W., Stirling, Y., and Barker, D. J. (1995b). Plasma concentrations of fibrinogen and factor VII in adult life and their relation to intra-uterine growth. *Br J Haematol*. **89**, 142–146.

Masliah, E., Mallory, M., Hansen, L., DeTeresa, R., and Terry, R. D. (1993). Quantitative synaptic alterations in the human neocortex during normal aging. *Neurology*. **43**, 192–197.

Masoro, E. J. (2005). Overview of caloric restriction and ageing. *Mech Ageing Dev*. **126**, 913–922.

Masoro, E. J., and Austad, S. N. (1996). The evolution of the antiaging action of dietary restriction: A hypothesis. *J Gerontol. A Biol Sci Med Sci*. **51**, B387–391.

Masoro, E. J., Iwasaki, K., Gleiser, C. A., McMahan, C. A., Seo, E. J., and Yu, B. P. (1989a). Dietary modulation of the progression of nephropathy in aging rats: An evaluation of the importance of protein. *Am J Clin Nutr*. **49**, 1217–1227.

Masoro, E. J., Katz, M. S., and McMahan, C. A. (1989bb). Evidence for the glycation hypothesis of aging from the food-restricted rodent model. *J Gerontol*. **44**, B20–22.

Masoro, E. J., McCarter, R. J., Katz, M. S., and McMahan, C. A. (1992). Dietary restriction alters characteristics of glucose fuel use. *J Gerontol*. **47**, B202–208.

Massion, P. B., Pelat, M., Belge, C., and Balligand, J. L. (2005). Regulation of the mammalian heart function by nitric oxide. *Comp Biochem Physiol A Mol Integr Physiol*. **142**, 144–150.

Masson, L. F., McNeill, G., and Avenell, A. (2003). Genetic variation and the lipid response to dietary intervention: A systematic review. *Am J Clin Nutr* **77**, 1098–1111.

Mastaitis, J. W., Wurmbach, E., Cheng, H., Sealfon, S. C., and Mobbs, C. V. (2005). Acute induction of gene expression in brain and liver by insulin-induced hypoglycemia. *Diabetes.* **54,** 952–958.

Mata, L. J. (1978). *The children of Santa Maria Cauque: A prospective field study of health and growth.* Cambridge, MA: MIT Press.

Mata, L. J., Jiménez, F., Cordón, M., Rosales, R., Prera, E., Schneider, R. E., and Viteri, F. (1972a). Gastrointestinal flora of children with protein-calorie malnutrition. *Am J Clin Nutr.* **25,** 118–126.

Mata, L. J., Urrutia, J. J., Albertazzi, C., Pellecer, O., and Arellano, E. (1972b). Influence of recurrent infections on nutrition and growth of children in Guatemala. *Am J Clin Nutr.* **25,** 1267–1275.

Matarese, G., Moschos, S., and Mantzoros, C. S. (2005). Leptin in immunology. *J Immunol.* **174,** 3137–3142.

Mateu, E., Calafell, F., Lao, O., Bonne-Tamir, B., Kidd, J. R., Pakstis, A., Kidd, K. K., and Bertranpetit, J. (2001). Worldwide genetic analysis of the CFTR region. *Am J Hum Genet.* **68,** 103–117.

Mateu, E., Calafell, F., Ramos, M. D., Casals, T., and Bertranpetit, J. (2002). Can a place of origin of the main cystic fibrosis mutations be identified? *Am J Hum Genet.* **70,** 257–264.

Mathers, C. D., Sadana, R., Salomon, J. A., Murray, C. J., and Lopez, A. D. (2001). Healthy life expectancy in 191 countries, 1999. *Lancet.* **357,** 1685–1691.

Matsumura, T., Hayashi, M., and Konishi, R. (1985). Immortalization in culture of rat cells: A genealogic study. *J Natl Cancer Inst.* **74,** 1223–1232.

Matsumura, T., Zerrudo, Z., and Hayflick, L. (1979). Senescent human diploid cells in culture: Survival, DNA synthesis and morphology. *J Gerontol.* **34,** 328–334.

Matsuzawa, Y. (1997). Pathophysiology and molecular mechanisms of visceral fat syndrome: the Japanese experience. *Diabetes/Metabolism Reviews.* **13,** 3–13.

Matthiesen, L., Berg, G., Ernerudh, J., Ekerfelt, C., Jonsson, Y., and Sharma, S. (2005). Immunology of preeclampsia. *Chem Immunol Allergy.* **89,** 49–61.

Mattson, M. P. (2004). Infectious agents and age-related neurodegenerative disorders. *Ageing Res Rev.* **3,** 105–120.

Mattson, M. P. (2005). Energy intake, meal frequency, and health: A neurobiological perspective. *Annu Rev Nutr.* **25,** 237–260.

Mattson, M. P., and Camandola, S. (2001). NF-kappaB in neuronal plasticity and neurodegenerative disorders. *J Clin Invest.* **107,** 247–254.

Mawdesley-Thomas, L. E. (1967). Discussion, p. 227. In E. Cotchin and C. Roe, Eds., *Pathology of laboratory rats and mice*, pp. (op. cit, p. 227). Oxford, UK: Blackwell.

May, P. C., and Finch, C. E. (1992). Sulfated glycoprotein 2: New relationships of this multifunctional protein to neurodegeneration. *Trends Neurosci.* **15,** 391–396.

May, P. C., Lampert-Etchells, M., Johnson, S. A., Poirier, J., Masters, J. N., and Finch, C. E. (1990). Dynamics of gene expression for a hippocampal glycoprotein elevated in Alzheimer's disease and in response to experimental lesions in rat. *Neuron.* **5,** 831–839.

May, P. C., Telford, N., Salo, D., Anderson, C., Kohama, S. G., Finch, C. E., Walford, R. L., and Weindruch, R. (1992). Failure of dietary restriction to retard age-related neuro-chemical changes in mice. *Neurobiol Aging.* **13,** 787–791.

Mayer, J., Roy, P., and Mitra, K. P. (1956). Relation between caloric intake, body weight, and physical work: Studies in an industrial male population in West Bengal. *Am J Clin Nutr.* **4,** 169–175.

Mayeux, R. (2003a). Apolipoprotein E, Alzheimer disease, and African Americans. *Archives of Neurology.* **60,** 161–163.

Mayeux, R. (2003b). Epidemiology of neurodegeneration. *Annu Rev Neurosci.* **26,** 81–104.

Maynard Smith, J. (1958). Prolongation of the life of *Drosophila subobscura* by a brief exposure of adults to a high temperature. *Nature.* **181,** 496–497.

Mayr, M., Kiechl, S., Tsimikas, S., Miller, E., Sheldon, J., Willeit, J., Witztum, J. L., and Xu, Q. (2006). Oxidized low-density lipoprotein autoantibodies, chronic infections, and carotid atherosclerosis in a population-based study. *J Am Coll Cardiol.* **47,** 2436–2443.

McCarron, M. O., Weir, C. J., Muir, K. W., Hoffmann, K. L., Graffagnino, C., Nicoll, J. A., Lees, K. R., and Alberts, M. J. (2003). Effect of apolipoprotein E genotype on in-hospital mortality following intracerebral haemorrhage. *Acta Neurol Scand.* **107,** 106–109.

McCarron, P., Okasha, M., McEwen, J., and Smith, G. D. (2002). Height in young adulthood and risk of death from cardiorespiratory disease: A prospective study of male former students of Glasgow University, Scotland. *Am J Epidemiol.* **155,** 683–687.

McCarter, R. J., Shimokawa, I., Ikeno, Y., Higami, Y., Hubbard, G. B., Yu, B. P., and McMahan, C. A. (1997). Physical activity as a factor in the action of dietary restriction on aging: Effects in Fischer 344 rats. *Aging (Milan, Italy).* **9,** 73–79.

McCarty, M. F. (1997). Up-regulation of IGF binding protein-1 as an anticarcinogenic strategy: Relevance to caloric restriction, exercise, and insulin sensitivity. *Med Hypotheses.* **48,** 297–308.

McCarty, M. F. (2004). Optimizing endothelial nitric oxide activity may slow endothelial aging. *Med Hypotheses.* **63,** 719–723.

McCay, C. M. (1947). Effect of restricted feeding upon aging and chronic diseases in rats and dogs. *Am J Public Health.* **37,** 521–528.

McCay, C. M., Crowell, M. F., and Maynard, L. A. (1935). Th effect of retarded growth upon the length of the life span and upon ultimate body size. *J Nutr* **13,** 669–679.

McCay, C. M., Ellis, G. H., Barnes, L. L., Smith, C. A. H., and Sperling, G. (1939a). Chemical and pathological changes in aging and after retarded growth. *J Nutr* **18,** 15–25.

McCay, C. M., L.A., M., Sperling, G., and Barnes, L. L. (1939b). Retarded growth, life span, ultimate body size and age changes in the albino rat after feeding diets restricted in calories. *J Nutr.* **18,** 1–13.

McCay, C. M., Sperling, G., and Barnes, C. (1943). Growth, ageing, chronic diseases, and life span in rats. *Arch Biochem.* **2,** 469–479.

McCurdy, S. A., Arretz, D. S., and Bates, R. O. (1997). Tuberculin reactivity among California Hispanic migrant farm workers. *Am J Ind Med.* **32,** 600–605.

McDade, T. W. (2001). Lifestyle incongruity, social integration, and immune function in Samoan adolescents. *Soc Sci Med.* **53,** 1351–1362.

McDade, T. W. (2003). Life history theory and the immune system: Steps toward a human ecological immunology. *Yearb Phys Anthropol.* **46,** 1–26.

McDade, T. W. (2005). Life history, maintenance, and the early origins of immune function. *Am J Hum Biol.* **17,** 81–94.

McDade, T. W., Beck, M. A., Kuzawa, C., and Adair, L. S. (2001a). Prenatal undernutrition, postnatal environments, and antibody response to vaccination in adolescence. *Am J Clin Nutr.* **74,** 543–548.

McDade, T. W., Beck, M. A., Kuzawa, C. W., and Adair, L. S. (2001b). Prenatal undernutrition and postnatal growth are associated with adolescent thymic function. *J Nutr.* **131,** 1225–1231.

McDade, T. W., Kuzawa, C. W., Adair, L. S., and Beck, M. A. (2004). Prenatal and early postnatal environments are significant predictors of total immunoglobulin E concentration in Filipino adolescents. *Clin Exp Allergy.* **34,** 44–50.

McDade, T. W., Leonard, W. R., Burhop, J., Reyes-García, V., Vadez, V., Huanca, T., and Godoy, R. A. (2005). Predictors of C-reactive protein in Tsimane' 2 to 15 year-olds in lowland Bolivia. *Am J Phys Anthropol.* **128,** 906–913.

McDermott, D. H., Yang, Q., Kathiresan, S., Cupples, L. A., Massaro, J. M., Keaney, J. F., Jr., Larson, M. G., Vasan, R. S., Hirschhorn, J. N., O'Donnell, C. J., Murphy, P. M., and Benjamin, E. J. (2005). CCL2 polymorphisms are associated with serum monocyte chemoattractant protein-1 levels and myocardial infarction in the Framingham Heart Study. *Circulation.* **112,** 1113–1120.

McDonagh, S., Maidji, E., Ma, W., Chang, H. T., Fisher, S., and Pereira, L. (2004). Viral and bacterial pathogens at the maternal-fetal interface. *J Infect Dis.* **190,** 826–834.

McDougall, I., Brown, F. H., and Fleagle, J. G. (2005). Stratigraphic placement and age of modern humans from Kibish, Ethiopia. *Nature.* **433,** 733–736.

McElhaney, J. E. (2005). The unmet need in the elderly: Designing new influenza vaccines for older adults. *Vaccine.* **23(Suppl 1),** S10–25.

McGeer, P.L., Akiyam, H. Itagaki, S., and McGeer, E.G. (1989). Activation of the classical complement pathway in brain tissue of Alzheimer patients. *Neurosci Lett* **107,** 341–346.

McGeer, P. L., Schulzer, M., and McGeer, E. G. (1996). Arthritis and anti-inflammatory agents as possible protective factors for Alzheimer's disease: A review of 17 epidemiologic studies. *Neurology.* **47,** 425–432.

McGill, H. C., Jr., Herderick, E. E., McMahan, C. A., Zieske, A. W., Malcolm, G. T., Tracy, R. E., and Strong, J. P. (2002). Atherosclerosis in youth. *Minerva Pediatrica.* **54,** 437–447.

McGrew, W. C. (2001). Human diet. Its origin and evolution. In C. B. Stanford and H. T. Bunn., Eds. *Meat eating and human evolution,* pp. 199–218. New York: Oxford University Press.

McGrew, W. C., Baldwin, P. J., Marchant, L. F., Pruetz, J. D., Scott, S. E., Tutin, C. E. G. (2003). Ethoarcheology and elementary technology of unhabituated wild chimpanzees at Assirik, Senegal West Africa. *Paleo Anthropol.* **1,** 1–20.

McKean, K. A., and Nunney, L. (2001). Increased sexual activity reduces male immune function in *Drosophila melanogaster. Proc Natl Acad Sci USA.* **98,** 7904–7909.

McKee, M., and Nolte, E. (2004). Lessons from health during the transition from communism. *Br Med J.* **329,** 1428–1429.

McKeown, T. (1976). *The modern rise of population.* New York: Academic Press

McMahon, M. M., Farnell, M. B., and Murray, M. J. (1993). Nutritional support of critically ill patients. *Mayo Clinic Proc.* **68,** 911–920.

McMinn, J., Wei, M., Schupf, N., Cusmai, J., Johnson, E. B., Smith, A. C., Weksberg, R., Thaker, H. M., and Tycko, B. (2006). Unbalanced placental expression of imprinted genes in human intrauterine growth restriction. *Placenta.* **27,** 540–549.

McNamara, J. J., Molot, M. A., Stremple, J. F., and Cutting, R. T. (1971). Coronary artery disease in combat casualties in Vietnam. *JAMA.* **216,** 1185–1187.

McQuarrie, I. G., Brady, S. T., and Lasek, R. J. (1989). Retardation in the slow axonal transport of cytoskeletal elements during maturation and aging. *Neurobiol Aging.* **10,** 359–365.

McShane, T. M., and Wise, P. M. (1996). Life-long moderate caloric restriction prolongs reproductive life span in rats without interrupting estrous cyclicity: Effects on the gonadotropin-releasing hormone/luteinizing hormone axis. *Biol Repro.* **54,** 70–75.

Mead, S., Stumpf, M. P. H., Whitfield, J., Beck, J. A., Poulter, M., Campbell, T., Uphill, J., Goldstein, D., Alpers, M., Fisher, E. M. C., and Collinge, J. (2003). Balancing selection at the prion protein gene consistent with prehistoric kurulike epidemics. *Science*. **300**, 640–643.

Meaney, M. J., Aitken, D. H., van Berkel, C., Bhatnagar, S., Sapolsky, R. M. (1988). Effect of neonatal handling on age-related impairments associated with the hippocampus. *Science*. **239**, 766–768.

Medzhitov, R., and Janeway, C. A., Jr. (2002). Decoding the patterns of self and nonself by the innate immune system. *Science*. **296**, 298–300.

Meek, R. L., Urieli-Shoval, S., and Benditt, E. P. (1994). Expression of apolipoprotein serum amyloid A mRNA in human atherosclerotic lesions and cultured vascular cells: Implications for serum amyloid A function. *Proc Natl Acad Sci USA*. **91**, 3186–3190.

Mekel-Bobrov, N., Gilbert, S. L., Evans, P. D., Vallender, E. J., Anderson, J. R., Hudson, R. R., Tishkoff, S. A., and Lahn, B. T. (2005). Ongoing adaptive evolution of ASPM, a brain size determinant in *Homo sapiens*. *Science*. **309**, 1720–1722.

Melamed, E., Lavy, S., Bentin, S., Cooper, G., and Rinot, Y. (1980). Reduction in regional cerebral blood flow during normal aging in man. *Stroke*. **11**, 31–35.

Mele, J., Van Remmen, H., Vijg, J., and Richardson, A. (2006). Characterization of transgenic mice that overexpress both copper zinc superoxide dismutase and catalase. *Antioxid Redox Signal*. **8**, 628–368.

Memon, R. A., Staprans, I., Noor, M., Holleran, W. M., Uchida, Y., Moser, A. H., Feingold, K. R., and Grunfeld, C. (2000). Infection and inflammation induce LDL oxidation *in vivo*. *Arterioscler Thromb Vasc Biol*. **20**, 1536–1542.

Mencacci, A., Romani, L., Mosci, P., Cenci, E., Tonnetti, L., Vecchiarelli, A., and Bistoni, F., (1993). Low-dose streptozotocin-induced diabetes in mice. II. Susceptibility to *Candida albicans* infection correlates with the induction of a biased Th2-like antifungal response. *Cell Immunol*. **150**, 36–44.

Mendez, G. F., and Cowie, M. R., (2001). The epidemiological features of heart failure in developing countries: A review of the literature. *Int J Cardiol*. **80**, 213–219.

Menendez, C. (1995). Malaria during pregnancy: A priority area of malaria research and control. *Parasitol Today*. **11**, 178–183.

Menendez, C., Todd, J., Alonso, P. L., Lulat, S., Francis, N., and Greenwood, B. M. (1994). Malaria chemoprophylaxis, infection of the placenta and birth weight in Gambian primigravidae. *J Trop Med Hyg*. **97**, 244–248.

Menetrez, M. Y., Foarde, K. K., and Ensor, D. S. (2001). An analytical method for the measurement of nonviable bioaerosols. *J Air Waste Manag Assoc*. **51**, 1436–1442.

Menotti, A., Kromhout, D., Blackburn, H., Jacobs, D., and Lanti, M. (2004). Forty-year mortality from cardiovascular diseases and all causes of death in the US Railroad cohort of the Seven Countries Study. *Eur J Epidemiol*. **19**, 417–424.

Merino, J., Martinez-Gonzalez, M. A., Rubio, M., Inoges, S., Sanchez-Ibarrola, A., and Subira, M. L. (1998). Progressive decrease of CD8high+ CD28+ CD57– cells with ageing. *Clin Exp Immunol*. **112**, 48–51.

Merry, B. J. (2002). Molecular mechanisms linking calorie restriction and longevity. *Int J Biochem Cell Biol*. **34**, 1340–1354.

Merry, B. J. (2004). Oxidative stress and mitochondrial function with aging—The effects of calorie restriction. *Aging Cell*. **3**, 7–12.

Merry, B. J. (2005). Dietary restriction in rodents—Delayed or retarded ageing? *Mech Ageing Dev*. **126**, 951–959.

Messaoudi, I., Warner, J., Nikolich-Zugich, D., Fischer, M., and Nikolich-Zugich, J. (2006). Molecular, cellular, and antigen requirements for development of age-associated T cell clonal expansions *in vivo*. *J Immunol.* **176,** 301–308.

Metchnikoff, E. (1901). Flora of the human body. The Wilde Medal and Lecture of the Manchester Literary and Philsophical Society. *Br Med J.* 1027–1028.

Meyer, A. A., Kundt, G., Steiner, M., Schuff-Werner, P., and Kienast, W. (2006a). Impaired flow-mediated vasodilation, carotid artery intima-media thickening, and elevated endothelial plasma markers in obese children: The impact of cardiovascular risk factors. *Pediatrics.* **117,** 1560–1567.

Meyer, C. G., Gallin, M., Erttmann, K. D., Brattig, N., Schnittger, L., Gelhaus, A., et al. (1994). HLA-D alleles associated with generalized disease, localized disease, and putative immunity in Onchocerca volvulus infection. *Proc. Nat Acad Sci.U.S.A.* **91,** 7515–7519.

Meyer, C. G., Schnittger, L., May, J. (1996). Met-11 of HLA class II DP alpha 1 first domain associated with onchocerciasis. *Exp Clin Immuno.* **13,** 12–19.

Meyer, J. M., and Breitner, J. C. (1998). Multiple threshold model for the onset of Alzheimer's disease in the NAS-NRC twin panel. *Am J Med Genet.* **81,** 92–97.

Meyer, J. S., and Shaw, T. G. (1984). Cerebral blood flow in aging. In *Clinical neurology of aging"* (M. L. Albert, Ed.), pp. 178–196. New York: Oxford University Press.

Meyer, K. C. (2005). Aging. *Proc Am Thorac Soc.* **2,** 433–439.

Meyer, M. R., Tschanz, J. T., Norton, M. C., Welsh-Bohmer, K. A., Steffens, D. C., Wyse, B. W., and Breitner, J. C. (1998). APOE genotype predicts when—not whether—one is predisposed to develop Alzheimer disease. *Nat Genet.* **19,** 321–322.

Meyer, T. E., Kovacs, S. J., Ehsani, A. A., Klein, S., Holloszy, J. O., and Fontana, L. (2006b). Long-term caloric restriction ameliorates the decline in diastolic function in humans. *J Am Coll Cardiol.* **47,** 398–402.

Meyers, D. G., Jensen, K. C., and Menitove, J. E. (2002). A historical cohort study of the effect of lowering body iron through blood donation on incident cardiac events. *Transfusion.* **42,** 1135–1139.

Michel, O., Nagy, A. M., Schroeven, M., Duchateau, J., Náeve, J., Fondu, P., and Sergysels, R. (1997). Dose-response relationship to inhaled endotoxin in normal subjects. *Am J Resp Crit Care Med.* **156,** 1157–1164.

Migliaccio, E., Giorgio, M., Mele, S., Pelicci, G., Reboldi, P., Pandolfi, P. P., Lanfrancone, L., and Pelicci, P. G. (1999). The p66shc adaptor protein controls oxidative stress response and life span in mammals. *Nature.* **402,** 309–313.

Miida, T., Yamada, T., Seino, U., Ito, M., Fueki, Y., Takahashi, A., Kosuge, K., Soda, S., Hanyu, O., Obayashi, K., Miyazaki, O., and Okada, M. (2006). Serum amyloid A (SAA)-induced remodeling of CSF-HDL. *Biochim Biophys Acta.* **1761,** 424–433.

Miller, J. L., Macedonia, C., and Sonies, B. C. (2006a). Sex differences in prenatal oral-motor function and development. *Dev Med Child Neurol.* **48,** 465–470.

Miller, L. M., Wang, Q., Telivala, T. P., Smith, R. J., Lanzirotti, A., and Miklossy, J. (2006b). Synchrotron-based infrared and X-ray imaging shows focalized accumulation of Cu and Zn co-localized with beta-amyloid deposits in Alzheimer's disease. *J Struct Biol.* **155,** 30–37.

Miller, R. A. (1991). Caloric restriction and immune function: Developmental mechanisms. *Aging.* **3,** 395–398.

Miller, R. A. (1997). Age-related changes in T cell surface markers: a longitudinal analysis in genetically heterogeneous mice. *Mech Ageing Devel.* **96,** 181–196.

Miller, R. A. (1999). Kleemeier Award lecture: Are there genes for aging? J. *Gerontol. Biol. Med. Sci.* **54A,** B297–307.

Miller, R. A. (2000a). Telomere diminution as a cause of immune failure in old age: An unfashionable demurral. *Biochem Soc Trans.* **28**, 241–245.

Miller, R. A. (2005a). Biomedicine. The anti-aging sweepstakes: Catalase runs for the ROSes. *Science.* **308**, 1875–1876.

Miller, R. A., Berger, S. B., Burke, D. T., Galecki, A., Garcia, G. G., Harper, J. M., and Sadighi Akha, A. A. (2005a). T cells in aging mice: Genetic, developmental, and biochemical analyses. *Immunol Rev.* **205**, 94–103.

Miller, R. A., Chang, Y., Galecki, A. T., Al-Regaiey, K., Kopchick, J. J., and Bartke, A. (2002a). Gene expression patterns in calorically restricted mice: Partial overlap with long-lived mutant mice. *Mol Endocrinol* **16**, 2657–2666.

Miller, R. A., Chrisp, C., and Atchley, W. (2000b). Differential longevity in mouse stocks selected for early life growth trajectory. *J Gerontol. A Biol Sci Med Sci.* **55**, B455–461.

Miller, R. A., Harper, J. M., Dysko, R. C., Durkee, S. J., and Austad, S. N. (2002a). Longer life spans and delayed maturation in wild-derived mice. *Expl Biol Med* **227**, 500–508.

Miller, R. A., Harper, J. M., Galecki, A., and Burke, D. T. (2002b). Big mice die young: Early life body weight predicts longevity in genetically heterogeneous mice. *Aging Cell.* **1**, 22–29.

Miller, R. A., and Nadon, N. L. (2000). Principles of animal use for gerontological research. *J Gerontol. Series A, Biol Sci Med Sci.* **55**, B117–123.

Miller, Y. I., Viriyakosol, S., Worrall, D. S., Boullier, A., Butler, S., and Witztum, J. L. (2005b). Toll-like receptor 4-dependent and -independent cytokine secretion induced by minimally oxidized low-density lipoprotein in macrophages. *Arterioscler Thromb Vasc Biol.* **25**, 1213–1219.

Millet, P., Lages, C. S., Haik, S., Nowak, E., Allemand, I., Granotier, C., and Boussin, F. D. (2005). Amyloid-beta peptide triggers Fas-independent apoptosis and differentiation of neural progenitor cells. *Neurobiol Dis.* **19**, 57–65.

Millonig, G., Malcom, G. T., and Wick, G. (2002). Early inflammatory-immunological lesions in juvenile atherosclerosis from the Pathobiological Determinants of Atherosclerosis in Youth (PDAY) -Study. *Atherosclerosis.* **160**, 441–448.

Mills, J., and Reiner, P. B. (1999). Regulation of amyloid precursor protein cleavage. *J Neurochem.* **72**, 443–460.

Milton, K. (1993). Diet and primate evolution. *Sci Am.* **269**, 86–93.

Milton, K. (1999a). A hypothesis to explain the role of meat-eating in human evolution. *Evol Anthrop.* **8**, 11–21.

Milton, K. (1999b). Nutritional characteristics of wild primate foods: Do the diets of our closest living relatives have lessons for us? *Nutrition.* **15**, 488–498.

Min, H., Montecino-Rodriguez, E., and Dorshkind, K. (2005). Effects of aging on early B- and T-cell development. *Immunol Rev.* **205**, 7–17.

Min, H., Montecino-Rodriguez, E., and Dorshkind, K. (2006a). Reassessing the role of growth hormone and sex steroids in thymic involution. *Clin Immunol.* **118**, 117–123.

Min, K. J., Hogan, M. F., Tatar, M., and O'Brien D, M. (2006b). Resource allocation to reproduction and soma in *Drosophila*: A stable isotope analysis of carbon from dietary sugar. *J Insect Physiol.* **52**, 763–770.

Min, K. J., and Tatar, M. (2006). *Drosophila* diet restriction in practice: Do flies consume fewer nutrients? *Mech Ageing Dev.* **127**, 93–96.

Min, K. T., and Benzer, S. (1997). Wolbachia, normally a symbiont of *Drosophila*, can be virulent, causing degeneration and early death. *Proc Natl Acad Sci USA.* **94**, 10792–10796.

Minamino, T., Miyauchi, H., Yoshida, T., Ishida, Y., Yoshida, H., and Komuro, I. (2002). Endothelial cell senescence in human atherosclerosis: Role of telomere in endothelial dysfunction. [see comment]. *Circulation.* **105,** 1541–1544.

Minamino, T., Miyauchi, H., Yoshida, T., Tateno, K., Kunieda, T., and Komuro, I. (2004). Vascular cell senescence and vascular aging. *J Mol Cell Cardiol.* **36,** 175–183.

Miquel, J., Bensch, K. G., Philpott, D. E., and Atlan, H. (1972). Natural aging and radiation-induced life shortening in *Drosophila melanogaster. Mech Ageing Dev.* **1,**71–97.

Mitch, W. E. (2005). Beneficial responses to modified diets in treating patients with chronic kidney disease. *Kidney Int Suppl.* **94,** S133–135.

Mitchell, E. A., Thompson, J. M., Robinson, E., Wild, C. J., Becroft, D. M., Clark, P. M., Glavish, N., Pattison, N. S., and Pryor, J. E. (2002). Smoking, nicotine and tar and risk of small for gestational age babies. [comment]. *Acta Paediatrica.* **91,** 323–328.

Mitrova, E., Mayer, V., Jovankovicova, V., Slivarichova, D., and Wsolova, L. (2005). Creutzfeldt-Jakob disease risk and PRNP codon 129 polymorphism: Necessity to revalue current data. *Eur J Neurol.* **12,** 998–1001.

Mitsumori, K., Maita, K., and Shirasu, Y. (1981). An ultrastructural study of spinal nerve roots and dorsal root ganglia in aging rats with spontaneous radiculoneuropathy. *Vet Pathol.* **18,** 714–726.

Miyasaka, K., Ichikawa, M., Kawanami, T., Kanai, S., Ohta, M., Sato, N., Ebisawa, H., and Funakoshi, A. (2003). Physical activity prevented age-related decline in energy metabolism in genetically obese and diabetic rats, but not in control rats. *Mech Ageing Dev.* **124,** 183–190.

Miyashita, M., Burns, S. F., and Stensel, D. J., Physical, A. (2006). Exercise and postprandial lipemia: Effect of continuous compared with intermittent activity patterns. *Am J Clin Nutr.* **83,** 24–29.

Miyashita, N., Fukano, H., Yoshida, K., Niki, Y., and Matsushima, T. (2002). Sero-epidemiology of *Chlamydia pneumoniae* in Japan between 1991 and 2000. *J Clin Pathol.* **55,** 115–117.

Miyata, T., Inagi, R., Iida, Y., Sato, M., Yamada, N., Oda, O., Maeda, K., and Seo, H. (1994). Involvement of beta 2-microglobulin modified with advanced glycation end products in the pathogenesis of hemodialysis-associated amyloidosis. Induction of human monocyte chemotaxis and macrophage secretion of tumor necrosis factor-alpha and interleukin-1. *J Clin Invest.* **93,** 521–528.

Miyata, T., Ueda, Y., Saito, A., and Kurokawa, K. (2000). 'Carbonyl stress' and dialysis-related amyloidosis. *Nephro Dialysis Transplant* **15,** 25–28.

Miyauchi, H., Minamino, T., Tateno, K., Kunieda, T., Toko, H., and Komuro, I. (2004). Akt negatively regulates the *in vitro* lifespan of human endothelial cells via a p53/p21-dependent pathway. *EMBO J.* **23,** 212–220.

Mizutani, T., and Shimada, H. (1992). Neuropathological background of twenty-seven centenarian brains. *J Neurol Sci.* **108,** 168–177.

Mo, R., Chen, J., Han, Y., Bueno-Cannizares, C., Misek, D. E., Lescure, P. A., Hanash, S., and Yung, R. L. (2003). T cell chemokine receptor expression in aging. *J Immunol (Baltimore, MD: 1950)* **170,** 895–904.

Modugno, F., Ness, R. B., Chen, C., and Weiss, N. S. (2005). Inflammation and endometrial cancer: A hypothesis. *Cancer Epidemiol Biomarkers Prev.* **14,** 2840–2847.

Moghadasian, M. H.(2002). Experimental atherosclerosis: A historical overview. *Life Sci.* **70,** 855–865.

Molleson, T., Andrews, P., Boz, B. (2005). Reconsrutction of the neolithic people at Çatalhöyük. *Inhabiting Çatalhöyük: Reports from the 1995-1999 Seasons by Members of the Çatalhöyük Teams.* pp 279–300. London: McDonald Institute Monographs.

Mombo, L. E., Ntoumi, F., Bisseye, C., Ossari, S., Lu, C. Y., Nagel, R. L., and Krishnamoorthy, R. (2003). Human genetic polymorphisms and asymptomatic *Plasmodium falciparum* malaria in Gabonese schoolchildren. *Am J Trop Med Hyg.* **68,** 186–190.

Monaco, C., and Paleolog, E. (2004). Nuclear factor kappaB: A potential therapeutic target in atherosclerosis and thrombosis. *Cardiovasc Res.* **61,** 671–682.

Monnier, V. M., Mustata, G. T., Biemel, K. L., Reihl, O., Lederer, M. O., Zhenyu, D., and Sell, D. R. (2005a). Cross-linking of the extracellular matrix by the Maillard reaction in aging and diabetes: An update on "A Puzzle Nearing Resolution." *Ann NY Acad Sci.* **1043,** 533–544.

Monnier, V. M., and Sell, D. R. (2006). Prevention and repair of protein damage by the Maillard reaction *in vivo. Rejuvenation Res.* **9,** 264–273.

Monnier, V. M., Sell, D. R., and Genuth, S. (2005b). Glycation products as markers and predictors of the progression of diabetic complications. *Ann NY Acad Sci.* **1043,** 567–581.

Moody, D. M., Brown, W. R., Challa, V. R., Ghazi-Birry, H. S., and Reboussin, D. M. (1997). Cerebral microvascular alterations in aging, leukoaraiosis, and Alzheimer's disease. *Ann NY Acad Sci.* **826,** 103–116.

Moon, M. K., Cho, Y. M., Jung, H. S., Park, Y. J., Yoon, K. H., Sung, Y. A., Park, B. L., Lee, H. K., Park, K. S., and Shin, H. D. (2005). Genetic polymorphisms in peroxisome proliferator-activated receptor gamma are associated with type 2 diabetes mellitus and obesity in the Korean population. *Diabetic Medicine.* **22,** 1161–1166.

Moore, J. E., Jr., Xu, C., Glagov, S., Zarins, C. K., and Ku, D. N. (1994). Fluid wall shear stress measurements in a model of the human abdominal aorta: Oscillatory behavior and relationship to atherosclerosis. *Atherosclerosis.* **110,** 225–240.

Moore, M., Gould, P., and Keary, B. S. (2003). Global urbanization and impact on health. *Int J Hyg Environ Health.* **206,** 269–278.

Moore, S., E, Collinson, A. C., Tamba N'gom, P., Aspinall, R., and Prentice, A. M. (2006). Early immunological development and mortality from infectious disease in later life. *Proc Nutr Soc.* **65,** 311–318.

Moore, S. E., Cole, T. J., Collinson, A. C., Poskitt, E. M., McGregor, I. A., and Prentice, A. M. (1999). Prenatal or early postnatal events predict infectious deaths in young adulthood in rural Africa. *Int J Epidemiol.* **28,** 1088–1095.

Moore, S. E., Cole, T. J., Poskitt, E. M., Sonko, B. J., Whitehead, R. G., McGregor, I. A., and Prentice, A. M. (1997). Season of birth predicts mortality in rural Gambia. *Nature.* **388,** 434.

Moore, S. E., Fulford, A. J., Streatfield, P. K., Persson, L. A., and Prentice, A. M. (2004a). Comparative analysis of patterns of survival by season of birth in rural Bangladeshi and Gambian populations. *Int J Epidemiol.* **33,** 137–143.

Moore, S. E., Halsall, I., Howarth, D., Poskitt, E. M., and Prentice, A. M. (2001). Glucose, insulin and lipid metabolism in rural Gambians exposed to early malnutrition. *Diabet Med.* **18,** 646–653.

Moore, S. E., Jalil, F., Ashraf, R., Szu, S. C., Prentice, A. M., and Hanson, L. A., (2004b). Birth weight predicts response to vaccination in adults born in an urban slum in Lahore, Pakistan. *Am J Clin Nutr.* **80,** 453–459.

Moore, S. E., Morgan, G., Collinson, A. C., Swain, J. A., O'Connell, M. A., and Prentice, A. M. (2002). Leptin, malnutrition, and immune response in rural Gambian children. *Arch Dis Child.* **87,** 192–197.

Moore, S. R., Lima, A. A., Conaway, M. R., Schorling, J. B., Soares, A. M., and Guerrant, R. L. (2001b). Early childhood diarrhoea and helminthiases associate with long-term linear growth faltering. *Int J Epidemiol.* **30,** 1457–1464.

Moormann, A. M., Sullivan, A. D., Rochford, R. A., Chensue, S. W., Bock, P. J., Nyirenda, T., and Meshnick, S. R. (1999). Malaria and pregnancy: Placental cytokine expression and its relationship to intrauterine growth retardation. *J Infect Dis.* **180,** 1987–1993.

Moreno, J. A., Pérez-Jiménez, F., Marín, C., Pérez-Martínez, P., Moreno, R., Gómez, P., Jiménez-Gómez, Y., Paniagua, J. A., Lairon, D., and López-Miranda, J. (2005). The apolipoprotein E gene promoter (-219G/T) polymorphism determines insulin sensitivity in response to dietary fat in healthy young adults. *J Nutr.* **135,** 2535–2540.

Moreschi, C. (1909). Beziehungen zwischen Ernährung und Tumorwachstum. *Zeitschrift fur Immunitätsforshung* **2,** 651–675.

Moret, Y., and Schmid-Hempel, P. (2000). Survival for immunity: The price of immune system activation for bumblebee workers. *Science.* **290,** 1166–1168.

Morgan, B. P. (1990a). *Complement. Clinical aspects and relevance to disease.* San Diego: Academic Press.

Morgan, D. G., Marcusson, J. O., Nyberg, P., Wester, P., Winblad, B., Gordon, M. N., and Finch, C. E. (1987a). Divergent changes in D-1 and D-2 dopamine binding sites in human brain during aging. *Neurobiol Aging.* **8,** 195–201.

Morgan, D. G., and May, P. C. (1990b). Age-related changes in synaptic neurochemistry. In E. L. Schneider and J. W. Rowe, Eds., *Handbook of the biology of aging, 3rd edition,*, pp. 219–254. San Diego: Academic Press.

Morgan, D. G., May, P. C., and Finch, C. E. (1987b). Dopamine and serotonin systems in human and rodent brain: Effects of age and neurodegenerative disease. *J Am Geriatr Soc.* **35,** 334–345.

Morgan, G. (2004). Aspirin and colorectal cancer? *Eur J Public Health.* **14,** 105–106.

Morgan, T. E., Rozovsky, I., Goldsmith, S. K., Stone, D. J., Yoshida, T., and Finch, C. E. (1997). Increased transcription of the astrocyte gene GFAP during middle-age is attenuated by food restriction: Implications for the role of oxidative stress. *Free Radic Biol Med.* **23,** 524–528.

Morgan, T. E., Rozovsky, I., Sarkar, D. K., Young-Chan, C. S., Nichols, N. R., Laping, N. J., and Finch, C. E. (2000). Transforming growth factor-beta1 induces transforming growth factor-beta1 and transforming growth factor-beta receptor messenger RNAs and reduces complement C1qB messenger RNA in rat brain microglia. *Neuroscience.* **101,** 313–321.

Morgan, T. E., Xie, Z., Goldsmith, S., Yoshida, T., Lanzrein, A. S., Stone, D., Rozovsky, I., Perry, G., Smith, M. A., and Finch, C. E. (1999). The mosaic of brain glial hyperactivity during normal ageing and its attenuation by food restriction. *Neuroscience.* **89,** 687–699.

Morihara, T., Teter, B., Yang, F., Lim, G. P., Boudinot, S., Boudinot, F. D., Frautschy, S. A., and Cole, G. M. (2005). Ibuprofen suppresses interleukin-1beta induction of pro-amyloido-genic alpha1-antichymotrypsin to ameliorate beta-amyloid (Abeta) pathology in Alzheimer's models. *Neuropsychopharmacology.* **30,** 1111–1120.

Morin, L. P. (1986). Environment and hamster reproduction: Responses to phase-specific starvation during estrous cycle. *Am J Physiol.* **251,** R663–669.

Morley, J. E., Haren, M. T., Kim, M. J., Kevorkian, R., and Perry, H. M., 3rd (2005). Testosterone, aging and quality of life. *J Endocrin Invest.* **28(3 Suppl),** 76–80.

Morley, J. F., and Morimoto, R. I. (2004). Regulation of longevity in *Caenorhabditis elegans* by heat shock factor and molecular chaperones. *Mol Biol Cell.* **15,** 657–664.

Morner, S., Hellman, U., Suhr, O. B., Kazzam, E., and Waldenstrom, A. (2005). Amyloid heart disease mimicking hypertrophic cardiomyopathy*. *J Intern Med.* **258,** 225–230.

Morohoshi, M., Fujisawa, K., Uchimura, I., and Numano, F. (1996). Glucose-dependent interleukin 6 and tumor necrosis factor production by human peripheral blood monocytes *in vitro. Diabetes.* **45,** 954–959.

Morris, J. C. (1999). Clinical presentation and course of Alzheimer disease. In R. D. Terry, R. Katzman, K. L. Bick, and S. S. Soisodia, Eds., *Alzheimer disease,* pp. 11–24. Philadelphia: Lippincott Williams & Wilkins

Morris, J. C., and Price, A. L. (2001). Pathologic correlates of nondemented aging, mild cognitive impairment, and early-stage Alzheimer's disease. *J Mol Neurosci.* **17,** 101–118.

Morris, J. Z., Tissenbaum, H. A., and Ruvkun, G. (1996). A phosphatidylinositol-3-OH kinase family member regulating longevity and diapause in *Caenorhabditis elegans. Nature.* **382,** 536–539.

Morse, A. D., Russell, J. C., Hunt, T. W., Wood, G. O., Epling, W. F., and Pierce, W. D. (1995). Diurnal variation of intensive running in food-deprived rats. *Can J Physiol and Pharmacology.* **73,** 1519–1523.

Mortimer, J. A., Snowdon, D. A., and Markesbery, W. R. (2003). Head circumference, education and risk of dementia: Findings from the Nun Study. *J Clin Exp Neuropsychol.* **25,** 671–679.

Mosci, P., Vecchiarelli, A., Cenci, E., Puliti, M., and Bistoni, F. (1993). Low-dose strepto-zotocin-induced diabetes in mice. I. Course of *Candida albicans* infection. *Cellular Immunology.* **150,** 27–35.

Moscrip, T. D., Ingram, D. K., Lane, M. A., Roth, G. S., and Weed, J. L., and Row Sciences, G. M. U. S. A. (2000). Locomotor activity in female rhesus monkeys: Assessment of age and calorie restriction effects. *J Gerontol. Series A, Biol Sci Med Sci.* **55,** B373–380.

Mosorin, M., Surcel, H. M., Laurila, A., Lehtinen, M., Karttunen, R., Juvonen, J., Paavonen, J., Morrison, R. P., Saikku, P., and Juvonen, T. (2000). Detection of *Chlamydia pneumo-niae*-reactive T lymphocytes in human atherosclerotic plaques of carotid artery. *Arterioscler Thromb Vasc Biol.* **20,** 1061–1067.

Mossey, J. M., and Shapiro, E. (1982). Self-rated health: A predictor of mortality among the elderly. *Am J Public Health.* **72,** 800–808.

Mostaghel, E., and Waters, D. (2003). Women do benefit from lipid lowering: Latest clinical trial data. *Cardiol Rev.* **11,** 4–12.

Motola, D. L., Cummins, C. L., Rottiers, V., Sharma, K. K., Li, T., Li, Y., Suino-Powell, K., Xu, H. E., Auchus, R. J., Antebi, A., and Mangelsdorf, D. J. (2006). Identification of ligands for DAF-12 that govern dauer formation and reproduction in *C. elegans. Cell.* **124,** 1209–1223.

Mounier, F., Bluet-Pajot, M. T., Durand, D., Kordon, C., Rasolonjanahary, R., and Epelbaum, J. (1989). Involvement of central somatostatin in the alteration of GH secretion in starved rats. *Horm Res.* **31,** 266–270.

Mucke, L., Masliah, E., Yu, G. Q., Mallory, M., Rockenstein, E. M., Tatsuno, G., Hu, K., Kholodenko, D., Johnson-Wood, K., and McConlogue, L. (2000). High-level neuronal expression of abeta 1–42 in wild-type human amyloid protein precursor transgenic mice: Synaptotoxicity without plaque formation. *J Neurosci.* **20,** 4050–4058.

Mucke, L., and Pitas, R. E. (2004). Food for thought: Essential fatty acid protects against neuronal deficits in transgenic mouse model of AD. [comment]. *Neuron.* **43,** 596–599.

Mueller, L. D., Graves, J. L., Rose, M. R. (1993). Interactions between density-dependent and age-specific selection in *Drosophila melanogaster. Functional Ecol.* **7,** 469–479.

Muhbock, O. (1959). Factors influencing the lifespan of inbred mice. *Gerontologia.* **3,** 177–183.

Muhlestein, J. B., Hammond, E. H., Carlquist, J. F., Radicke, E., Thomson, M. J., Karagounis, L. A., Woods, M. L., and Anderson, J. L. (1996). Increased incidence of *Chlamydia* species within the coronary arteries of patients with symptomatic atherosclerotic versus other forms of cardiovascular disease. *J Am Coll Cardiol.* **27,** 1555–1561.

Mukherjee, T. K., Mukhopadhyay, S., and Hoidal, J. R. (2005). The role of reactive oxygen species in TNFalpha-dependent expression of the receptor for advanced glycation end products in human umbilical vein endothelial cells. *Biochimica et Biophysica Acta.* **1744,** 213–223.

Muller, C. (1938). Xanthomata, hypercholesterolemia, and angina pectoris. *Acta Med Scand.* **89 ,** 75–84.

Muller, Y. L., Bogardus, C., Beamer, B. A., Shuldiner, A. R., and Baier, L. J. (2003). A functional variant in the peroxisome proliferator-activated receptor gamma2 promoter is associated with predictors of obesity and type 2 diabetes in Pima Indians. *Diabetes.* **52,** 1864–1871.

Mulligan, J. D., Gonzalez, A. A., Kumar, R., Davis, A. J., and Saupe, K. W. (2005). Aging elevates basal adenosine monophosphate-activated protein kinase (AMPK) activity and eliminates hypoxic activation of AMPK in mouse liver. *J Gerontol. A Biol Sci Med Sci.* **60,** 21–27.

Mullin, J. M., Agostino, N., Rendon-Huerta, E., and Thornton, J. J. (2005). Keynote review: Epithelial and endothelial barriers in human disease. *Drug Discov Today.* **10,** 395–408.

Mullin, J. M., Valenzano, M. C., Verrecchio, J. J., and Kothari, R. (2002). Age- and diet-related increase in transepithelial colon permeability of Fischer 344 rats. *Dig Dis Sci.* **47,** 2262–2270.

Mulvihill, N. T., and Foley, J. B. (2002). Inflammation in acute coronary syndromes. *Heart.* **87,** 201–204.

Munch, G., Apelt, J., Rosemarie Kientsch, E., Stahl, P., Luth, H. J., and Schliebs, R. (2003). Advanced glycation endproducts and pro-inflammatory cytokines in transgenic Tg2576 mice with amyloid plaque pathology. *J Neurochem.* **86,** 283–289.

Murasawa, S., Kawamoto, A., Horii, M., Nakamori, S., and Asahara, T. (2005). Niche-dependent translineage commitment of endothelial progenitor cells, not cell fusion in general, into myocardial lineage cells. *Arterioscler Thromb Vasc Biol.* **25,** 1388–1394.

Murin, S., and Bilello, K. S. (2005). Respiratory tract infections: Another reason not to smoke. *Cleve Clin J Med.* **72,** 916–920.

Murphy, C. T., McCarroll, S. A., Bargmann, C. I., Fraser, A., Kamath, R. S., Ahringer, J., Li, H., and Kenyon, C. (2003). Genes that act downstream of DAF-16 to influence the lifespan of *Caenorhabditis elegans. Nature.* **424,** 277–283.

Murphy, W. A., Jr., zur Nedden, D., Gostner, P., Knapp, R., Recheis, W., and Seidler, H. (2003b). The iceman: Discovery and imaging. *Radiology.* **226,** 614–629.

Murray, J., and Murray, A. (1981). Toward a nutritional concept of host resistance to malignancy and intracellular infection. *Perspect Biol Med.* **24,** 290–301.

Murray, J., Murray, A., and Murray, N. (1978a). Anorexia: Sentinel of host defense? *Perspect Biol Med.* **22,** 134–142.

Murray, M. J., and Murray, A. B. (1979). Anorexia of infection as a mechanism of host defense. *Am J Clin Nutr.* **32,** 593–596.

Murray, M. J., and Murray, A. B. (1979b). Suppression of intracellular infection by serum from undernourished animals. *Clin Res.* **26,** 718A.

Murray, M. J., Murray, A. B., and Murray, C. J. (1980a). An ecological interdependence of diet and disease? A study of infection in one tribe consuming two different diets. *Am J Clin Nutr.* **33(3),** 697–701.

Murray, M. J., Murray, A. B., Murray, M. B., and Murray, C. J. (1978b). The adverse effect of iron repletion on the course of certain infections. *Br Med J.* **2,** 1113–1115.

Murray, M. J., Murray, A. B., and Murray, N. J. (1980b). The ecological interdependence of diet and disease in tribal societies. *Yale J Biol Med.* **53,** 295–306.

Murray, M. J., Murray, A. B., Murray, N. J., and Murray, M. B. (1978c). Diet and cerebral malaria: The effect of famine and refeeding. *Am J Clin Nutr.* **31,** 57–61.

Murray, M. J., Murray, A. B., Murray, N. J., and Murray, M. B. (1978d). The effect of iron status of Nigeriaen mothers on that of their infants at birth and 6 months, and on the concentration of Fe in breast milk. *Br J Nutr.* **39,** 627–630.

Murray, M. J., Murray, A. B., Murray, N. J., and Murray, M. B. (1995). Infections during severe primary undernutrition and subsequent refeeding: Paradoxical findings. *Aust N Z J Med.* **25,** 507–511.

Murray, M. J., Murray, A. B., Murray, N. J., Murray, M. B., and Murray, C. J. (1980). *Molluscum contagiosum* and herpes simplex in Maasai pastoralists; Refeeding activation of virus infection following famine? *Trans Roy Soc Trop Med Hygiene.* **74,** 371–374.

Mustafa, A., Lannfelt, L., Lilius, L., Islam, A., Winblad, B., and Adem, A. (1999). Decreased plasma insulin-like growth factor-I level in familial Alzheimer's disease patients carrying the Swedish APP 670/671 mutation. *Dementia Geriatr Cogn Disord* **10,** 446–451.

Mylonakis, E., and Aballay, A. (2005). Worms and flies as genetically tractable animal models to study host-pathogen interactions. *Infect Immun.* **73,** 3833–3841.

Mylonakis, E., Ausubel, F. M., Perfect, J. R., Heitman, J., and Calderwood, S. B.. (2002a). Killing of *Caenorhabditis elegans* by *Cryptococcus neoformans* as a model of yeast pathogenesis. *Proc Natl Acad Sci USA.* **99,** 15675–15680.

Mylonakis, E., Paliou, M., Hohmann, E. L., Calderwood, S. B., and Wing, E. J. (2002b). Listeriosis during pregnancy: A case series and review of 222 cases. *Medicine.* **81,** 260–269.

Nadeau, S., and Rivest, S. (2003). Glucocorticoids play a fundamental role in protecting the brain during innate immune response. *J Neurosci.* **23,** 5536–5544.

Naeye, R. L. (1981). Influence of maternal cigarette smoking during pregnancy on fetal and childhood growth. *Obstet Gynecol.* **57,** 18–21.

Nagai, Y., Metter, E. J., Earley, C. J., Kemper, M. K., Becker, L. C., Lakatta, E. G., and Fleg, J. L. (1998). Increased carotid artery intimal-medial thickness in asymptomatic older subjects with exercise-induced myocardial ischemia. *Circulation.* **98,** 1504–1509.

Nagata, T., Kiriike, N., Tobitani, W., Kawarada, Y., Matsunaga, H., and Yamagami, S. (1999a). Lymphocyte subset, lymphocyte proliferative response, and soluble interleukin-2 receptor in anorexic patients. *Biol Psychiatry.* **45,** 471–474.

Nagata, T., Tobitani, W., Kiriike, N., Iketani, T., and Yamagami, S. (1999b). Capacity to produce cytokines during weight restoration in patients with anorexia nervosa. *Psychosom Med.* **61,** 371–377.

Najjar, S. S., Scuteri, A., and Lakatta, E. G. (2005). Arterial aging: Is it an immutable cardiovascular risk factor? *Hypertension.* **46,** 464–462.

Naka, Y., Bucciarelli, L. G., Wendt, T., Lee, L. K., Rong, L. L., Ramasamy, R., Yan, S. F., and Schmidt, A. M. (2004). RAGE axis: Animal models and novel insights into the vascular complications of diabetes. *Arterioscler Thromb Vasc Biol.* **24,** 1342–1349.

Nakada, T. A., Hirasawa, H., Oda, S., Shiga, H., Matsuda, K., Nakamura, M., Watanabe, E., Abe, R., Hatano, M., and Tokuhisa, T. (2005). Influence of Toll-like receptor 4, CD14, tumor necrosis factor, and interleukine-10 gene polymorphisms on clinical outcome in Japanese critically ill patients. *J Surg Res.* **129,** 322–328.

Nakajima, T., Schulte, S., Warrington, K. J., Kopecky, S. L., Frye, R. L., Goronzy, J. J., and Weyand, C. M. (2002). T-cell-mediated lysis of endothelial cells in acute coronary syndromes. *Circulation.* **105,** 570–575.

Nakamura, H., De Rosa, S., Roederer, M., Anderson, M. T., Dubs, J. G., Yodoi, J., Holmgren, A., Herzenberg, L. A. (1996). Elevation of plasma thioredoxin levels in HIV-infected individuals. *Int Immunol.* **8,** 603–611.

Nan, B., Yang, H., Yan, S., Lin, P. H., Lumsden, A. B., Yao, Q., and Chen, C. (2005). C-reactive protein decreases expression of thrombomodulin and endothelial protein C receptor in human endothelial cells. *Surgery.* **138,** 212–222.

Napoli, C., D'Armiento, F. P., Mancini, F. P., Postiglione, A., Witztum, J. L., Palumbo, G., and Palinski, W. (1997). Fatty streak formation occurs in human fetal aortas and is greatly enhanced by maternal hypercholesterolemia. Intimal accumulation of low density lipoprotein and its oxidation precede monocyte recruitment into early atherosclerotic lesions. *J Clin Invest.* **100,** 2680–2690.

Napoli, C., de Nigris, F., Welch, J. S., Calara, F. B., Stuart, R. O., Glass, C. K., and Palinski, W. (2002). Maternal hypercholesterolemia during pregnancy promotes early atherogenesis in LDL receptor-deficient mice and alters aortic gene expression determined by microarray. *Circulation.* **105,** 1360–1367.

Napoli, C., Glass, C. K., Witztum, J. L., Deutsch, R., D'Armiento, F. P., and Palinski, W. (1999a). Influence of maternal hypercholesterolaemia during pregnancy on progression of early atherosclerotic lesions in childhood: Fate of Early Lesions in Children (FELIC) Study. *Lancet.* **354,** 1234–1241.

Napoli, C., Martin-Padura, I., de Nigris, F., Giorgio, M., Mansueto, G., Somma, P., Condorelli, M., Sica, G., De Rosa, G., and Pelicci, P. (2003a). Deletion of the p66Shc longevity gene reduces systemic and tissue oxidative stress, vascular cell apoptosis, and early atherogenesis in mice fed a high-fat diet. *Proc Natl Acad Sci USA.* **100,** 2112–2116.

Napoli, C., Martin-Padura, I., de Nigris, F., Giorgio, M., Mansueto, G., Somma, P., Condorelli, M., Sica, G., De Rosa, G., and Pelicci, P. (2003b). Deletion of the p66Shc longevity gene reduces systemic and tissue oxidative stress, vascular cell apoptosis, and early atherogenesis in mice fed a high-fat diet. *Proc Natl Acad Sci USA.* **100,** 2112–2116.

Napoli, C., and Palinski, W. (2001). Maternal hypercholesterolemia during pregnancy influences the later development of atherosclerosis: Clinical and pathogenic implications. *Eur Heart J.* **22,** 4–9.

Napoli, C., Witztum, J. L., de Nigris, F., Palumbo, G., D'Armiento, F. P., and Palinski, W. (1999b). Intracranial arteries of human fetuses are more resistant to hypercholesterolemia-induced fatty streak formation than extracranial arteries. *Circulation.* **99,** 2003–2010.

Napolitano, G., Bucci, I., Giuliani, C., Massafra, C., Di Petta, C., Devangelio, E., Singer, D. S., Monaco, F., and Kohn, L. D. (2002). High glucose levels increase major histocompatibility complex class I gene expression in thyroid cells and amplify interferon-gamma action. *Endocrinology.* **143,** 1008–1017.

Nappo, F., Esposito, K., Cioffi, M., Giugliano, G., Molinari, A. M., Paolisso, G., Marfella, R., and Giugliano, D. (2002). Postprandial endothelial activation in healthy subjects and in type 2 diabetic patients: Role of fat and carbohydrate meals. *J Am Coll Cardiol.* **39,** 1145–1150.

Nardone, G., and Rocco, A. (2004). Chemoprevention of gastric cancer: Role of COX-2 inhibitors and other agents. *Digest Dis.* **22,** 320–326.

Nassar, T., Sachais, B. S., Akkawi, S., Kowalska, M. A., Bdeir, K., Leitersdorf, E., Hiss, E., Ziporen, L., Aviram, M., Cines, D., Poncz, M., and Higazi, A. A. (2003). Platelet factor 4 enhances the binding of oxidized low-density lipoprotein to vascular wall cells. *J Biol Chem.* **278,** 6187–6193.

Nassel, D. R. (2002). Neuropeptides in the nervous system of *Drosophila* and other insects: Multiple roles as neuromodulators and neurohormones. *Progr Neurobiol.* **68,** 1–84.

Nathan, B. P., Jiang, Y., Wong, G. K., Shen, F., Brewer, G. J., and Struble, R. G. (2002). Apolipoprotein E4 inhibits, and apolipoprotein E3 promotes neurite outgrowth in cultured adult mouse cortical neurons through the low-density lipoprotein receptor-related protein. *Brain Res.* **928,** 96–105.

Nathan, C. (2002). Points of control in inflammation. *Nature.* **420,** 846–852.

National Cholesterol Education Program. (2001). Executive summary of the Third Report of the National Cholesterol Education Program (NCEP) Expert Panel on Detection, Diagnosis, and Treatment of High Blood Cholesterol in Adults (Adult Treatment Panel III). *JAMA.* **285,** 539–553.

National Institute on Aging, and Reagan Institute Working Group on Diagnostic Criteria for the Neuropathological Assessment of Alzheimer's Disease . (1997). Consensus recommendations for the postmortem diagnosis of Alzheimer's disease. The National Institute on Aging, and Reagan Institute Working Group on Diagnostic Criteria for the Neuropathological Assessment of Alzheimer's Disease. *Neurobiol Aging.* **18,** S1–2.

Neel, J. V. (1962). Diabetes mellitus: A "thrifty" genotype rendered detrimental by "progress"? *Am J Hum Genet.* **14,** 238–239.

Neel, J. V. (1999). The "thrifty genotype" in 1998. *Nutr Rev.* **57,** S2–9.

Nekhaeva, E., Bodyak, N. D., Kraytsberg, Y., McGrath, S. B., Van Orsouw, N. J., Pluzhnikov, A., Wei, J. Y., Vijg, J., and Khrapko, K. (2002). Clonally expanded mtDNA point mutations are abundant in individual cells of human tissues. *Proc Natl Acad Sci USA.* **99,** 5521–5526.

Nelson, J. B. (1940). Infectious catarrh of the albino rat. II. The causal relation of the coccobacilliform bodies. J. *Exp. Med.* **72,** 645–662.

Nelson, J. B. (1963). Chronic respiratory disease in mice and rats. *Lab An Care.* **13,** 137–143.

Nelson, J. B. (1967). Respiratory infections of rats and mice with emphasis on indigenous mycoplasms. In E. Cotchin and F. Roe, J. C., Eds., *Pathology of laboratory rats and mice,* pp. 259–294. Oxford: Blackwell Scientific Publications.

Nelson, J. F., and Felicio, L. S. (1986). Radical ovarian resection advances the onset of persistent vaginal cornification but only transiently disrupts hypothalamic-pituitary regulation of cyclicity in C57BL/6J mice. *Biol Reprod* **35,** 957–64.

Nelson, J. F., Gosden, R. G., and Felicio, L. S. (1985). Effect of dietary restriction on estrous cyclicity and follicular reserves in aging C57BL/6J mice. *Biol Reprod.* **32,** 515–522.

Nelson, J. F., Karelus, K., Bergman, M. D., and Felicio, L. S. (1995). Neuroendocrine involvement in aging: Evidence from studies of reproductive aging and caloric restriction. *Neurobiol Aging.* **16,** 837–843.

Nemoto, S., and Finkel, T.. (2002). Redox regulation of forkhead proteins through a p66shc-dependent signaling pathway. *Science.* **295,** 2450–2452.

Nemoto, S., and Finkel, T. (2004). Ageing and the mystery at Arles. *Nature.* **429,** 149–152.

Netea, M. G., Van Der Graaf, C., Van Der Meer, J. W., and Kullberg, B. J. l. (2004). Toll-like receptors and the host defense against microbial pathogens: Bringing specificity to the innate-immune system. *J Leukocyte Biol.* **75,** 749–755.

Newman, A. B., and Brach, J. S. (2001). Gender gap in longevity and disability in older persons. *Epidemiol Rev.* **23,** 343–350.

Newsome, C. A., Shiell, A. W., Fall, C. H., Phillips, D. I., Shier, R., and Law, C. M. (2003). Is birth weight related to later glucose and insulin metabolism?—A systematic review. *Diabet Med.* **20,** 339–348.

Ng, P. M., Jin, Z., Tan, S. S., Ho, B., and Ding, J. L. (2004). C-reactive protein: A predominant LPS-binding acute phase protein responsive to *Pseudomonas* infection. *J Endotoxin Research.* **10,** 163–174.

Nicholas, H. R., and Hodgkin, J. (2004). Responses to infection and possible recognition strategies in the innate immune system of *Caenorhabditis elegans. Mol Immunol.* **41,** 479–493.

Nichols, N. R., Day, J. R., Laping, N. J., Johnson, S. A., and Finch, C. E. (1993). GFAP mRNA increases with age in rat and human brain. *Neurobiol Aging.* **14,** 421–429.

Nichols, S. M., Bavister, B. D., Brenner, C. A., Didier, P. J., Harrison, R. M., and Kubisch, H. M. (2005). Ovarian senescence in the rhesus monkey (*Macaca mulatta*). *Human Reproduction (Oxford, England).* **20,** 79–83.

Nichols, W. W., and O'Rourke, M. F. (2005). "McDonald's blood flow in arteries." London: Arnold.

Nicholson, D. A., Yoshida, R., Berry, R. W., Gallagher, M., and Geinisman, Y. (2004). Reduction in size of perforated postsynaptic densities in hippocampal axospinous synapses and age-related spatial learning impairments. *J Neurosci.* **24,** 7648–7653.

Niculescu, F., Niculescu, T., and Rus, H. (2004). C5b-9 terminal complement complex assembly on apoptotic cells in human arterial wall with atherosclerosis. *Exp Mol Pathol* **76,** 17–23.

Nilsson, K., Liu, A., Pahlson, C., and Lindquist, O. (2005). Demonstration of intracellular microorganisms (*Rickettsia spp., Chlamydia pneumoniae, Bartonella spp.*) in pathological human aortic valves by PCR. *J Infect.* **50,** 46–52.

Nilsson, S. E., Johansson, B., Takkinen, S., Berg, S., Zarit, S., McClearn, G., and Melander, A. (2003). Does aspirin protect against Alzheimer's dementia? A study in a Swedish population-based sample aged > or = 80 years. *Eur J Clin Pharm.* **59,** 313–319.

Niro, G. A., Fontana, R., Gioffreda, D., Valvano, M. R., Lacobellis, A., Facciorusso, D., and Andriulli, A. (2005). Tumor necrosis factor gene polymorphisms and clearance or progression of hepatitis B virus infection. *Liver Int.* **25,** 1175–1181.

Nishikawa, T., Edelstein, D., Du, X. L., Yamagishi, S., Matsumura, T., Kaneda, Y., Yorek, M. A., Beebe, D., Oates, P. J., Hammes, H. P., Giardino, I., and Brownlee, M. (2000). Normalizing mitochondrial superoxide production blocks three pathways of hyperglycaemic damage. *Nature.* **404,** 787–790.

Niwa, K., Kazama, K., Younkin, S. G., Carlson, G. A., and Iadecola, C. (2002). Alterations in cerebral blood flow and glucose utilization in mice overexpressing the amyloid precursor protein. *Neurobiol Dis.* **9,** 61–68.

Nixon, R. A. (2005). Endosome function and dysfunction in Alzheimer's disease and other neurodegenerative diseases. *Neurobiol Aging.* **26,** 373–382.

Nochlin, D., Shaw, C. M., Campbell, L. A., and Kuo, C. C. (1999). Failure to detect *Chlamydia pneumoniae* in brain tissues of Alzheimer's disease. *Neurology.* **53,** 1888.

Noguchi, H., Ohta, M., Wakasugi, S., Noguchi, K., Nakamura, N., Nakamura, O., Miyakawa, K., Takeya, M., Suzuki, M., Nakagata, N., Urano, T., Ono, T., and Yamamura, K. (2002). Effect of the intestinal flora on amyloid deposition in a transgenic mouse model of familial amyloidotic polyneuropathy. *Exp An.* **51,** 309–316.

Nørrelund, H. (2005). The metabolic role of growth hormone in humans with particular reference to fasting. *Growth Horm IGF Res.* **15,** 95–122.

Norry, F. M., and Loeschcke, V. (2003). Heat-induced expression of a molecular chaperone decreases by selecting for long-lived individuals. *Exp Gerontol.* **38,** 673–681.

Nowakowska, D., Kurnatowska, A., Stray-Pedersen, B., and Wilczynski, J. (2004). Prevalence of fungi in the vagina, rectum and oral cavity in pregnant diabetic women: Relation to gestational age and symptoms. *Acta Obstet Gynecol Scand.* **83,** 251–256.

Nursten, H. (2005). *The Maillard reaction. Chemistry, biochemistry, and implications.* Cambridge UK: Royal Society of Chemistry.

Nusbaum, T. J., Mueller, L. D., and Rose, M. R. (1996). Evolutionary patterns among measures of aging. *Exp Gerontol.* **31,** 507–516.

Nwasokwa, O. N., Weiss, M., Gladstone, C., and Bodenheimer, M. M. (1996). Effect of coronary artery size on the prevalence of atherosclerosis. *Am J Cardiol.* **78,** 741–746.

Nwasokwa, O. N., Weiss, M., Gladstone, C., and Bodenheimer, M. M. (1997). Higher prevalence and greater severity of coronary disease in short versus tall men referred for coronary arteriography. *Am Heart J.* **133,** 147–152.

Nystrom-Rosander, C., Lindh, U., Ilback, N. G., Hjelm, E., Thelin, S., Lindqvist, O., and Friman, G. (2003). Interactions between *Chlamydia pneumoniae* and trace elements: A possible link to aortic valve sclerosis. *Biol Trace Elem Res.* **91,** 97–110.

Obermayr, R. P., Mayerhofer, L., Knechtelsdorfer, M., Mersich, N., Huber, E. R., Geyer, G., and Tragl, K. H. (2005). The age-related down-regulation of the growth hormone/insulin-like growth factor-1 axis in the elderly male is reversed considerably by donepezil, a drug for Alzheimer's disease. *Exp Gerontol.* **40,** 157–63.

O'Brien, K. D., McDonald, T. O., Kunjathoor, V., Eng, K., Knopp, E. A., Lewis, K., Lopez, R., Kirk, E. A., Chait, A., Wight, T. N., deBeer, F. C., and LeBoeuf, R. C. (2006). Serum amyloid A and lipoprotein retention in murine models of atherosclerosis. *Arterioscler Thromb Vasc Biol.* **25,** 785–790.

O'Connell, J., Hawkes, K., and Blurton-Jones, N. (2002). Meat-eating, grandmothering, and the evolution of early human diets. In P. S. Ungar and M. F. Teafordm, Eds., *Human diet: Its origins and evolution*, pp. 49–60. Westport, CT: Bergman and Garvey.

Oda, K., and Kitano, H. (2006). A comprehensive map of the Toll-like receptor signaling network. *Mol Syst Biol.* **2.** on line

Oda, T., Pasinetti, G. M., Osterburg, H. H., Anderson, C., Johnson, S. A., and Finch, C. E. (1994). Purification and characterization of brain clusterin. *Biochem Biophys Res Comm.* **204,** 1131–1136.

Oda, T., Wals, P., Osterburg, H. H., Johnson, S. A., Pasinetti, G. M., Morgan, T. E., Rozovsky, I., Stine, W. B., Snyder, S. W., Holzman, T. F., Krafft, G., and Finch, C.E. (1995). Clusterin (apoJ) alters the aggregation of amyloid beta-peptide (A beta 1–42) and forms slowly sedimenting A beta complexes that cause oxidative stress. *Exp Neurol.* **136,** 22–31.

Oddo, S., Caccamo, A., Kitazawa, M., Tseng, B. P., and LaFerla, F. M. (2003a). Amyloid deposition precedes tangle formation in a triple transgenic model of Alzheimer's disease. *Neurobiol Aging.* **24,** 1063–1070.

Oddo, S., Caccamo, A., Shepherd, J. D., Murphy, M. P., Golde, T. E., Kayed, R., Metherate, R., Mattson, M. P., Akbari, Y., and LaFerla, F. M. (2003b). Triple-transgenic model of Alzheimer's disease with plaques and tangles: Intracellular Abeta and synaptic dysfunction. *Neuron.* **39,** 409–421.

Oeppen, J., and Vaupel, J. W. (2002). Demography. Broken limits to life expectancy. *Science.* **296,** 1029–1031.

Offenbacher, S., Riché, E. L., Barros, S. P., Bobetsis, Y. A., Lin, D., and Beck, J. D. (2005). Effects of maternal *Campylobacter rectus* infection on murine placenta, fetal and neonatal survival, and brain development. *J Periodontol.* **76,** 2133–2143.

Ogasawara, K., Mashiba, S., Wada, Y., Sahara, M., Uchida, K., Aizawa, T., and Kodama, T. (2004). A serum amyloid A and LDL complex as a new prognostic marker in stable coronary artery disease. *Atherosclerosis.* **174,** 349–356.

Ogden, C. L., Carroll, M. D., Curtin, L. R., McDowell, M. A., Tabak, C. J., and Flegal, K. M. (2006). Prevalence of overweight and obesity in the United States, 1999–2004. *JAMA.* **295,** 1549–1555.

Oh, J., Wunsch, R., Turzer, M., Bahner, M., Raggi, P., Querfeld, U., Mehls, O., and Schaefer, F. (2002). Advanced coronary and carotid arteriopathy in young adults with childhood-onset chronic renal failure. *Circulation.* **106,** 100–105.

Ohlstein, B., and Spradling, A., (2006). The adult *Drosophila* posterior midgut is maintained by pluripotent stem cells. *Nature.* **439,** 470–474.

Ohm, T. G., Muller, H., Braak, H., and Bohl, J. (1995). Close-meshed prevalence rates of different stages as a tool to uncover the rate of Alzheimer's disease-related neurofibrillary changes. *Neuroscience.* **64,** 209–217.

Ohsuzu, F. (2004). The roles of cytokines, inflammation and immunity in vascular diseases. *J Atheroscler Thromb.* **11,** 313–321.

O'Huigin, C., Satta, Y., Hausmann, A., Dawkins, R. L., and Klein, J. (2000). The implications of intergenic polymorphism for major histocompatibility complex evolution. *Genetics.* **156,** 867–877.

Oken, E., and Gillman, M. W. (2003). Fetal origins of obesity. *Obes Res.* **11,** 496–506.

Oken, E., Huh, S. Y., Taveras, E. M., Rich-Edwards, J. W., and Gillman, M. W., (2005). Associations of maternal prenatal smoking with child adiposity and blood pressure. *Obes Res.* **13,** 2021–2028.

Okuda, K., Khan, M. Y., Skurnick, J., Kimura, M., Aviv, H., and Aviv, A. (2000). Telomere attrition of the human abdominal aorta: Relationships with age and atherosclerosis. *Atherosclerosis.* **152,** 391–398.

O'Leary, D. H., Polak, J. F., Kronmal, R. A., Manolio, T. A., Burke, G. L., and Wolfson, S. K., Jr. (1999). Carotid-artery intima and media thickness as a risk factor for myocardial infarction and stroke in older adults. Cardiovascular Health Study Collaborative Research Group. *New Engl J Med.* **340,** 14–22.

O'Leary, V. B., Marchetti, C. M., Krishnan, R. K., Stetzer, B. P., CGonzalez, F., and Kirwan, J. P. (2006). Exercise-induced reversal of insulin resistance in obese elderly is associated with reduced visceral fat. *J Appl Physiol.* **100,** 1584–1589

Olsen, A., Vantipalli, M. C., and Lithgow, G. J. (2006a). Lifespan extension of *Caenorhabditis elegans* following repeated mild hormetic heat treatments. *Biogerontology.* **7,** 221–230

Olsen, A., Vantipalli, M. C., and Lithgow, G. J. (2006). Using *Caenorhabditis elegans* as a model for aging and age-related diseases. *Ann NY Acad Sci.* **1067,** 120–128.

Olsen, N. J., and Kovacs, W. J. (1996). Gonadal steroids and immunity. *Endocr Rev.* **17,** 369–384.

Olshansky, S. J., Hayflick, L., and Carnes, B. A. (2002). Position statement on human aging. *The J Gerontol. Series A, Biol Sci Med Sci.* **57,** B292–297.

Olshansky, S. J., Passaro, D. J., Hershow, R. C., Layden, J., Carnes, B. A., Brody, J., Hayflick, L., Butler, R. N., Allison, D. B., and Ludwig, D. S. (2005). A potential decline in life expectancy in the United States in the 21st century. *New Engl J Med.* **352,** 1138–1145.

Olshansky, S. J., and Rattan, S. I. (2005). At the heart of aging: Is it metabolic rate or stability? *Biogerontology.* **6,** 291–295.

Olsson, J., Wikby, A., Johansson, B., Lofgren, S., Nilsson, B. O., and Ferguson, F. G. (2000). Age-related change in peripheral blood T-lymphocyte subpopulations and cytomegalovirus infection in the very old: The Swedish longitudinal OCTO immune study. *Mech Ageing Dev.* **121,** 187–201.

O'Mahony, L., Holland, J., Jackson, J., Feighery, C., Hennessy, T. P., and Mealy, K. (1998). Quantitative intracellular cytokine measurement: Age-related changes in proinflammatory cytokine production. *Clin Exp Immunol.* **113,** 213–219.

O'Meara, E. S., White, M., Siscovick, D. S., Lyles, M. F., and Kuller, L. H. (2005). Hospitalization for pneumonia in the Cardiovascular Health Study: Incidence, mortality, and influence on longer-term survival. *J Am Geriatr Soc.* **53,** 1108–1116.

Ong, K. K. (2006). Size at birth, postnatal growth and risk of obesity. *Horm Res.* **65,** 65–69.

Ophir, E., Oettinger, M., Nisimov, J., Hirsch, Y., Fait, V., Dourleshter, G., Shnaider, O., Snitkovsky, T., and Bornstein, J. (2004). Cord blood lipids concentrations and their relation to body size at birth: Possible link between intrauterine life and adult diseases. *Am J Perinatol.* **21,** 35–40.

Orchard, T. J., Temprosa, M., Goldberg, R., Haffner, S., Ratner, R., Marcovina, S., and Fowler, S. (2005). The effect of metformin and intensive lifestyle intervention on the metabolic syndrome: The Diabetes Prevention Program randomized trial. *Ann Intern Med.* **142,** 611–619.

Ordovas, J. M. (2002). Gene-diet interaction and plasma lipid responses to dietary intervention. *Biochem Soc Trans.* **30,** 68–73.

Oria, R. B., Patrick, P. D., Zhang, H., Lorntz, B., de Castro Costa, C. M., Brito, G. A., Barrett, L. J., Lima, A. A., and Guerrant, R. L. (2005). APOE4 protects the cognitive development in children with heavy diarrhea burdens in Northeast Brazil. *Pediatric Research.* **57,** 310–316.

Orlandi, A., Marcellini, M., and Spagnoli, L. G. (2000). Aging influences development and progression of early aortic atherosclerotic lesions in cholesterol-fed rabbits. *Arterioscler Thromb Vasc Biol.* **20,** 1123–1136.

O'Rourke, M. F. (1976). Pulsatile arterial haemodynamics in hypertension. *Aust N Z J Med.* **6,** 40–48.

O'Rourke, M. F., and Nichols, W. W. (2005). Aortic diameter, aortic stiffness, and wave reflection increase with age and isolated systolic hypertension. *Hypertension.* **45,** 652–658.

O'Rourke, M. F., Nichols, W. W., and Safar, M. E. (2004). Pulse waveform analysis and arterial stiffness: Realism can replace evangelism and scepticism. *J Hypertension.* **22,** 1633–1634.

Orsini, F., Migliaccio, E., Moroni, M., Contursi, C., Raker, V. A., Piccini, D., Martin-Padura, I., Pelliccia, G., Trinei, M., Bono, M., Puri, C., Tacchetti, C., Ferrini, M., Mannucci, R.,

Nicoletti, I., Lanfrancone, L., Giorgio, M., and Pelicci, P. G. (2004). The life span determinant p66Shc localizes to mitochondria where it associates with mitochondrial heat shock protein 70 and regulates trans-membrane potential. *J Biol Chem.* **279,** 25689–25695.

Osaki, M., Oshimura, M., and Ito, H. (2004). PI3K-Akt pathway: Its functions and alterations in human cancer. *Apoptosis: An International Journal on Programmed Cell Death.* **9,** 667–676.

Osborne, T. B., and Mendel, L. B. (1914). The supression of growth and capacity to grow. *J Biol Chem.* **18,** 95.

Osborne, T. B., and Mendel, L. B. (1993). Amino-acids in nutrition and growth. 1914. *J Am Coll Nutrition.* **12,** 484–485.

Osborne, T. B., Mendel, L. B., and Ferry, E. L. (1917). The effect of retardation of growth upon the breeding period and duration of life in rats. *Science.* **45,** 294–295.

Ose, L., and Tolleshaug, H. (1989). Familial hypercholesterolemia. 50 years of research. *Arteriosclerosis.* **9,** 11–12.

Osler, W. (1892). *The principles and practice of medicine.* New York: Appleton.

Osmond, C., Kajantie, E., Forsen, T. J., Eriksson, J. G., Barker, D. J. (2007). Infant Growth and Stroke in Adult Life. The Helsinki Birth Cohort Study. *Stroke.* **38,** 264–270.

Ostergard, T., Ek, J., Hamid, Y., Saltin, B., Pedersen, O. B., Hansen, T., and Schmitz, O. (2005). Influence of the PPAR-gamma2 Pro12Ala and ACE I/D polymorphisms on insulin sensitivity and training effects in healthy offspring of type 2 diabetic subjects. *Horm Metab Res.* **37,** 99–105.

Ott, A., Breteler, M. M., van Harskamp, F., Stijnen, T., and Hofman, A. (1998). Incidence and risk of dementia. The Rotterdam Study. *Am J Epidemiology.* **147,** 574–580.

Oudejans, C. B., Mulders, J., Lachmeijer, A. M., van Dijk, M., Kèonst, A. A., Westerman, B. A., van Wijk, I. J., Leegwater, P. A., Kato, H. D., Matsuda, T., Wake, N., Dekker, G. A., Pals, G., ten Kate, L. P., and Blankenstein, M. A. (2004). The parent-of-origin effect of 10q22 in pre-eclamptic females coincides with two regions clustered for genes with down-regulated expression in androgenetic placentas. *Mol Hum Reprod.* **10,** 589–598.

Ounsted, M. (1986). Transmission through the female line of fetal growth constraint. *Early Hum Dev.* **13,** 339–341.

Ounsted, M. (1988). Small-for-dates babies: Heterogeneity and the concept of 'brain sparing'. *Paediatr Perinat Epidemiol.* **2,** 365–370.

Ounsted, M., Moar, V. A., and Scott, A. (1986b). Growth and proportionality in early childhood. I. Within population variations. *Early Hum Dev.* **13,** 27–36.

Ounsted, M., Scott, A., and Ounsted, C. (1986a). Transmission through the female line of a mechanism constraining human fetal growth. *Ann Hum Biol.* **13,** 143–151.

Overton, J. M., and Williams, T. D. (2004). Behavioral and physiologic responses to caloric restriction in mice. *Physiol Behav.* **81,** 749–754.

Owen-Ashley, N. T., Turner, M., Hahn, T. P., and Wingfield, J. C. (2006). Hormonal, behavioral, and thermoregulatory responses to bacterial lipopolysaccharide in captive and free-living white-crowned sparrows (*Zonotrichia leucophrys gambelii*). *Horm Behav.* **49,** 15–29.

Packer, C., Tatar, M., and Collins, A. (1998). Reproductive cessation in female mammals. *Nature.* **392,** 807–811.

Pagel, M. D. and Harvey, P. H. (1988). Recent developments in the analysis of comparative data. *Q Rev Biol.* **63,** 413–440.

Paglia, D. E., and Walford, R. L. (2005). Atypical hematological response to combined calorie restriction and chronic hypoxia in Biosphere 2 crew: A possible link to latent features of hibernation capacity. *Habitation*. **10**, 79–85.

Pahlavani, M. A. (2000). Caloric restriction and immunosenescence: A current perspective. *Front Biosci*. **5**, D580–587.

Pahlavani, M. A., and Vargas, D. M. (2000). Influence of aging and caloric restriction on activation of Ras/MAPK, calcineurin, and CaMK-IV activities in rat T cells. *Proc Soc Exp Biol Med*. **223**, 163–169.

Paine, R. R., Boldsen, J. L. (2006). Paleodemographic data and why understanding holocene demography is essential to understanding human life history evolution in the Pleistocene. In: The Evolution of Human Life History (Hawkes, K., Paine, R. R., eds), pp. 307–331. Sante Fe: School for American Research Press.

Painter, R. C., Roseboom, T. J., and Bleker, O. P. (2005a). Prenatal exposure to the Dutch famine and disease in later life: An overview. *Reprod Toxicol*. **20**, 345–352.

Painter, R. C., Roseboom, T. J., Bossuyt, P. M., Osmond, C., Barker, D. J., and Bleker, O. P. (2005b). Adult mortality at age 57 after prenatal exposure to the Dutch famine. *Eur J Epidemiol*. **20**, 673–676.

Painter, R. C., Roseboom, T. J., van Montfrans, G. A., Bossuyt, P. M., Krediet, R. T., Osmond, C., Barker, D. J., and Bleker, O. P. (2005c). Microalbuminuria in adults after prenatal exposure to the Dutch famine. *J Am Soc Nephrol*. **16**, 189–194.

Palinski, W. (2004). Aneurysms: Leukotrienes weaken aorta from the outside. *Nature Med*. **10**, 896–898.

Palinski, W., and Napoli, C. (2002a). The fetal origins of atherosclerosis: Maternal hypercholesterolemia, and cholesterol-lowering or antioxidant treatment during pregnancy influence in utero programming and postnatal susceptibility to atherogenesis. *FASEB J*. **16**, 1348–1360.

Palinski, W., and Tsimikas, S. (2002b). Immunomodulatory effects of statins: Mechanisms and potential impact on arteriosclerosis. *J Am Soc Nephrol*. **13**, 1673–1681.

Pampel, F. (2002). Cigarette use and the narrowing sex differential in mortality. *Popul Devel Rev*. **28**, 77–104.

Panagiotakos, D. B., Pitsavos, C., Chrysohoou, C., Skoumas, J., Masoura, C., Toutouzas, P., and Stefanadis, C. (2004). Effect of exposure to secondhand smoke on markers of inflammation: The ATTICA Study. *Am J Medicine*. **116**, 145–150.

Panagiotakos, D. B., Pitsavos, C. E., Chrysohoou, C. A., Skoumas, J., Toutouza, M., Belegrinos, D., Toutouzas, P. K., and Stefanadis, C. (2004b). The association between educational status and risk factors related to cardiovascular disease in healthy individuals: The ATTICA Study. *Ann Epidemiol*. **14**, 188–194.

Paneth, N., Ahmed, F., and Stein, A. D. (1996). Early nutritional origins of hypertension: A hypothesis still lacking support. *J Hypertens Suppl*. **14**, S121–129.

Paneth, N., and Susser, M. (1995). Early origin of coronary heart disease (the "Barker hypothesis"). *Br Med J*. **310**, 411–412.

Panza, F., Solfrizzi, V., Colacicco, A., Basile, A., D'Introno, A., Capurso, C., Sabba, M., Capurso, S., and Capurso, A. (2003). Apolipoprotein E (APOE) polymorphism influences serum APOE levels in Alzheimer's disease patients and centenarians. *Neuroreport*. **14**, 605–608.

Paolisso, G., Ammendola, S., Del Buono, A., Gambardella, A., Riondino, M., Tagliamonte, M. R., Rizzo, M. R., Carella, C., and Varricchio, M. (1997). Serum levels of insulin-like growth factor-I (IGF-I) and IGF-binding protein-3 in healthy centenarians: Relationship with plasma leptin and lipid concentrations, insulin action, and cognitive function. *J Clin Endocrinol Metab.* **82,** 2204–2209.

Paolisso, G., Barbieri, M., Bonafáe, M., and Franceschi, C., (2000). Metabolic age modelling: The lesson from centenarians. *Eur J Clin Invest.* **30,** 888–894.

Paolisso, G., Barbieri, M., Rizzo, M. R., Carella, C., Rotondi, M., Bonafáe, M., Franceschi, C., Rose, G., and De Benedictis, G. (2001). Low insulin resistance and preserved beta-cell function contribute to human longevity but are not associated with TH-INS genes. *Exp Gerontol.* **37,** 149–156.

Paolisso, G., Gambardella, A., Ammendola, S., D'Amore, A., Balbi, V., Varricchio, M., and D'Onofrio, F. (1996). Glucose tolerance and insulin action in healty centenarians. *Am J Physiol.* **270,** E2890–E894.

Paolisso, G., Tagliamonte, M. R., Rizzo, M. R., and Giugliano, D. (1999). Advancing age and insulin resistance: New facts about an ancient history. *Eur J Clin Invest.* **29,** 758–769.

Pardio, V. T., Landin, L. A., Waliszewski, K. N., Perez-Gil, F., Diaz, L., and Hernandez, B. (2005). The effect of soybean soapstock on the quality parameters and fatty acid composition of the hen egg yolk. *Poultry Sci.* **84,** 148–157.

Pardo Silva, M. C., De Laet, C., Nusselder, W. J., Mamun, A. A., and Peeters, A., (2006). Adult obesity and number of years lived with and without cardiovascular disease. *Obesity.* **14,** 1264–1273.

Park, I. H., Hwang, E. M., Hong, H. S., Boo, J. H., Oh, S. S., Lee, J., Jung, M. W., Bang, O. Y., Kim, S. U., and Mook-Jung, I. (2003). Lovastatin enhances Abeta production and senile plaque deposition in female Tg2576 mice. *Neurobiol Aging.* **24,** 637–643.

Parker, D. C., Rossman, L. G., and VanderLaan, E. F. (1972). Persistence of rhythmic human growth hormone release during sheep in fasted and nonisocalorically fed normal subjects. *Metabolism.* **21,** 241–252.

Parkin, D. M., Bray, F., Ferlay, J., and Pisani, P. (2005). Global cancer statistics, 2002. *CA Cancer J Clin.* **55,** 74–108.

Parrinello, S., Coppe, J. P., Krtolica, A., and Campisi, J. (2005). Stromal-epithelial interactions in aging and cancer: Senescent fibroblasts alter epithelial cell differentiation. *J Cell Sci.* **118,** 485–496.

Parrinello, S., Samper, E., Krtolica, A., Goldstein, J., Melov, S., and Campisi, J. (2003). Oxygen sensitivity severely limits the replicative lifespan of murine fibroblasts. *Nat Cell Biol.* **5,** 741–747.

Partridge, L., Piper, M. D., and Mair, W. (2005a). Dietary restriction in *Drosophila. Mech Ageing Dev.* **12,** 938–950.

Partridge, L., Pletcher, S. D., and Mair, W. (2005b). Dietary restriction, mortality trajectories, risk and damage. *Mech Ageing Dev.* **126,** 35–41.

Pasche, B., Kalaydjiev, S., Franz, T. J., Kremmer, E., Gailus-Durner, V., Fuchs, H., Hrabé de Angelis, M., Lengeling, A., and Busch, D. H. (2005). Sex-dependent susceptibility to *Listeria monocytogenes* infection is mediated by differential interleukin-10 production. *Infect Immun.* **73,** 5952–5960.

Pashko, L. L., and Schwartz, A. G. (1992). Reversal of food restriction-induced inhibition of mouse skin tumor promotion by adrenalectomy. *Carcinogenesis.* **13,** 1925–1928.

Pashko, L. L., and Schwartz, A. G. (1996). Inhibition of 7,12–dimethylbenz[a]anthracene-induced lung tumorigenesis in A/J mice by food restriction is reversed by adrenalectomy. *Carcinogenesis.* **17,** 209–212.

Pasinetti, G. M., Hassler, M., Stone, D., and Finch, C. E. (1999). Glial gene expression during aging in rat striatum and in long-term responses to 6-OHDA lesions. *Synapse.* **31,** 278–284.

Pasinetti, G. M., Johnson, S. A., Rozovsky, I., Lampert-Etchells, M., Morgan, D. G., Gordon, M. N., Morgan, T. E., Willoughby, D., and Finch, C. E. s. (1992). Complement C1qB and C4 mRNAs responses to lesioning in rat brain. *Exp Neurol.* **118,** 117–125.

Pasinetti, G. M., Tocco, G., Sakhi, S., Musleh, W. D., DeSimoni, M. G., Mascarucci, P., Schreiber, S., Baudry, M., and Finch, C. E. (1996). Hereditary deficiencies in complement C5 are associated with intensified neurodegenerative responses that implicate new roles for the C-system in neuronal and astrocytic functions. *Neurobiol Dis.* **3,** 197–204.

Passerini, A. G., Polacek, D. C., Shi, C., Francesco, N. M., Manduchi, E., Grant, G. R., Pritchard, W. F., Powell, S., Chang, G. Y., Stoeckert, C. J., Jr., and Davies, P. F. (2004). Coexisting proinflammatory and antioxidative endothelial transcription profiles in a disturbed flow region of the adult porcine aorta. *Proc Natl Acad Sci USA.* **101,** 2482–2487.

Patel, A. C., Nunez, N. P., Perkins, S. N., Barrett, J. C., and Hursting, S. D. (2004). Effects of energy balance on cancer in genetically altered mice. *J Nutr.* **134,** 3394S–3398S.

Patel, A. V., Press, M. F., Meeske, K., Calle, E. E., and Bernstein, L. (2003). Lifetime recreational exercise activity and risk of breast carcinoma *in situ. Cancer.* **98,** 2161–2169.

Patel, A. V., Rodriguez, C., Bernstein, L., Chao, A., Thun, M. J., Calle, E. E., (2005). Obesity, recreational physical activity, and risk of pancreatic cancer in a large U.S. Cohort. *Cancer Epidemiol Biomarkers Prev.* **14,** 459–466.

Patel, N. V., and Finch, C. E. (2002). The glucocorticoid paradox of caloric restriction in slowing brain aging. *Neurobiol Aging.* **23,** 707–717.

Patel, N. V., Gordon, M. N., Connor, K. E., Good, R. A., Engelman, R. W., Mason, J., Morgan, D. G., Morgan, T. E., and Finch, C. E. (2005). Caloric restriction attenuates Abeta -deposition in Alzheimer transgenic models. *Neurobiol Aging.* **26,** 995–1000.

Paterson, J. R., and Lawrence, J. R. (2001). Salicylic acid: A link between aspirin, diet and the prevention of colorectal cancer. *Qjm.* **94,** 445–448.

Paterson, T. J., Baxter, G., Lawrence, J., and Duthie, G. (2006). Is there a role for dietary salicylates in health? *Proc Nutr Soc* **65,** 93–96.

Patronek, G. J., Waters, D. J., and Glickman, L. T. (1997). Comparative longevity of pet dogs and humans: Implications for gerontology research. *J Gerontol. A Biol Sci Med Sci.* **52,** B171–178.

Pavlidis, P., Qin, J., Arango, V., Mann, J. J., and Sibille, E. (2004). Using the gene ontology for microarray data mining: A comparison of methods and application to age effects in human prefrontal cortex. *Neurochem Res.* **29,** 1213–1222.

Pavlov, D. V. (1965). *Leningrad 1941: The blockade.* Chicago: University of Chicago Press.

Pawelec, G., Akbar, A., Caruso, C., Solana, R., Grubeck-Loebenstein, B., and Wikby, A. (2005). Human immunosenescence: Is it infectious? *Immunol Rev.* **205,** 257–268.

Pawelec, G., Barnett, Y., Forsey, R., Frasca, D., Globerson, A., McLeod, J., Caruso, C., Franceschi, C., Fulop, T., Gupta, S., Mariani, E., Mocchegiani, E., and Solana, R. (2002). T cells and aging, January 2002 update. *Front Biosci.* **7,** d1056–1183.

Pearce-Duvet, J. M. (2006). The origin of human pathogens: evalUating the role of agriculture and domestic animals in the evolution of human disease. *Biol Rev Camb Philos Soc.* **81,** 369–382.

Peccei, J. S. (2001). A critique of the grandmother hypotheses: old and new. *Am J Hum Biol.* **13,** 434–452.

Peden, D. B (2005). The epidemiology and genetics of asthma risk associated with air pollution. *J Allergy Clin Immunol.* **115,** 213–219.

Pedersen, B. K., Steensberg, A., Keller, P., Keller, C., Fischer, C., Hiscock, N., van Hall, G., Plomgaard, P., and Febbraio, M. A. (2003). Muscle-derived interleukin-6: Lipolytic, anti-inflammatory and immune regulatory effects. *Pflugers Archiv: Eur J Physiol.* **446,** 9–16.

Peeling, R. W., Wang, S. P., Grayston, J. T., Blasi, F., Boman, J., Clad, A., Freidank, H., Gaydos, C. A., Gnarpe, J., Hagiwara, T., Jones, R. B., Orfila, J., Persson, K., Puolakkainen, M., Saikku, P., and Schachter, J. (2000). *Chlamydia pneumoniae* serology: Interlaboratory variation in microimmunofluorescence assay results. *J Infect Dis.* **181,** S426–429.

Peila, R., White, L. R., Petrovich, H., Masaki, K., Ross, G. W., Havlik, R. J., and Launer, L. J. (2001). Joint effect of the APOE gene and midlife systolic blood pressure on late-life cognitive impairment: The Honolulu-Asia Aging Study. *Stroke.* **32,** 2882–2889.

Pelletier, D. L. (1994). The potentiating effects of malnutrition on child mortality: Epidemiologic evidence and policy implications. *Nutr Rev.* **52,** 409–415.

Peng, J., Zipperlen, P., and Kubli, E. (2005a). *Drosophila* sex-peptide stimulates female innate immune system after mating via the Toll and Imd pathways. *Curr Biol.* **15,** 1690–11694.

Peng, S., Glennert, J., and Westermark, P. (2005b). Medin-amyloid: A recently characterized age-associated arterial amyloid form affects mainly arteries in the upper part of the body. *Amyloid: Int J Exp Clin Invest.* **12,** 96–102.

Peng, S., Westermark, G. T., Nèaslund, J., Hèaggqvist, B., Glennert, J., and Westermark, P. (2002). Medin and medin-amyloid in ageing inflamed and non-inflamed temporal arteries. *J Pathol.* **196,** 91–96.

Penta, R., De Falco, M., Iaquinto, G., and De Luca, A. (2005). *Helicobacter pylori* and gastric epithelial cells: From gastritis to cancer. *J Exp Clin Cancer Res.* **24,** 337–345.

Pepys, M. B. (2006). Amyloidosis. *Annu Rev Med.* **57,** 223–241.

Pepys, M. B., and Hirschfield, G. M. (2003). C-reactive protein: A critical update. [erratum appears in *J Clin Invest.* **112,** 299] *J Clin Invest.* **111,** 1805–1812.

Perillo, N.L., Walford, R.L., Newman, M.A., Effros, R.B. (1989). Human T lymphocytes possess a limited in vitro life span. *Exp Gerontol.* **24,** 177–187.

Perkins, S. N., Hursting, S. D., Phang, J. M., and Haines, D. C. (1998). Calorie restriction reduces ulcerative dermatitis and infection-related mortality in p53-deficient and wild-type mice. *J Invest Dermatol.* **111,** 292–296.

Perlmutter, L. S., Chui, H. C., Saperia, D., and Athanikar, J. (1990). Microangiopathy and the colocalization of heparan sulfate proteoglycan with amyloid in senile plaques of Alzheimer's disease. *Brain Res.* **508,** 13–19.

Perron, L., Bairati, I., Moore, L., and Meyer, F. (2003). Dosage, duration and timing of nonsteroidal antiinflammatory drug use and risk of prostate cancer. *Int J Cancer.* **106,** 409–515.

Perry, H. M., Jr., Davis, B. R., Price, T. R., Applegate, W. B., Fields, W. S., Guralnik, J. M., Kuller, L., Pressel, S., Stamler, J., and Probstfield, J. L. (2000). Effect of treating isolated systolic hypertension on the risk of developing various types and subtypes of stroke: The Systolic Hypertension in the Elderly Program (SHEP). *JAMA.* **284,** 465–471.

Peters, C. R. (2007). Theoretical and actualistic ecobotanical perspectives on early hominin diets and paleocology. *The evolution of human life history,* pp. 233–261. Sante Fe: School for American Research Press.

Petersen, R. C. (2004). Mild cognitive impairment as a diagnostic entity. *J Intern Med.* **256,** 183–194.

Peto R, D. S., Deo H, Silcocks P, Whitley E, Doll R. (2000). Smoking, smoking cessation, and lung cancer in the UK since 1950: Combination of national statistics with two case-control studies. *Br Med J.* **321,** 323–329.

Petot, G. J., Debanne, S. M., Traore, F., Fritsch, T., and Lerner, A. J. (2002). Dietary patterns during mid-adult life and risk for Alzheimer's disease. *Neurobiol Aging* , abstract 1124.

Petot, G. J., and Friedland, R. P. (2004). Lipids, diet and Alzheimer disease: An extended summary. *J Neurol Sci.* **226,** 31–33.

Petronio, A. S., Amoroso, G., Limbruno, U., Papini, B., De Carlo, M., Micheli, A., Ciabatti, N., and Mariani, M. (2005). Simvastatin does not inhibit intimal hyperplasia and restenosis but promotes plaque regression in normocholesterolemic patients undergoing coronary stenting: A randomized study with intravascular ultrasound. *Am Heart J.* **149,** 520–526.

Petruska, J., and Goodman, M. F. (1995). Enthalpy-entropy compensation in DNA melting thermodynamics. *J Biol Chem.* **270,** 746–750.

Pettus, B. J., Kitatani, K., Chalfant, C. E., Taha, T. A., Kawamori, T., Bielawski, J., Obeid, L. M., and Hannun, Y. A. (2005). The coordination of prostaglandin E2 production by sphingosine-1-phosphate and ceramide-1-phosphate. *Mol Pharmacol.* **68,** 330–335.

Pfister, G., Stroh, C. M., Perschinka, H., Kind, M., Knoflach, M., Hinterdorfer, P., and Wick, G. (2005). Detection of HSP60 on the membrane surface of stressed human endothelial cells by atomic force and confocal microscopy. *J Cell Sci.* **118,** 1587–1594.

Phelan, J. P., and Austad, S. N. (1994). Selecting animal models of human aging: Inbred strains often exhibit less biological uniformity than F1 hybrids. *J Gerontol.* **49,** B1–11.

Phelan, J. P., and Rose, M. R. (2005). Why dietary restriction substantially increases longevity in animal models but won't in humans. *Ageing Res Rev.* **4,** 339–350.

Phillips, D. I., Davies, M. J., and Robinson, J. S. (2001). Fetal growth and the fetal origins hypothesis in twins—Problems and perspectives. *Twin Res* **4,** 327–331.

Picken, M. M. (2001). The changing concepts of amyloid. [comment]. *Arch Pathol Lab Med.* **125,** 38–43.

Pickford, M. (2005). Incisor-molar relationships in chimpanzees and other hominoids: Implications for diet and phylogeny. *Primates.* **46,** 21–32.

Piconi, L., Quagliaro, L., Assaloni, R., Da Ros, R., Maier, A., Zuodar, G., and Ceriello, A. (2006). Constant and intermittent high glucose enhances endothelial cell apoptosis through mitochondrial superoxide overproduction. *Diabetes Metab Res Rev.* **22,** 198–203.

Pierpaoli, W., Baroni, C., Fabris, N., and Sorkin, E. (1969). Hormones and immunological capacity. II. Reconstitution of antibody production in hormonally deficient mice by somatotropic hormone, thyrotropic hormone and thyroxin. *Immunology.* **16,** 217–230.

Pierri, H., Higuchi-Dos-Santos, M. H., Higuchi, M. D., Palomino, S., Sambiase, N. V., Demarchi, L. M., Rodrigues, G. H., Nussbacher, A., Ramires, J. A., and Wajngarten, M. (2005). Density of *Chlamydia pneumoniae* is increased in fibrotic and calcified areas of degenerative aortic stenosis. *Int J Cardiol.* **108,** 43–47.

Piers, L. S., Diggavi, S. N., Thangam, S., van Raaij, J. M., Shetty, P. S., and Hautvast, J. G. (1995). Changes in energy expenditure, anthropometry, and energy intake during the course of pregnancy and lactation in well-nourished Indian women. *Am J Clin Nutr.* **61,** 501–513.

Pike, C. J. (1999). Estrogen modulates neuronal Bcl-xL expression and beta-amyloid-induced apoptosis: Relevance to Alzheimer's disease. *J Neurochem.* **72,** 1552–1563.

Pike, M. C., Krailo, M. D., Henderson, B. E., Casagrande, J. T., and Hoel, D. G. (1983). 'Hormonal' risk factors, 'breast tissue age' and the age-incidence of breast cancer. *Nature.* **303,** 767–770.

Pimentel, M., Chow, E. J., and Lin, H. C. (2000). Eradication of small intestinal bacterial overgrowth reduces symptoms of irritable bowel syndrome. *Am J Gastroenterology.* **95,** 3503–3506.

Piper, P. W. (2006). Long-lived yeast as a model for ageing research. *Yeast.* **23(3),** 215–226.

Pitkanen, K. J. (1993). *Deprivation and disease. Mortality during the Great Finnish Famine of the 1860s.* Helsinki: Finnish Demographic Society.

Pitsikas, N., Carli, M., Fidecka, S., and Algeri, S. (1990). Effect of life-long hypocaloric diet on age-related changes in motor and cognitive behavior in a rat population. *Neurobiol Aging.* **11,** 417–423.

Plageman, T. F., Jr., and Yutzey, K. E. (2005). T-box genes and heart development: putting the "T" in heart. *Dev Dyn.* **232,** 11–20.

Plagemann, A. (2005). Perinatal programming and functional teratogenesis: Impact on body weight regulation and obesity. *Physiol Behav.* **86,** 661–668.

Plagemann, A., Davidowa, H., Harder, T., and Dudenhausen, J. W. (2006). Developmental programming of the hypothalamus: A matter of insulin. [A comment on: Horvath, T. L., Bruning, J. C.: Developmental programming of the hypothalamus: A matter of fat. *Nat. Med.* (2006) 12:52–53.] *Neuro Endocrinol Lett.* **27,** 70–72.

Plank, L. D., and Hill, G. L. (2003). Energy balance in critical illness. *Proc Nutr Soc.* **62,** 545–552.

Plaschke, K. (2005). Aspects of ageing in chronic cerebral oligaemia. Mechanisms of degeneration and compensation in rat models. *J Neural Transm.* **112,** 393–413.

Plata-Salaman, C. R. (1996). Anorexia during acute and chronic disease. *Nutrition.* **12,** 69–78.

Pletcher, S. D., Khazaeli, A. A., and Curtsinger, J. W. (2000). Why do life spans differ? Partitioning mean longevity differences in terms of age-specific mortality parameters. *J Gerontol. Series A, Biol Sci Med Sci.* **55,** B381–389.

Pletcher, S. D., Macdonald, S. J., Marguerie, R., Certa, U., Stearns, S. C., Goldstein, D. B., and Partridge, L. (2002). Genome-wide transcript profiles in aging and calorically restricted *Drosophila melanogaster. Curr Biol.* **12,** 712–723.

Plotnick, G. D., Corretti, M. C., and Vogel, R. A. (1997). Effect of antioxidant vitamins on the transient impairment of endothelium-dependent brachial artery vasoactivity following a single high-fat meal. *JAMA.* **278,** 1682–1686.

Plytycz, B., and Seljelid, R. (2003). From inflammation to sickness: Historical perspective. *Arch Immunol Ther Exp (Warsz).* **51,** 105–109.

Pocai, A., Obici, S., Schwartz, G. J., and Rossetti, L. (2005). A brain-liver circuit regulates glucose homeostasis. **1,** 53–61.

Podewils, L. J., Guallar, E., Kuller, L. H., Fried, L. P., Lopez, O. L., Carlson, M., and Lyketsos, C. G. (2005). Physical activity, APOE genotype, and dementia risk: Findings from the Cardiovascular Health Cognition Study. *Am J Epidemiol.* **161,** 639–651.

Podlutsky, A. J., Khritankov, A. M., Ovodov, N. D., and Austad, S. N. (2005). A new field record for bat longevity. *J Gerontol. A Biol Sci Med Sci.* **60,** 1366–1368.

Podolsky, S. (1998). Cultural divergence: Elie Metchnikoff's *Bacillus bulgaricus* therapy and his underlying concept of health. *Bull Hist Med.* **72,** 1–27.

Poehlman, E. T., Turturro, A., Bodkin, N., Cefalu, W., Heymsfield, S., Holloszy, J., and Kemnitz, J. (2001). Caloric restriction mimetics: Physical activity and body composition changes. *J Gerontol. Series A, Biol Sci Med Sci.* **56,** 45–54.

Poirier, J. (2005). Apolipoprotein E, cholesterol transport, and synthesis in sporadic Alzheimer's disease. *Neurobiol Aging.* **26,** 355–361

Poirier, J., Davignon, J., Bouthillier, D., Kogan, S., Bertrand, P., and Gauthier, S. (1993). Apolipoprotein E polymorphism and Alzheimer's disease. *Lancet.* **342,** 697–699.

Poirier, J., Delisle, M. C., Quirion, R., Aubert, I., Farlow, M., Lahiri, D., Hui, S., Bertrand, P., Nalbantoglu, J., Gilfix, B. M., and Gauthier, S.. (1995). Apolipoprotein E4 allele as a predictor of cholinergic deficits and treatment outcome in Alzheimer disease. *Proc Natl Acad Sci USA.* **92,** 12260–12264.

Pollard, K. S., Salama, S. R., Lambert, N., Lambot, M. A., Coppens, S., Pedersen, J. S., Katzman, S., King, B., Onodera, C., Siepel, A., Kern, A. D., Dehay, C., Igel, H., Ares, M. J., Vanderhaeghen, P., and Haussler, D. (2006). An RNA gene expressed during cortical development evolved rapidly in humans. *Nature.* **443,** 167–172.

Pomposelli, J. J., Baxter, J. K., 3rd, Babineau, T. J., Pomfret, E. A., Driscoll, D. F., Forse, R. A., and Bistrian, B. R. (1998). Early postoperative glucose control predicts nosocomial infection rate in diabetic patients. *J Parent Ent Nutrit.* **22,** 77–81.

Pond, C. M. (2003). Paracrine interactions of mammalian adipose tissue. *J Exp Zoolog A Comp Exp Biol.* **295,** 99–110.

Pond, C. M. (2005). Adipose tissue and the immune system. *Prostaglandins Leukot Essent Fatty Acids.* **73,** 17–30.

Poppitt, S. D., Prentice, A. M., Goldberg, G. R., and Whitehead, R. G. (1994). Energy-sparing strategies to protect human fetal growth. *Am J Obstet Gynecol.* **171,** 118–125.

Poppitt, S. D., Prentice, A. M., Jéquier, E., Schutz, Y., and Whitehead, R. G. (1993). Evidence of energy sparing in Gambian women during pregnancy: A longitudinal study using whole-body calorimetry. *Am J Clin Nutr.* **57,** 353–364.

Porte, D., Jr., Baskin, D. G., and Schwartz, M. W. (2005). Insulin signaling in the central nervous system: A critical role in metabolic homeostasis and disease from *C. elegans* to humans. *Diabetes.* **54,** 1264–1276.

Porto, I., Maria Leone, A., Crea, F., and Andreotti, F. (2005). Inflammation, genetics, and ischemic heart disease: Focus on the major histocompatibility complex (MHC) genes. *Cytokine.* **29,** 187–196.

Poskitt, E. M., Cole, T. J., and Whitehead, R. G. (1999). Less diarrhoea but no change in growth: 15 years' data from three Gambian villages. *Arch Dis Childhd.* **80,** 115–119; discussion, 119–120.

Posnett, D. N., Edinger, J. W., Manavalan, J. S., Irwin, C., and Marodon, G. (1999). Differentiation of human CD8 T cells: Implications for *in vivo* persistence of CD8+ CD28– cytotoxic effector clones. *Int Immunol.* **11,** 229–241.

Potten, C. S., Booth, C., and Hargreaves, D. (2003). The small intestine as a model for evaluating adult tissue stem cell drug targets. *Cell Prolif.* **36,** 115–129.

Potten, C. S., Martin, K., and Kirkwood, T. B. (2001). Ageing of murine small intestinal stem cells. *Novartis Found Symp.* **235,** 66–79.

Poullis, A. P., Zar, S., Sundaram, K. K., Moodie, S. J., Risley, P., Theodossi, A., and Mendall, M. A. (2002). A new, highly sensitive assay for C-reactive protein can aid the differentiation of inflammatory bowel disorders from constipation- and diarrhoea-predominant functional bowel disorders. *Eur J Gastroenterol Hepatol.* **14,** 409–412.

Powell, J. T., Vine, N., and Crossman, M. (1992). On the accumulation of D-aspartate in elastin and other proteins of the ageing aorta. *Atherosclerosis.* **97**, 201–208.

Powell, L. A., Nally, S. M., McMaster, D., Catherwood, M. A., and Trimble, E. R. (2001). Restoration of glutathione levels in vascular smooth muscle cells exposed to high glucose conditions. *Free Radic Biol Med.* **31**, 1149–1155.

Powers, R. W., 3rd, Kaeberlein, M., Caldwell, S. D., Kennedy, B. K., and Fields, S. (2006a). Extension of chronological life span in yeast by decreased TOR pathway signaling. *Genes Dev.* **20**, 174–184.

Powers, R. W. 3rd, Harrison, D. E., and Flurkey, K. (2006b). Pituitary removal in adult mice increases life span. *Mech Ageing Dev.* **127**, 658–659.

Prasher, V. P., Farrer, M. J., Kessling, A. M., Fisher, E. M., West, R. J., Barber, P. C., and Butler, A. C. (1998). Molecular mapping of Alzheimer-type dementia in Down's syndrome. Ann Neurol. **43**, 380–383.

Prentice, A. M., Cole, T. J., Foord, F. A., Lamb, W. H., and Whitehead, R. G. (1987). Increased birthweight after prenatal dietary supplementation of rural African women. *Am J Clin Nutr.* **46**, 912–925.

Prentice, A. M., and Goldberg, G. R. (2000). Energy adaptations in human pregnancy: Limits and long-term consequences. *Am J Clin Nutr.* **71**, 1226S–1232S.

Prentice, R. L., Caan, B., Chlebowski, R. T., Patterson, R., Kuller, L. H., Ockene, J. K., Margolis, K. L., Limacher, M. C., Manson, J. E., Parker, L. M., Paskett, E., Phillips, L., Robbins, J., Rossouw, J. E., Sarto, G. E., Shikany, J. M., Stefanick, M. L., Thomson, C. A., Van Horn, L., Vitolins, M. Z., Wactawski-Wende, J., Wallace, R. B., Wassertheil-Smoller, S., Whitlock, E., Yano, K., Adams-Campbell, L., Anderson, G. L., Assaf, A. R., Beresford, S. A., Black, H. R., Brunner, R. L., Brzyski, R. G., Ford, L., Gass, M., Hays, J., Heber, D., Heiss, G., Hendrix, S. L., Hsia, J., Hubbell, F. A., Jackson, R. D., Johnson, K. C., Kotchen, J. M., LaCroix, A. Z., Lane, D. S., Langer, R. D., Lasser, N. L., and Henderson, M. M. (2006). Low-fat dietary pattern and risk of invasive breast cancer: The Women's Health Initiative Randomized Controlled Dietary Modification Trial. *JAMA.* **295**, 629–642.

Prescott, G. J., Cohen, G. R., Elton, R. A., Fowkes, F. G., and Agius, R. M. (1998). Urban air pollution and cardiopulmonary ill health: A 14.5 year time series study. *Occup Environ Med.* **55**, 697–704.

Preston, S. H. (1976). *Mortality pattterns in national populations.* New York: Academic Press.

Preston, S. H., Kayfitz, N., and Schoen, R. (1972). Causes of death, life tables for national population. In *Causes of death, life tables for national population,* pp. 1–8. New York: Seminar Press Inc.

Price, J. L., Ko, A. I., Wade, M. J., Tsou, S. K., McKeel, D. W., and Morris, J. C. (2001). Neuron number in the entorhinal cortex and CA1 in preclinical Alzheimer disease. *Arch Neurol.* **58**, 1395–1402.

Price, J. L., and Morris, J. C. (1999). Tangles and plaques in nondemented aging and "pre-clinical" Alzheimer's disease. *Ann Neurol.* **45**, 358–368.

Price, K. C., and Coe, C. L. (2000). Maternal constraint on fetal growth patterns in the rhesus monkey (*Macaca mulatta*): The intergenerational link between mothers and daughters. *Hum Repro.* **15**, 452–457.

Price, K. C., Hyde, J. S., and Coe, C. L. (1999a). Matrilineal transmission of birth weight in the rhesus monkey (*Macaca mulatta*) across several generations. *Obstet Gynecol.* **94**, 128–134.

Price, P., Witt, C., Allcock, R., Sayer, D., Garlepp, M., Kok, C. C., French, M., Mallal, S., and Christiansen, F. (1999b). The genetic basis for the association of the 8.1 ancestral haplotype (A1, B8, DR3) with multiple immunopathological diseases. *Immunological Reviews.* **167,** 257–274.

Pries, A. R., Secomb, T. W., and Gaehtgens, P. (1996). Relationship between structural and hemodynamic heterogeneity in microvascular networks. *Am J Physiol.* **270,** H545–553.

Probst-Hensch, N. M., Pike, M. C., McKean-Cowdin, R., Stanczyk, F. Z., Kolonel, L. N., and Henderson, B. E. (2000). Ethnic differences in post-menopausal plasma oestrogen levels: High oestrone levels in Japanese-American women despite low weight. *Br J Cancer.* **82,** 1867–1870.

Prolla, T. A., and Mattson, M. P. (2001). Molecular mechanisms of brain aging and neurodegenerative disorders: Lessons from dietary restriction. *Trends Neurosci.* **24 (Suppl),** S21–31.

Promislow, D. E., and Haselkorn, T. S. (2002). Age-specific metabolic rates and mortality rates in the genus *Drosophila*. *Aging Cell.* **1,** 66–74.

Proud, C. G. (2004). mTOR-mediated regulation of translation factors by amino acids. *Biochem Biophys Res Comm.* **313,** 429–436.

Prusiner, S. B., and Hsiao, K. K. (1994). Human prion diseases. *Ann Neurol.* **35,** 385–395.

Prusiner, S. B., Safar, J., Cohen, F. E., DeArmond, S. J.(1999).The prion diseases, 2nd ed Edition. Philadelphia: Lippencott Williams and Wilkins.

Puchner, M. J., Lohmann, F., Valdueza, J. M., Siepmann, G., and Freckmann, N. (1994). Monozygotic twins not identical with respect to the existence of intracranial aneurysms: A case report. *Surg Neurol.* **41,** 284–289.

Puglielli, L., Konopka, G., Pack-Chung, E., Ingano, L. A., Berezovska, O., Hyman, B. T., Chang, T. Y., Tanzi, R. E., and Kovacs, D. M. (2001). Acyl-coenzyme A: Cholesterol acyltransferase modulates the generation of the amyloid beta-peptide. *Nature Cell Biology.* **3,** 905–912.

Pujol, N., Link, E. M., Liu, L. X., Kurz, C. L., Alloing, G., Tan, M. W., Ray, K. P., Solari, R., Johnson, C. D., and Ewbank, J. J. (2001). A reverse genetic analysis of components of the Toll signaling pathway in *Caenorhabditis elegans*. *Curr Biol.* **11,** 809–821.

Qi, L., van Dam, R. M., Meigs, J. B., Manson, J. E., Hunter, D., and Hu, F. B. (2006). Genetic variation in IL6 gene and type 2 diabetes: Tagging-SNP haplotype analysis in large-scale case-control study and meta-analysis. *Hum Mol Genet.* **15,** 1914–1920.

Qiu, C., Luthy, D. A., Zhang, C., Walsh, S. W., Leisenring, W. M., and Williams, M. A. (2004). A prospective study of maternal serum C-reactive protein concentrations and risk of preeclampsia. *Am J Hypertens.* **17,** 154–160.

Qiu, C., Winblad, B., and Fratiglioni, L. (2005). The age-dependent relation of blood pressure to cognitive function and dementia. *Lancet Neurol.* **4,** 487–499.

Quintanilla, R. A., Muänoz, F. J., Metcalfe, M. J., Hitschfeld, M., Olivares, G., Godoy, J. A., and Inestrosa, N. C. (2005). Trolox and 17beta-estradiol protect against amyloid beta-peptide neurotoxicity by a mechanism that involves modulation of the Wnt signaling pathway. *J Biol Chem.* **280,** 11615–11625.

Quinton, P. M. (1994). Human genetics. What is good about cystic fibrosis? *Curr Biol.* **4,** 742–743.

Rad, R., Dossumbekova, A., Neu, B., Lang, R., Bauer, S., Saur, D., Gerhard, M., and Prinz, C. (2004). Cytokine gene polymorphisms influence mucosal cytokine expression, gastric inflammation, and host specific colonisation during *Helicobacter pylori* infection. *Gut.* **53,** 1082–1089.

Radaelli, T., Uvena-Celebrezze, J., Minium, J., Huston-Presley, L., Catalano, P., and Hauguel-de Mouzon, S. (2006). Maternal interleukin-6: Marker of fetal growth and adiposity. *J Soc Gynecol Investig.* **13,** 53–57.

Radak, Z., Chung, H. Y., Naito, H., Takahashi, R., Jung, K. J., Kim, H. J., and Goto, S. (2004). Age-associated increase in oxidative stress and nuclear factor kappaB activation are attenuated in rat liver by regular exercise. *FASEB J.* **18,** 749–750.

Radak, Z., Naito, H., Kaneko, T., Tahara, S., Nakamoto, H., Takahashi, R., Cardozo-Pelaez, F., and Goto, S. (2002a). Exercise training decreases DNA damage and increases DNA repair and resistance against oxidative stress of proteins in aged rat skeletal muscle. *Pflugers Archiv: Eur J Physiol.* **445,** 273–278.

Radak, Z., Takahashi, R., Kumiyama, A., Nakamoto, H., Ohno, H., Ookawara, T., and Goto, S. (2002b). Effect of aging and late onset dietary restriction on antioxidant enzymes and proteasome activities, and protein carbonylation of rat skeletal muscle and tendon. *Exp Gerontol.* **37,** 1423–1430.

Radak, Z., Taylor, A. W., Ohno, H., and Goto, S. (2001). Adaptation to exercise-induced oxidative stress: From muscle to brain. *Exerc Immunol Rev.* **7,** 90–107.

Radu, D. L., Weksler, M. E., and Bona, C. A. (2001). Maintenance of size and function of influenza virus hemagglutinin specific transgenic T-cell clone during life. *J Cell Mol Med.* **5,** 388–396.

Raffai, R. L., Dong, L. M., Farese, R. V., Jr., and Weisgraber, K. H. (2001). Introduction of human apolipoprotein E4 "domain interaction" into mouse apolipoprotein E. *Proc Natl Acad Sci USA.* **98,** 11587–11591.

Raisz, L. G.(2005) Pathogenesis of osteoporosis: Concepts, conflicts, and prospects. *J Clin Invest.* **115,** 3318–3325.

Rajah, M. N., and D'Esposito, M. (2005). Region-specific changes in prefrontal function with age: A review of PET and fMRI studies on working and episodic memory. *Brain.* **128,** 1964–1983.

Ramakrishnan, U. (2004). Nutrition and low birth weight: From research to practice. *Am J Clin Nutr.* **79,** 17–21.

Ramalingam, T. S., Chakrabarti, A., and Edidin, M. (1997). Interaction of class I human leukocyte antigen (HLA-I) molecules with insulin receptors and its effect on the insulin-signaling cascade. *Mol Biol Cell.* **8,** 2463–2474.

Ramana, C. V., Boldogh, I., Izumi, T., and Mitra, S. (1998). Activation of apurinic/apyrimidinic endonuclease in human cells by reactive oxygen species and its correlation with their adaptive response to genotoxicity of free radicals. *Proc Natl Acad Sci USA.* **95,** 5061–5066.

Ramasamy, R., Vannucci, S. J., Yan, S. S., Herold, K., Yan, S. F., and Schmidt, A. M. (2005). Advanced glycation end products and RAGE: A common thread in aging, diabetes, neurodegeneration, and inflammation. *Glycobiology.* **15,** 16R–28R.

Ramirez, I., and Sprott, R. L. (1978). Hunger and satiety in genetically obese mice (C57BL/6J-ob/ob). *Physiol Behav.* **20,** 257–264.

Ramos, E., Gaudier, F. L., Hearing, L. R., Del Valle, G. O., Jenkins, S., and Briones, D. (1997). Group B *Streptococcus* colonization in pregnant diabetic women. *Obstet Gynecol.* **89,** 257–260.

Ramsay, J. E., Ferrell, W. R., Crawford, L., Wallace, A. M., Greer, I. A., and Sattar, N. (2002). Maternal obesity is associated with dysregulation of metabolic, vascular, and inflammatory pathways. *J Clin Endocrinol Metab.* **87,** 4231–4237.

Ramsey, M. M., Ingram, R. L., Cashion, A. B., Ng, A. H., Cline, J. M., Parlow, A. F., and Sonntag, W. E. (2002). Growth hormone-deficient dwarf animals are resistant to dimethylbenzanthracine (DMBA)-induced mammary carcinogenesis. *Endocrinology.* **143,** 4139–4142.

Rapp, P. R. and M. Gallagher (1996). Preserved neuron number in the hippocampus of aged rats with spatial learning deficits. *Proc Natl Acad Sci USA*. **93**, 9926-9930.

Rasmussen, T., Schliemann, T., Sørensen, J. C., Zimmer, J., and West, M. J. (1996). Memory impaired aged rats: No loss of principal hippocampal and subicular neurons. *Neurobiol Aging*. **17**, 143–147.

Rathod, M., Vangipuram, S. D., Krishnan, B., Heydari, A. R., Holland, T. C., and Dhurandhar, N. V. (2007). Viral mRNA expression but not DNA replication is required for lipogenic effect of human adenovirus Ad-36 in preadipocytes. *Int J Obes*. **31**, 78–86

Rauscher, F. M., Goldschmidt-Clermont, P. J., Davis, B. H., Wang, T., Gregg, D., Ramaswami, P., Pippen, A. M., Annex, B. H., Dong, C., and Taylor, D. A. (2003). Aging, progenitor cell exhaustion, and atherosclerosis. [see comment]. *Circulation*. **108**, 457–463.

Rauser, C. L., Mueller, L. D., and Rose, M. R. (2004). Dietary restriction in *Drosophila*. *Science*. **303**, 1610–1612.

Ravelli, G. P., Stein, Z. A., and Susser, M. W. (1976). Obesity in young men after famine exposure in utero and early infancy. *New Engl J Med*. **295**, 349–353.

Raxter, M. H., Ruff, C. B., Auerbach, B. M. (2007). Technical note: Revised Fully stature estimation technique. *Am J Phys Anthropol*. http://dx.doi.org/10.1002/ajpa.20588

Ray, N., Currat, M., Berthier, P., and Excoffier, L. (2005). Recovering the geographic origin of early modern humans by realistic and spatially explicit simulations. *Genome Res*. **15**, 1161–1167.

Rayco-Solon, P., Fulford, A. J., and Prentice, A. M. (2005). Differential effects of seasonality on preterm birth and intrauterine growth restriction in rural Africans. *Am J Clin Nutr*. **81**, 134–139.

Rea, I., McKeown, P., McMaster, D., Young, I., Patterson, C., Savage, M., Belton, C., Marchegiani, F., Olivieri, F., Bonafe, M., and Franceschi, C. (2004). Paraoxonase polymorphisms PON1 192 and 55 and longevity in Italian centenarians and Irish nonagenarians. A pooled analysis. *Exp Gerontol*. **39**, 629–635.

Rea, S. L., Wu, D., Cypser, J. R., Vaupel, J. W., and Johnson, T. E. (2005). A stress-sensitive reporter predicts longevity in isogenic populations of *Caenorhabditis elegans*. *Nat Genet*. **37**, 894–898.

Read, J. S., Troendle, J. F., and Klebanoff, M. A. (1997). Infectious disease mortality among infants in the United States, 1983 through 1987. *Am J Public Health*. **87**, 192–198.

Reading, P. C., Allison, J., Crouch, E. C., and Anders, E. M. (1998). Increased susceptibility of diabetic mice to influenza virus infection: Compromise of collectin-mediated host defense of the lung by glucose? *J Virol*. **72**, 6884–6887.

Reading, P. C., Morey, L. S., Crouch, E. C., and Anders, E. M. (1997). Collectin-mediated antiviral host defense of the lung: Evidence from influenza virus infection of mice. *J Virol*. **71**, 8204–8212.

Reaven, P., Merat, S., Casanada, F., Sutphin, M., and Palinski, W. (1997). Effect of streptozotocin-induced hyperglycemia on lipid profiles, formation of advanced glycation endproducts in lesions, and extent of atherosclerosis in LDL receptor-deficient mice. *Arterioscler Thromb Vasc Biol*. **17**, 2250–2256.

Rebrin, I., Bayne, A. C., Mockett, R. J., Orr, W. C., and Sohal, R. S. (2004). Free aminothiols, glutathione redox state and protein mixed disulphides in aging *Drosophila melanogaster*. *Biochem J*. **382**, 131–136.

Rebrin, I., Kamzalov, S., and Sohal, R. S. (2003). Effects of age and caloric restriction on glutathione redox state in mice. *Free Radic Biol Med*. **35**, 626–635.

Rebrin, I., and Sohal, R. S. (2004). Comparison of thiol redox state of mitochondria and homogenates of various tissues between two strains of mice with different longevities. *Exp Gerontol.* **39,** 1513–1519.

Reddy, V. P., Obrenovich, M. E., Atwood, C. S., Perry, G., and Smith, M. A. (2002). Involvement of Maillard reactions in Alzheimer disease. *Neurotox Res.* **4,** 191–209.

Reed, B. R., Mungas, D. M., Kramer, J. H., Betz, B. P., Ellis, W., Vinters, H. V., Zarow, C., Jagust, W. J., and Chui, H. C. (2004a). Clinical and neuropsychological features in autopsy-defined vascular dementia. *Clin Neuropsychol.* **18,** 63–74.

Reed, J. R., Vukmanovic-Stejic, M., Fletcher, J. M., Soares, M. V., Cook, J. E., Orteu, C. H., Jackson, S. E., Birch, K. E., Foster, G. R., Salmon, M., Beverley, P. C., Rustin, M. H., and Akbar, A. N. (2004b). Telomere erosion in memory T cells induced by telomerase inhibition at the site of antigenic challenge *in vivo. J Exp Med.* **199,** 1433–1443.

Reed, M. J., Penn, P. E., Li, Y., Birnbaum, R., Vernon, R. B., Johnson, T. S., Pendergrass, W. R., Sage, E. H., Abrass, I. B., and Wolf, N. S. (1996). Enhanced cell proliferation and biosynthesis mediate improved wound repair in refed, caloric-restricted mice. *Mech Ageing Devel.* **89,** 21–43.

Reeves, S., Bench, C., and Howard, R. (2002). Ageing and the nigrostriatal dopaminergic system. *Int J Geriatric Psychiatry.* **17,** 359–370.

Reff, M. E., and Schneider, E. L. (1982). Biological markers of aging. *NIH Publication 82–2221. USDHHS.*

Refojo, D., Liberman, A. C., Giacomini, D., Carbia Nagashima, A., Graciarena, M., Echenique, C., Paez Pereda, M., Stalla, G., Holsboer, F., and Arzt, E. (2003). Integrating systemic information at the molecular level: Cross-talk between steroid receptors and cytokine signaling on different target cells. *Ann NY Acad Sci.* **992,** 196–204.

Refolo, L. M., Malester, B., LaFrancois, J., Bryant-Thomas, T., Wang, R., Tint, G. S., Sambamurti, K., Duff, K., and Pappolla, M. A. (2000). Hypercholesterolemia accelerates the Alzheimer's amyloid pathology in a transgenic mouse model. *Neurobiol Dis.* **7,** 321–331.

Refolo, L. M., Pappolla, M. A., LaFrancois, J., Malester, B., Schmidt, S. D., Thomas-Bryant, T., Tint, G. S., Wang, R., Mercken, M., Petanceska, S. S., and Duff, K. E. (2001). A cholesterol-lowering drug reduces beta-amyloid pathology in a transgenic mouse model of Alzheimer's disease. *Neurobiol Dis* **8,** 890–899.

Regnault, T. R. H., Marconi, A. M., Smith, C. H., Glazier, J. D., Novak, D. A., Sibley, C. P., and Jansson, T. (2005). Placental amino acid transport systems and fetal growth restriction—A workshop report. *Placenta.* **26,** S76–80.

Reik, W., Constãancia, M., Fowden, A., Anderson, N., Dean, W., Ferguson-Smith, A., Tycko, B., and Sibley, C. (2003). Regulation of supply and demand for maternal nutrients in mammals by imprinted genes. *J Physiol.* **547,** 35–44.

Reiman, E. M., Chen, K., Alexander, G. E., Caselli, R. J., Bandy, D., Osborne, D., Saunders, A. M., and Hardy, J. (2004). Functional brain abnormalities in young adults at genetic risk for late-onset Alzheimer's dementia. *Proc Natl Acad Sci USA.* **101,** 284–289.

Reiman, E. M., Chen, K., Alexander, G. E., Caselli, R. J., Bandy, D., Osborne, D., Saunders, A. M., and Hardy, J. (2005). Correlations between apolipoprotein E epsilon4 gene dose and brain-imaging measurements of regional hypometabolism. *Proc Natl Acad Sci USA.* **102,** 8299–8302.

Reines, S. A., Block, G. A., Morris, J. C., Liu, G., Nessly, M. L., Lines, C. R., Norman, B. A., and Baranak, C. C. (2004). Rofecoxib: No effect on Alzheimer's disease in a 1-year, randomized, blinded, controlled study. *Neurology.* **62,** 66–71.

Reisin, E., and Alpert, M. A. (2005). Definition of the metabolic syndrome: Current proposals and controversies. *Am J Med. Sci* **330,** 269–272.

Reixach, N., Deechongkit, S., Jiang, X., Kelly, J. W., and Buxbaum, J. N. (2004). Tissue damage in the amyloidoses: Transthyretin monomers and nonnative oligomers are the major cytotoxic species in tissue culture. *Proc Natl Acad Sci USA.* **101,** 2817–2822.

Rempel, H. C., and Pulliam, L. (2005). HIV-1 Tat inhibits neprilysin and elevates amyloid beta. *AIDS (London, England).* **19,** 127–135.

Remuzzi, G., Benigni, A., and Remuzzi, A. (2006). Mechanisms of progression and regression of renal lesions of chronic nephropathies and diabetes. *J Clin Invest.* **116,** 288–296.

Ren, C., Webster, P., Finkel, S. E., and Tower, J. (2007). Lack of effect of microbial load on *Drosophila* life span, In prep.

Renaud, S. C. (2001). Diet and stroke. *J Nutr Health Aging.* **5,** 167–172.

Renier, G., Clément, I., Desfaits, A. C., and Lambert, A. (1996). Direct stimulatory effect of insulin-like growth factor-I on monocyte and macrophage tumor necrosis factor-alpha production. *Endocrinology.* **137,** 4611–4618.

Ressler S, B. J., Niederegger H, Bartek J, Scharffetter-Kochanek K, Jansen-Durr P, Wlaschek M. (2006). p16 is a robust *in vivo* biomarker of cellular aging in human skin. *Aging Cell.* **5,** 379–389.

Reuben, D. B., Judd-Hamilton, L., Harris, T. B., and Seeman, T. E. (2003). The associations between physical activity and inflammatory markers in high-functioning older persons: MacArthur Studies of Successful Aging. *J Am Geriatr Soc.* **51,** 1125–1130.

Reusens, B., and Remacle, C. (2006). Programming of the endocrine pancreas by the early nutritional environment. *Int J Biochem Cell Biol.* **38,** 913–922.

Reynolds, K., and He, J. (2005). Epidemiology of the metabolic syndrome. *Am J Med Sci.* **330,** 273–279.

Reznick, A. Z., and Gershon, D. (1979). The effect of age on the protein degradation system in the nematode *Turbatrix aceti. Mech Ageing Dev.* **11,** 403–415.

Reznick, A. Z., Lavie, L., Gershon, H. E., and Gershon, D. (1981). Age-associated accumulation of altered FDP aldolase B in mice. Conditions of detection and determination of aldolase half life in young and old animals. *FEBS Lett.* **128,** 221–224.

Reznick, D., Bryant, M., and Holmes, D. (2006). The evolution of senescence and post-reproductive lifespan in guppies (*Poecilia reticulata*). *Plos Biology.* **4,** e7.

Reznick, D., Buckwalter, G., Groff, J., and Elder, D. (2001). The evolution of senescence in natural populations of guppies (*Poecilia reticulata*): A comparative approach. *Exp Gerontol.* **36,** 791–812.

Reznik, Y., Morello, R., Pousse, P., Mahoudeau, J., and Fradin, S. (2002). The effect of age, body mass index, and fasting triglyceride level on postprandial lipemia is dependent on apolipoprotein E polymorphism in subjects with non-insulin-dependent diabetes mellitus. *Metabolism.* **51,** 1088–1092.

Riad, M., Mogos, M., Thangathurai, D., and Lumb, P. D. (2002). Steroids. *Curr Opin Crit Care.* **8,** 281–284.

Ribelin, W. I., and McCoy, J. B. (1965). *Pathology of laboratory animals.* Springfield, IL: C.C. Thomas.

Ricci, R., Sumara, G., Sumara, I., Rozenberg, I., Kurrer, M., Akhmedov, A., Hersberger, M., Eriksson, U., Eberli, F. R., Becher, B., Borén, J., Chen, M., Cybulsky, M. I., Moore, K. J., Freeman, M. W., Wagner, E. F., Matter, C. M., and Lèuscher, T. F. (2004). Requirement of JNK2 for scavenger receptor A-mediated foam cell formation in atherogenesis. *Science.* **306,** 1558–1561.

Rich, S. M., Licht, M. C., Hudson, R. R., and Ayala, F. J. (1998). Malaria's Eve: Evidence of a recent population bottleneck throughout the world populations of *Plasmodium falciparum. Proc Natl Acad Sci USA.* **95,** 4425–4430.

Richard, D., and Rivest, S. (1989). The role of exercise in thermogenesis and energy balance. *Can J Physiol Pharm.* **67,** 402–409.

Richards, M. P., Pettitt, P. B., Trinkaus, E., Smith, F. H., Paunovic, M., and Karavanic, I. (2000). Neanderthal diet at Vindija and Neanderthal predation: The evidence from stable isotopes. *Proc Natl Acad Sci USA.* **97,** 7663–7666.

Richardson, A., Liu, F., Adamo, M. L., Remmen, H. V., and Nelson, J. F. (2004). The role of insulin and insulin-like growth factor-I in mammalian ageing. *Best Pract Res Clin Endocrinol Metab.* **18,** 393–406.

Ricklefs, R. E., Scheuerlein, A. (2002). Biological implications of the Weibull and Gompertz models of aging. *J Gerontol A Biol Sci Med Sci.* **57,** B69–76.

Ridker, P. M. (1998). Inflammation, infection, and cardiovascular risk: How good is the clinical evidence? *Circulation.* **97,** 1671–1674.

Ridker, P. M. (2002). On evolutionary biology, inflammation, infection, and the causes of atherosclerosis. *Circulation.* **105,** 2–4.

Ridker, P. M., Glynn, R. J., and Hennekens, C. H. (1998a). C-reactive protein adds to the predictive value of total and HDL cholesterol in determining risk of first myocardial infarction. *Circulation.* **97,** 2007–2011.

Ridker, P. M., Hennekens, C. H., Buring, J. E. a., and Rifai, N. (2000). C-reactive protein and other markers of inflammation in the prediction of cardiovascular disease in women. *New Engl J Med.* **342,** 836–843.

Ridker, P. M., Hennekens, C. H., Stampfer, M. J., and Wang, F. (1998b). Prospective study of herpes simplex virus, cytomegalovirus, and the risk of future myocardial infarction and stroke. *Circulation.* **98,** 2796–2799.

Ridker, P. M., Rifai, N., Rose, L., Buring, J. E., and Cook, N. R. (2002). Comparison of C-reactive protein and low-density lipoprotein cholesterol levels in the prediction of first cardiovascular events. *New Engl J Med.* **347,** 1557–1565.

Rightmire, G. P. (2004). Brain size and encephalization in early to Mid-Pleistocene *Homo. Am J Phys Anthropol.* **124,** 109–123.

Rightmire, G. P., Lordkipanidze, D., and Vekua, A. (2006). Anatomical descriptions, comparative studies and evolutionary significance of the hominin skulls from Dmanisi, Republic of Georgia. *J Hum Evol.* **50,** 115–141.

Rikke, B. A., Yerg, J. E., 3rd, Battaglia, M. E., Nagy, T. R., Allison, D. B., and Johnson, T. E. (2003). Strain variation in the response of body temperature to dietary restriction. *Mech Ageing Dev.* **124,** 663–678.

Riley, J. C. (2001). *"Rising life expectancy. A global history."* New York: Cambridge University Press, New York.

Rimoin, D. L., Merimee, T. J., and Mc Kusick, V. A. (1966). Growth-hormone deficiency in man: An isolated, recessively inherited defect. *Science.* **152,** 1635–1637.

Rinaldi, S., et al. (2006). IGF-1, IGFBP-3 and breast cancer risk in women. *Endocrine-Related Cancer.* **13,** 593–605.

Rincon, M., Muzumdar, R., Atzmon, G., and Barzilai, N. (2004). The paradox of the insulin/IGF-1 signaling pathway in longevity. *Mech Ageing Dev.* **125,** 379–403.

Ring, R. H., and Lyons, J. M. (2000). Failure to detect *Chlamydia pneumoniae* in the late-onset Alzheimer's brain. *J Clin Microbiol.* **38,** 2591–2594.

Ringheim, G. E., and Conant, K. (2004). Neurodegenerative disease and the neuroimmune axis (Alzheimer's and Parkinson's disease, and viral infections). [see comment]. *J Neuroimmunol* **147,** 43–49.

Ritz, P., Dumas, J. F., Ducluzeau, P. H., and Simard, G. (2005). Hormonal regulation of mitochondrial energy production. *Curr Opin Clin Nutrit Metabol Care.* **8,** 415–418.

Rivera, J., and Ruel, M. T. (1997). Growth retardation starts in the first three months of life among rural Guatemalan children. *Eur J Clin Nutr.* **51,** 92–96.

Rivest, D. R.. (1989). The role of exercise in thermogenesis and energy balance. *Can. J. Physiol. Pharm* **67,** 402–409.

Rivest, S., and Richard, D. (1990). Involvement of corticotropin-releasing factor in the anorexia induced by exercise. *Brain Res Bull.* **25,** 169–172.

Roach, J. (2003). Tarzan's Cheeta's life as a retired movie star. In *National Geographic News.* http://news.nationalgeographic.com/news/2003/05/0509_cheeta.html

Robbesyn, F., Salvayre, R., and Negre-Salvayre, A. (2004). Dual role of oxidized LDL on the NF-kappaB signaling pathway. *Free Radic Res.* **38,** 541–551.

Robert, L. (1996). Aging of the vascular wall and atherogenesis: Role of the elastin-laminin receptor. *Atherosclerosis.* **123,** 169–179.

Roberts, J. M., and Gammill, H. (2005). Pre-eclampsia and cardiovascular disease in later life. *Lancet.* **366,** 961–962.

Robertson, T. B., and Ray, L. A. (1920). On the growth of relatively long-lived compared with that of relatively short-lived animals. *J Biol Chem.* **42,** 71–107.

Robine, J.-M., and Caselli, G. (2005). An unprecedented increase in the number of centenarians. *Genus.* **LXI,** 57–82.

Robine, J., and Vaupel, J. W. (2001). Supercentenarians: Slower ageing individuals or senile elderly? *Exp Gerontol.* **36,** 915–930.

Robine, J. M., Caselli, G., Rasulo, D., and Cournil, A. (2006). Differentials in the femininity ratio among centenarians: Variations between northern and southern Italy from 1870. *Popul Stud (Camb).* **60,** 99–113.

Robinson, S. R., Dobson, C., and Lyons, J. (2004). Challenges and directions for the pathogen hypothesis of Alzheimer's disease. *Neurobiol Aging.* **25,** 629–637.

Robles de Medina, P. G., Visser, G. H., Huizink, A. C., Buitelaar, J. K., and Mulder, E. J. (2003). Fetal behaviour does not differ between boys and girls. *Early Hum Dev.* **73,** 17–26.

Robson, S. L., van Schaik, C. P., and Hawkes, K. (2006). The derived features of human life history. In K. Hawkes and R. R. Paine, Eds., *The evolution of human life history,* pp. 17–44. Santa Fe, NM: School for American Research Press.

Roderick, T. H., and Storer, J. H. (1961). Correlation between mean size and mean lifespan among 12 inbred strains of mice. *Science.* **134,** 48–49.

Rodriguez, E., Mateo, I., Infante, J., Llorca, J., Berciano, J., and Combarros, O. (2006). Cholesteryl ester transfer protein (CETP) polymorphism modifies the Alzheimer's disease risk associated with APOE epsilon4 allele. *J Neurol.* **253,** 181–185.

Roe, C., and Kinney, J. (1965). The caloric equivalent of fever. Influence of major trauma. *Annals of Surgery.* **161,** 140–148.

Roecker, E. B., Kemnitz, J. W., Ershler, W. B., and Weindruch, R. (1996). Reduced immune responses in rhesus monkeys subjected to dietary restriction. *J Gerontol. Series A, Biol Sci Med Sci.* **51,** B276–279.

Rogers, J., Cooper, N. R., Webster, S., Schultz, J., McGeer, P. L., Styren, S. D., Civin, W. H., Brachova, L., Bradt, B., Ward, P., et al. (1992a). Complement activation by beta-amyloid in Alzheimer disease. *Proc Natl Acad Sci USA.* **89,** 10016–10020.

Rogers, J., Kirby, L. C., Hempelman, S. R., Berry, D. L., McGeer, P. L., Kaszniak, A. W., Zalinski, J., Cofield, M., Mansukhani, L., Willson, P., et al. (1993). Clinical trial of indomethacin in Alzheimer's disease. *Neurology.* **43,** 1609–1611.

Rogers, J., and Lue, L. F. (2001). Microglial chemotaxis, activation, and phagocytosis of amyloid beta-peptide as linked phenomena in Alzheimer's disease. *Neurochem Int.* **39,** 333–340.

Rogers, J., Schultz, J., Brachova, L., Lue, L. F., Webster, S., Bradt, B., Cooper, N. R., and Moss, D. E. (1992b). Complement activation and beta-amyloid-mediated neurotoxicity in Alzheimer's disease. *Res Immunol.* **143,** 624–630.

Rogers, J. T., Randall, J. D., Cahill, C. M., Eder, P. S., Huang, X., Gunshin, H., Leiter, L., McPhee, J., Sarang, S. S., Utsuki, T., Greig, N. H., Lahiri, D. K., Tanzi, R. E., Bush, A. I., Giordano, T., and Gullans, S. R. (2002). An iron-responsive element type II in the 5'-untranslated region of the Alzheimer's amyloid precursor protein transcript. *J Biol Chem.* **277,** 45518–45528.

Roggia, C., Gao, Y., Cenci, S., Weitzmann, M. N., Toraldo, G., Isaia, G., and Pacifici, R. (2001). Up-regulation of TNF-producing T cells in the bone marrow: A key mechanism by which estrogen deficiency induces bone loss *in vivo. Proc Natl Acad Sci USA.* **98,** 13960–13965.

Rogina, B., and Helfand, S. L. (2004). Sir2 mediates longevity in the fly through a pathway related to calorie restriction. *Proc Natl Acad Sci USA.* **101,** 15998–16003.

Rolfe, D. F., Newman, J. M., Buckingham, J. A., Clark, M. G., and Brand, M. D. (1999). Contribution of mitochondrial proton leak to respiration rate in working skeletal muscle and liver and to SMR. *Am J Physiol.* **276,** C692–699.

Rollo, C. D. (2002). Growth negatively impacts the life span of mammals. *Evol Devel.* **4,** 55–61.

Rolph, M. S., Zimmer, S., Bottazzi, B., Garlanda, C., Mantovani, A., and Hansson, G. K. (2002). Production of the long pentraxin PTX3 in advanced atherosclerotic plaques. *Arterioscler Thromb Vasc Biol.* **22,** e10–14.

Roman, G. C. (2004). Facts, myths, and controversies in vascular dementia. *J Neurol Sci.* **226,** 49–52.

Roman, G. C., Erkinjuntti, T., Wallin, A., Pantoni, L., and Chui, H. C. (2002). Subcortical ischaemic vascular dementia. *Lancet Neurol.* **1,** 426–436.

Roman, G. C., Sachdev, P., Royall, D. R., Bullock, R. A., Orgogozo, J. M., Lopez-Pousa, S., Arizaga, R., and Wallin, A. (2004). Vascular cognitive disorder: A new diagnostic category updating vascular cognitive impairment and vascular dementia. *J Neurol Sci.* **226,** 81–87.

Roncarati, R., Sestan, N., Scheinfeld, M. H., Berechid, B. E., Lopez, P. A., Meucci, O., McGlade, J. C., Rakic, P., and D'Adamio, L. (2002). The gamma-secretase-generated intracellular domain of beta-amyloid precursor protein binds Numb and inhibits Notch signaling. *Proc Natl Acad Sci USA.* **99,** 7102–7107.

Ronti, T., Lupattelli, G., and Mannarino, E. (2006). The endocrine function of adipose tissue: An update. *Clin Endocrinol.* **64,** 355–365.

Rontu, R., Ojala, P., Hervonen, A., Goebeler, S., Karhunen, P. J., Nikkilèa, M., Kunnas, T., Jylhä, M., Eklund, C., Hurme, M., and Lehtimèaki, T. (2006). Apolipoprotein E genotype is related to plasma levels of C-reactive protein and lipids and to longevity in nonagenarians. *Clin Endocrinol.* **64,** 265–270.

Rooth, G. (1980). Low birthweight revised. *Lancet.* **1,** 639–641.

Rooth, G., and Ericson, A. (1980). Perinatal mortality in Sweden. *Lancet.* **1,** 371.

Rose, M. R. (1984). Laboratory evolution of postponed senescence in *Drosophila melanogaster. Genetics.* **38,** 1004–1010.

Rose, M. R. (1991). *The evolutionary biology of aging.* New York: Oxford University Press.

Rose, M.R., Passananti, H.B., Matos, M., (2004). Methuselah Flies, A Case Study in the Evolution of Aging. Singapore: World Scientific.

Roseboom, T. J., van der Meulen, J. H., Osmond, C., Barker, D. J., Ravelli, A. C., and Bleker, O. P. (2001a). Adult survival after prenatal exposure to the Dutch famine 1944–45. *Paediatr Perinat Epidemiol.* **15,** 220–225.

Roseboom, T. J., van der Meulen, J. H., Osmond, C., Barker, D. J., Ravelli, A. C., and Bleker, O. P. (2000). Plasma lipid profiles in adults after prenatal exposure to the Dutch famine. *Am J Clin Nutr.* **72,** 1101–1106.

Roseboom, T. J., van der Meulen, J. H., Osmond, C., Barker, D. J., Ravelli, A. C., Schroeder-Tanka, J. M., van Montfrans, G. A., Michels, R. P., and Bleker, O. P (2000b). Coronary heart disease after prenatal exposure to the Dutch famine, 1944–45. *Heart.* **84,** 595–598.

Roseboom, T. J., van der Meulen, J. H., Ravelli, A. C., Osmond, C., Barker, D. J., and Bleker, O. P. (2001b). Effects of prenatal exposure to the Dutch famine on adult disease in later life: An overview. *Mol Cell Endocrinol.* **185,** 93–98.

Roseboom, T. J., Van Der Meulen, J. H., Ravelli, A. C., Osmond, C., Barker, D. J., and Bleker, O. P. (2003). Perceived health of adults after prenatal exposure to the Dutch famine. *Paediatr Perinat Epidemiol.* **17,** 391–397.

Roseboom, T. J., van der Meulen, J. H., Ravelli, A. C., van Montfrans, G. A., Osmond, C., Barker, D. J., and Bleker, O. P. (1999). Blood pressure in adults after prenatal exposure to famine. *J Hypertens.* **17,** 325–330.

Roseboom, T. J., van der Meulen, J. H., van Montfrans, G. A., Ravelli, A. C., Osmond, C., Barker, D. J., and Bleker, O. P. (2001c). Maternal nutrition during gestation and blood pressure in later life. *J Hypertens.* **19,** 29–34.

Rosello-Soberon, M. E., Fuentes-Chaparro, L., and Casanueva, E. (2005). Twin pregnancies: Eating for three? Maternal nutrition update. *Nutr Rev.* **63,** 295–302.

Rosenberg, K. and Trevathan, W. (2002). Birth, obstetrics and human evolution. *Brit J Obstet Gyn .***109,** 1199–1206.

Rosenberg, K. and Trevethan, W. (1996). Bipedalism and human birth: the obstetrical dilemma revisited. *Evol Anthropol.* **4,** 61–68.

Rosenberg, K. R., Zunâe, L., Ruff, C. B. (2006). Body size, body proportions, and encephalization in a Middle Pleistocene archaic human from northern China. *Proc Natl Acad Sci USA.* **103,** 3552–3556.

Rosenbloom, A. L., Guevara-Aguirre, J., Rosenfeld, R. G., and Francke, U. (1999). Growth hormone receptor deficiency in Ecuador. *J Clin Endocrinol Metab.* **84,** 4436–4443.

Rosenzweig, E. S., and Barnes, C. A. (2003). Impact of aging on hippocampal function: Plasticity, network dynamics, and cognition. *Prog Neurobiol.* **69,** 143–179.

Roses, A. D. (2006). On the discovery of the genetic association of apolipoprotein E genotypes and common late-onset Alzheimer disease. *J Alzheimers Dis.* **9,** 361–366.

Ross, G. W., Petrovitch, H., White, L. R., Masaki, K. H., Li, C. Y., Curb, J. D., Yano, K., Rodriguez, B. L., Foley, D. J., Blanchette, P. L., and Havlik, R. (1999). Characterization of risk factors for vascular dementia: The Honolulu-Asia Aging Study. *Neurology.* **53,** 337–343.

Ross, M. H. (1959). Protein, calories and life expectancy. *Fed Proc.* **18,** 1190–1207.

Ross, R. (1995). Cell biology of atherosclerosis. *Annu Rev Physiol.* **57,** 791–804.

Ross, R. (1999). Atherosclerosis—An inflammatory disease. *New Engl J Med.* **340,** 115–126.

Rossi, G. P., Cavallin, M., Belloni, A. S., Mazzocchi, G., Nussdorfer, G. G., Pessina, A. C., and Sartore, S. (2002). Aortic smooth muscle cell phenotypic modulation and fibrillar collagen deposition in angiotensin II-dependent hypertension. *Cardiovascular Research.* **55,** 178–189.

Rost, N. S., Wolf, P. A., Kase, C. S., Kelly-Hayes, M., Silbershatz, H., Massaro, J. M., D'Agostino, R. B., Franzblau, C., and Wilson, P. W. (2001). Plasma concentration of C-reactive protein and risk of ischemic stroke and transient ischemic attack: The Framingham Study. *Stroke.* **32,** 2575–2579.

Roth, G. S., Ingram, D. K., and Joseph, J. A. (1984). Delayed loss of striatal dopamine receptors during aging of dietarily restricted rats. *Brain Res.* **300,** 27–32.

Roth, G. S., Kowatch, M. A., Hengemihle, J., Ingram, D. K., Spangler, E. L., Johnson, L. K., and Lane, M. A. (1997). Effect of age and caloric restriction on cutaneous wound closure in rats and monkeys. *J Gerontol. Series A, Biol Sci Med Sci.* **52,** B98–102.

Rothenbacher, D., Winkler, M., Gonser, T., Adler, G., and Brenner, H. (2002). Role of infected parents in transmission of *Helicobacter pylori* to their children. *Pediatr Infect Dis J.* **21,** 674–679.

Rother, K., and Till, G. O. (1988). *The complement system.* New York: Springer-Verlag.

Rottiers, V., Motola, D. L., Gerisch, B., Cummins, C. L., Nishiwaki, K., Mangelsdorf, D. J., and Antebi, A. (2006). Hormonal control of *C. elegans* dauer formation and life span by a Rieske-like oxygenase. *Dev Cell.* **10,** 473–482.

Rotwein, P. (1999). Human growth disorders: Molecular genetics of the growth hormone-insulin-like growth factor I axis. *Acta Paediatr Suppl.* **88,** 148–151.

Rous, P. (1914). The influence of diet on transplanted and spontaneous mouse tumors. *J Exp Med.* **20,** 433–451.

Routtenberg, A. (1968). "Self-starvation" of rats living in activity wheels: Adaptation effects. *J Comp Physiol Psychol.* **66,** 234–238.

Routtenberg, A., and Kuznesof, A. W. (1967). Self-starvation of rats living in activity wheels on a restricted feeding schedule. *J CompPhysiol Psychol.* **64,** 414–421.

Rowland, M. G., Cole, T. J., and Whitehead, R. G. (1977). A quantitative study into the role of infection in determining nutritional status in Gambian village children. *Br J Nutr.* **37,** 441–450.

Rozovsky, I., Hoving, S., Anderson, C. P., O'Callaghan, J., and Finch, C. E. (2002a). Equine estrogens induce apolipoprotein E and glial fibrillary acidic protein in mixed glial cultures. *Neuroscience Lett.* **323,** 191–194.

Rozovsky, I., Wei, M., Morgan, T. E., and Finch, C. E. (2005). Reversible age impairments in neurite outgrowth by manipulations of astrocytic GFAP. *Neurobiol Aging.* **26,** 705–715.

Rozovsky, I., Wei, M., Stone, D. J., Zanjani, H., Anderson, C. P., Morgan, T. E., and Finch, C. E. (2002b). Estradiol (E2) enhances neurite outgrowth by repressing glial fibrillary acidic protein expression and reorganizing laminin. *Endocrinology.* **143,** 636–646.

Rubenstein, A. H. (2005). Obesity: A modern epidemic. *Trans Am Clin Climatol Assoc.* **116,** 103–111.

Rubinstein, A., Mizrachi, Y., Bernstein, L., Shliozberg, J., Golodner, M., Liu, G. Q., and Ochs, H. D. (2000). Progressive specific immune attrition after primary, secondary and tertiary immunizations with bacteriophage phi X174 in asymptomatic HIV-1 infected patients. *AIDS.* **14,** F55–62.

Rubner, M. (1908). *Das Problem det Lebensdaur und seiner beziehunger zum Wachstum und Ernarnhung.* Munich: Oldenberg.

Ruder, A. M., Hein, M. J., Nilsen, N., Waters, M. A., Laber, P., Davis-King, K., Prince, M. M., and Whelan, E. (2006). Mortality among workers exposed to polychlorinated biphenyls (PCBs) in an electrical capacitor manufacturing plant in Indiana: An update. *Environ Health Perspect.* **114,** 18–23.

Rudman, D., Kutner, M. H., Rogers, C. M., Lubin, M. F., Fleming, G. A., and Brain, R. P. (1981). Impaired growth hormone secretion in the adult population: Relation to age and adiposity. *J Clin Invest.* **67,** 1361–1369.

Ruff, C. B. (1995). Biomechanics of the hip and birth in early Homo. *Am J Phys Anthropol.* **98,** 527–574.

Ruff, C. B., Holt, B. M., Sladek, V., Berner, M., Murphy, W. A., Jr., zur Nedden, D., Seidler, H., and Recheis, W. (2006). Body size, body proportions, and mobility in the Tyrolean "Iceman.". *J Hum Evol.* **51,** 91–101.

Ruff, C. B., Trinkaus, E., and Holliday, T. W. (1997). Body mass and encephalization in Pleistocene *Homo. Nature* **387,** 173–176.

Ruffer, M. (1911). On arterial lesions found in Egyptian mummies. *J Pathol Bacteriol.* **15,** 453–462.

Ruiz-Torres, A., Gimeno, A., Melon, J., Mendez, L., Munoz, F. J., and Macia, M. (1999). Age-related loss of proliferative activity of human vascular smooth muscle cells in culture. *Mech Ageing Dev.* **110,** 49–55.

Ruiz-Torres, A., Lozano, R., Melón, J., and Carraro, R. (2003). Age-dependent decline of *in vitro* migration (basal and stimulated by IGF-1 or insulin) of human vascular smooth muscle cells. *J Gerontol. Series A, Biol Sci Med Sci.* **58,** B1074–1077.

Ruiz-Torres, A., Lozano, R., Melon, J., and Carraro, R. (2005). On how insulin may influence ageing and become atherogenic throughout the insulin-like growth factor-1 receptor pathway: *In vitro* studies with human vascular smooth muscle cells. *Gerontology.* **51,** 225–230.

Rullan, E., and Sigal, L. H. (2001). Rheumatic fever. *Curr Rheumatol Rep.* **3,** 445–452.

Rus, H. G., Vlaicu, R., and Niculescu, F. (1996). Interleukin-6 and interleukin-8 protein and gene expression in human arterial atherosclerotic wall. *Atherosclerosis.* **127,** 263–271.

Rusche, L. N., Kirchmaier, A. L., and Rine, J. (2003). The establishment, inheritance, and function of silenced chromatin in Saccharomyces cerevisiae. *Annu Rev Biochem.* **72,** 481–516.

Russell, E. S. (1957). Study of life span and pathology tendencies of breeding mice from ten inbred strains. *Proc Am Soc Canc Res.* **2,** 245.

Russell, E. S. (1966). Lifespan and aging patterns. In E. L. Green, Ed., *The biology of the laboratory mouse,* pp. 511–520. New York: McGraw-Hill.

Russell, J. C., Epling, W. F., Pierce, D., Amy, R. M., and Boer, D. P. (1987). Induction of voluntary prolonged running by rats. *J Appl Physiol.* **63,** 2549–2553.

Russo, V. C., Gluckman, P., Feldman, E. L., and Werther, G. A. (2005). The insulin-like growth factor system and its pleiotropic functions in brain. *Endocr Rev.* **26,** 913–943.

Rylander, R., Andersson, K., Belin, L., Berglund, G., Bergstrom, R., Hanson, L., Lundholm, M., and Mattsby, I. (1977). Studies on humans exposed to airborne sewage sludge. *J Suisse Med.* **107,** 182–184.

Saarelainen, H., Laitinen, T., Raitakari, O. T., Juonala, M., Heiskanen, N., Lyyra-Laitinen, T., Viikari, J. S., Vanninen, E., and Heinonen, S. (2006). Pregnancy-related hyperlipidemia and endothelial function in healthy women. *Circ J.* **70,** 768–772.

Sabatino, F., Masoro, E. J., McMahan, C. A., and Kuhn, R. W. (1991). Assessment of the role of the glucocorticoid system in aging processes and in the action of food restriction. *J Gerontol.* **46,** B171–179.

Sabbagh, M. N., Tyas, S. L., Emery, S. C., Hansen, L. A., Alford, M. F., Reid, R. T., Tiraboschi, P., and Thal, L. J. (2005). Smoking affects the phenotype of Alzheimer disease. *Neurology.* **64,** 1301–1303.

Sacher, G. (1977). Life table modification and life prolongation. In C. E. Finch and L. Hayflick, Eds., *Handbook of the biology of aging,* pp. 582–638. New York: Van Nostrand Rheinhold.

Sack, M. N., Rader, D. J., and Cannon, R. O., 3rd. (1994). Oestrogen and inhibition of oxidation of low-density lipoproteins in postmenopausal women. *Lancet.* **343,** 269–270.

Safar, M. E. (2005). Systolic hypertension in the elderly: Arterial wall mechanical properties and the renin-angiotensin-aldosterone system. *J Hypertension.* **23,** 673–681.

Sagie, A., Larson, M. G., and Levy, D. (1993). The natural history of borderline isolated systolic hypertension. *New Engl J Med.* **329,** 1912–1917.

Sagie, A., Larson, M. G., and Levy, D. (1993b). The natural history of borderline isolated systolic hypertension. [see comment]. *New Engl J Med.* **329,** 1912–7.

Saikku, P., Leinonen, M., Mattila, K., Ekman, M. R., Nieminen, M. S., Makela, P. H., Huttunen, J. K., and Valtonen, V. (1988). Serological evidence of an association of a novel *Chlamydia,* TWAR, with chronic coronary heart disease and acute myocardial infarction. *Lancet.* **2,** 983–986.

Saito, H., Dhanasekaran, P., Baldwin, F., Weisgraber, K. H., Phillips, M. C., and Lund-Katz, S. (2003a). Effects of polymorphism on the lipid interaction of human apolipoprotein E. *J Biol Chem.* **278,** 40723–40729.

Saito, K., Nakaji, S., Umeda, T., Shimoyama, T., Sugawara, K., and Yamamoto, Y. (2003). Development of predictive equations for body density of sumo wrestlers using B-mode ultrasound for the determination of subcutaneous fat thickness. *Br J Sports Medicine.* **37,** 144–148.

Saito, M., Eto, M., Nitta, H., Kanda, Y., Shigeto, M., Nakayama, K., Tawaramoto, K., Kawasaki, F., Kamei, S., Kohara, K., Matsuda, M., Matsuki, M., and Kaku, K., (2004). Effect of apolipoprotein E4 allele on plasma LDL cholesterol response to diet therapy in type 2 diabetic patients. *Diabetes Care.* **27,** 1276–1280.

Sakaguchi, S. (2004). Naturally arising CD4+ regulatory T Cells for immunologic self-tolerance and negative control of immune responses. *Annu Rev Immunol.* **22,** 531–562.

Salas, M., John, R., Saxena, A., Barton, S., Frank, D., Fitzpatrick, G., Higgins, M. J., and Tycko, B. (2004). Placental growth retardation due to loss of imprinting of Phlda2. *Mech Dev.* **121,** 1199–1210.

Salmon, A. B., Murakami, S., Bartke, A., Kopchick, J., Yasumura, K., and Miller, R. A. (2005). Fibroblast cell lines from young adult mice of long-lived mutant strains are resistant to multiple forms of stress. *Am J Physiol Endocrinol Metab.* **289,** E23–29.

Salmon, G. K., Leslie, G., Roe, F. J., and Lee, P. N. (1990). Influence of food intake and sexual segregation on longevity, organ weights and the incidence of non-neoplastic and neoplastic diseases in rats. *Food Chem Toxicol.* **28,** 39–48.

Samaras, T. T., and Elrick, H. (1999). Height, body size and longevity. *Acta Med Okayama.* **53,** 149–169.

Samaras, T. T., Elrick, H., and Storms, L. H. (2003a). Birthweight, rapid growth, cancer, and longevity: A review. *J Natl Med Assoc.* **95**, 1170–1183.

Samaras, T. T., Elrick, H., and Storms, L. H. (2003b). Is height related to longevity? *Life Sci.* **72**, 1781–1802.

Sampath, H., and Ntambi, J. M. (2004). Polyunsaturated fatty acid regulation of gene expression. *Nutrit Rev.* **62**, 333–339.

Sampson, M. J., Davies, I. R., Brown, J. C., Ivory, K., and Hughes, D. A. (2002). Monocyte and neutrophil adhesion molecule expression during acute hyperglycemia and after antioxidant treatment in type 2 diabetes and control patients. *Arterioscler Thromb Vasc Biol.* **22**, 1187–1193.

Sanchez, D., López-Arias, B., Torroja, L., Canal, I., Wang, X., Bastiani, M. J., and Ganfornina, M. D. (2006). Loss of glial lazarillo, a homolog of apolipoprotein D, reduces lifespan and stress resistance in *Drosophila. Curr Biol.* **16**, 680–686.

Sanders, A. E., Scarborough, C., Layen, S. J., Kraaijeveld, A. R., and Godfray, H. C. (2005). Evolutionary change in parasitoid resistance under crowded conditions in *Drosophila melanogaster. Evolution Int J Org Evolution.* **59**, 1292–1299.

Sandhu, R. S., Petroni, D. H., and George, W. J. (2005). Ambient particulate matter, C-reactive protein, and coronary artery disease. *Inhal Toxicol.* **17**, 409–413.

Sandu, O., Song, K., Cai, W., Zheng, F., Uribarri, J., and Vlassara, H. (2005). Insulin resistance and type 2 diabetes in high-fat-fed mice are linked to high glycotoxin intake. *Diabetes.* **54**, 2314–2319.

Sangiorgi, G., Rumberger, J. A., Severson, A., Edwards, W. D., Gregoire, J., Fitzpatrick, L. A., and Schwartz, R. S. (1998). Arterial calcification and not lumen stenosis is highly correlated with atherosclerotic plaque burden in humans: A histologic study of 723 coronary artery segments using nondecalcifying methodology. *J Am Coll Cardiol.* **31**, 126–33.

Sanna, V., Di Giacomo, A., La Cava, A., Lechler, R. I., Fontana, S., Zappacosta, S., and Matarese, G. (2003). Leptin surge precedes onset of autoimmune encephalomyelitis and correlates with development of pathogenic T cell responses. *J Clin Invest.* **111**, 241–250.

Santini, G., Patrignani, P., Sciulli, M. G., Seta, F., Tacconelli, S., Panara, M. R., Ricciotti, E., Capone, M. L., and Patrono, C. (2001). The human pharmacology of monocyte cyclooxygenase 2 inhibition by cortisol and synthetic glucocorticoids. *Clinl Pharmacol Therap.* **70**, 475–483.

Sanz, C., Morgan, D., and Gulick, S. (2004). New insights into chimpanzees, tools, and termites from the Congo Basin. *Am Nat.* **16**, 567–581.

Sapolsky, R. M. (2005). The influence of social hierarchy on primate health. *Science.* **308**, 648–652.

Sarbassov dos, D., Ali, S. M., and Sabatini, D. M. (2005). Growing roles for the mTOR pathway. *Curr Opin Cell Biol.* **17**, 596–603.

Sarkar, D., and Fisher, P. B. (2005). Molecular mechanisms of aging-associated inflammation. *Cancer Lett.*, 1–11.

Sato, Y., Inoue, F., Yoshimura, A., Fukui, T., Imazeki, T., Kato, M., Ono, H., Yoda, S., Mitsui, M., Matsumoto, N., Furuhashi, S., Takahashi, M., and Kanmatsuse, K. (2003). Regression of an atherosclerotic coronary artery plaque demonstrated by multislice spiral computed tomography in a patient with stable angina pectoris. *Heart Vessels.* **18**, 224–226.

Sattar, N., McConnachie, A., O'Reilly, D., Upton, M. N., Greer, I. A., Davey Smith, G., and Watt, G. (2004). Inverse association between birth weight and C-reactive protein concentrations in the MIDSPAN Family Study. *Arterioscler Thromb Vasc Biol.* **24,** 583–587.

Saurwein-Teissl M., Lung, T. L., Marx, F., Gschosser, C., Asch, E., Blasko, I., Parson, W., Bock, G., Schonitzer, D., Trannoy, E., and Grubeck-Loebenstein, B. (2002). Lack of antibody production following immunization in old age: association with CD8(+) CD28(−) T cell clonal expansions and an imbalance in the production of Th1 and Th2 cytokines. *J Immunol.* **168,** 5893–5899.

Savin, J. A. (1974). Bacterial infections in diabetes mellitus. *Br J Dermatology.* **91,** 481–484.

Savino, W. (2006). The thymus is a common target organ in infectious diseases. *PLoS Pathog.* **2,** e62.

Savion, W. (2006). The thymus is a common target organ in infectious diseases. *PLoS Pathogens* **2,** e62.

Saxton, J. A., Barnes, L. L., and Sperling, G. (1946). The study of the pathogenesis of chronic pulmonary disease (bronchiectasis) of old rats. *J Gerontol.* **1,** 165–178.

Sbrana, E., Paladini, A., Bramanti, E., Spinetti, M. C., and Raspi, G. (2004). Quantitation of reduced glutathione and cysteine in human immunodeficiency virus-infected patients. *Electrophoresis.* **25,** 1522–1529.

Scarpace, P. J., Matheny, M., Moore, R. L., and Tèumer, N. (2000a). Impaired leptin responsiveness in aged rats. *Diabetes.* **49,** 431–435.

Scarpace, P. J., Matheny, M., and Shek, E. W. (2000b). Impaired leptin signal transduction with age-related obesity. *Neuropharmacology.* **39,** 1872–1879.

Schachter, F., Faure-Delanef, L., Guénot, F., Rouger, H., Froguel, P., Lesueur-Ginot, L., and Cohen, D. (1994). Genetic associations with human longevity at the APOE and ACE loci. *Nat Genet.* **6,** 29–32.

Schaedler, R. W., and Dubos, R. J. (1956). Reversible changes in the susceptibility of mice to bacterial infections. II. Changes brought about by nutritional disturbances. *J Exp Med.* **104,** 67–84.

Scharff, C., and Haesler, S. (2005). An evolutionary perspective on FoxP2: Strictly for the birds? *Curr Opin Neurobiol.* **15,** 694–703.

Schatzl, H. M., Da Costa, M., Taylor, L., Cohen, F. E., Prusiner, S. B. (1995). Prion protein gene variation among primates. *J Mol Bio.* **245,** 362–374.

Scheidegger, K. J., James, R. W., Delafontaine, P. (2000). Differential effects of low density lipoproteins on insulin-like growth factor-1 (IGF-1) and IGF-1 receptor expression in vascular smooth muscle cells. *J Biol Chem.* **275,** 26864–26869.

Schieberle, P. (2005). The carbon module labeling (CAMOLA) technique: A useful tool for identifying transient intermediates in the formation of Maillard-type target molecules. *Ann NY Acad Sci.* **1043,** 236–248.

Schmechel, D., Mace, B., Sawyer, J., Rudel, L., and Sullivan., P. (2002). High saturated fat diets are associated with Abeta deposition in primates. *8th Int Conf Alz Dis Related Disord. Abst 1202. Neurobiol Aging,* **23 (Suppl 1),** 323.

Schmidt, P. S., Duvernell, D. D., and Eanes, W. F. (2000). Adaptive evolution of a candidate gene for aging in *Drosophila. Proc Natl Acad Sci USA.* **97,** 10861–10865.

Schmidt, P. S., Matzkin, L., Ippolito, M., and Eanes, W. F. (2005). Geographic variation in diapause incidence, life-history traits, and climatic adaptation in *Drosophila melanogaster. Evolution Int J Org Evolution.* **59,** 1721–1732.

Schmidt, R., Schmidt, H., Curb, J. D., Masaki, K., White, L. R., and Launer, L. J. (2002). Early inflammation and dementia: A 25-year follow-up of the Honolulu-Asia Aging Study. *Ann Neurol.* **52,** 168–174.

Schmitt, A., Bigl, K., Meiners, I., and Schmitt, J. (2006). Induction of reactive oxygen species and cell survival in the presence of advanced glycation end products and similar structures. *Biochim Biophys Acta. Mol. Cell Res.* **1763,** 927–936.

Schneider, J. A., Wilson, R. S., Bienias, J. L., Evans, D. A., and Bennett, D. A. (2004). Cerebral infarctions and the likelihood of dementia from Alzheimer disease pathology. *Neurology.* **62,** 1148–1155.

Schneider, L. S. (2004). Estrogen and dementia: Insights from the Women's Health Initiative Memory Study. *JAMA.* **291,** 3005–3007.

Schoeb, T. R., Kervin, K. C., and Lindsey, J. R. (1985). Exacerbation of murine respiratory mycoplasmosis in gnotobiotic F344/N rats by Sendai virus infection. *Veterinary Pathology.* **22,** 272–282.

Schoenemann, P. T., Sheehan, M. J., and Glotzer, L. D. (2005). Prefrontal white matter volume is disproportionately larger in humans than in other primates. *Nat Neurosci.* **8,** 242–252.

Schonbeck, U., and Libby, P. (2004). Inflammation, immunity, and HMG-CoA reductase inhibitors: Statins as antiinflammatory agents? *Circulation.* **109(Suppl 1),** II18–26.

Schreider, J. P., Culbertson, M. R., and Raabe, O. G. (1985). Comparative pulmonary fibrogenic potential of selected particles. *Environ Res.* **38,** 256–274.

Schriner, S. E., Linford, N. J., Martin, G. M., Treuting, P., Ogburn, C. E., Emond, M., Coskun, P. E., Ladiges, W., Wolf, N., Van Remmen, H., Wallace, D. C., and Rabinovitch, P. S. (2005). Extension of murine life span by overexpression of catalase targeted to mitochondria. *Science.* **308,** 1909–1911.

Schroder, J., Kahlke, V., Staubach, K. H., Zabel, P., and Stuber, F. (1998). Gender differences in human sepsis. *Arch Surg.* **133,** 1200–1205.

Schroeder, D. G. (1995). Malnutrition. In R. D. Semboa and M. W. Bloem, Eds., *Nutrition and health in developing countries*, pp. 393–426. Totowa NJ: Human Press Inc.

Schroeder, D. G., Martorell, R., Rivera, J. A., Ruel, M. T., and Habicht, J. P. (1995). Age differences in the impact of nutritional supplementation on growth. *J Nutr.* **125 (Suppl),** 1051S–1059S.

Schultz, A. H. (1969). The Life of Primates. London: Weidenfeld and Nicholson.

Schulz, H., Harder, V., Ibald-Mulli, A., Khandoga, A., Koenig, W., Krombach, F., Radykewicz, R., Stampfl, A., Thorand, B., and Peters, A. (2005). Cardiovascular effects of fine and ultrafine particles. *J Aerosol Med.* **18,** 1–22.

Schupf, N., Pang, D., Patel, B. N., Silverman, W., Schubert, R., Lai, F., Kline, J. K., Stern, Y., Ferin, M., Tycko, B., and Mayeux, R. (2003). Onset of dementia is associated with age at menopause in women with Down's syndrome. *Ann Neurol.* **54,** 433–438.

Schwab, S. R., Pereira, J. P., Matloubian, M., Xu, Y., Huang, Y., and Cyster, J. G. (2005). Lymphocyte sequestration through S1P lyase inhibition and disruption of S1P gradients. [see comment]. *Science* **309,** 1735–1739.

Schwahn, C., Volzke, H., Robinson, D. M., Luedemann, J., Bernhardt, O., Gesch, D., John, U., and Kocher, T. (2004). Periodontal disease, but not edentulism, is independently associated with increased plasma fibrinogen levels. Results from a population-based study. *Thromb Haemost.* **92,** 244–252.

Schwartz, A. G., and Pashko, L. L. (1994). Role of adrenocortical steroids in mediating cancer-preventive and age-retarding effects of food restriction in laboratory rodents. *J Gerontol.* **49,** B37–41.

Schwartz, J. H. (2004). Barking up the wrong ape—Australopiths and the quest for chimpanzee characters in hominid fossils. *Coll Antropol.* **28(Suppl 2),** 87–101.

Schwartz, P. (1970). *Amyloidosis: Cause and manifestation of senile deterioration."* Springfield, ILL C.C. Thomas.

Schwartz, R. S., Bayes-Genis, A., Lesser, J. R., Sangiorgi, M., Henry, T. D., and Conover, C. A. (2003). Detecting vulnerable plaque using peripheral blood: Inflammatory and cellular markers. *J Intervent Cardiol.* **16,** 231–242.

Scott, L. K., Vachharajani, V., Mynatt, R. L., Minagar, A., and Conrad, S. A. (2004). Brain RNA expression in obese vs lean mice after LPS-induced systemic inflammation. *Front Biosci.* **9,** 2686–2696.

Scrimshaw, N. S. (1959). Protein malnutrition and infection. *Federation Proceedings.* **18,** 1207–1211.

Scrimshaw, N. S. (2003). Historical concepts of interactions, synergism and antagonism between nutrition and infection. *J Nutr.* **133,** 316S–321S.

Scrimshaw, N. S., and Guzman, M. (1995). A comparison of supplementary feeding and medical care of preschool children in Guatemala, 1959–1964. In N. S. Schrimshaw, Ed., *Community-based longitudinal nutrition and health studies: Classical examples from Guatemala, Haiti, and Mexico.,* pp. 1–28. Boston: International Foundation for Developing Countries (INDFC).

Scrimshaw, N. S., Salomon, J. B., Bruch, H. A., and Gordon, J. E. (1966). Studies of diarrheal disease in Central America. 8. Measles, diarrhea, and nutritional deficiency in rural Guatemala. *Am J Trop Med Hyg.* **15,** 625–631.

Scrimshaw, N. S., Taylor, A. W., and Gordon, J. E. (1968). *Interaction of nutrition and infection.* Geneva: World Health Organization.

Scrimshaw, N. S., Taylor, C. E., and Gordon, J. E. (1959). Interactions of nutrition and infection. *Am J Med Sci.* **Monograph 57,** 367–403.

Sebire, N. J., Jolly, M., Harris, J. P., Wadsworth, J., Joffe, M., Beard, R. W., Regan, L., and Robinson, S., (2001). Maternal obesity and pregnancy outcome: A study of 287, 213 pregnancies in London. *Int J Obes Relat Metab Disord.* **25,** 1175–1182.

Seckler, D. (1984). Malnutrition: An intellectual odyssey. In K. T. Achaya, Ed., *Interfaces between agriculture, nutrition, and food science,* pp. 418. Tokyo: United Nations University Press.

Seed, M., Ayres, K. L., Humphries, S. E., Miller, G. J. (2001), Lipoprotein (a) as a predictor of myocardial infarction in middle-aged men. *Am J Med.* **110,** 22–27.

Seehuus, S. C., Norberg, K., Gimsa, U., Krekling, T., and Amdam, G. V., (2006). Reproductive protein protects functionally sterile honey bee workers from oxidative stress. *Proc Natl Acad Sci USA.* **103,** 962–967.

Seeland, U., Haeuseler, C., Hinrichs, R., Rosenkranz, S., Pfitzner, T., Scharffetter-Kochanek, K., and Bèohm, M. (2002). Myocardial fibrosis in transforming growth factor-beta(1) - (TGF-beta(1)) transgenic mice is associated with inhibition of interstitial collagenase. *Eur J Clin Invest.* **32,** 295–303.

Segall, P. E., and Timiras, P. S. (1976). Patho-physiologic findings after chronic tryptophan deficiency in rats: A model for delayed growth and aging. *Mech Ageing Dev.* **5,** 109–124.

Selkoe, D. J. (2000). Toward a comprehensive theory for Alzheimer's disease. Hypothesis: Alzheimer's disease is caused by the cerebral accumulation and cytotoxicity of amyloid beta-protein. *Ann NY Acad Sci.* **924,** 17–25.

Sell, D. R., Biemel, K. M., Reihl, O., Lederer, M. O., Strauch, C. M., and Monnier, V. M. (2005). Glucosepane is a major protein cross-link of the senescent human extracellular matrix. Relationship with diabetes. *J Biol Chem*. **280**, 12310–12315.

Sell, D. R., Lane, M. A., Obrenovich, M. E., Mattison, J. A., Handy, A., Ingram, D. K., Cutler, R. G., Roth, G. S., Monnier, V. M. (2003). The effect of caloric restriction on glycation and glycoxidation in skin collagen of nonhuman primates. *J Gerontol A Biol Sci Med Sci*. **58**, 508–516.

Sell, D. R., and Monnier, V. M. (1989). Structure elucidation of a senescence cross-link from human extracellular matrix. Implication of pentoses in the aging process. *J Biol Chem*. **264**, 21597–21602.

Sell, D. R., and Monnier, V. M. (1990). End-stage renal disease and diabetes catalyze the formation of a pentose-derived crosslink from aging human collagen. *J Clin Invest*. **85**, 380–384.

Sellen, D. W. (2001). Comparison of infant feeding patterns reported for nonindustrial populations with current recommendations. *J Nutrit*. **131**, 2707–2715.

Sellen, D. W. (2006). Lactation, complementary feding, and human life history. In K. Hawkes and R. R. Paine, Eds., *The evolution of human life history*, pp. 155–197. Santa Fe, NM: School for American Research Press.

Selling, K. E., Carstensen, J., Finnströem, O., and Sydsjèo, G. (2006). Intergenerational effects of preterm birth and reduced intrauterine growth: A population-based study of Swedish mother-offspring pairs. *Bjog*. **113**, 430–440.

Selnes, O. A. (2005). Memory loss in persons with HIV/AIDS: Assessment and strategies for coping. *AIDS Read*. **15**, 289–292.

Selsby, J. T., Judge, A. R., Yimlamai, T., Leeuwenburgh, C., and Dodd, S. L. (2005). Life long calorie restriction increases heat shock proteins and proteasome activity in soleus muscles of Fisher 344 rats. *Exp Gerontol*. **40**, 37–42.

Seng, J. E., Gandy, J., Turturro, A., Lipman, R., Bronson, R. T., Parkinson, A., Johnson, W., Hart, R. W., and Leakey, J. E. (1996). Effects of caloric restriction on expression of testicular cytochrome P450 enzymes associated with the metabolic activation of carcinogens. *Arch Biochem Biophys*. **335**, 42–52.

Senger, K., Harris, K., Levine, M. (2006). GATA factors participate in tissue-specific immune responses in Drosophila larvae. *Proc Natl Acad Sci USA*. **103**, 15957–15962.

Senior, K. (2003). Aspirin withdrawal increases risk of heart problems. *Lancet*. **362**, 1558.

Sentinelli, F., Romeo, S., Barbetti, F., Berni, A., Filippi, E., Fanelli, M., Fallarino, M., and Baroni, M. G. (2006). Search for genetic variants in the p66Shc longevity gene by PCR-single strand conformational polymorphism in patients with early-onset cardiovascular disease. *BMC Genet*. **7**, 14.

Sept, J. (2007). Modeling the significance of paleoenvironmental context for early human diets. *Evolution of the human diet. The known, unknown, and the unknowable*., pp 289–309. New York: Oxford U Press.

Seroude, L., Brummel, T., Kapahi, P., and Benzer, S. (2002). Spatio-temporal analysis of gene expression during aging in *Drosophila melanogaster*. *Aging Cell*. **1**, 47–56.

Serra, V., von Zglinicki, T., Lorenz, M., and Saretzki, G. (2003). Extracellular superoxide dismutase is a major antioxidant in human fibroblasts and slows telomere shortening. *J Biol Chem*. **278**, 6824–6830.

Setse, R. W., Cutts, F., Monze, M., Ryon, J. J., Quinn, T. C., Griffin, D. E., and Moss, W. J. (2006). HIV-1 infection as a risk factor for incomplete childhood immunization in Zambia. *J Trop. Pediatr*. **5**, 324–328.

Shamsuzzaman, A. S., Winnicki, M., Wolk, R., Svatikova, A., Phillips, B. G., Davison, D. E., Berger, P. B., and Somers, V. K. (2004). Independent association between plasma leptin and C-reactive protein in healthy humans. *Circulation.* **109,** 2181–2185.

Shapiro, S. D., Endicott, S. K., Province, M. A., Pierce, J. A., and Campbell, E. J. (1991). Marked longevity of human lung parenchymal elastic fibers deduced from prevalence of D-aspartate and nuclear weapons-related radiocarbon. *J Clin Invest.* **87,** 1828–1834.

Sharapov, V. M. (1984). Influence of animal hibernation on the development of mycoses. *Mycopathologia.* **84,** 77–80.

Sharma, R. A., Gescher, A. J., and Steward, W. P. (2005). Curcumin: The story so far. *Eur J Cancer.* **41,** 1955–1968.

Sharrett, A. R., Ballantyne, C. M., Coady, S. A., Heiss, G., Sorlie, P. D., Catellier, D., Patsch, W. (2001). Coronary heart disease prediction from lipoprotein cholesterol levels, triglycerides, lipoprotein(a), apolipoproteins A-I and B, and HDL density subfractions: The Atherosclerosis Risk in Communities (ARIC) Study. *Circulation.* **104,** 1108–1113.

Shashkin, P., Dragulev, B., and Ley, K. (2005). Macrophage differentiation to foam cells. *Curr Pharmaceut Design.* **11,** 3061–3072.

Shea, J. L. (2007). Lithic archeology, or what stone tools can (and can't) tell us about early hominin diets. *Evolution of the Human Diet. The known, unknown, and the unknowable.*, pp 212–229. New York: Oxford U Press.

Sheng, J. G., Bora, S. H., Xu, G., Borchelt, D. R., Price, D. L., and Koliatsos, V. E. A. (2003). Lipopolysaccharide-induced-neuroinflammation increases intracellular accumulation of amyloid precursor protein and amyloid beta peptide in APPswe transgenic mice. *Neurobiol Dis.* **14,** 133–145.

Sheng, J. G., Price, D. L., and Koliatsos, V. E. (2002). Disruption of corticocortical connections ameliorates amyloid burden in terminal fields in a transgenic model of Abeta amyloidosis. *J Neurosci.* **22,** 9794–9799.

Sheridan, J. F., Stark, J. L., Avitsur, R., and Padgett, D. A. (2000). Social disruption, immunity, and susceptibility to viral infection. Role of glucocorticoid insensitivity and NGF. *Ann NY Acad Sci.* **917,** 894–905.

Sherwin, B. B. (2005). Estrogen and memory in women: How can we reconcile the findings? *Horm Behav.* **47,** 371–375.

Sheu, M. L., Chao, K. F., Sung, Y. J., Lin, W. W., Lin-Shiau, S. Y., and Liu, S. H. (2005). Activation of phosphoinositide 3-kinase in response to inflammation and nitric oxide leads to the up-regulation of cyclooxygenase-2 expression and subsequent cell proliferation in mesangial cells. *Cellular Signalling.* **17,** 975–984.

Shevah, O., Kornreich, L., Galatzer, A., and Laron, Z. (2005). The intellectual capacity of patients with Laron syndrome (LS) differs with various molecular defects of the growth hormone receptor gene. Correlation with CNS abnormalities. *Horm Metab Res.* **37,** 757–760.

Shie, F. S., Jin, L. W., Cook, D. G., Leverenz, J. B., and LeBoeuf, R. C. (2002). Diet-induced hypercholesterolemia enhances brain A beta accumulation in transgenic mice. *Neuroreport.* **13,** 455–459.

Shimizu, K., Mitchell, R. N., and Libby, P. (2006). Inflammation and cellular immune responses in abdominal aortic aneurysms. *Arterioscler Thromb Vasc Biol.* **26,** 987–994.

Shimoda, T., Ozawa, R., Sano, K., Yano, E., and Takabayashi, J. (2005). The involvement of volatile infochemicals from spider mites and from food-plants in prey location of the generalist predatory mite *Neoseiulus californicus. J Chem Ecol.* **31,** 2019–2032.

Shimokawa, I., Fukuyama, T., Yanagihara-Outa, K., Tomita, M., Komatsu, T., Higami, Y., Tuchiya, T., Chiba, T., and Yamaza, Y. (2003). Effects of caloric restriction on gene expression in the arcuate nucleus. *Neurobiol Aging*. **24,** 117–123.

Shimokawa, I., Higami, Y., Hubbard, G. B., McMahan, C. A., Masoro, E. J., and Yu, B. P. (1993a). Diet and the suitability of the male Fischer 344 rat as a model for aging research. *J Gerontol*. **48,** B27–32.

Shimokawa, I., Higami, Y., Utsuyama, M., Tuchiya, T., Komatsu, T., Chiba, T., and Yamaza, H. (2002). Life span extension by reduction in growth hormone-insulin-like growth factor-1 axis in a transgenic rat model. *Am J Pathol*. **160,** 2259–2265.

Shimokawa, I., Yu, B. P., Higami, Y., Ikeda, T., and Masoro, E. J. (1993b). Dietary restriction retards onset but not progression of leukemia in male F344 rats. *J Gerontol*. **48,** B68–73.

Shipman, P. (1986). Scavenging or hunting in early hominids: Theoretical framework and tests. *Am Anthropol*. **88,** 27–43.

Shire, J. G. (1973). Growth hormone and premature ageing. *Nature*. **245,** 215–216.

Shishehbor, M. H., Litaker, D., Pothier, C. E., and Lauer, M. S. (2006). Association of socioeconomic status with functional capacity, heart rate recovery, and all-cause mortality. *JAMA*. **295,** 784–792.

Shor, A. (2001). A pathologist's view of organisms and human atherosclerosis. *J Infect Dis*. **183,** 1428–1429.

Shor, A., Phillips, J. I., Ong, G., Thomas, B. J., and Taylor-Robinson, D. (1998). *Chlamydia pneumoniae* in atheroma: Consideration of criteria for causality. *J Clin Pathol*. **51,** 812–817.

Shpitz, B., Bomstein, Y., Mekori, Y., Cohen, R., Kaufman, Z., Neufeld, D., Galkin, M., and Bernheim, J. (1998). Aberrant crypt foci in human colons: Distribution and histomorphologic characteristics. *Hum Pathol*. **29,** 469–475.

Shrive, A. K., Metcalfe, A. M., Cartwright, J. R., and Greenhough, T. J. (1999). C-reactive protein and SAP-like pentraxin are both present in *Limulus polyphemus haemolymph*: Crystal structure of Limulus SAP. *J Mol Biol*. **290,** 997–1008.

Shumaker, S. A., Legault, C., Kuller, L., Rapp, S. R., Thal, L., Lane, D. S., Fillit, H., Stefanick, M. L., Hendrix, S. L., Lewis, C. E., Masaki, K., and Coker, L. H. (2004). Conjugated equine estrogens and incidence of probable dementia and mild cognitive impairment in postmenopausal women: Women's Health Initiative Memory Study. *JAMA*. **291,** 2947–2958.

Siegel, A. J., Stec, J. J., Lipinska, I., Van Cott, E. M., Lewandrowski, K. B., Ridker, P. M., and Tofler, G. H. (2001). Effect of marathon running on inflammatory and hemostatic markers. *Am J Cardiol*. **88,** 918–920, A9.

Siervo, M., Grey, P., Nyan, O. A., and Prentice, A. M. (2006). Urbanization and obesity in The Gambia: A country in the early stages of the demographic transition. *Eur J Clin Nutr*. **60,** 455–463.

Sies, H. (1999). Glutathione and its role in cellular functions. *Free Radic Biol Med*. **27,** 916–921.

Silberberg, R. (1972). Articular aging and osteoarthrosis in dwarf mice. *Pathol Microbiol*. **38,** 17–33.

Silberberg, R. (1973). Vertebral aging in hypopituitary dwarf mice. *Gerontologia*. **19,** 281–294.

Silventoinen, K., Kaprio, J., Koskenvuo, M., and Lahelma, E. (2003a). The association between body height and coronary heart disease among Finnish twins and singletons. *Int J Epidemiol*. **32,** 78–82.

Silventoinen, K., Kaprio, J., Lahelma, E., and Koskenvuo, M. (2000). Relative effect of genetic and environmental factors on body height: Differences across birth cohorts among Finnish men and women. *Am J Public Health*. **90,** 627–630.

Silventoinen, K., Sammalisto, S., Perola, M., Boomsma, D. I., Cornes, B. K., Davis, C., Dunkel, L., De Lange, M., Harris, J. R., Hjelmborg, J. V., Luciano, M., Martin, N. G., Mortensen, J., Nisticáo, L., Pedersen, N. L., Skytthe, A., Spector, T. D., Stazi, M. A., Willemsen, G., and Kaprio, J. (2003b). Heritability of adult body height: A comparative study of twin cohorts in eight countries. *Twin Res*. **6,** 399–408.

Silver, M. H., Newell, K., Brady, C., Hedley-White, E. T., and Perls, T. T. (2002). Distinguishing between neurodegenerative disease and disease-free aging: Correlating neuropsychological evaluations and neuropathological studies in centenarians. *Psychosom Mede*. **64,** 493–501.

Simerly, R. B. (2005). Wired on hormones: Endocrine regulation of hypothalamic development. *Curr Opin Neurobiol*. **15,** 81–85.

Simms, H. S., and Berg, B. N. (1957). Longevity and the onset of lesions in male rats. *J Gerontol*. **12,** 244–252.

Simms, H. S., and Berg, B. N. (1962). Longevity in relation to lesion onset. *Geriatrics*. **17,** 235–242.

Simon, A. F., Shih, C., Mack, A., and Benzer, S. (2003). Steroid control of longevity in *Drosophila melanogaster. Science*. **299,** 1407–1410.

Simoni, R. D., Hill, R. L., and Vaughan, M. (2002). The amino-acid minimum for maintenance and growth, as exemplified by further experiments with lysine and tryptophane (Osborne, T. B., and Mendel, L. B. (1916) *J Biol Chem*. 25, 1–12) and The role of vitamins in the diet (Osborne, T. B., and Mendel, L. B. (1917) *J Biol Chem*. 31, 149–163). *J Biol Chem*. **277,** E7.

Simpkins, J. W., Yang, S. H., Wen, Y., and Singh, M. (2005). Estrogens, progestins, menopause and neurodegeneration: Basic and clinical studies. *Cell Mol Life Sci*. **62,** 271–280.

Sims, E. A. (2001). Are there persons who are obese, but metabolically healthy? [erratum appears in *Metabolism* 2002 Apr; 51(4):536]. *Metab: Clin Exp*. **50,** 1499–1504.

Sims, F. H. (2000). The initiation of intimal thickening in human arteries. *Pathology*. **32,** 171–175.

Sims, F. H., Gavin, J. B., Edgar, S., and Koelmeyer, T. (2001). Diffusion of gamma globulin into the arterial wall identifies localized entry of lipid and cells in atherosclerosis. *Coronary Artery Dis*. **12,** 21–30.

Sims, F. H., Gavin, J. B., Edgar, S., and Koelmeyer, T. D. (2002). Comparison of the endothelial surface and subjacent elastic lamina of anterior descending coronary arteries at the location of atheromatous lesions with internal thoracic arteries of the same subjects: A scanning electron microscopic study. *Pathology*. **34,** 433–441.

Sinclair, D., Mills, K., and Guarente, L. (1998). Aging in *Saccharomyces cerevisiae. Annu Rev Microbiol*. **52,** 533–560.

Sinclair, D. A. (2005). Toward a unified theory of caloric restriction and longevity regulation. *Mech Ageing Dev*. **126,** 987–1002.

Sing, C. F., and Davignon, J. (1985). Role of the apolipoprotein E polymorphism in determining normal plasma lipid and lipoprotein variation. *Am J Hum Genet*. **37,** 268–285.

Singh, A. K., and Jiang, Y. (2004). How does peripheral lipopolysaccharide induce gene expression in the brain of rats? *Toxicology*. **201,** 197–207.

Singh, B. S., Westfall, T. C., and Devaskar, S. U. (1997). Maternal diabetes-induced hyper-glycemia and acute intracerebral hyperinsulinism suppress fetal brain neuropeptide Y concentrations. *Endocrinology.* **138,** 963–969.

Singh, N., and Davis, G. S. (2002). Review: Occupational and environmental lung disease. *Curr Opin Pulm Med.* **8,** 117–125.

Singh, P. P., Singh, M., Mastana, S. S.(2006). APOE distribution in world populations with new data from India and the UK. *Ann Hum Biol.* **33,** 279–308.

Singh, R. K., McMahon, A. D., Patel, H., Packard, C. J., Rathbone, B. J., and Samani, N. J. (2002). Prospective analysis of the association of infection with CagA bearing strains of *Helicobacter pylori* and coronary heart disease. *Heart.* **88,** 43–46.

Singhrao, S. K., Morgan, B. P., Neal, J. W., and Newman, G. R. (1995). A functional role for corpora amylacea based on evidence from complement studies. *Neurodegeneration.* **4,** 335–345.

Sipahi, T., Pocan, H., and Akar, N. (2006). Effect of various genetic polymorphisms on the incidence and outcome of severe sepsis. *Clin Appl Thromb Hemost.* **12,** 47–54.

Sipe, J. D. (1994). Amyloidosis. *Crit Rev Clin Lab Sci.* **31,** 325–354.

Sipe, J. D., and Cohen, A. S. (2000). Review: History of the amyloid fibril. *J Struct Biol* **130,** 88–98.

Sitte, N., Saretzki, G., and von Zglinicki, T. (1998). Accelerated telomere shortening in fibroblasts after extended periods of confluency. *Free Radic Biol Med.* **24,** 885–893.

Siwik, D. A., and Colucci, W. S. (2004). Regulation of matrix metalloproteinases by cytokines and reactive oxygen/nitrogen species in the myocardium. *Heart Fail Rev.* **9,** 43–51.

Skilton, M. R., Evans, N., Griffiths, K. A., Harmer, J. A., and Celermajer, D. S. (2005). Aortic wall thickness in newborns with intrauterine growth restriction. *Lancet.* **365,** 1484–1486.

Skinner, M. M., and Wood, B. (2006). The evolution of modern life history. A paleonto-logical perspective. In K. Hawkes and R. R. Paine, Eds., *The evolution of human life history,* pp. 331–364. Santa Fe, NM: School for American Research Press.

Skog, K. I., Johansson, M. A., and Jagerstad, M. I. (1998). Carcinogenic heterocyclic amines in model systems and cooked foods: A review on formation, occurrence and intake. *Food Chem Toxicol.* **36,** 879–896.

Skold, P. (2000). The key to success: The role of local government in the organization of smallpox vaccination in Sweden. *Med Hist.* **44,** 201–226.

Skytthe, A., Pedersen, N. L., Kaprio, J., Stazi, M. A., Hjelmborg, J. V., Iachine, I., Vaupel, J. W., and Christensen, K. (2003). Longevity studies in genomEUtwin. *Twin Res.* **6,** 448–454.

Slade, G. D., Ghezzi, E. M., Heiss, G., Beck, J. D., Riche, E., and Offenbacher, S. (2003). Relationship between periodontal disease and C-reactive protein among adults in the Atherosclerosis Risk in Communities Study. *Arch Intern Med.* **163,** 1172–1179.

Slager, C. J., Wentzel, J. J., Gijsen, F. J., Schuurbiers, J. C., van der Wal, A. C., van der Steen, A. F., and Serruys, P. W. (2005a). The role of shear stress in the generation of rupture-prone vulnerable plaques. *Nat Clin Pract Cardiovasc Med.* **2,** 401–407.

Slager, C. J., Wentzel, J. J., Gijsen, F. J., Thury, A., van der Wal, A. C., Schaar, J. A., and Serruys, P. W. (2005b). The role of shear stress in the destabilization of vulnerable plaques and related therapeutic implications. *Nat Clin Pract Cardiovasc Med.* **2,** 456–464.

Slattery, M. L., Samowitz, W., Hoffman, M., Ma, K. N., Levin, T. R., and Neuhausen, S. (2004). Aspirin, NSAIDs, and colorectal cancer: Possible involvement in an insulin-related pathway. *Canc Epidemiol Biomarkers Prevent.* **13,** 538–545.

Slauson, D. O., and Hahn, F. F. (1980). Criteria for development of animal models of diseases of the respiratory system: The comparative approach in respiratory disease model development. *Am J Pathol.* **101,** S103–122.

Slonaker, J. R. (1912). The normal activity of the albino rat from birth to natural death, its rate of growth, and duration of life. *J Anim Behavior.* **2,** 20–42.

Slots, J. (2003). Update on general health risk of periodontal disease. *Int Dent J.* **53,** 200–207.

Small, G. W., Ercoli, L. M., Silverman, D. H., Huang, S. C., Komo, S., Bookheimer, S. Y., Lavretsky, H., Miller, K., Siddarth, P., Rasgon, N. L., Mazziotta, J. C., Saxena, S., Wu, H. M., Mega, M. S., Cummings, J. L., Saunders, A. M., Pericak-Vance, M. A., Roses, A. D., Barrio, J. R., and Phelps, M. E. (2000). Cerebral metabolic and cognitive decline in persons at genetic risk for Alzheimer's disease. *Proc Natl Acad Sci USA.* **97,** 6037–6042.

Smith, D. E., Roberts, J., Gage, F. H., and Tuszynski, M. H. (1999). Age-associated neuronal atrophy occurs in the primate brain and is reversible by growth factor gene therapy. *Proc Natl Acad Sci USA.* **96,** 10893–10898.

Smith, F. M., Garfield, A. S., and Ward, A. (2006). Regulation of growth and metabolism by imprinted genes. *Cytogenet Genome Res.* **113,** 279–291.

Smith, G. D. (2002). The conundrum of height and mortality. *West J Med.* **176,** 209.

Smith, J. M., and Dubos, R. J. (1956). The effect of nutritional disturbances on the susceptibility of mice to staphylococcal infections. *J Exp Med.* **103,** 109–118.

Smith, J. R., Venable, S., Roberts, T. W., Metter, E. J., Monticone, R., Schneider, E. L., and Roy, M. (2002). Relationship between *in vivo* age and *in vitro* aging: Assessment of 669 cell cultures derived from members of the Baltimore Longitudinal Study of Aging. *J Gerontol. Series A, Biol Sci Med Sci.* **57,** B239–246.

Smith, M. A., Taneda, S., Richey, P. L., Miyata, S., Yan, S. D., Stern, D., Sayre, L. M., Monnier, V. M., and Perry, G. (1994). Advanced Maillard reaction end products are associated with Alzheimer disease pathology. *Proc Natl Acad Sci USA.* **91,** 5710–5714.

Smith, N. L., Psaty, B. M., Heckbert, S. R., Tracy, R. P., and Cornell, E. S. (1999). The reliability of medication inventory methods compared to serum levels of cardiovascular drugs in the elderly. *J Clin Epidemiol.* **52,** 143–146.

Snell, G. D. (1929). Dwarf, a new mendelian recessive character of the house mouse. *Proc Natl Acad Sci USA.* **15,** 733–734.

Sobel, E., Louhija, J., Sulkava, R., Davanipour, Z., Kontula, K., Miettinen, H., Tikkanen, M., Kainulainen, K., and Tilvis, R. (1995). Lack of association of apolipoprotein E allele epsilon 4 with late-onset Alzheimer's disease among Finnish centenarians. *Neurology.* **45,** 903–907.

Soffer, O., Adovasio, J. M., Hyland, D. C., Gvozdover, M. D., Habu, J., Kozlowski, J. K., McDermott, L., Mussi, M., Owen, L. R., Svoboda, J., and Zilhão, J. (2000). The 'Venus' figurines. *Curr Anthropol.* **41,** 511–537.

Sohal, R. S. (1981). Relationship between metabolic rate, lipofuscin accumulation and lysosomal enzyme activity during aging in the adult housefly *Musca domestica. Exp Gerontol.* **16,** 347–355.

Sohal, R. S., and Allison, V. F. (1971a). Age-related changes in the fine structure of the flight muscle in the house fly. *Exp Gero.* **6,** 167–172.

Sohal, R. S., and Allison, V. F. (1971b). Senescent changes in the cardiac myofiber of the house fly, *Musca domestica.* An electron microscopic study. *J Gerontol.* **26,** 167–172.

Sohal, R. S., McCarthy, J. L., and Allison, V. F. (1972). The formation of 'giant' mitochondria in the fibrillar flight muscles of the house fly, *Musca domestica L. J Ultrastruct Res.* **39,** 484–495.

Sohal, R. S., Peters, T. A., and Hall, T. A. (1977). Origin, structure, composition and age-dependence of mineralized dense bodies (concretins) in the midgut epithelium of the adult housefly *Musca domestica. Tissue & Cell.* **9,** 87–102.

Sohal, R. S., and Weindruch, R. (1996). Oxidative stress, caloric restriction, and aging. *Science.* **273,** 59–63.

Solter, D. (1988). Imprinting *Int J Dev Biol.* **42,** 951–954.

Song, W., Ranjan, R., Dawson-Scully, K., Bronk, P., Marin, L., Seroude, L., Lin, Y. J., Nie, Z., Atwood, H. L., Benzer, S., and Zinsmaier, K. E. (2002). Presynaptic regulation of neurotransmission in *Drosophila* by the g protein-coupled receptor Methuselah. *Neuron.* **36,** 105–119.

Song, Y., Stampfer, M. J., and Liu, S. (2004). Meta-analysis: Apolipoprotein E genotypes and risk for coronary heart disease. *Ann Intern Med.* **141,** 137–147.

Sonntag, W. E. (2005). Adult-onset growth hormone and IGF-1 deficiency modulates age-relalted pathology and increases life span. *Endocrinology* **146,** 2920–2932.

Sonntag, W. E., Carter, C. S., Ikeno, Y., Ekenstedt, K., Carlson, C. S., Loeser, R. F., Chakrabarty, S., Lee, S., Bennett, C., Ingram, R., Moore, T., and Ramsey, M. (2005). Adult-onset growth hormone and insulin-like growth factor I deficiency reduces neoplastic disease, modifies age-related pathology, and increases life span. *Endocrinology.* **146,** 2920–2932.

Sonntag, W. E., Lynch, C., Thornton, P., Khan, A., Bennett, S., and Ingram, R. (2000). The effects of growth hormone and IGF-1 deficiency on cerebrovascular and brain ageing. *J Anat.* **197,** 575–585.

Sonntag, W. E., Lynch, C. D., Cooney, P. T., and Hutchins, P. M. (1997). Decreases in cerebral microvasculature with age are associated with the decline in growth hormone and insulin-like growth factor 1. *Endocrinology.* **138,** 3515–3520.

Sonntag, W. E., Ramsey, M., and Carter, C. S. (2005b). Growth hormone and insulin-like growth factor-1 (IGF-1) and their influence on cognitive aging. *Ageing Res Rev.* **4,** 195–212.

Sotiriou, S. N., Orlova, V. V., Al-Fakhri, N., Ihanus, E., Economopoulou, M., Isermann, B., Bdeir, K., Nawroth, P. P., Preissner, K. T., Gahmberg, C. G., Koschinsky, M. L., and Chavakis, T. (2006). Lipoprotein(a) in atherosclerotic plaques recruits inflammatory cells through interaction with Mac-1 integrin. *FASEB J.* **20,** 559–561.

Soucy, G., Boivin, G., Labrie, F., and Rivest, S. (2005). Estradiol is required for a proper immune response to bacterial and viral pathogens in the female brain. *J Immunol.* **174,** 6391–6398.

Souza, S. C., Palmer, H. J., Kang, Y. H., Yamamoto, M. T., Muliro, K. V., Paulson, K. E., and Greenberg, A. S. (2003). TNF-alpha induction of lipolysis is mediated through activation of the extracellular signal related kinase pathway in 3T3–L1 adipocytes. *J Cell Biochem.* **89,** 1077–1086.

Sowell, E. R., Thompson, P. M., Tessner, K. D., Toga, A. W. (2001). Mapping continued brain growth and gray matter density reduction in dorsal frontal cortex: Inverse relationships during postadolescent brain maturation. *J Neuro.* **21,** 8819–8829.

Sparen, P., Vagero, D., Shestov, D. B., Plavinskaja, S., Parfenova, N., Hoptiar, V., Paturot, D., and Galanti, M. R. (2004). Long term mortality after severe starvation during the siege of Leningrad: Prospective cohort study. *Br Med J.* **328,** 11.

Sparks, D. L. (1996). Intraneuronal beta-amyloid immunoreactivity in the CNS. *Neurobiol Aging.* **17,** 291–299.

Sparks, D. L., Connor, D. J., Sabbagh, M. N., Petersen, R. B., Lopez, J., and Browne, P. (2006a). Circulating cholesterol levels, apolipoprotein E genotype and dementia severity influence the benefit of atorvastatin treatment in Alzheimer's disease: Results of the Alzheimer's Disease Cholesterol-Lowering Treatment (ADCLT) trial. *Acta Neurol Scand Suppl.* **185,** 3–7.

Sparks, D. L., Friedland, R., Petanceska, S., Schreurs, B. G., Shi, J., Perry, G., Smith, M. A., Sharma, A., Derosa, S., Ziolkowski, C., and Stankovic, G. (2006b). Trace copper levels in the drinking water, but not zinc or aluminum influence CNS Alzheimer-like pathology. *J Nutr Health Aging.* **10,** 247–254.

Sparmann, A., and Bar-Sagi, D. (2004). Ras-induced interleukin-8 expression plays a critical role in tumor growth and angiogenesis. *Cancer Cell.* **6,** 447–458.

Spaulding, C. C., Walford, R. L., and Effros, R. B. (1997). The accumulation of non-replicative, non-functional, senescent T cells with age is avoided in calorically restricted mice by an enhancement of T cell apoptosis. *Mech Ageing Dev.* **93,** 25–33.

Speakman, J. R. (2005). Body size, energy metabolism and lifespan. *J Exp Biol.* **208,** 1717–1730.

Speakman, J. R., and Krol, E. (2005). Limits to sustained energy intake IX: A review of hypotheses. *J Comp Physiol [B].* **175,** 375–394.

Speidl, W. S., Exner, M., Amighi, J., Kastl, S. P., Zorn, G., Maurer, G., Wagner, O., Huber, K., Minar, E., Wojta, J., and Schillinger, M. (2005). Complement component C5a predicts future cardiovascular events in patients with advanced atherosclerosis. *Eur Heart J.* **26,** 2294–2299.

Speir, E., Yu, Z. X., Takeda, K., Ferrans, V. J., and Cannon, R. O., 3rd. (2000). Antioxidant effect of estrogen on cytomegalovirus-induced gene expression in coronary artery smooth muscle cells. *Circulation.* **102,** 2990–2996.

Spencer, C. C., Howell, C. E., Wright, A. R., and Promislow, D. E. (2003). Testing an 'aging gene' in long-lived *Drosophila* strains: Increased longevity depends on sex and genetic background. *Aging Cell.* **2,** 123–130.

Spindler, S. R., Crew, M. D., Mote, P. L., Grizzle, J. M., and Walford, R. L. (1990). Dietary energy restriction in mice reduces hepatic expression of glucose-regulated protein 78 (BiP) and 94 mRNA. *J Nutr.* **120,** 1412–1417.

Spinetti, G., Wang, M., Monticone, R., Zhang, J., Zhao, D., and Lakatta, E. G. (2004). Rat aortic MCP-1 and its receptor CCR2 increase with age and alter vascular smooth muscle cell function. *Arterioscler Thromb Vasc Biol.* **24,** 1397–402.

Spirduso, W. W., and Clifford, P. (1978). Replication of age and physical activity effects on reaction and movement time. *J Gerontol.* **33,** 26–30.

Spires, T. L., Meyer-Luehmann, M., Stern, E. A., McLean, P. J., Skoch, J., Nguyen, P. T., Bacskai, B. J., and Hyman, B. T. (2005). Dendritic spine abnormalities in amyloid precursor protein transgenic mice demonstrated by gene transfer and intravital multiphoton microscopy. *J Neurosci.* **25,** 7278–7287.

Sponheimer, M., and Lee-Thorp, J. A. (1999). Isotopic evidence for the diet of an early hominid, *Australopithecus africanus. Science.* **283,** 368–370.

Sponheimer, M., Lee-Thorp, J. A., De Ruiter, D. (2007). Icarus, isotopes, and autralopith diets. *The Evolution of Human Life.* pp. 132–149. Sante Fe: School for American Research Press.

Sponheimer, M., Reed, K. E., and Lee-Thorp, J. A. (1999). Combining isotopic and ecomorphological data to refine bovid paleodietary reconstruction: A case study from the Makapansgat Limeworks hominin locality. *J Hum Evol.* **36,** 705–718.

Sprott, R. L., and Eleftheriou, B. E. (1974). Open-field behavior in aging inbred mice. *Gerontologia.* **20,** 155–162.

Spyridopoulos, I., Haendeler, J., Urbich, C., Brummendorf, T. H., Oh, H., Schneider, M. D., Zeiher, A. M., and Dimmeler, S. (2004). Statins enhance migratory capacity by upregulation of the telomere repeat-binding factor TRF2 in endothelial progenitor cells. *Circulation.* **110,** 3136–3142.

Srinivasan, S. R., Radhakrishnamurthy, B., Smith, C. C., Wolf, R. H., Berenson, G. S. (1976b). Serum lipid and lipoprotein responses of six nonhuman primate species to dietary changes in cholesterol levels. *J Nut.* **106,** 1757–1767.

Srinivasan, S. R., Smith, C. C., Radhakrishnamurthy, B., Wolf, R. H., Berenson, G. S. (1976a). Phylogenetic variability of serum lipids and lipoproteins in non-human primates fed diets with different contents of dietary cholesterol. *Adv Exp Med Biol.* **67,** 65–75.

Staats, J. (1985). Standardized nomenclature for inbred strains of mice: Eighth listing. *Cancer Res.* **45,** 954–977.

Stadler, N., Lindner, R. A., and Davies, M. J. (2004). Direct detection and quantification of transition metal ions in human atherosclerotic plaques: Evidence for the presence of elevated levels of iron and copper. *Arterioscler Thromb Vasc Biol.* **24,** 949–954.

Stadtman, E. R., and Levine, R. L. (2003). Free radical-mediated oxidation of free amino acids and amino acid residues in proteins. *Amino Acids.* **25,** 207–218.

Stalder, M., Deller, T., Staufenbiel, M., and Jucker, M. (2001). 3D-reconstruction of microglia and amyloid in APP23 transgenic mice: No evidence of intracellular amyloid. *Neurobiol Aging.* **22,** 427–434.

Stampfer, M., Colditz, G., and Willett, W. (1990). Menopause and heart disease: A review. *Ann NY Acad Sci.* **592,** 193–203.

Stanford, C. B. (1998). *Chimpanzee and red colobus.* Cambridge MA: Harvard University Press.

Stanford, C. B. (1999). *The hunting apes."* Princeton: Princeton University Press.

Stanford, C. B. (2006). Arboreal bipedalism in wild chimpanzees: Implications for the evolution of hominid posture and locomotion. *Am J Phys Anthropol.* **129,** 225–231.

Stanner, S. A., Bulmer, K., Andráes, C., Lantseva, O. E., Borodina, V., Poteen, V. V., and Yudkin, J. S. (1997). Does malnutrition in utero determine diabetes and coronary heart disease in adulthood? Results from the Leningrad Siege Study, a cross sectional study. *Br Med J.* **315,** 1342–1348.

Stanner, S. A., and Yudkin, J. S. (2001). Fetal programming and the Leningrad Siege Study. *Twin Res.* **4,** 287–292.

Starkie, R., Ostrowski, S. R., Jauffred, S., Febbraio, M., and Pedersen, B. K. (2003). Exercise and IL-6 infusion inhibit endotoxin-induced TNF-alpha production in humans. *FASEB J.* **17,** 884–886.

Stary, H. C. (2000). Lipid and macrophage accumulations in arteries of children and the development of atherosclerosis. *Am J Clin Nutr.* **72,** 1297S–1306S.

Stary, H. C. (2000b). Natural history and histological classification of atherosclerotic lesions: An update. *Arterioscler Thromb Vasc Biol.* **20,** 1177–1178.

Stary, H. C., Chandler, A. B., Glagov, S., Guyton, J. R., Insull, W., Jr., Rosenfeld, M. E., Schaffer, S. A., Schwartz, C. J., Wagner, W. D., and Wissler, R. W. (1994). A definition of initial, fatty streak, and intermediate lesions of atherosclerosis. A report from the Committee on Vascular Lesions of the Council on Arteriosclerosis, American Heart Association. *Circulation.* **89,** 2462–2478.

Stassen, F. R., Vega-Córdova, X., Vliegen, I., and Bruggeman, C. A. (2006). Immune activation following cytomegalovirus infection: More important than direct viral effects in cardiovascular disease? *J Clin Virol.* **35,** 349–353.

Stearns, S. C., and Koella, J. C. (1986). The evolution of phenotypic plasticity in life-history traits: Predictions of reaction norms for age and size at maturity. *Evolution.* **40,** 893–913.

Steen, E., Terry, B. M., Rivera, E. J., Cannon, J. L., Neely, T. R., Tavares, R., Xu, X. J., Wands, J. R., and de la Monte, S. M. (2005). Impaired insulin and insulin-like growth factor expression and signaling mechanisms in Alzheimer's disease—Is this type 3 diabetes? *J Alzheimers Dis.* **7,** 63–80.

Steenland, K., Hein, M. J., Cassinelli, R. T., 2nd, Prince, M. M., Nilsen, N. B., Whelan, E. A., Waters, M. A., Ruder, A. M., and Schnorr, T. M. (2006). Polychlorinated biphenyls and neurodegenerative disease mortality in an occupational cohort. *Epidemiology.* **17,** 8–13.

Steger, R. W., Bartke, A., and Cecim, M. (1993). Premature ageing in transgenic mice expressing different growth hormone genes. *J Reprod Fertil.* **46(Suppl),** 61–75.

Stein, A. D., Ravelli, A. C., and Lumey, L. H. (1995). Famine, third-trimester pregnancy weight gain, and intrauterine growth: The Dutch Famine Birth Cohort Study. *Hum Biol.* **67,** 135–150.

Stein, A. D., Zybert, P. A., and Lumey, L. H. (2004a). Acute undernutrition is not associated with excess of females at birth in humans: The Dutch hunger winter. *Proc Biol Sci.* **271 (Suppl 4),** S138–141.

Stein, A. D., Zybert, P. A., van de Bor, M., and Lumey, L. H. (2004b). Intrauterine famine exposure and body proportions at birth: the Dutch Hunger Winter. [see comment]. *Int J Epidemiol.* **33,** 831–836.

Stein, C. E., Fall, C. H., Kumaran, K., Osmond, C., Cox, V., and Barker, D. J. (1996). Fetal growth and coronary heart disease in south India. *Lancet.* **348,** 1269–1273.

Stein, Z., and Susser, M. (1975a). The Dutch famine, 1944–1945, and the reproductive process. I. Effects or six indices at birth. *Pediatr Res.* **9,** 70–76.

Stein, Z., and Susser, M. (1975b). The Dutch famine, 1944–1945, and the reproductive process. II. Interrelations of caloric rations and six indices at birth. *Pediatr Res.* **9,** 76–83.

Stein, Z., and Susser, M. (1975c). Fertility, fecundity, famine: Food rations in the Dutch famine 1944/5 have a causal relation to fertility, and probably to fecundity. *Hum Biol.* **47,** 131–154.

Stein, Z., Susser, M., Saenger, G., and Marolla, F. (1975). *Famine and human development: The Dutch hunger winter of 1944–1944.* New York: Oxford.

Steiner, M. S., Couch, R. C., Raghow, S., and Stauffer, D. (1999). The chimpanzee as a model of human benign prostatic hyperplasia. *J Urology.* **162,** 1454–1461.

Steiner, S., Schaller, G., Puttinger, H., Fodinger, M., Kopp, C. W., Seidinger, D., Grisar, J., Horl, W. H., Minar, E., Vychytil, A., Wolzt, M., and Sunder-Plassmann, G. (2005). History of cardiovascular disease is associated with endothelial progenitor cells in peritoneal dialysis patients. *Am J Kidney Diseases.* **46,** 520–528.

Steinetz, B. G., Randolph, C., Cohn, D., and Mahoney, C. J. (1996). Lipoprotein profiles and glucose tolerance in lean and obese chimpanzees. *J Med Primatol.* **25,** 17–25.

Steinman, L., Conlon, P., Maki, R., and Foster, A. (2003). The intricate interplay among body weight, stress, and the immune response to friend or foe. *J Clin Invest.* **111,** 183–185.

Steinmann, G. G. (1986). Changes in the human thymus during aging. *Curr Topics Pathol.* **75,** 43–48.

Steiper, M. E. and Young, N. M. (2006). Primate molecular divergence dates. *Mol Phylogenet Evol.* **41**, 384–394.

Stengard, J. H., Kardia, S. L., Hamon, S. C., Frikke-Schmidt, R., Tybjaerg-Hansen, A., Salomaa, V., Boerwinkle, E., and Sing, C. F. (2006). Contribution of regulatory and structural variations in APOE to predicting dyslipidemia. *J Lipid Res.* **47**, 318–328.

Stengard, J. H., Weiss, K. M., Sing, C. F. (1998). An ecological study of association between coronary heart disease mortality rates in men and the relative frequencies of common allelic variations in the gene coding for apolipoprotein E. *Hum Genet.* **103**, 234–241.

Stollerman, G. H. (1997). Rheumatic fever. *Lancet.* **349**, 935–942.

Storer, J. H. (1966). Longevity and gross pathology at death in 22 inbred mouse strains. *J Gerontol.* **21**, 537–547.

Storer, J. H. (1971). Chemical protection of the mouse against radiation-induced life shortening. *Rad Res.* **47**, 537–547.

Stout, R. D., and Suttles, J. (2005). Immunosenescence and macrophage functional plasticity: Dysregulation of macrophage function by age-associated microenvironmental changes. *Immunol Rev.* **205**, 60–71.

Strachan, D. P. (1989). Hay fever, hygiene, and household size. *Br Med J.* **299**, 1259–1260.

Stratton, C. W., and Sriram, S. (2003). Association of *Chlamydia pneumoniae* with central nervous system disease. *Microbes Infect.* **5**, 1249–1253.

Strauss, H. W., Dunphy, M., and Tokita, N. (2004). Imaging the vulnerable plaque: A scintillating light at the end of the tunnel? *J Nucl Med.* **45**, 1106–1107.

Strehler, B. L. (1977). *Time, cells, and aging.* New York: Academic Press.

Strehlow, K., Werner, N., Berweiler, J., Link, A., Dirnagl, U., Priller, J., Laufs, K., Ghaeni, L., Milosevic, M., Bèohm, M., and Nickenig, G. (2003). Estrogen increases bone marrow-derived endothelial progenitor cell production and diminishes neointima formation. *Circulation.* **107**, 3059–3065.

Strom, A., and Jensen, R. A. (1951). Mortality from circulatory diseases in Norway 1940–1945. *Lancet.* **1**, 126–129.

Strong, J. P., Malcom, G. T., McMahan, C. A., Tracy, R. E., Newman, W. P., 3rd, Herderick, E. E., and Cornhill, J. F. (1999). Prevalence and extent of atherosclerosis in adolescents and young adults: Implications for prevention from the Pathobiological Determinants of Atherosclerosis in Youth Study. *JAMA.* **281**, 727–735.

Stuart, J. A., Bourque, B. M., de Souza-Pinto, N. C., and Bohr, V. A. (2005). No evidence of mitochondrial respiratory dysfunction in OGG1-null mice deficient in removal of 8-oxodeoxyguanine from mitochondrial DNA. *Free Radic Biol Med.* **38**, 737–745.

Stuart, J. A., and Brown, M. F. (2005). Energy, quiescence, and the cellular basis of animal life spans. *Comp Biochem Physiol A.* **143**, 12–23.

Stuesse, S. L., Cruce, W. L., Lovell, J. A., McBurney, D. L., and Crisp, T. (2000). Microglial proliferation in the spinal cord of aged rats with a sciatic nerve injury. *Neuroscience Lett.* **287**, 121–124.

Stuve, O., Youssef, S., Steinman, L., Zamvil, S. S. (2003). Statins as potential therapeutic agents in neuroinflammatory disorders. *Curr Opin Neurol.* **16**, 393–401.

Sugishita, K., Li, F., Su, Z., and Barry, W. H. (2003). Anti-oxidant effects of estrogen reduce [Ca2+]i during metabolic inhibition. *J Mol Cell Cardiol.* **35**, 331–336.

Sugiyama, T., and Asaka, M. (2004). *Helicobacter pylori* infection and gastric cancer. *Medical Electron Microscopy.* **37**, 149–157.

Suh, W., Kim, K. L., Choi, J. H., Lee, Y. S., Lee, J. Y., Kim, J. M., Jang, H. S., Shin, I. S., Lee, J. S., Byun, J., Jeon, E. S., and Kim, D. K. (2004). C-reactive protein impairs angiogenic functions and decreases the secretion of arteriogenic chemo-cytokines in human endothelial progenitor cells. *Biochem Biophys Res Comm.* **321,** 65–71.

Suh, Y., Vijg, J. (2006). Maintaining genetic integrity in aging: a zero sum game. *Antioxid Redox Signal.* **8,** 559–571.

Suhara, T., Okubo, Y., Yasuno, F., Sudo, Y., Inoue, M., Ichimiya, T., Nakashima, Y., Nakayama, K., Tanada, S., Suzuki, K., Halldin, C., and Farde, L. (2002). Decreased dopamine D2 receptor binding in the anterior cingulate cortex in schizophrenia. *Arch Gen Psychiatry* **59,** 25–30.

Sukupolvi, S., Lorenz, R. G., Gordon, J. I., Bian, Z., Pfeifer, J. D., Normark, S. J., and Rhen, M. (1997). Expression of thin aggregative fimbriae promotes interaction of *Salmonella typhimurium* SR-11 with mouse small intestinal epithelial cells. *Infect Immunity.* **65,** 5320–5325.

Sullivan, D. H., Morley, J. E., Johnson, L. E., Barber, A., Olson, J. S., Stevens, M. R., Yamashita, B. D., Reinhart, S. P., Trotter, J. P., and Olave, X. E. (2002). The GAIN (Geriatric Anorexia Nutrition) registry: The impact of appetite and weight on mortality in a long-term care population. *J Nutr Health Aging.* **6,** 275–281.

Sun, D., Muthukumar, A. R., Lawrence, R. A., and Fernandes, G. (2001). Effects of calorie restriction on polymicrobial peritonitis induced by cecum ligation and puncture in young C57BL/6 mice. *Clin Diagn Lab Immunol.* **8,** 1003–1011.

Sun, L. Y., Al-Regaiey, K., Masternak, M. M., Wang, J., and Bartke, A. (2005a). Local expression of GH and IGF-1 in the hippocampus of GH-deficient long-lived mice. *Neurobiol Aging.* **26,** 929–937.

Sun, L. Y., Evans, M. S., Hsieh, J., Panici, J., and Bartke, A. (2005b). Increased neurogenesis in dentate gyrus of long-lived Ames dwarf mice. *Endocrinology.* **146,** 1138–1144.

Sun, P., Dwyer, K. M., Merz, C. N., Sun, W., Johnson, C. A., Shircore, A. M., and Dwyer, J. H. (2000). Blood pressure, LDL cholesterol, and intima-media thickness: A test of the "response to injury" hypothesis of atherosclerosis. *Arterioscler Thromb Vasc Biol.* **20,** 2005–2010.

Sun, Y., and Weber, K. T. (2005). Animal models of cardiac fibrosis. In J. Varga, D. A. Brenner, and S. H. Phan, Eds., *Methods in molecular medicine. Fibrosis Research: methods and protocols*, Vol. 117, pp. 273–290. Totowa, NJ: Humana Press.

Sunder, M. (2005). Toward generation XL: Anthropometrics of longevity in late 20th-century United States. *Econ Hum Biol.* **3,** 271–295.

Susser, M. (1991). Maternal weight gain, infant birth weight, and diet: causal sequences. *Am J Clin Nutr.* **53,** 1384–1396.

Suthers, K., Kim, J. K., and Crimmins, E. (2003). Life expectancy with cognitive impairment in the older population of the United States. *J Gerontol. B Psychol Sci Soc Sci.* **58,** S179–186.

Suttie, A. W., Dinse, G. E., Nyska, A., Moser, G. J., Goldsworthy, T. L., and Maronpot, R. R. (2005). An investigation of the effects of late-onset dietary restriction on prostate cancer development in the TRAMP mouse. *Toxicol Pathol.* **33,** 386–397.

Suwa, T., Hogg, J. C., Quinlan, K. B., Ohgami, A., Vincent, R., and van Eeden, S. F. (2002). Particulate air pollution induces progression of atherosclerosis. *J Am Coll Cardiol.* **39,** 935–942.

Suzuki, H., Kurihara, Y., Takeya, M., Kamada, N., Kataoka, M., Jishage, K., Ueda, O., Sakaguchi, H., Higashi, T., Suzuki, T., Takashima, Y., Kawabe, Y., Cynshi, O., Wada, Y., Honda, M., Kurihara, H., Aburatani, H., Doi, T., Matsumoto, A., Azuma, S., Noda, T., Toyoda, Y., Itakura, H., Yazaki, Y., Kodama, T., et al. (1997). A role for macrophage scavenger receptors in atherosclerosis and susceptibility to infection. *Nature.* **386,** 292–296.

Svensson, A. C., Pawitan, Y., Cnattingius, S., Reilly, M., and Lichtenstein, P. (2006). Familial aggregation of small-for-gestational-age births: The importance of fetal genetic effects. *Am J Obstet Gynecol.* **194,** 475–479.

Swallow, D. M. (2003). Genetics of lactase persistence and lactose intolerance. *Annu Rev Genet.* **37,** 197–219.

Swartz, M. (2003). Galapagos turtles can lay eggs at ages of 100 years or more. *Exp Gerontol.* **38,** 721.

Szalai, A. J. (2002a). The antimicrobial activity of C-reactive protein. *Microbes and Infection/Institut Pasteur.* **4(2),** 201–205.

Szalai, A. J. (2002b). The biological functions of C-reactive protein. *Vascul Pharmacol.* **39(3),** 105–107.

Szalai, A. J., McCrory, M. A., Cooper, G. S., Wu, J., and Kimberly, R. P. (2002). Association between baseline levels of C-reactive protein (CRP) and a dinucleotide repeat polymorphism in the intron of the CRP gene. *Genes Immun.* **3,** 14–19.

Tabet, N. (2005). Obesity in middle age and future risk of dementia: Dietary fat and sugar may hold the clue. *Br Med J.* **331,** 454–455.

Taddei, S., Virdis, A., Ghiadoni, L., Salvetti, G., Bernini, G., Magagna, A., and Salvetti, A. (2001). Age-related reduction of NO availability and oxidative stress in humans. *Hypertension.* **38,** 274–279.

Tai, L. K., Zheng, Q., Pan, S., Jin, Z. G., and Berk, B. C. (2005). Flow activates ERK1/2 and eNOS via a pathway involving PECAM1, SHP2, and Tie2. *J Biol Chem.* **280,** 29620–29624.

Takayama, T., Katsuki, S., Takahashi, Y., Ohi, M., Nojiri, S., Sakamaki, S., Kato, J., Kogawa, K., Miyake, H., and Niitsu, Y. (1998). Aberrant crypt foci of the colon as precursors of adenoma and cancer. *New Engl J Med.* **339,** 1277–1284.

Takeda, T., Hosokawa, M., Takeshita, S., Irino, M., Higuchi, K., Matsushita, T., Tomita, Y., Yasuhira, K., Hamamoto, H., Shimizu, K., Ishii, M., Yamamuro, T. (1981). A new murine model of accelerated senescence. *Mech Ageing Dev.* **17,** 183–194.

Talmud, P. J., Stephens, J. W., Hawe, E., Demissie, S., Cupples, L. A., Hurel, S. J., Humphries, S. E., and Ordovas, J. M. (2005). The significant increase in cardiovascular disease risk in APOE epsilon4 carriers is evident only in men who smoke: Potential relationship between reduced antioxidant status and ApoE4. *Annals of Human Genetics.* **69,** 613–622.

Tan, S. Y., and Pepys, M. B. (1994). Amyloidosis. *Histopathology.* **25,** 403–414.

Tanaka, M., Gong, J., Zhang, J., Yamada, Y., Borgeld, H. J., and Yagi, K. (2000a). Mitochondrial genotype associated with longevity and its inhibitory effect on mutagenesis. *Mech Ageing Dev.* **116,** 65–76.

Tanaka, S., Segawa, T., Tamaya, N., and Ohno, T. (2000). Establishment of an aging farm of F344/N rats and C57BL/6 mice at the National Institute for Longevity Sciences (NILS). *Arch Gerontol Geriatr.* **30,** 215–223.

Tanaka, Y., Nakayamada, S., and Okada, Y. (2005). Osteoblasts and osteoclasts in bone remodeling and inflammation. *Current Drug Targets. Inflammation and Allergy.* **4,** 325–328.

Tangkijvanich, P., Vimolket, T., Theamboonlers, A., Kullavanijaya, P., Suwangool, P., and Poovorawan, Y. (2000). Serum interleukin-6 and interferon-gamma levels in patients with hepatitis B-associated chronic liver disease. *Asian Pac J Allergy Immunol.* **18,** 109–114.

Tannenbaum, B. M., Brindley, D. N. Tannenbaum, G. S., Dallman, M. F., McArthur, M. D., Meaney, M. J. (1997). High-fat feeding alters both basal and stress-induced hypothalamic-pituitary-adrenal activity in the rat. *Am J Physiol.* **273,** E1168–E1177.

Tanner, J. M. (1962). *Growth at adolescence.* Oxford: Blackwell Scientific Publications.

Tanner, J. M. (1981). *A history of the study of human growth.* Cambridge: Cambridge University Press.

Tantisira, K. G., and Weiss, S. T. (2001). Childhood infections and asthma: At the crossroads of the hygiene and Barker hypotheses. *Respir Res.* **2(6),** 324–327.

Tapia, P. C. (2006). RhoA, Rho kinase, JAK2, and STAT3 may be the intracellular determinants of longevity implicated in the progeric influence of obesity: Insulin, IGF-1, and leptin may all conspire to promote stem cell exhaustion. *Med Hypoth.* **66,** 832–843.

Tappen, M., and Wrangham, R. (2000). Recognizing hominoid-modified bones: The taphonomy of colobus bones partially digested by free-ranging chimpanzees in the Kibale Forest, Uganda. *Am J Phys Anthropol.* **113,** 217–234.

Tarim, E., Yigit, F., Kilicdag, E., Bagis, T., Demircan, S., Simsek, E., Haydardedeoglu, B., and Yanik, F. (2006). Early onset of subclinical atherosclerosis in women with gestational diabetes mellitus. *Ultrasound Obstet Gynecol.* **27,** 177–182.

Tarkowski, E., Issa, R., Sjèogren, M., Wallin, A., Blennow, K., Tarkowski, A., and Kumar, P. (2002). Increased intrathecal levels of the angiogenic factors VEGF and TGF-beta in Alzheimer's disease and vascular dementia. *Neurobiol Aging.* **23,** 237–243.

Tatar, M., Bartke, A., and Antebi, A. (2003). The endocrine regulation of aging by insulin-like signals. *Science.* **299,** 1346–1351.

Tatar, M., Kopelman, A., Epstein, D., Tu, M. P., Yin, C. M., and Garofalo, R. S. (2001). A mutant *Drosophila* insulin receptor homolog that extends life-span and impairs neuroendocrine function. *Science.* **292,** 107–110.

Tatar, M., and Yin, C. (2001). Slow aging during insect reproductive diapause: Why butterflies, grasshoppers and flies are like worms. *Exp Gerontol.* **36,** 723–738.

Taylor, D. M. (1999). Inactivation of prions by physical and chemical means. *J Hospital Infection.* **43,** S69–S76.

Taylor, R. J. (1974). The bacteriological status of a specific-pathogen-free animal production building and of its staff and the microbiological integrity of the animals one year after the building was commissioned. *J Hygiene.* **73,** 271–276.

Taylor, R. J., and Doy, T. G. (1975). The microbiological and parasitological colonisation of specified-pathogen-free mice maintained in a conventional animal house. *Laboratory Animals.* **9,** 99–104.

Tazume, S., Umehara, K., Matsuzawa, H., Aikawa, H., Hashimoto, K., and Sasaki, S. (1991a). Effects of germfree status and food restriction on longevity and growth of mice. *Jikken Dobutsu. Exp Anim.* **40,** 517–522.

Tazume, S., Umehara, K., Matsuzawa, H., Yoshida, T., Hashimoto, K., and Sasaki, S. (1991b). Immunological function of food-restricted germfree and specific pathogen-free mice. *Jikken Dobutsu. Experimental Animals.* **40,** 523–528.

Technau, G. M. (1984). Fiber number in the mushroom bodies of adult *Drosophila melanogaster* depends on age, sex and experience. *J Neurogenetics.* **1,** 113–126.

Teleman, A. A., Chen, Y. W., and Cohen, S. M. (2005). 4E-BP functions as a metabolic brake used under stress conditions but not during normal growth. *Genes Dev.* **19,** 1844–1848.

Telling, G. C., Haga, T., Torchia, M., Tremblay, P., DeArmond. S. J., Prusiner, S. B. (1996). Interactions between wild-type and mutant prion proteins modulate, neurodegeneration in transgenic mice. *Gen Dev.* **10,** 1736–1750.

Tempel, D. L., McEwen, B. S., and Leibowitz, S. F. (1992). Effects of adrenal steroid ago-nists on food intake and macronutrient selection. *Physiol Behav.* **52,** 1161–1166.

Tempfer, C. B., Riener, E. K., Keck, C., Grimm, C., Heinze, G., Huber, J. C., Gitsch, G., and Hefler, L. A. (2005). Polymorphisms associated with thrombophilia and vascular homeostasis and the timing of menarche and menopause in 728 white women. *Menopause.* **12,** 325–330.

Teo, J. L., Ma, H., Nguyen, C., Lam, C., and Kahn, M. (2005). Specific inhibition of CBP/{beta}-catenin interaction rescues defects in neuronal differentiation caused by a presenilin-1 mutation. *Proc Natl Acad Sci USA.* **102,** 12171–12176.

Teotonio, H., Matos, M., Rose, M. (2002). Reverse evolution of fitness in *Drosophila melanogaster. J Evol Biol.* **15,** 608–617.

Terao, A., Apte-Deshpande, A., Dousman, L., Morairty, S., Eynon, B. P., Kilduff, T. S., and Freund, Y. R. (2002). Immune response gene expression increases in the aging murine hippocampus. *J Neuroimmunol.* **132,** 99–112.

Teriokhin, A. T., Budilova, E. V., Thomas, F., and Guegan, J. F. (2004). Worldwide varia-tion in life-span sexual dimorphism and sex-specific environmental mortality rates. *Hum Biol.* **76,** 623–641.

Ternak, G. (2004). Antibiotics may act as growth/obesity promoters in humans as an inadvertent result of antibiotic pollution? *Med Hypotheses.* **64,** 14–16.

Terry, M. B., Gammon, M. D., Zhang, F. F., Tawfik, H., Teitelbaum, S. L., Britton, J. A., Subbaramaiah, K., Dannenberg, A. J., and Neugut, A. I. (2004). Association of fre-quency and duration of aspirin use and hormone receptor status with breast cancer risk. *JAMA.* **291,** 2433–2440.

Terry, R. D., DeTeresa, R., and Hansen, L. A. (1987). Neocortical cell counts in normal human adult aging. *Ann Neurol.* **21,** 530–539.

Terry, R. D., Masliah, E., and Hansen, L. A. (1999). The neuropathology of Alzheimer disease and the structural basis of its cognitive alterations. In R. D. Terry, R. Katzman, K. L. Bick, and S. S. Sisodia, Eds., *Alzheimer disease*, pp. 187–206. Philadelphia: Lippincott Williams & Wilkens.

Terry, R. D., Masliah, E., Salmon, D. P., Butters, N., DeTeresa, R., Hill, R., Hansen, L. A., and Katzman, R. (1991). Physical basis of cognitive alterations in Alzheimer's disease: Synapse loss is the major correlate of cognitive impairment. *Ann Neurol.* **30,** 572–580.

Tesfaigzi, Y., Singh, S. P., Foster, J. E., Kubatko, J., Barr, E. B., Fine, P. M., McDonald, J. D., Hahn, F. F., and Mauderly, J. L. (2002). Health effects of subchronic exposure to low levels of wood smoke in rats. *Toxicological Sciences.* **65,** 115–125.

Teter, B., and Finch, C. E. (2004). Caliban's heritance and the genetics of neuronal aging. *Trends in Neurosciences.* **27,** 627–632.

Teunissen, C. E., Lutjohann, D., von Bergmann, K., Verhey, F., Vreeling, F., Wauters, A., Bosmans, E., Bosma, H., van Boxtel, M. P. J., and Maes, M. (2003a). Combination of serum markers related to several mechanisms in Alzheimer's disease. *Neurobiol Aging.* **24,** 893–902.

Teunissen, C. E., van Boxtel, M. P., Bosma, H., Bosmans, E., Delanghe, J., De Bruijn, C., Wauters, A., Maes, M., Jolles, J., Steinbusch, H. W., and de Vente, J. (2003). Inflammation markers in relation to cognition in a healthy aging population. *J Neuroimmunol.* **134,** 142–150.

Thal, D. R., Schultz, C., Dehghani, F., Yamaguchi, H., Braak, H., and Braak, E. (2000). Amyloid beta-protein (Abeta)-containing astrocytes are located preferentially near N-terminal-truncated Abeta deposits in the human entorhinal cortex. *Acta Neuropathologica.* **100,** 608–617.

Thapar, N., and Sanderson, I. R. (2004). Diarrhoea in children: An interface between developing and developed countries. *Lancet.* **363,** 641–653.

Thieme, H. (1997). Lower Palaeolithic hunting spears from Germany. *Nature.* **385,** 807–810.

Thomas, D. P., McCormick, R. J., Zimmerman, S. D., Vadlamudi, R. K., and Gosselin, L. E. (1992). Aging- and training-induced alterations in collagen characteristics of rat left ventricle and papillary muscle. *Am J Physiol.* **263,** H778–783.

Thomas, J. E., Dale, A., Bunn, J. E., Harding, M., Coward, W. A., Cole, T. J., and Weaver, L. T. (2004). Early *Helicobacter pylori* colonisation: The association with growth faltering in The Gambia. *Arch Dis Child.* **89,** 1149–1154.

Thomas, T. N., Rhodin, J. A., Clark, L., Garces, A., and Bryant, M. (2003). A comparison of the anti-inflammatory activities of conjugated estrogens and 17-beta estradiol. *Inflamm Res.* **52,** 452–460.

Thompson, H. J., McGinley, J. N., Spoelstra, N. S., Jiang, W., Zhu, Z., and Wolfe, P. (2004a). Effect of dietary energy restriction on vascular density during mammary carcinogenesis. *Cancer Res.* **64,** 5643–5650.

Thompson, H. J., Zhu, Z., and Jiang, W. (2004b). Identification of the apoptosis activation cascade induced in mammary carcinomas by energy restriction. *Cancer Res.* **64,** 1541–1545.

Thomson, A. M., Billewicz, W. Z., and Hytten, F. E. (1968). The assessment of fetal growth. *J Obstet Gynaecol.* **75,** 903–916.

Thomson, C. A., LeWinn, K., Newton, T. R., Alberts, D. S., and Martinez, M. E. (2003). Nutrition and diet in the development of gastrointestinal cancer. *Curr Oncol Reps.* **5,** 192–202.

Thorn, J. (2001). The inflammatory response in humans after inhalation of bacterial endotoxin: A review. *Inflamm Res.* **50,** 254–261.

Thornalley, P. J. (2003). Protecting the genome: Defence against nucleotide glycation and emerging role of glyoxalase I overexpression in multidrug resistance in cancer chemotherapy. *Biochem Soc Trans.* **31,** 1372–1377.

Tice, J. A., Browner, W., Tracy, R. P., and Cummings, S. R. (2003). The relation of C-reactive protein levels to total and cardiovascular mortality in older U.S. women. *Am J Med.* **114,** 199–205.

Tilvis, R. S., Kèahèonen-Vèare, M. H., Jolkkonen, J., Valvanne, J., Pitkala, K. H., and Strandberg, T. E. (2004). Predictors of cognitive decline and mortality of aged people over a 10-year period. *J Gerontol. Series A, Biol Sci Med Sci.* **59,** 268–274.

Timiras, P. S., Yaghmaie, F., Saeed, O., Thung, E., and Chinn, G. (2005). The ageing phenome: Caloric restriction and hormones promote neural cell survival, growth, and de-differentiation. *Mech Ageing Dev.* **126,** 3–9.

Tintut, Y., Patel, J., Territo, M., Saini, T., Parhami, F., and Demer, L. L. (2002). Monocyte/macrophage regulation of vascular calcification *in vitro*. *Circulation.* **105,** 650–655.

Tishkoff, S. A., Reed, F. A., Ranciaro, A., Voight, B. F., Babbitt, C. C., Silverman, J. S., et al (2006). Convergent adaptation of human lactase persistence in Africa and Europe. *Nature Genet.* **39,** 31–40.

Tofighi, R., Tillmark, N., Daré, E., Aberg, A. M., Larsson, J. E., and Ceccatelli, S. (2006). Hypoxia-independent apoptosis in neural cells exposed to carbon monoxide *in vitro*. *Brain Res.* **1098,** 1–8.

Tokishita, S., Kato, Y., Kobayashi, T., Nakamura, S., Ohta, T., and Yamagata, H. (2006). Organization and repression by juvenile hormone of a vitellogenin gene cluster in the crustacean, *Daphnia magna*. *Biochem Biophys Res Commun.* **345,** 362–370.

Tomasch, J. (1971). Comments on "neuromythology." *Nature.* **233,** 60.

Tomlinson, B. E., Blessed, G., and Roth, M. (1968). Observations on the brains of non-demented old people. *J Neurol Sci.* **7,** 331–356.

Tomlinson, B. E., Blessed, G., and Roth, M. (1970). Observations on the brains of demented old people. *J Neurol Sci.* **11,** 205–242.

Tomlinson, J. W., Holden, N., Hills, R. K., Wheatley, K., Clayton, R. N., Bates, A. S., Sheppard, M. C., and Stewart, P. M. (2001). Association between premature mortality and hypopituitarism. West Midlands Prospective Hypopituitary Study Group. *Lancet.* **357,** 425–431.

Ton, J., Van Pelt, J. A., Van Loon, L. C., and Pieterse, C. M. (2002). Differential effectiveness of salicylate-dependent and jasmonate/ethylene-dependent induced resistance in *Arabidopsis. Mol Plant-Microbe Interact.* **15,** 27–34.

Toni, R., Malaguti, A., Castorina, S., Roti, E., and Lechan, R. M. (2004). New paradigms in neuroendocrinology: Relationships between obesity, systemic inflammation and the neuroendocrine system. *J Endocrinol Invest.* **27,** 182–186.

Torella, D., Leosco, D., Indolfi, C., Curcio, A., Coppola, C., Ellison, G. M., Russo, V. G., Torella, M., Li Volti, G., Rengo, F., and Chiariello, M. (2004). Aging exacerbates negative remodeling and impairs endothelial regeneration after balloon injury. *Am J Physiol Heart Circ Physiol.* **287,** H2850–2860.

Torella, D., Rota, M., Nurzynska, D., Musso, E., Monsen, A., Shiraishi, I., Zias, E., Walsh, K., Rosenzweig, A., Sussman, M. A., Urbanek, K., Nadal-Ginard, B., Kajstura, J., Anversa, P., and Leri, A. (2004b). Cardiac stem cell and myocyte aging, heart failure, and insulin-like growth factor-1 overexpression. [see comment]. *Circ Res.* **94,** 514–524.

Torroja, L., Packard, M., Gorczyca, M., White, K., and Budnik, V. (1999). The *Drosophila* beta-amyloid precursor protein homolog promotes synapse differentiation at the neuromuscular junction. *J Neurosci.* **19,** 7793–7803.

Tortoriello, D. V., McMinn, J., and Chua, S. C. (2004). Dietary-induced obesity and hypothalamic infertility in female DBA/2J mice. *Endocrinology.* **145,** 1238–1247.

Torzewski, J., Torzewski, M., Bowyer, D. E., Frohlich, M., Koenig, W., Waltenberger, J., Fitzsimmons, C., and Hombach, V. (1998). C-reactive protein frequently colocalizes with the terminal complement complex in the intima of early atherosclerotic lesions of human coronary arteries. [comment]. *Arterioscler Thromb Vasc Biol.* **18,** 1386–1392.

Toungoussova, O. S., Bjune, G., and Caugant, D. A. (2006). Epidemic of tuberculosis in the former Soviet Union: Social and biological reasons. *Tuberculosis (Edinb).* **86,** 1–10.

Tower, J. (2006). Sex-specific regulation of aging and apoptosis. *Mech Ageing Dev.* **127,** 705–718.

Townsend, P., and Davidson, N. (1982). *Inequalities in health. The Black Report.* Hammondsworth: Penguin.

Tracey, K. J. (2002). The inflammatory reflex. *Nature.* **420,** 853–859.

Tracy, R. P. (2002). Inflammation in cardiovascular disease: Cart, horse or both—Revisited. *Arterioscler Thromb Vasc Biol.* **22,** 1514–1515.

Traub, O., and Berk, B. C. (1998). Laminar shear stress: Mechanisms by which endothelial cells transduce an atheroprotective force. *Arterioscler Thromb Vasc Biol.* **18,** 677–685.

Traw, M. B., Kim, J., Enright, S., Cipollini, D. F., and Bergelson, J. (2003). Negative cross-talk between salicylate- and jasmonate-mediated pathways in the Wassilewskija ecotype of *Arabidopsis thaliana*. *Mol Ecol* **12**, 1125–1135.

Trayhurn, P., and Wood, I. S. (2004). Adipokines: Inflammation and the pleiotropic role of white adipose tissue. *Br J Nutr.* **92**, 347–355.

Trevathan, W. and Rosenberg, K. (2000). The shoulders follow the head: postcranial constraints on human childbirth. *J Hum Evol.* **39**, 583–586.

Trevilatto, P. C., Scarel-Caminaga, R. M., de Brito, R. B., de Souza, A. P., and Line, S. R. (2003). Polymorphism at position -174 of IL-6 gene is associated with susceptibility to chronic periodontitis in a Caucasian Brazilian population. *J Clin Periodontol.* **30**, 438–442.

Triantafilou, M., and Triantafilou, K. (2003). Receptor cluster formation during activation by bacterial products. *J Endotoxin Res.* **9**, 331–335.

Trienekens, G. M. T. (1985). *"Tussen ons voilk en de honger de voedselvoorziening."* Utrecht, Netherlands: Matrijs Publ.

Trinei, M., Giorgio, M., Cicalese, A., Barozzi, S., Ventura, A., Migliaccio, E., Milia, E., Padura, I. M., Raker, V. A., Maccarana, M., Petronilli, V., Minucci, S., Bernardi, P., Lanfrancone, L., and Pelicci, P. G. (2002). A p53-p66Shc signalling pathway controls intracellular redox status, levels of oxidation-damaged DNA and oxidative stress-induced apoptosis. *Oncogene.* **21**, 3872–3878.

Truman, J. W., and Riddiford, L. M. (2002). Endocrine insights into the evolution of metamorphosis in insects. *Annu Rev Entomol.* **47**, 467–500.

Trzonkowski, P., Mysliwska, J., Szmit, E., Wieckiewicz, J., Lukaszuk, K., Brydak, L. B., Machala, M., and Mysliwski, A. (2003). Association between cytomegalovirus infection, enhanced proinflammatory response and low level of anti-hemagglutinins during the anti-influenza vaccination—an impact of immunosenescence. *Vaccine.* **21**, 3826–3836.

Tschanz, J. T., Welsh-Bohmer, K. A., Lyketsos, C. G., Corcoran, C., Green, R. C., Hayden, K., Norton, M. C., Zandi, P. P., Toone, L., West, N. A., and Breitner, J. C. (2006). Conversion to dementia from mild cognitive disorder: The Cache County Study. *Neurology.* **67**, 229–234.

Tsegaye, A., Wolday, D., Otto, S., Petros, B., Assefa, T., Alebachew, T., Hailu, E., Adugna, F., Measho, W., Dorigo, W., Fontanet, A. L., van Baarle, D., and Miedema, F. (2003). Immunophenotyping of blood lymphocytes at birth, during childhood, and during adulthood in HIV-1–uninfected Ethiopians. *Clin Immunol.* **109**, 338–346.

Tsigos, C., Papanicolaou, D. A., Kyrou, I., Defensor, R., Mitsiadis, C. S., and Chrousos, G. P. (1997). Dose-dependent effects of recombinant human interleukin-6 on glucose regulation. *J Clin Endocrinol Metab.* **82**, 4167–4170.

Tsuchiya, T., Dhahbi, J. M., Cui, X., Mote, P. L., Bartke, A., and Spindler, S. R. (2004). Additive regulation of hepatic gene expression by dwarfism and caloric restriction. *Physiol Genom.* **17**, 307–315.

Tsuchiya, T., Higami, Y., Komatsu, T., Tanaka, K., Honda, S., Yamaza, H., Chiba, T., Ayabe, H., and Shimokawa, I. (2005). Acute stress response in calorie-restricted rats to lipopolysaccharide-induced inflammation. *Mech Ageing Dev.* **126**, 568–579.

Tsujinaka, T., Ebisui, C., Fujita, J., Kishibuchi, M., Morimoto, T., Ogawa, A., Katsume, A., Ohsugi, Y., Kominami, E., and Monden, M. (1995). Muscle undergoes atrophy in association with increase of lysosomal cathepsin activity in interleukin-6 transgenic mouse. *Biochem Biophys Res Commun.* **207**, 168–174.

Tu, M. P., Epstein, D., and Tatar, M. (2002a). The demography of slow aging in male and female *Drosophila* mutant for the insulin-receptor substrate homologue chico. *Aging Cell.* **1**, 75–80.

Tu, M. P., Yin, C. M., and Tatar, M. (2002b). Impaired ovarian ecdysone synthesis of *Drosophila melanogaster* insulin receptor mutants. *Aging Cell.* **1**, 158–160.

Tuazon, M. A., van Raaij, J. M., Hautvast, J. G., and Barba, C. V. (1987). Energy requirements of pregnancy in the Philippines. *Lancet.* **2**, 1129–1131.

Tuppo, E. E., and Arias, H. R. (2005). The role of inflammation in Alzheimer's disease. *Int J Biochemistry & Cell Biology.* **37**, 289–305.

Turrin, N. P., and Rivest, S. (2004). Unraveling the molecular details involved in the intimate link between the immune and neuroendocrine systems. *Exp Biol Med.* **229**, 996–1006.

Turturro, A., Duffy, P., Hass, B., Kodell, R., and Hart, R. (2002). Survival characteristics and age-adjusted disease incidences in C57BL/6 mice fed a commonly used cereal-based diet modulated by dietary restriction. *J Gerontol. Series A, Biol Sci Med Sci.* **57**, B379–389.

Tuya, C., Mutch, W. J., Haggarty, P., Campbell, D. M., Cumming, A., Kelly, K., Broom, I., and McNeill, G. (2006). The influence of birth weight and genetic factors on lipid levels: A study in adult twins. *Br J Nutr.* **95**, 504–510.

Tuzcu, E. M., Kapadia, S. R., Tutar, E., Ziada, K. M., Hobbs, R. E., McCarthy, P. M., Young, J. B., and Nissen, S. E. (2001). High prevalence of coronary atherosclerosis in asymptomatic teenagers and young adults: Evidence from intravascular ultrasound. *Circulation.* **103**, 2705–2710.

Tycko, B. (2006). Imprinted genes in placental growth and obstetric disorders. *Cytogenet Genome Res.* **113**, 271–278.

Tycko, B., and Efstratiadis, A. (2002). Genomic imprinting: Piece of cake. *Nature.* **417**, 913–914.

Tyner, S. D., Venkatachalam, S., Choi, J., Jones, S., Ghebranious, N., Igelmann, H., Lu, X., Soron, G., Cooper, B., Brayton, C., Hee Park, S., Thompson, T., Karsenty, G., Bradley, A., and Donehower, L. A. (2002). p53 mutant mice that display early ageing-associated phenotypes. *Nature.* **415**, 45–53.

Ubalee, R., Tsukahara, T., Kikuchi, M., Lum, J. K., Dzodzomenyo, M., and Kaneko, A. (2005). Associations between frequencies of a susceptible TNF-alpha promoter allele and protective alpha-thalassaemias and malaria parasite incidence in Vanuatu. *Trop Med Int Health.* **10**, 544–549.

Uddin, M., Wildman, D. E., Liu, G., Xu, W., Johnson, R. M., Hof, P. R., Kapatos, G., Grossman, L. I., and Goodman, M. (2004). Sister grouping of chimpanzees and humans as revealed by genome-wide phylogenetic analysis of brain gene expression profiles. *Proc Natl Acad Sci USA.* **101**, 2957–2962.

Uemura, S., Matsushita, H., Li, W., Glassford, A. J., Asagami, T., Lee, K. H., Harrison, D. G., and Tsao, P. S. (2001). Diabetes mellitus enhances vascular matrix metalloproteinase activity: Role of oxidative stress. *Circulation Research.* **88**, 1291–1298.

Undie, A. S., and Friedman, E. (1993). Diet restriction prevents aging-induced deficits in brain phosphoinositide metabolism. *J Gerontol.* **48**, B62–67.

Ungvari, Z., Csiszar, A., and Kaley, G. (2004). Vascular inflammation in aging. *Herz.* **29**, 733–740.

UNICEF. (2004). Low birthweight—Country, regional, and global estimates, UNICEF/WHO 2004. www.childinfo.org/areas/birthweight.

Urban, B. A., Fishman, E. K., Goldman, S. M., Scott, W. W., Jr., Jones, B., Humphrey, R. L., and Hruban, R. H. (1993). CT evaluation of amyloidosis: Spectrum of disease. *Radiographics.* **13**, 1295–1308.

Urbich, C., and Dimmeler, S. (2005). Risk factors for coronary artery disease, circulating endothelial progenitor cells, and the role of HMG-CoA reductase inhibitors. *Kidney Int.* **67,** 1672–1676.

Uribarri, J., Peppa, M., Cai, W., Goldberg, T., Lu, M., Baliga, S., Vassalotti, J. A., and Vlassara, H. (2003). Dietary glycotoxins correlate with circulating advanced glycation end product levels in renal failure patients. *Am J Kidney Diseases.* **42,** 532–538.

Ursin, G., Bernstein, L., and Pike, M. C. (1994). Breast cancer. In R. Doll, J. Fraumeni, C. S. Muir, Eds. *Trends in cancer incidence and mortality: Cancer survey,* pp. 19–20.

Urvater, J. A., McAdam, S. N., Loehrke, J. H., Allen, T. M., Moran, J. L., Rowell, T. J. et al. (2000). A high incidence of Shigella-induced arthritis in a primate species: major histocompatibility complex class I molecules associated with resistance and susceptibility, and their relationship to HLA-B27. *Immunogenetics.* **51,** 314–325.

U.S. Surgeon General. (1990). *The health benefits of smoking cessation: A report of the Surgeon General.* Rockville, MD: U.S. Department of Health and Human Services.

Uzun, H., Benian, A., Madazli, R., Topcuoglu, M. A., Aydin, S., and Albayrak, M. (2005). Circulating oxidized low-density lipoprotein and paraoxonase activity in preeclampsia. *Gynecol Obstet Invest.* **60,** 195–200.

Vagnucci, A. H., Jr., and Li, W. W. (2003). Alzheimer's disease and angiogenesis. *Lancet.* **361,** 605–608.

Valdes, A. M., Andrew, T., Gardner, J. P., Kimura, M., Oelsner, E., Cherkas, L. F., Aviv, A., and Spector, T. D. (2005). Obesity, cigarette smoking, and telomere length in women. *Lancet.* **366,** 662–664.

Valledor, A. F. (2005). The innate immune response under the control of the LXR pathway. *Immunobiology.* **210,** 127–132.

van Baarle, D., Tsegaye, A., Miedema, F., and Akbar, A. (2005). Significance of senescence for virus-specific memory T cell responses: Rapid ageing during chronic stimulation of the immune system. *Immunol Lett.* **97,** 19–29.

Van den Brink, D. M. and Wanders, R. J. A., (2006). Phytanic acid: production from phytol, its breakdown and role in human disease. *Cell Mol Life Sci.* **63,** 1752–1765.

van den Elzen, P., Garg, S., León, L., Brigl, M., Leadbetter, E. A., Gumperz, J. E., Dascher, C. C., Cheng, T. Y., Sacks, F. M., Illarionov, P. A., Besra, G. S., Kent, S. C., Moody, D. B., and Brenner, M. B. (2005). Apolipoprotein-mediated pathways of lipid antigen presentation. *Nature.* **437,** 906–910.

van der Loo, B., Labugger, R., Skepper, J. N., Bachschmid, M., Kilo, J., Powell, J. M., Palacios-Callender, M., Erusalimsky, J. D., Quaschning, T., Malinski, T., Gygi, D., Ullrich, V., and Lèuscher, T. F. (2000). Enhanced peroxynitrite formation is associated with vascular aging. *J Exp Med.* **192,** 1731–1744.

van der Sande, M. A., Ceesay, S. M., Milligan, P. J., Nyan, O. A., Banya, W. A., Prentice, A., McAdam, K. P., and Walraven, G. E. (2001). Obesity and undernutrition and cardiovascular risk factors in rural and urban Gambian communities. *Am J Public Health.* **91,** 1641–1644.

Van Dorpe, J., Smeijers, L., Dewachter, I., Nuyens, D., Spittaels, K., Van Den Haute, C., Mercken, M., Moechars, D., Laenen, I., Kuiperi, C., Bruynseels, K., Tesseur, I., Loos, R., Vanderstichele, H., Checler, F., Sciot, R., and Van Leuven, F. (2000). Prominent cerebral amyloid angiopathy in transgenic mice overexpressing the London mutant of human APP in neurons. *Am J Pathol.* **157,** 1283–1298.

Van Dusseldorp, M., Schneede, J., Refsum, H., Ueland, P. M., Thomas, C. M., de Boer, E., and van Staveren, W. A. (1999). Risk of persistent cobalamin deficiency in adolescents fed a macrobiotic diet in early life. *Am J Clin Nutr.* **69,** 664–671.

Vane, J. R., and Botting, R. M. (2003). The mechanism of action of aspirin. *Thromb Res.* **110,** 255–258.

van Exel, E., Gussekloo, J., de Craen, A. J., Frèolich, M., Bootsma-Van Der Wiel, A., and Westendorp, R. G. (2002). Low production capacity of interleukin-10 associates with the metabolic syndrome and type 2 diabetes: The Leiden 85-Plus Study. *Diabetes.* **51,** 1088–1092.

Vanfleteren, J. R., DeVreese, A., and Braeckman, B. P. (1998). Two-parameter logistic and Weibull equations provide better fits to survival data from isogenic populations of *Caenorhabditis elegans* in axenic culture than does the Gompertz model. J. *Gerontol.* **53,** B393–B403.

van Gijn, J., and Algra, A. (2002). Aspirin and stroke prevention. *Thromb Res.* **110,** 349–353.

van Heemst, D., Beekman, M., Mooijaart, S. P., Heijmans, B. T., Brandt, B. W., Zwaan, B. J., Slagboom, P. E., and Westendorp, R. G. (2005a). Reduced insulin/IGF-1 signalling and human longevity. *Aging Cell.* **4,** 79–85.

van Heemst, D., Mooijaart, S., Beekman, M., Schreuder, J., de Craen, A., Brandt, B., Slagboom, P., and Westendorp, R. (2005b). Variation in the human TP53 gene affects old age survival and cancer mortality. *Exp Gerontol.* **40,** 11–15.

Van Lenten, B. J., Hama, S. Y., de Beer, F. C., Stafforini, D. M., McIntyre, T. M., Prescott, S. M., La Du, B. N., Fogelman, A. M., and Navab, M. (1995). Anti-inflammatory HDL becomes pro-inflammatory during the acute phase response. Loss of protective effect of HDL against LDL oxidation in aortic wall cell cocultures. *J Clin Invest.* **96,** 2758–2767.

Van Lenten, B. J., Reddy, S. T., Navab, M., and Fogelman, A. M. (2006). Understanding changes in high density lipoproteins during the acute phase response. *Arterioscler Thromb Vasc Biol.* **26,** 1687–1688.

van Noord, P. A. (2004). Breast cancer and the brain: A neurodevelopmental hypothesis to explain the opposing effects of caloric deprivation during the Dutch famine of 1944–1945 on breast cancer and its risk factors. *J Nutr.* **134,** 3399S–3406S.

van Noord, P. A., and Kaaks, R. (1991). The effect of wartime conditions and the 1944–45 'Dutch famine' on recalled menarcheal age in participants of the DOM breast cancer screening project. *Ann Hum Biol.* **18,** 57–70.

Van Nostrand, W. E., Schmaier, A. H., and Wagner, S. L. (1992). Potential role of protease nexin-2/amyloid beta-protein precursor as a cerebral anticoagulant. *Ann NY Acad Sci.* **674,** 243–252.

van Praag, H., Christie, B. R., Sejnowski, T. J., and Gage, F. H. (1999). Running enhances neurogenesis, learning, and long-term potentiation in mice. *Proc Natl Acad Sci USA.* **96,** 13427–13431.

van Praag, H., Shubert, T., Zhao, C., and Gage, F. H. (2005). Exercise enhances learning and hippocampal neurogenesis in aged mice. *J Neurosci.* **25,** 8680–8685.

Van Remmen, H., Ikeno, Y., Hamilton, M., Pahlavani, M., Wolf, N., Thorpe, S. R., Alderson, N. L., Baynes, J. W., Epstein, C. J., Huang, T. T., Nelson, J., Strong, R., and Richardson, A. (2003). Life-long reduction in MnSOD activity results in increased DNA damage and higher incidence of cancer but does not accelerate aging. *Physiological Genomics.* **16,** 29–37.

Van Remmen, H., and Richardson, A. (2001). Oxidative damage to mitochondria and aging. *Exp Gerontol.* **36,** 957–968.

Van Voorhies, W., Fuchs, J., and Thomas, S. (2005). The longevity of *Caenorhaabditis elegans* in soil. *Biol Lett.* **1**, 247–249.

Varki, A. (2001). Loss of N-glycolylneuraminic acid in humans: Mechanisms, consequences, and implications for hominid evolution. *Am J Phys Anthropol.* (**Suppl 33**), 54–69.

Vasa, M., Fichtlscherer, S., Adler, K., Aicher, A., Martin, H., Zeiher, A. M., and Dimmeler, S. (2001a). Increase in circulating endothelial progenitor cells by statin therapy in patients with stable coronary artery disease. *Circulation.* **103**, 2885–2890.

Vasa, M., Fichtlscherer, S., Aicher, A., Adler, K., Urbich, C., Martin, H., Zeiher, A. M., and Dimmeler, S. (2001b). Number and migratory activity of circulating endothelial progenitor cells inversely correlate with risk factors for coronary artery disease. *Circulation Research.* **89**, E1–7.

Vasan, R. S., Sullivan, L. M., D'Agostino, R. B., Roubenoff, R., Harris, T., Sawyer, D. B., Levy, D., and Wilson, P. W. (2003). Serum insulin-like growth factor I and risk for heart failure in elderly individuals without a previous myocardial infarction: The Framingham Heart Study. [see comment]. *Ann Intern Med.* **139**, 642–648.

Vassalle, C., Masini, S., Bianchi, F., and Zucchelli, G. C. (2004). Evidence for association between hepatitis C virus seropositivity and coronary artery disease. *Heart.* **90**, 565–566.

Vastesaeger, M., and Delcourt, R. (1961). Spontaneous atherosclerosis and diet in captive animals. *Nutritio et Dieta.* **3**, 174–188.

Vatay, A., Yang, Y., Chung, E. K., Zhou, B., Blanchong, C. A., Kovacs, M., Karadi, I., Fèust, G., Romics, L. L., Varga, L., Yu, C. Y., and Szalai, C. (2003). Relationship between complement components C4A and C4B diversities and two TNF alpha promoter polymorphisms in two healthy Caucasian populations. *Hum Immunol.* **64**, 543–552.

Vater, R., Cullen, M. J., Nicholson, L. V., and Harris, J. B. (1992). The fate of dystrophin during the degeneration and regeneration of the soleus muscle of the rat. *Acta Neuropathol (Berl).* **83**, 140–148.

Vaughan, C. H., and Rowland, N. E. (2003). Meal patterns of lean and leptin-deficient obese mice in a simulated foraging environment. *Physiol Behav.* **79**, 275–279.

Vaughan, D. W., and Peters, A. (1974). Neuroglial cells in the cerebral cortex of rats from young adulthood to old age: An electron microscope study. *J Neurocytology.* **3**, 405–429.

Vaupel, J. W., Baudisch, A., Dolling, M., Roach, D. A., and Gampe, J. (2004). The case for negative senescence. *Theoret Pop Biol.* **65**, 339–351.

Vaupel, J. W., Carey, J. R., Christensen, K., Johnson, T. E., Yashin, A. I., Holm, N. V., Iachine, I. A., Kannisto, V., Khazaeli, A. A., Liedo, P., Longo, V. D., Zeng, Y., Manton, K. G., and Curtsinger, J. W. (1998). Biodemographic trajectories of longevity. *Science.* **280**, 855–860.

Vaynman, S., Ying, Z., and Gómez-Pinilla, F. (2004). Exercise induces BDNF and synapsin I to specific hippocampal subfields. *J Neurosci Res.* **76**, 356–362.

Vaziri, H., Dessain, S. K., Ng Eaton, E., Imai, S. I., Frye, R. A., Pandita, T. K., Guarente, L., and Weinberg, R. A. (2001). hSIR2(SIRT1) functions as an NAD-dependent p53 deacetylase. *Cell.* **107**, 149–159.

Veerhuis, R., Janssen, I., De Groot, C. J., Van Muiswinkel, F. L., Hack, C. E., and Eikelenboom, P. (1999). Cytokines associated with amyloid plaques in Alzheimer's disease brain stimulate human glial and neuronal cell cultures to secrete early complement proteins, but not C1–inhibitor. *Exp Neurol.* **160**, 289–299.

Veerhuis, R., Van Breemen, M. J., Hoozemans, J. M., Morbin, M., Ouladhadj, J., Tagliavini, F., and Eikelenboom, P. (2003). Amyloid beta plaque-associated proteins C1q and SAP enhance the Abeta1–42 peptide-induced cytokine secretion by adult human microglia *in vitro. Acta Neuropath.* **105,** 135–144.

Velando, A., Drummond, H., Torres, R. (2006). Senescent birds redouble reproductive effort when ill: confirmation of the terminal investment hypothesis. *Proc Roy Soc London Series B.* **273,** 1443–1448.

Vellai, T., Takacs-Vellai, K., Zhang, Y., Kovacs, A. L., Orosz, L., and Muller, F. (2003). Genetics: Influence of TOR kinase on lifespan in *C. elegans. Nature.* **426,** 620.

Venditti, C. P., Lawlor, D. A., Sharma, P., and Chorney, M. J. (1996). Structure and content of the major histocompatibility complex (MHC) class I regions of the great anthropoid apes. *Hum Immunol.* **49,** 71–84.

Veneti, Z., Toda, M. J., and Hurst, G. D. (2004). Host resistance does not explain variation in incidence of male-killing bacteria in *Drosophila* bifasciata. *BMC Evol Biol.* **4,** 52.

Verdery, R. B., and Walford, R. L. (1998). Changes in plasma lipids and lipoproteins in humans during a 2-year period of dietary restriction in Biosphere 2. *Archives of Internal Medicine.* **158,** 900–906.

Vergani, C., Lucchi, T., Caloni, M., Ceconi, I., Calabresi, C., Scurati, S., and Arosio, B. (2006). I405V polymorphism of the cholesteryl ester transfer protein (CETP) gene in young and very old people. *Arch Gerontol Geriatr.* **43,** 213–221.

Vergara, M., Smith-Wheelock, M., Harper, J. M., Sigler, R., and Miller, R. A. (2004). Hormone-treated Snell dwarf mice regain fertility but remain long lived and disease resistant. *J Gerontol. A Biol Sci Med Sci* **59,** 1244–1250.

Verhaeghen, P., and Cerella, J. (2002). Aging, executive control, and attention: A review of meta-analyses. *Neuroscience Biobehavioral Reviews.* **26,** 849–857.

Verheye, S., De Meyer, G. R., Van Langenhove, G., Knaapen, M. W., and Kockx, M. M. (2002). *In vivo* temperature heterogeneity of atherosclerotic plaques is determined by plaque composition. *Circulation.* **105,** 1596–1601.

Verma, S., Kuliszewski, M. A., Li, S. H., Szmitko, P. E., Zucco, L., Wang, C. H., Badiwala, M. V., Mickle, D. A., Weisel, R. D., Fedak, P. W., Stewart, D. J., and Kutryk, M. J. (2004). C-reactive protein attenuates endothelial progenitor cell survival, differentiation, and function: Further evidence of a mechanistic link between C-reactive protein and cardiovascular disease. *Circulation.* **109,** 2058–2067.

Verreault, R., Laurin, D., Lindsay, J., and De Serres, G. (2001). Past exposure to vaccines and subsequent risk of Alzheimer's disease. *Can Med Assoc J.* **165,** 1495–1498.

Verzijl, N., DeGroot, J., Thorpe, S. R., Bank, R. A., Shaw, J. N., Lyons, T. J., Bijlsma, J. W., Lafeber, F. P., Baynes, J. W., and TeKoppele, J. M. (2000). Effect of collagen turnover on the accumulation of advanced glycation end products. *J Biol Chem.* **275,** 39027–39031.

Vickers, M. A., Green, F. R., Terry, C., Mayosi, B. M., Julier, C., Lathrop, M., Ratcliffe, P. J., Watkins, H. C., and Keavney, B. (2002). Genotype at a promoter polymorphism of the interleukin-6 gene is associated with baseline levels of plasma C-reactive protein. *Cardiovasc Res.* **53,** 1029–1034.

Vickers, M. H., Gluckman, P. D., Coveny, A. H., Hofman, P. L., Cutfield, W. S., Gertler, A., Breier, B. H., and Harris, M. (2005). Neonatal leptin treatment reverses developmental programming. *Endocrinology.* **146,** 4211–4216.

Videan, E.N., Fritz, J., Heward, C.B., Murphy, J. (2006). The effects of aging on hormone and reproductive cycles in female chimpanzees (Pan troglodytes). *Comp Med.* **56,** 291–299.

Vigen, C., Hodis, H. N., Selzer, R. H., Mahrer, P. R., and Mack, W. J. (2005). Relation of progression of coronary artery atherosclerosis to risk of cardiovascular events (from the Monitored Atherosclerosis Regression Study). *Am J Cardiol.* **95,** 1277–1282.

Viitanen, L., Pihlajamèaki, J., Miettinen, R., Karkkainen, P., Vauhkonen, I., Halonen, P., Kareinen, A., Lehto, S., and Laakso, M. (2001). Apolipoprotein E gene promoter (-219G/T) polymorphism is associated with premature coronary heart disease. *J Mol Med.* **79,** 732–737.

Vijayamalini, M., and Manoharan, S. (2004). Lipid peroxidation, vitamins C, E and reduced glutathione levels in patients with pulmonary tuberculosis. *Cell Biochem Funct.* **22,** 19–22.

Villar, J., and Belizan, J. M. (1982). The relative contribution of prematurity and fetal growth retardation to low birth weight in developing and developed societies. *Am J Obstet Gynecol.* **143,** 793–798.

Vineis, P., Alavanja, M., Buffler, P., Fontham, E., Franceschi, S., Gao, Y. T., Gupta, P. C., Hackshaw, A., Matos, E., Samet, J., Sitas, F., Smith, J., Stayner, L., Straif, K., Thun, M. J., Wichmann, H. E., Wu, A. H., Zaridze, D., Peto, R., and Doll, R. (2004). Tobacco and cancer: Recent epidemiological evidence. *J Natl Canc Inst.* **96,** 99–106.

Virmani, R., Burke, A. P., Kolodgie, F. D., and Farb, A. (2003). Pathology of the thin-cap fibroatheroma: A type of vulnerable plaque. *J Intervent Cardiol.* **16,** 267–272.

Visscher, T. L., and Seidell, J. C. (2001). The public health impact of obesity. *Annu Rev Public Health.* **22,** 355–375.

Vlassara, H. (2005). Advanced glycation in health and disease: Role of the modern environment. *Ann NY Acad Sci.* **1043,** 452–460.

Vlassara, H., Cai, W., Crandall, J., Goldberg, T., Oberstein, R., Dardaine, V., Peppa, M., and Rayfield, E. J. (2002). Inflammatory mediators are induced by dietary glycotoxins, a major risk factor for diabetic angiopathy. [erratum appears in *Proc Natl Acad Sci USA.* 2003;100(2):763.]. *Proc Natl Acad Sci USA.* **99,** 15596–15601.

Volkow, N. D., Logan, J., Fowler, J. S., Wang, G. J., Gur, R. C., Wong, C., Felder, C., Gatley, S. J., Ding, Y. S., Hitzemann, R., and Pappas, N. (2000). Association between age-related decline in brain dopamine activity and impairment in frontal and cingulate metabolism. *Am J Psychiatry.* **157,** 75–80.

vom Saal, F., Finch C. E., and Nelson, J. (1994). The natural history of reproductive aging in humans, laboratory rodents, and selected other vertebrates. In E. Knobil, Ed., *Physiology of reproduction*, Vol. 2, pp. 1213–1314. New York: Raven Press.

vom Saal, F. S. (1989). The production of and sensitivity to cues that delay puberty and prolong subsequent oestrous cycles in female mice are influenced by prior intrauterine position. *J Reprod Fert.* **86,** 457–471.

von Hundelshausen, P., Weber, K. S., Huo, Y., Proudfoot, A. E., Nelson, P. J., Ley, K., and Weber, C. (2001). RANTES deposition by platelets triggers monocyte arrest on inflamed and atherosclerotic endothelium. *Circulation.* **103,** 1772–1777.

Von Kanel, R., Dimsdale, J. E., Mills, P. J., Ancoli-Israel, S., Patterson, T. L., Mausbach, B. T., Grant, I. (2006). Effect of Alzheimer caregiving stress and age on frailty markers inter-leukin-6, C-reactive protein, and D-dimer. *J Gerontol A Biol Sci Med Sci.* **61,** 963–969.

von Schacky, C., and Dyerberg, J. (2001). Omega 3 fatty acids. From Eskimos to clinical cardiology—What took us so long? *World Review of Nutrition and Dietetics.* **88,** 90–99.

von Zglinicki, T., and Martin-Ruiz, C. M. (2005). Telomeres as biomarkers for ageing and age-related diseases. *Curr Mol Med.* **5,** 197–203.

von Zglinicki, T., Serra, V., Lorenz, M., Saretzki, G., Lenzen-Grossimlighaus, R., Gessner, R., Risch, A., and Steinhagen-Thiessen, E. (2000). Short telomeres in patients with vascular dementia: An indicator of low antioxidative capacity and a possible risk factor? *Lab Invest.* **80,** 1739–1747.

Voravuthikunchai, S. P., Chaowana, C., Perepat, P., Iida, T., and Honda, T. (2005). Antibodies among healthy population of developing countries against enterohaemorrhagic *Escherichia coli* O157:H7. *J Health Popul Nutr.* **23,** 305–310.

Vuorinen, H. S. (2006). *Tautinen Suomi 1857–1865.* Tampere, Finland: Tampere University Press.

Waaler, H. T. (1984). Height, weight and mortality. The Norwegian experience. *Acta Med Scand. Suppl.* **679,** 1–56

Wade, S., Bleiberg, F., Mossé, A., Lubetzki, J., Flavigny, H., Chapuis, P., Roche, D., Lemonnier, D., and Dardenne, M. (1985). Thymulin (Zn-facteur thymique serique) activity in anorexia nervosa patients. *Am J Clin Nutr.* **42,** 275–280.

Wadham, C., Albanese, N., Roberts, J., Wang, L., Bagley, C. J., Gamble, J. R., Rye, K. A., Barter, P. J., Vadas, M. A., and Xia, P. (2004). High-density lipoproteins neutralize C-reactive protein proinflammatory activity. *Circulation.* **109,** 2116–2122.

Wagner, J. D., and Clarkson, T. B. (2005). The applicability of hormonal effects on atherosclerosis in animals to heart disease in postmenopausal women. *Seminars in Reproductive Medicine.* **23,** 149–156.

Wald, N. J., and Law, M. R. (2003). A strategy to reduce cardiovascular disease by more than 80%. *Br Med J.* **326,** 1419.

Waldron, I. (1985). What do we know about causes of sex differences in mortality? A review of the literature. *Popul Bull United Nations.* **18,** 59–76.

Walford, R. L. (1969). *The immunological theory of aging.* Copenhagen: Munksgaard.

Walford, R. L., Bechtel, R., MacCallum, T., Paglia, D. E., and Weber, L. J. (1996). "Biospheric medicine" as viewed from the two-year first closure of Biosphere 2. *Aviat Space Environ Med.* **67,** 609–617.

Walford, R. L., Harris, S. B., and Gunion, M. W. (1992). The calorically restricted low-fat nutrient-dense diet in Biosphere 2 significantly lowers blood glucose, total leukocyte count, cholesterol, and blood pressure in humans. *Proc Natl Acad Sci USA.* **89,** 11533–11537.

Walford, R. L., Mock, D., MacCallum, T., and Laseter, J. L. (1999). Physiologic changes in humans subjected to severe, selective calorie restriction for two years in Biosphere 2: Health, aging, and toxicological perspectives. *Toxicol Sci.* **52,** 61–65.

Walford, R. L., Mock, D., Verdery, R., and MacCallum, T. (2002). Calorie restriction in Biosphere 2: Alterations in physiologic, hematologic, hormonal, and biochemical parameters in humans restricted for a 2-year period. *J Gerontol. A Biol Sci Med Sci.* **57,** B211–224.

Walford, R. L., and Sjaarda, J. R. (1964). Increase of Thioflavine-T-staining material (amyloid) in human tissues with age. *J Gerontol.* **19,** 57–61.

Walford, R. L., and Spindler, S. R. (1997). The response to calorie restriction in mammals shows features also common to hibernation: A cross-adaptation hypothesis. *J Gerontol. A Biol Sci Med Sci.* **52,** B179–183.

Walker, D. G., and McGeer, P. L. (1992). Complement gene expression in human brain: Comparison between normal and Alzheimer disease cases. *Brain Res. Mol Brain Res.* **14,** 109–116.

Walker, D. W., Muffat, J., Rundel, C., and Benzer, S. (2006b). Overexpression of a *Drosophila* homolog of apolipoprotein D leads to increased stress resistance and extended lifespan. *Curr Biol.* **16,** 674–679.

Walker, G., Houthoofd, K., Vanfleteren, J. R., and Gems, D. (2005). Dietary restriction in *C. elegans*: From rate-of-living effects to nutrient sensing pathways. *Mech Ageing Dev.* **126,** 929–937.

Walker, N. J., Crockett, P. W., Nyska, A., Brix, A. E., Jokinen, M. P., Sells, D. M., Hailey, J. R., Easterling, M., Haseman, J. K., Yin, M., Wyde, M. E., Bucher, J. R., and Portier, C. J. (2005). Dose-additive carcinogenicity of a defined mixture of "dioxin-like compounds". *Environ Health Perspect.* **113,** 43–48.

Walker, R., Gurven, M., Hill, K., Migliano, A., Chagnon, N., De Souza, R., Djurovic, G., Hames, R., Hurtado, A. M., Kaplan, H., Kramer, K., Oliver, W. J., Valeggia, C., and Yamauchi, T. (2006a). Growth rates and life histories in twenty-two small-scale societies. *Am J Hum Biol.* **18,** 295–311.

Wallace, D. C. (2005). A mitochondrial paradigm of metabolic and degenerative diseases, aging, and cancer: A dawn for evolutionary medicine. *Annu Rev Genetics.* **39,** 359–407.

Walsh, D. M., Townsend, M., Podlisny, M. B., Shankar, G. M., Fadeeva, J. V., Agnaf, O. E., Hartley, D. M., and Selkoe, D. J. (2005). Certain inhibitors of synthetic amyloid beta-peptide (Abeta) fibrillogenesis block oligomerization of natural Abeta and thereby rescue long-term potentiation. *J Neurosci.* **25,** 2455–2462.

Walter, D. H., Dimmeler, S., and Zeiher, A. M. (2004). Effects of statins on endothelium and endothelial progenitor cell recruitment. *Seminars in Vascular Medicine.* **4,** 385–393.

Walters, M. J., Paul-Clark, M. J., McMaster, S. K., Ito, K., Adcock, I. M., and Mitchell, J. A. (2005). Cigarette smoke activates human monocytes by an oxidant-AP-1 signaling pathway: Implications for steroid resistance. *Mol Pharmacol.* **68,** 1343–1353.

Wang, C., Wilson, W. A., Moore, S. D., Mace, B. E., Maeda, N., Schmechel, D. E., and Sullivan, P. M. (2005a). Human apoE4-targeted replacement mice display synaptic deficits in the absence of neuropathology. *Neurobiol Dis.* **18,** 390–398.

Wang, J., Ho, L., Qin, W., Rocher, A. B., Seror, I., Humala, N., Maniar, K., Dolios, G., Wang, R., Hof, P. R., and Pasinetti, G. M. (2005b). Caloric restriction attenuates beta-amyloid neuropathology in a mouse model of Alzheimer's disease. *FASEB J.* **19,** 659–661.

Wang, L., Wang, X., Laird, N., Zuckerman, B., Stubblefield, P., and Xu, X. (2006). Polymorphism in maternal LRP8 gene is associated with fetal growth. *Am J Hum Genet.* **78,** 770–777.

Wang, M., and Lakatta, E. G. (2006). Central arterial aging: Humans to molecules. In M. Safar, Ed., *Handbook of hypertension,* **23, pp. 137-160**. London: Elsevier.

Wang, M., Takagi, G., Asai, K., Resuello, R. G., Natividad, F. F., Vatner, D. E., Vatner, S. F., and Lakatta, E. G. (2003a). Aging increases aortic MMP-2 activity and angiotensin II in nonhuman primates. *Hypertension.* **41,** 1308–1316.

Wang, M., Zhang, J., Spinetti, G., Jiang, L. Q., Monticone, R., Zhao, D., Cheng, L., Krawczyk, M., Talan, M., Pintus, G., and Lakatta, E. G. (2005d). Angiotensin II activates matrix metalloproteinase type II and mimics age-associated carotid arterial remodeling in young rats. *Am J Pathol.* **167,** 1429–1442.

Wang, W. H., Huang, J. Q., Zheng, G. F., Lam, S. K., Karlberg, J., and Wong, B. C. (2003b). Non-steroidal anti-inflammatory drug use and the risk of gastric cancer: A systematic review and meta-analysis. *J Natl Can Inst.* **95,** 1784–1791.

Wang, W. H., Wong, W. M., Dailidiene, D., Berg, D. E., Gu, Q., Lai, K. C., Lam, S. K., and Wong, B. C. (2003c). Aspirin inhibits the growth of *Helicobacter pylori* and enhances its susceptibility to antimicrobial agents. *Gut.* **52,** 490–495.

Wang, X. Y., Hurme, M., Jylhèa, M., and Hervonen, A. (2001). Lack of association between human longevity and polymorphisms of IL-1 cluster, IL-6, IL-10 and TNF-alpha genes in Finnish nonagenarians. *Mech Ageing Dev.* **123,** 29–38.

Wang, Y., Michikawa, Y., Mallidis, C., Bai, Y., Woodhouse, L., Yarasheski, K. E., Miller, C. A., Askanas, V., Engel, W. K., Bhasin, S., and Attardi, G. (2001b). Muscle-specific mutations accumulate with aging in critical human mtDNA control sites for replication. *Proc Natl Acad Sci USA*. **98,** 4022–4027.

Wang, Y. X. (2005). Cardiovascular functional phenotypes and pharmacological responses in apolipoprotein E deficient mice. *Neurobiol Aging*. **26,** 309–316.

Wang, Z., Zeng, Y., Jeune, B., and Vaupel, J. W. (1998). Age validation of Han Chinese centenarians. *Genus*. **54,** 123–141.

Wanhainen, A., Bergqvist, D., Boman, K., Nilsson, T. K., Rutegard, J., and Bjorck, M. (2005). Risk factors associated with abdominal aortic aneurysm: A population-based study with historical and current data. *J Vascular Surgery*. **41,** 390–396.

Wardle, J., Guthrie, C., Sanderson, S., Birch, L., and Plomin, R. (2001). Food and activity preferences in children of lean and obese parents. *Int J Obesity and Related Metabolic Disorders*. **25,** 971–977.

Warner, H. R. (2004). Current status of efforts to measure and modulate the biological rate of aging. *J Gerontol*. **59,** 692–696.

Waterland, R. A., Lin, J. R., Smith, C. A., and Jirtle, R. L. (2006). Post-weaning diet affects genomic imprinting at the insulin-like growth factor 2 (Igf2) locus. *Hum Mol Genet*. **15,** 705–716.

Waterlow, J. C. (1984). Protein turnover with special reference to man. *Q J Exp Physiol*. **69,** 409–438.

Waters, A. P., Higgins, D. G., and McCutchan, T. F. (1993). Evolutionary relatedness of some primate models of *Plasmodium*. *Mol Biol Evol*. **10,** 914–923.

Waters, A. P., Higgins, D. G., and McCutchan, T. F. (1991). *Plasmodium falciparum* appears to have arisen as a result of lateral transfer between avian and human hosts. *Proc Natl Acad Sci USA*. **88,** 3140–3144.

Wautier, M. P., Chappey, O., Corda, S., Stern, D. M., Schmidt, A. M., and Wautier, J. L. (2001). Activation of NADPH oxidase by AGE links oxidant stress to altered gene expression via RAGE. *Am J Physiol. Endocrinol Metab*. **280,** E685–694.

Waxman, A. B., Mahboubi, K., Knickelbein, R. G., Mantell, L. L., Manzo, N., Pober, J. S., and Elias, J. A. (2003). IL-11 and IL-6 protect cultured human endothelial cells from H2O2-induced cell death. *Am J Respir Cell Mol Biol*. **29,** 513–522

Weaver, I. C., D'Alessio, A. C., Brown, S. E., Hellstromm, I. C., Dymov, S., Sharma, S., Szyf, M., Meaney, M. J. (2007). The transcription factor nerve growth factor-inducible protein a mediates epigenetic programming: altering epigenetic marks by immediate-early genes. *J Neurosci*. **27,** 1756–1768.

Weaver, J. D., Huang, M. H., Albert, M., Harris, T., Rowe, J. W., and Seeman, T. E. (2002). Interleukin-6 and risk of cognitive decline: MacArthur studies of successful aging. *Neurology*. **59,** 371–378.

Webb, P. M., Knight, T., Greaves, S., Wilson, A., Newell, D. G., Elder, J., and Forman, D. (1994). Relation between infection with *Helicobacter pylori* and living conditions in childhood: Evidence for person to person transmission in early life. *Br Med J*. **308,** 750–753.

Webster, P. (2003). Infant mortality is falling in Russia, latest figures suggest. *Lancet*. **361,** 758.

Webster, R. G., and Virology. (2000). Immunity to influenza in the elderly. *Vaccine*. **18,** 1686–1689.

Webster, S. D., Yang, A. J., Margol, L., Garzon-Rodriguez, W., Glabe, C. G., and Tenner, A. J. (2000). Complement component C1q modulates the phagocytosis of Abeta by microglia. *Exp Neurol*. **161,** 127–138.

Weggen, S., Eriksen, J. L., Sagi, S. A., Pietrzik, C. U., Ozols, V., Fauq, A., Golde, T. E., and Koo, E. H. (2003). Evidence that nonsteroidal anti-inflammatory drugs decrease amyloid beta 42 production by direct modulation of gamma-secretase activity. *J Biol Chem.* **278,** 31831–31837.

Wegiel, J., Imaki, H., Wang, K. C., Wronska, A., Osuchowski, M., and Rubenstein, R. (2003). Origin and turnover of microglial cells in fibrillar plaques of APPsw transgenic mice. *Acta Neuropath.* **105,** 393–402.

Wegner, K. M., Kalbe, M., Schaschl, H., and Reusch, T. B. (2004). Parasites and individual major histocompatibility complex diversity—An optimal choice? *Microbes Infect.* **6,** 1110–1116.

Weight, L. M., Alexander, D., and Jacobs, P. (1991). Strenuous exercise: Analogous to the acute-phase response? *Clin Sci.* **81,** 677–683.

Weindruch, R. (1992). Effect of caloric restriction on age-associated cancers. *Exp Gerontol.* **27,** 575–581.

Weindruch, R., Gottesman, S. R., and Walford, R. L. (1982). Modification of age-related immune decline in mice dietarily restricted from or after midadulthood. *Proc Natl Acad Sci USA.* **79,** 898–902.

Weindruch, R., Kayo, T., Lee, C. K., and Prolla, T. A. (2002). Gene expression profiling of aging using DNA microarrays. *Mech Ageing Dev.* **123,** 177–193.

Weindruch, R., Keenan, K. P., Carney, J. M., Fernandes, G., Feuers, R. J., Floyd, R. A., Halter, J. B., Ramsey, J. J., Richardson, A., Roth, G. S., and Spindler, S. R. (2001). Caloric restriction mimetics: Metabolic interventions. *J Gerontol. A Biol Sci Med Sci.* **56,** 20–33.

Weindruch, R., Lane, M. A., Ingram, D. K., Ershler, W. B., and Roth, G. S. (1997). Dietary restriction in rhesus monkeys: Lymphopenia and reduced mitogen-induced proliferation in peripheral blood mononuclear cells. *Aging.* **9,** 304–308.

Weindruch, R., and Prolla, T. A. (2002). Gene expression profile of the aging brain. *Arch Neurol.* **59,** 1712–1714.

Weindruch, R., and Walford, R. L. (1982). Dietary restriction in mice beginning at 1 year of age: Effect on life-span and spontaneous cancer incidence. *Science.* **215,** 1415–1418.

Weindruch, R. H., and Walford, R. L. (1988). *The retardation of aging and disease by dietary restriction.* Springfield, IL: C.C. Thomas.

Weisberg, S. P., McCann, D., Desai, M., Rosenbaum, M., Leibel, R. L., and Ferrante, A. W., Jr. (2003). Obesity is associated with macrophage accumulation in adipose tissue. *J Clin Invest.* **112,** 1796–1808.

Weiss, R., Taksali, S. E., and Caprio, S. (2006). Development of type 2 diabetes in children and adolescents. *Curr Diab Rep.* **6,** 182–187.

Weksler, M. E., and Goodhardt, M. (2002). Do age-associated changes in 'physiologic' autoantibodies contribute to infection, atherosclerosis, and Alzheimer's disease? *Exp Gerontol.* **37,** 971–979.

Wells, J. C. (2007). The thrifty phenotype as an adaptive maternal effect. *Biol Rev Camb Philos Soc.* **82,** 143–172.

Wells, J. C. K. (2000). Natural selection and sex differences in morbidity and mortality in early life. *J Theor Biol.* **202,** 65–76.

Weltman, A., Weltman, J. Y., Roy, C. P., Wideman, L., Patrie, J., Evans, W. S., and Veldhuis, J. D. (2006). The growth hormone (GH) response to graded exercise intensities is attenuated and the gender difference abolished in older adults. *J Appl Physiol.* **100,** 1623–1629.

Wen, J. J., Yachelini, P. C., Sembaj, A., Manzur, R. E., and Garg, N. J. (2006). Increased oxidative stress is correlated with mitochondrial dysfunction in chagasic patients. *Free Radic Biol Med.* **41,** 270–276.

Wertheim, B., Kraaijeveld, A. R., Schuster, E., Blanc, E., Hopkins, M., Pletcher, S. D., Strand, M. R., Partridge, L., and Godfray, H. C. (2005). Genome-wide gene expression in response to parasitoid attack in *Drosophila. Genome Biol.* **6,** R94.

Wessells, R. J., Fitzgerald, E., Cypser, J. R., Tatar, M., and Bodmer, R. (2004). Insulin regulation of heart function in aging fruit flies. *Nature Genet.* **36,** 1275–1281.

West, A. P., Jr., Llamas, L. L., Snow, P. M., Benzer, S., and Bjorkman, P. J. (2001). Crystal structure of the ectodomain of Methuselah, a *Drosophila* G protein-coupled receptor associated with extended lifespan. *Proc Natl Acad Sci USA.* **98,** 3744–3749.

West, M. D., Pereira-Smith, O. M., and Smith, J. R. (1989). Replicative senescence of human skin fibroblasts correlates with a loss of regulation and overexpression of collagenase activity. *Exp Cell Res.* **184,** 138–147.

Westendorp, R. G., Langermans, J. A., Huizinga, T. W., Elouali, A. H., Verweij, C. L., Boomsma, D. I., and Vandenbroucke, J. P. (1997a). Genetic influence on cytokine production and fatal meningococcal disease. *Lancet.* **349,** 170–173.

Westendorp, R. G., Langermans, J. A., Huizinga, T. W., Verweij, C. L., and Sturk, A. (1997b). Genetic influence on cytokine production in meningococcal disease. *Lancet.* **349,** 1912–1913.

Wexler, B. C. (1964). Spontaneous coronary arteriosclerosis in repeatedly bred male and female rats. *Circ Res.* **14,** 32–43.

Wexler, B. C. (1976). Comparative aspects of hyperadrenocorticism and aging. In *Hypothalamus, pituitary, and aging,* A. V. Everitt and J. A. Burgess, Eds., pp. 333–361. Springfield, IL: C. C. Thomas.

Wexler, B. C., Brown, T. E., and Miller, B. F. (1960). Atherosclerosis in rats induced by repeated breedings, ACTH and unilateral nephrectomy. Acid mucopolysaccharides, fibroplasia, elastosis and other changes in early lesions. *Circ Res.* **8,** 278–286.

Wexler, B. C., and Miller, B. F. (1958). Severe arteriosclerosis and other diseases in the rat produced by corticotrophin. *Science.* **127,** 590–591.

Wexler, B. C., and True, C. W. (1963). Carotid and cerebral arteriosclerosis in the rat. *Circulation Research.* **12,** 659–666.

Weyer, C., Walford, R. L., Harper, I. T., Milner, M., MacCallum, T., Tataranni, P. A., and Ravussin, E. (2000). Energy metabolism after 2 y of energy restriction: The biosphere 2 experiment. *Am J Clin Nutr.* **72,** 946–953.

Wheeler, J. C., Bieschke, E. T., and Tower, J. (1995). Muscle-specific expression of *Drosophila* hsp70 in response to aging and oxidative stress. *Proc Natl Acad Sci USA.* **92,** 10408–10412.

Wheeler, J. C., King, V., and Tower, J. (1999). Sequence requirements for upregulated expression of *Drosophila* hsp70 transgenes during aging. *Neurobiol Aging.* **20,** 545–553.

Whitaker, H. A., and Selnes, O. A. (1975). Anatomic variations in the cortex. Individual variations and the problem of localization of language functions. *Ann NY Acad Sci.* **280,** 844–854.

Whitcombe, C. (2003). //witcombe.sbc.edu/willendorf/willendorfdiscovery.

White, J. G., Southgate, E., Thomson, J. N., and Brenner, S. (1976). The structure of the ventral nerve cord of *Caenorhabditis elegans. Philos Trans R Soc Lond B Biol Sci.* **275,** 327–348.

White, T. D., WoldeGabriel, G., Asfaw, B., Ambrose, S., Beyene, Y., Bernor, R. L., Boisserie, J. R., Currie, B., Gilbert, H., Haile-Selassie, Y., Hart, W. K., Hlusko, L. J., Howell, F. C., Kono, R. T., Lehmann, T., Louchart, A., Lovejoy, C. O., Renne, P. R., Saegusa, H., Vrba, E. S., Wesselman, H., and Suwa, G. (2006). Asa Issie, Aramis and the origin of *Australopithecus. Nature.* **440,** 883–889.

Whiten, A., Goodall, J., McGrew, W. C., Nishida, T., Reynolds, V., Sugiyama, Y., Tutin, C. E., Wrangham, R. W., and Boesch, C. (1999). Cultures in chimpanzees. *Nature.* **399,** 682–685.

Whitten, P. L. (1987). Infants and adult males. In: *Primate Societies* (Smuts, B. B., Cheney, D. L., Seyfarth, R. M., Wrangham, R. W., Struhsaker, T. T., eds), pp. 343–357. Chicago: U Chicago Press.

Wich, S. A., Utami-Atmoko, S. S., Setia, T. M., Rijksen, H. D., Schurmann, C., van Hooff, J. A., van Schaik, C. P. (2004). Life history of wild Sumatran orangutans (Pongo abelii). *J Hum Evol.* **47,** 385–398.

Wichmann, M. W., Inthorn, D., Andress, H. J., and Schildberg, F. W. (2000). Incidence and mortality of severe sepsis in surgical intensive care patients: The influence of patient gender on disease process and outcome. *Intensive Care Med.* **26,** 167–172.

Widdowson, E. M., Mavor, W. O., and McCance, R. A. (1964). The effect of undernutrition and rehabilitation on the development of the reproductive organs: Rats. *J Endocrinol.* **29,** 119–126.

Widdowson, E. M., and McCance, R. A. (1959). The effect of food and growth on the metabolism of phosphorus in the newly born. *Acta Paediatr.* **48,** 383–387.

Widdowson, E. M., and McCance, R. A. (1975). A review: New thoughts on growth. *Pediatr Res.* **9,** 154–156.

Wiersma, P., Salomons, H. M., and Verhulst, S. (2005). Metabolic adjustments to increasing foraging costs of starlings in a closed economy. *J Exp Biol.* **208,** 4099–4108.

Wiersma, P., and Verhulst, S. (2005). Effects of intake rate on energy expenditure, somatic repair and reproduction of zebra finches. *J Exp Biol.* **208,** 4091–4098.

Wierzbicki, A. S., Poston, R., and Ferro, A. (2003). The lipid and non-lipid effects of statins. *Pharmacol Therap.* **99,** 95–112.

Wikby, A., Ferguson, F., Forsey, R., Thompson, J., Strindhall, J., Lèofgren, S., Nilsson, B. O., Ernerudh, J., Pawelec, G., and Johansson, B. (2005). An immune risk phenotype, cognitive impairment, and survival in very late life: Impact of allostatic load in Swedish octogenarian and nonagenarian humans. *J Gerontol. A Biol Sci Med Sci.* **60,** 556–565.

Wilcox, J. N., Subramanian, R. R., Sundell, C. L., Tracey, W. R., Pollock, J. S., Harrison, D. G., and Marsden, P. A. (1997). Expression of multiple isoforms of nitric oxide synthase in normal and atherosclerotic vessels. *Arterioscler Thromb Vasc Biol.* **17,** 2479–2488.

Wildman, D. E., Uddin, M., Liu, G., Grossman, L. I., and Goodman, M. (2003). Implications of natural selection in shaping 99.4% nonsynonymous DNA identity between humans and chimpanzees: Enlarging genus *Homo. Proc Natl Acad Sci USA.* **100,** 7181–7188.

Wilens, S. L., and Sproul, E. E. (1938a). Spontaneous cardiovascular disease in the rat. I. Lesions of the heart. *Am J Pathol.* **14,** 177–200.

Wilens, S. L., and Sproul, E. E. (1938b). Spontaneous cardiovascular disease in the rat. II. Lesions of the vascular system. *Am J Pathol.* **14,** 201–216.

Wilgram, G. F., and Ingle, D. J. (1959). Renal-cardiovascular pathologic changes in aging female breeder rats. *Arch Pathol.* **68,** 690—703.

Wilkinson, G. S., and South, J. M. (2002). Life history, ecology and longevity in bats. *Aging Cell.* **1,** 124–131.

Wilkinson, P., Leach, C., Ah-Sing, E. E., Hussain, N., Miller, G. J., Millward, D. J., and Griffin, B. A. (2005). Influence of alpha-linolenic acid and fish-oil on markers of cardiovascular risk in subjects with an atherogenic lipoprotein phenotype. *Atherosclerosis.* **181,** 115–124.

Williams, C. E., Davenport, E. S., Sterne, J. A., Sivapathasundaram, V., Fearne, J. M., and Curtis, M. A. (2000). Mechanisms of risk in preterm low-birthweight infants. *Periodontol.* **23,** 142–150.

Williams, G. C. (1957). Pleiotropy, natural selection, and the evolution of senescence. *Evolution.* **11,** 398–411.

Williams, G. C., and Nesse, R. M. (1998). Evolution and the origins of disease. *Scientific American.* **279,** 86–93.

Williams, P. T., Blanche, P. J., and Krauss, R. M. (2005a). Behavioral versus genetic correlates of lipoproteins and adiposity in identical twins discordant for exercise. *Circulation.* **112,** 350–356.

Williams, P. T., Blanche, P. J., Rawlings, R., and Krauss, R. M. (2005b). Concordant lipoprotein and weight responses to dietary fat change in identical twins with divergent exercise levels 1. *Am J Clin Nutr.* **82,** 181–187.

Wilson, C. J., Finch, C. E., and Cohen, H. J. (2002). Mechanisms of cognitive impairment. Cytokines and cognition—The case for a head-to-toe inflammatory paradigm. *J Am Geriatr Soc.* **50,** 2041–2056.

Wilson, M. G. (1940). *Rheumatic Fever. Studies of the epidemiology, manifestations, diagnosis, and treatment of the disease, pp.* 272–281.

Wilson, P. W., Myers, R. H., Larson, M. G., Ordovas, J. M., Wolf, P. A., and Schaefer, E. J. (1994). Apolipoprotein E alleles, dyslipidemia, and coronary heart disease. The Framingham Offspring Study. *JAMA.* **272,** 1666–1671.

Wimmer, R., Kirsch, S., Rappold, G. A., and Schempp, W. (2005). Evolutionary breakpoint analysis on Y chromosomes of higher primates provides insight into human Y evolution. *Cytogenet Genome Res.* **108,** 204–210.

Wing, E. J., and Barczynski, L. K. (1984). Effect of acute nutritional deprivation on immune function in mice. II. Response to sublethal radiation. *Clin Immunol Immunopath.* **30,** 479–487.

Wing, E. J., Barczynski, L. K., and Boehmer, S. M. (1983a). Effect of acute nutritional deprivation on immune function in mice. I. Macrophages. *Immunology.* **48,** 543–550.

Wing, E. J., Barczynski, L. K., and Sherbondy, J. M. (1986). Effect of acute nutritional deprivation on macrophage colony-stimulating factor and macrophage progenitor cells in mice. *Infect Immun* **54,** 245–249.

Wing, E. J., Stanko, R. T., Winkelstein, A., and Adibi, S. A. (1983b). Fasting-enhanced immune effector mechanisms in obese subjects. *Am J Medicine.* **75,** 91–96.

Wing, E. J., and Young, J. B. (1980). Acute starvation protects mice against *Listeria monocytogenes. Infect Immun.* **28,** 771–776.

Winick, M. (1968). Cellular response with increased feeding in pituitary dwarf mice. *J Nutr.* **94,** 121–124.

Wise, P. M., Dubal, D. B., Rau, S. W., Brown, C. M., and Suzuki, S. (2005). Are estrogens protective or risk factors in brain injury and neurodegeneration? Reevaluation after the Women's Health Initiative. *Endocr Rev.* **26,** 308–312.

Wise, P. M., Smith, M. J., Dubal, D. B., Wilson, M. E., Krajnak, K. M., and Rosewell, K. L. (1999). Neuroendocrine influences and repercussions of the menopause. *Endocr Rev* **20**, 243–248.

Wisniewski, H. M., and Terry, R. D. (1973). Morphology of the aging brain, human and animal. In D. H. Ford, Ed., *Neurobiological aspects of maturation and aging*, Vol. 40, pp. 167–186. Amsterdam: Elsevier.

Wissler, R. W., Eilert, M. L., Schroeder, M. A., and Cohen, L. (1954). Production of lipomatous and atheromatous arterial lesions in the albino rat. *Arch Pathol.* **57**, 333–351.

Wit, J. M., Balen, H. V., Kamp, G. A., Oostdijk, W. (2004). Benefit of postponing normal puberty for improving final height. *Eur J Endocrinol Suppl.* **1**, S41–45.

Witcombe, L. C. E. (2005). *Venus of Willendorf. http://witcombe.sbc.edu/willendorf/.*

Wolday, D., Mayaan, S., Mariam, Z. G., Berhe, N., Seboxa, T., Britton, S., Galai, N., Landay, A., and Bentwich, Z. (2002). Treatment of intestinal worms is associated with decreased HIV plasma viral load. *J Acquir Immune Defic Syndr.* **31**, 56–62.

Wolf, G. (2006). Calorie restriction increases life span: A molecular mechanism. *Nutr Rev.* **64**, 89–92.

Wolf, G. (2006b). Gut microbiota: A factor in energy regulation. *Nutr Rev.* **64**, 47–50.

Wolf, M. J., Amrein, H., Izatt, J. A., Choma, M. A., Reedy, M. C., and Rockman, H. A. (2006). *Drosophila* as a model for the identification of genes causing adult human heart disease. *Proc Natl Acad Sci USA.* **103**, 1394–1399.

Wolff, S., Ma, H., Burch, D., Maciel, G. A., Hunter, T., and Dillin, A. (2006). SMK-1, an essential regulator of DAF-16–mediated longevity. *Cell.* **124**, 1039–1053.

Wolfner, M. F. (2002). The gifts that keep on giving: Physiological functions and evolutionary dynamics of male seminal proteins in *Drosophila. Heredity.* **88**, 85–93.

Wolkow, C. A., Kimura, K. D., Lee, M. S., and Ruvkun, G. (2000). Regulation of *C. elegans* life-span by insulinlike signaling in the nervous system. *Science.* **290**, 147–150.

Wolozin, B., Kellman, W., Ruosseau, P., Celesia, G. G., and Siegel, G. (2000). Decreased prevalence of Alzheimer disease associated with 3-hydroxy-3-methyglutaryl coenzyme A reductase inhibitors. *Arch Neurol.* **57**, 1439–1443.

Wong, A., Luth, H. J., Deuther-Conrad, W., Dukic-Stefanovic, S., Gasic-Milenkovic, J., Arendt, T., and Munch, G. (2001). Advanced glycation endproducts co-localize with inducible nitric oxide synthase in Alzheimer's disease. *Brain Res.* **920**, 32–40.

Wong, D. F., Young, D., Wilson, P. D., Meltzer, C. C., and Gjedde, A. (1997). Quantification of neuroreceptors in the living human brain: III. D2-like dopamine receptors: Theory, validation, and changes during normal aging. *J Cereb Blood Flow Metab.* **17**, 316–330.

Wood, J. G., Rogina, B., Lavu, S., Howitz, K., Helfand, S. L., Tatar, M., and Sinclair, D. (2004). Sirtuin activators mimic caloric restriction and delay ageing in metazoans. *Nature.* **430**, 686–689.

Woodruff-Pak, D. S. (2001). Eyeblink classical conditioning differentiates normal aging from Alzheimer's disease. *Integr Physiol Behav Sci.* **36**, 87–108.

Woollett, L. A. (2005). Maternal cholesterol in fetal development: Transport of cholesterol from the maternal to the fetal circulation. *Am J Clin Nutr.* **82**, 1155–1161.

Wootton, D. M., and Ku, D. N. (1999). Fluid mechanics of vascular systems, diseases and thrombosis. *Annu Rev Biomed Eng.* **1**, 299–329.

World Health Organization. (2002). Reducing risks, promoting healthy life style. Geneva: World Health Organization.

World Health Organization. (2005a). Low Birthweight. Country, regional, and global estimates. Geneva: UNICEF.

World Health Organization. (2005b). Major causes of death among children under five and neonates, worldwide, 2000–2003, Vol. 2006. Geneva: World Health Organization.

Wouters, K., Shiri-Sverdlov, R., van Gorp, P. J., van Bilsen, M., and Hofker, M. H. (2005). Understanding hyperlipidemia and atherosclerosis: Lessons from genetically modified apoe and ldlr mice. *Clin Chem Lab Med.* **43,** 470–479.

Wozniak, M. A., Cookson, A., Wilcock, G. K., and Itzhaki, R. F. (2003). Absence of *Chlamydia pneumoniae* in brain of vascular dementia patients. *Neurobiol Aging.* **24,** 761–765.

Wozniak, M. A., Itzhaki, R. F., Faragher, E. B., James, M. W., Ryder, S. D., and Irving, W. L. (2002). Apolipoprotein E-epsilon 4 protects against severe liver disease caused by hepatitis C virus. *Hepatology.* **36,** 456–463.

Wozniak, M. A., Shipley, S. J., Combrinck, M., Wilcock, G. K., and Itzhaki, R. F. (2005). Productive herpes simplex virus in brain of elderly normal subjects and Alzheimer's disease patients. *J Med Virol.* **75,** 300–306.

Wrangham, R. W., Conklin-Brittain, N. L. (2003). The biological significance of cooking in human evolution. *Comp Biochem Physiol A.* **135,** 35–46.

Wrangham, R. W. (2007). The cooking enigma. *Evolution of the human diet.* pp. 308–323. New York: Oxford U Press.

Wright, J. R., Calkins, E., Breen, W. J., Stolte, G., and Schultz, R. T. (1969). Relationship of amyloid to aging. Review of the literature and systematic study of 83 patients derived from a general hospital population. *Medicine.* **48,** 39–60.

Wright, L. (1960). *Clean and decent. The Fascinating History of the Bathroom and the Water-Closet.* London: Penguin Books.

Wright, S. (1920). The relative importance of heridity and enviroment in determining the piebald pattern of guinea pigs. *PNAS.* **6,** 321–332.

Wright, S. (1978). Variability Within and Between Populations. Chicago: University of Chicago Press.

Wrigley, E. A., Schofeld, R. S. (1989). The Population History of England 1541–1871: A Reconstruction. Cambridge: Cambridge University Press.

Writing Group for the Women's Health Initiative Investigators. (2002). Risks and benefits of estrogen plus progestin in healthy postmenopausal women. *JAMA.* **288,** 321–333.

Wu, D., and Meydani, S. N. (2004). Mechanism of age-associated up-regulation in macrophage PGE2 synthesis. *Brain Behav Immun.* **18,** 487–494.

Wu, K., Higashi, N., Hansen, E. R., Lund, M., Bang, K., and Thestrup-Pedersen, K. (2000). Telomerase activity is increased and telomere length shortened in T cells from blood of patients with atopic dermatitis and psoriasis. *J Immunol.* **165,** 4742–4747.

Wu, Q., and Brown, M. R. (2006). Signaling and function of insulin-like peptides in insects. *Annu Rev Entomol.* **51,** 1–24.

Wu, Q., Kumagai, T., Kawahara, M., Ogawa, H., Hiura, H., Obata, Y., Takano, R., and Kono, T. (2006a). Regulated expression of two sets of paternally imprinted genes is necessary for mouse parthenogenetic development to term. *Reproduction.* **131,** 481–488.

Wu, X., Schepartz, L. A., Falk, D., and Liu, W. (2006). Endocranial cast of *Hexian Homo erectus* from South China. *Am J Phys Anthropol.* **130,** 445–454.

Wu, X., Zhao, H., Suk, R., and Christiani, D. C. (2004). Genetic susceptibility to tobacco-related cancer. *Oncogene.* **23,** 6500–6523.

Wyss-Coray, T., Lin, C., Sanan, D. A., Mucke, L., and Masliah, E. (2000a). Chronic overproduction of transforming growth factor-beta1 by astrocytes promotes Alzheimer's disease-like microvascular degeneration in transgenic mice. *Am J Pathol.* **156,** 139–150.

Wyss-Coray, T., Lin, C., von Euw, D., Masliah, E., Mucke, L., and Lacombe, P. (2000b). Alzheimer's disease-like cerebrovascular pathology in transforming growth factor-beta 1 transgenic mice and functional metabolic correlates. *Ann NY Acad Sci.* **903,** 317–323.

Wyss-Coray, T., Loike, J. D., Brionne, T. C., Lu, E., Anankov, R., Yan, F., Silverstein, S. C., and Husemann, J. (2003). Adult mouse astrocytes degrade amyloid-beta *in vitro* and *in situ. Nature Med.* **9,** 453–457.

Xiang, M., Alfven, G., Blennow, M., Trygg, M., and Zetterstrom, R. (2000). Long-chain polyunsaturated fatty acids in human milk and brain growth during early infancy. *Acta Paediat.* **89,** 142–147.

Xie, Z., Morgan, T. E., Rozovsky, I., and Finch, C. E. (2003). Aging and glial responses to lipopolysaccharide *in vitro*: Greater induction of IL-1 and IL-6, but smaller induction of neurotoxicity. *Exp Neurol.* **182,** 135–141.

Xiong, X., Buekens, P., Fraser, W. D., Beck, J., and Offenbacher, S. (2006). Periodontal disease and adverse pregnancy outcomes: A systematic review. *Brit J Obstet Gyn.* **113,** 135–143.

Xu, B., Kalra, P. S., Farmerie, W. G., and Kalra, S. P. (1999). Daily changes in hypothalamic gene expression of neuropeptide Y, galanin, proopiomelanocortin, and adipocyte leptin gene expression and secretion: Effects of food restriction. *Endocrinology.* **140,** 2868–2875.

Xu, C., Zarins, C. K., and Glagov, S. (2002). Gene expression of tropoelastin is enhanced in the aorta proximal to the coarctation in rabbits. *Experimental and Molecular Pathology.* **72,** 115–123.

Xu, C., Zarins, C. K., Pannaraj, P. S., Bassiouny, H. S., and Glagov, S. (2000a). Hypercholesterolemia superimposed by experimental hypertension induces differential distribution of collagen and elastin. *Arterioscler Thromb Vasc Biol.* **20,** 2566–2572.

Xu, D., and Kyriakis, J. M. (2003). Phosphatidylinositol 3'-kinase-dependent activation of renal mesangial cell Ki-Ras and ERK by advanced glycation end products. *J Biol Chem.* **278,** 39349–39355.

Xu, D. X., Chen, Y. H., Wang, H., Zhao, L., Wang, J. P., and Wei, W. (2006). Tumor necrosis factor alpha partially contributes to lipopolysaccharide-induced intra-uterine fetal growth restriction and skeletal development retardation in mice. *Toxicol Lett.* **163,** 20–29.

Xu, J., Thornburg, T., Turner, A. R., Vitolins, M., Case, D., Shadle, J., et al (2005). Serum levels of phytanic acid are associated with prostate cancer risk. *Prostate.* **63,** 209–214.

Xu, Q., Schett, G., Perschinka, H., Mayr, M., Egger, G., Oberhollenzer, F., Willeit, J., Kiechl, S., and Wick, G. (2000b). Serum soluble heat shock protein 60 is elevated in subjects with atherosclerosis in a general population. *Circulation.* **102,** 14–20.

Xu, X., and Sonntag, W. E. (1996). Moderate caloric restriction prevents the age-related decline in growth hormone receptor signal transduction. *J Gerontol. Series A, Biol Sci Med Sci.* **51,** B167–174.

Xu, Y., Szalai, A. J., Zhou, T., Zinn, K. R., Chaudhuri, T. R., Li, X., Koopman, W. J., and Kimberly, R. P. (2003). Fc gamma Rs modulate cytotoxicity of anti-Fas antibodies: Implications for agonistic antibody-based therapeutics. *J Immunol.* **171,** 562–568.

Yaffe, K., Kanaya, A., Lindquist, K., Simonsick, E. M., Harris, T., Shorr, R. I., Tylavsky, F. A., and Newman, A. B. (2004). The metabolic syndrome, inflammation, and risk of cognitive decline. *JAMA.* **292,** 2237–2242.

Yaffe, K., Lindquist, K., Penninx, B. W., Simonsick, E. M., Pahor, M., Kritchevsky, S., Launer, L., Kuller, L., Rubin, S., and Harris, T. (2003). Inflammatory markers and cognition in well-functioning African-American and white elders. *Neurology.* **61,** 76–80.

Yajnik, C. S. (2004a). Early life origins of insulin resistance and type 2 diabetes in India and other Asian countries. *J Nutr.* **134(1),** 205–210.

Yajnik, C. S. (2004b). Obesity epidemic in India: Intrauterine origins? *Proc Nutr Soc.* **63,** 387–396.

Yajnik, C. S., Fall, C. H., Coyaji, K. J., Hirve, S. S., Rao, S., Barker, D. J., Joglekar, C., and Kellingray, S. (2003). Neonatal anthropometry: The thin-fat Indian baby. The Pune Maternal Nutrition Study. *Int J Obes Relat Metab Disord.* **27,** 173–180.

Yamada, M., Kubo, H., Ishizawa, K., Kobayashi, S., Shinkawa, M., and Sasaki, H. (2005). Increased circulating endothelial progenitor cells in patients with bacterial pneumonia: Evidence that bone marrow derived cells contribute to lung repair. *Thorax.* **60,** 410–413.

Yamada, T., Kakihara, T., Kamishima, T., Fukuda, T., and Kawai, T. (1996). Both acute phase and constitutive serum amyloid A are present in atherosclerotic lesions. *Pathology International.* **46,** 797–800.

Yamamoto, H., Watanabe, T., Miyazaki, A., Katagiri, T., Idei, T., Iguchi, T., Mimura, M., and Kamijima, K. (2005). High prevalence of *Chlamydia pneumoniae* antibodies and increased high-sensitive C-reactive protein in patients with vascular dementia. *J Am Geriatr Soc.* **53,** 583–589.

Yamaoka, K., and Tango, T. (2005). Efficacy of lifestyle education to prevent type 2 diabetes: A meta-analysis of randomized controlled trials. *Diabetes Care.* **28,** 2780–2786.

Yamashita, T., Freigang, S., Eberle, C., Pattison, J., Gupta, S., Napoli, C., and Palinski, W. (2006). Maternal immunization programs postnatal immune responses and reduces atherosclerosis in offspring. *Circ Res.* **99,** e51–64.

Yamawaki, H., Lehoux, S., and Berk, B. C. (2003). Chronic physiological shear stress inhibits tumor necrosis factor-induced proinflammatory responses in rabbit aorta perfused *ex vivo. Circulation.* **108,** 1619–1625.

Yamawaki, H., Pan, S., Lee, R. T., and Berk, B. C. (2005). Fluid shear stress inhibits vascular inflammation by decreasing thioredoxin-interacting protein in endothelial cells. *J Clin Invest.* **115,** 733–738.

Yamaza, H., Komatsu, T., Chiba, T., Toyama, H., To, K., Higami, Y., and Shimokawa, I. (2004). A transgenic dwarf rat model as a tool for the study of calorie restriction and aging. *Exp Gerontol.* **39,** 269–272.

Yan, S. D., Yan, S. F., Chen, X., Fu, J., Chen, M., Kuppusamy, P., Smith, M. A., Perry, G., Godman, G. C., Nawroth, P., et al. (1995). Non-enzymatically glycated tau in Alzheimer's disease induces neuronal oxidant stress resulting in cytokine gene expression and release of amyloid beta-peptide. *Nature Med.* **1,** 693–699.

Yang, C. Y., Tseng, Y. T., and Chang, C. C. (2003). Effects of air pollution on birth weight among children born between 1995 and 1997 in Kaohsiung, Taiwan. *J Toxicol Env Health Part A.* **66,** 807–816.

Yang, F., Lim, G. P., Begum, A. N., Ubeda, O. J., Simmons, M. R., Ambegaokar, S. S., Chen, P. P., Kayed, R., Glabe, C. G., Frautschy, S. A., and Cole, G. M. (2005). Curcumin inhibits formation of amyloid beta oligomers and fibrils, binds plaques, and reduces amyloid *in vivo. J Biol Chem.* **280,** 5892–5901.

Yang, H., Roberts, L. J., Shi, M. J., Zhou, L. C., Ballard, B. R., Richardson, A., and Guo, Z. M. (2004a). Retardation of atherosclerosis by overexpression of catalase or both Cu/Zn-super-oxide dismutase and catalase in mice lacking apolipoprotein E. *Circ Res.* **95,** 1075–1081.

Yang, H., Shi, M., Story, J., Richardson, A., and Guo, Z. (2004b). Food restriction attenu-ates age-related increase in the sensitivity of endothelial cells to oxidized lipids. *J Gerontol. A Biol Sci Med Sci.* **59**, 316–323.

Yang, T., Fu, M., Pestell, R., and Sauve, A. A. (2006). SIRT1 and endocrine signaling. *Trends Endocrinol Metab.* **17**, 186–191.

Yang, X. J., Kow, L. M., Pfaff, D. W., and Mobbs, C. V. (2004c). Metabolic pathways that mediate inhibition of hypothalamic neurons by glucose. *Diabetes.* **53**, 67–73.

Yang, Y., Mufson, E. J., and Herrup, K. (2003b). Neuronal cell death is preceded by cell cycle events at all stages of Alzheimer's disease. *J Neurosci.* **23**, 2557–2563.

Yankner, B. A. (2000). The pathogenesis of Alzheimer's disease. Is amyloid beta-protein the beginning or the end? *Ann NY Acad Sci.* **924**, 26–28.

Yankner, B. A., Dawes, L. R., Fisher, S., Villa-Komaroff, L., Oster-Granite, M. L., and Neve, R. L. (1989). Neurotoxicity of a fragment of the amyloid precursor associated with Alzheimer's disease. *Science.* **245**, 417–420.

Yanni, A. E. (2004). The laboratory rabbit: An animal model of atherosclerosis research. *Lab Ani.* **38**, 246–256.

Yasojima, K., Schwab, C., McGeer, E. G., and McGeer, P. L. (2000). Human neurons gen-erate C-reactive protein and amyloid P: Upregulation in Alzheimer's disease. *Brain Res.* **887**, 80–89.

Yasojima, K., Schwab, C., McGeer, E. G., and McGeer, P. L. (2001a). Complement com-ponents, but not complement inhibitors, are upregulated in atherosclerotic plaques. *Arterioscler Thromb Vasc Biol.* **21**, 1214–1219.

Yasojima, K., Schwab, C., McGeer, E. G., and McGeer, P. L. (2001b). Generation of C-reac-tive protein and complement components in atherosclerotic plaques. *Am J Pathol.* **158**, 1039–1051.

Ye, S. M., and Johnson, R. W. (1999). Increased interleukin-6 expression by microglia from brain of aged mice. *J Neuroimmunol.* **93**, 139–148.

Yearsley, J. M., Kyriazakis, I., Gordon, I. J., Johnston, S. L., Speakman, J. R., Tolkamp, B. J., and Illius, A. W. (2005). A life history model of somatic damage associated with resource acquisition: Damage protection or prevention? *J Theor Biol.* **235**, 305–317.

Yeomans, L. (2005). Discard and disposal practices at Çatalhöyük: *Inhabiting Çatalhöyük: Reports from the 1995-1999 Seasons by Members of the Çatalhöyük Teams.* pp 573–586. London: McDonald Institute Monographs.

Yesilbursa, D., Serdar, Z., Serdar, A., Sarac, M., Coskun, S., and Jale, C. (2005). Lipid per-oxides in obese patients and effects of weight loss with orlistat on lipid peroxides levels. *International Journal of Obesity (London).* **29**, 142–145.

Yeung, C. Y., Lee, H. C., Lin, S. P., Fang, S. B., Jiang, C. B., Huang, F. Y., and Chuang, C. K. (2004). Serum cytokines in differentiating between viral and bacterial enterocolitis. *Ann Trop Paediat.* **24**, 337–343.

Yilmaz, V., Yentèur, S. P., and Saruhan-Direskeneli, G. (2005). IL-12 and IL-10 polymor-phisms and their effects on cytokine production. *Cytokine.* **30**, 188–194.

Ying, S. C., Marchalonis, J. J., Gewurz, A. T., Siegel, J. N., Jiang, H., Gewurz, B. E., and Gewurz, H. (1992). Reactivity of anti-human C-reactive protein (CRP) and serum amyloid P component (SAP) monoclonal antibodies with limulin and pentraxins of other species. *Immunology.* **76**, 324–330.

Ylikoski, R., Ylikoski, A., Erkinjuntti, T., Sulkava, R., Raininko, R., and Tilvis, R. (1993). White matter changes in healthy elderly persons correlate with attention and speed of mental processing. *Arch Neurol.* **50**, 818–824.

Yonekura, H., Yamamoto, Y., Sakurai, S., Watanabe, T., and Yamamoto, H. (2005). Roles of the receptor for advanced glycation endproducts in diabetes-induced vascular injury. *J Pharmacol Sci.* **97,** 305–311.

Yoshida, K., Inoue, T., Hirabayashi, Y., Matsumura, T., Nemoto, K., and Sado, T. (1997). Radiation-induced myeloid leukemia in mice under calorie restriction. *Leukemia.* **11,** 410–412.

Yu, B. P., Masoro, E. J., Murata, I., Bertrand, H. A., and Lynd, F. T. (1982). Life span study of SPF Fischer 344 male rats fed ad libitum or restricted diets: Longevity, growth, lean body mass and disease. *Jf Gerontol.* **37,** 130–141.

Zamaria, N. (2004). Alteration of polyunsaturated fatty acid status and metabolism in health and disease. *Reprod Nutrit Devel.* **44,** 273–282.

Zamenhof, S., Van Marthens, E., and Grauel, L. (1971a). DNA (cell number) and protein in neonatal rat brain: Alteration by timing of maternal dietary protein restriction. *J Nutrit.* **101,** 1265–1269.

Zamenhof, S., Van Marthens, E., and Grauel, L. (1971b). DNA (cell number) and protein in rat brain. Second generation (F2) alteration by maternal (F0) dietary protein restriction. *Science.* **172,** 850–851.

Zamenhof, S., Van Marthens, E., Grauel, L. (1972). DNA (cell number) and protein in rat brain. Second generation (F2) alteration by maternal (F0) dietary protein restriction. *Nutr Metab.* **14,** 262–270.

Zanjani, H., Finch, C. E., Kemper, C., Atkinson, J. P., McKeel Jr., D. W., Morris, J. C., and Price, J. L. (2005). Complement activation in very early Alzheimer's disease. *Alzheimer Disease Assoc Disord.* **19,** 55–66.

Zannad, F., and Radauceanu, A. (2005). Effect of MR blockade on collagen formation and cardiovascular disease with a specific emphasis on heart failure. *Heart Failure Rev.* **10,** 71–78.

Zaretsky, M. V., Alexander, J. M., Byrd, W., and Bawdon, R. E. (2004). Transfer of inflammatory cytokines across the placenta. *Obstet Gynecol.* **103,** 546–550.

Zee, R. Y., and Ridker, P. M. (2002). Polymorphism in the human C-reactive protein (CRP) gene, plasma concentrations of CRP, and the risk of future arterial thrombosis. *Atherosclerosis.* **162,** 217–219.

Zeinoaldini, S., Swarts, J. J., and Van de Heijning, B. J. (2006). Chronic leptin infusion advances, and immunoneutralization of leptin postpones puberty onset in normally fed and feed restricted female rats. *Peptides.* **27,** 1652–1658.

Zeng, G., McCue, H. M., Mastrangelo, L., and Millis, A. J. (1996). Endogenous TGF-beta activity is modified during cellular aging: Effects on metalloproteinase and TIMP-1 expression. *Exp Cell Res.* **228,** 271–276.

Zerofsky, M., Harel, E., Silverman, N., and Tatar, M. (2005). Aging of the innate immune response in *Drosophila melanogaster.* *Aging Cell.* **4,** 103–108.

Zerr, K. J., Furnary, A. P., Grunkemeier, G. L., Bookin, S., Kanhere, V., and Starr, A. (1997). Glucose control lowers the risk of wound infection in diabetics after open heart operations. *Ann Thorac Surg.* **63,** 356–361.

Zhang, H., and Burrows, F. (2004). Targeting multiple signal transduction pathways through inhibition of Hsp90. *J Mol Med.* **82,** 488–499.

Zhang, J., and Smith, K. R. (2003). Indoor air pollution: A global health concern. *Brit Med Bull.* **68,** 209–225.

Zhang, R., Becnel, L., Li, M., Chen, C., Yao, Q. (2006). C-reactive protein impairs human CD14+ monocyte-derived dendritic cell differentiation, maturation and function. *Eur J Immunol.* **36,** 2993–3006.

Zhang, Y. (2004). Molecular biology: No exception to reversibility. *Nature.* **431,** 637–639.

Zhang, Y., Coogan, P. F., Palmer, J. R., Strom, B. L., and Rosenberg, L. (2005). Use of non-steroidal antiinflammatory drugs and risk of breast cancer: The Case-Control Surveillance Study revisited. *Am J Epidemiol.* **162,** 165–70.

Zhao, L., Moos, M. P., Grèabner, R., Pédrono, F., Fan, J., Kaiser, B., John, N., Schmidt, S., Spanbroek, R., Lèotzer, K., Huang, L., Cui, J., Rader, D. J., Evans, J. F., Habenicht, A. J., and Funk, C. D. (2004). The 5-lipoxygenase pathway promotes pathogenesis of hyperlipidemia-dependent aortic aneurysm. *Nature Med.* **10,** 966–973.

Zheng, F., Cheng, Q. L., Plati, A. R., Ye, S. Q., Berho, M., Banerjee, A., Potier, M., Jaimes, E. A., Yu, H., Guan, Y. F., Hao, C. M., Striker, L. J., and Striker, G. E. (2004). The glomerulosclerosis of aging in females: Contribution of the proinflammatory mesangial cell phenotype to macrophage infiltration. *Am J Pathol.* **165,** 1789–1798.

Zheng, J., Edelman, S. W., Tharmarajah, G., Walker, D. W., Pletcher, S. D., and Seroude, L. (2005). Differential patterns of apoptosis in response to aging in *Drosophila. Proc Natl Acad Sci USA.* **102,** 12083–12088.

Zheng, W. H., Kar, S., Dore, S., and Quirion, R. (2000). Insulin-like growth factor-1 (IGF-1): A neuroprotective trophic factor acting via the Akt kinase pathway. *J Neural Transmiss.* **Suppl,** 261–272.

Zhu, B. Q., Sun, Y. P., Sudhir, K., Sievers, R. E., Browne, A. E., Gao, L., Hutchison, S. J., Chou, T. M., Deedwania, P. C., Chatterjee, K., Glantz, S. A., and Parmley, W. W. (1997a). Effects of second-hand smoke and gender on infarct size of young rats exposed in utero and in the neonatal to adolescent period. *J Am Coll Cardiol.* **30,** 1878–1885.

Zhu, J., Quyyumi, A. A., Norman, J. E., Csako, G., Waclawiw, M. A., Shearer, G. M., and Epstein, S. E. (2000). Effects of total pathogen burden on coronary artery disease risk and C-reactive protein levels. *Am J Cardiol.* **85,** 140–146.

Zhu, Z., Haegele, A. D., and Thompson, H. J. (1997b). Effect of caloric restriction on pre-malignant and malignant stages of mammary carcinogenesis. *Carcinogenesis.* **18,** 1007–1012.

Zhu, Z., Jiang, W., and Thompson, H. J. (1999). Effect of energy restriction on the expression of cyclin D1 and p27 during premalignant and malignant stages of chemically induced mammary carcinogenesis. *Mol Carcinogen.* **24,** 241–245.

Zin Thet, K., Khin Maung, U., Myo, K., Yi Yi, M., Myat, T., and Kyi Kyi, M. (1992). Sodium balance during acute diarrhoea in malnourished children. *J Trop Pediatr.* **38,** 153–157.

Zlokarnik, G., Negulescu, P. A., Knapp, T. E., Mere, L., Burres, N., Feng, L., Whitney, M., Roemer, K., and Tsien, R. Y. (1998). Quantitation of transcription and clonal selection of single living cells with beta-lactamase as reporter. *Science.* **279,** 84–88.

Zou, G. M., and Tam, Y. K. (2002). Cytokines in the generation and maturation of dendritic cells: Recent advances. *Europ Cytokine Netw.* **13,** 186–199.

Zou, Y., Jung, K. J., Kim, J. W., Yu, B. P., and Chung, H. Y. (2004). Alteration of soluble adhesion molecules during aging and their modulation by calorie restriction. *FASEB Journal.* **18,** 320–322.

Zwaka, T. P., Hombach, V., and Torzewski, J. (2001). C-reactive protein-mediated low density lipoprotein uptake by macrophages: Implications for atherosclerosis. *Circulation.* **103,** 1194–1197.

—

NAME INDEX

Note: b, box; f, figure; t, table

SUBJECT INDEX

Note: b, box; f, figure; t, table